Nutritional Intervention in Metabolic Syndrome

Edited by
Isaias Dichi
University of Londrina
Paraná, Brazil

Andréa Name Colado Simão
University of Londrina
Paraná, Brazil

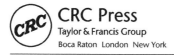

CRC Press
Taylor & Francis Group
Boca Raton London New York

CRC Press is an imprint of the
Taylor & Francis Group, an **informa** business

First published 2016 by CRC Press

Published 2019 by CRC Press
Taylor & Francis Group
6000 Broken Sound Parkway NW, Suite 300
Boca Raton, FL 33487-2742

First issued in paperback 2021

© 2016 by Taylor & Francis Group, LLC
CRC Press is an imprint of the Taylor & Francis Group, an informa business

No claim to original U.S. Government works

ISBN 13: 978-1-03-209831-9 (pbk)
ISBN 13: 978-1-4665-5682-9 (hbk)

Visit the Taylor & Francis Web site at
http://www.taylorandfrancis.com

and the CRC Press Web site at
http://www.crcpress.com

Contents

SECTION I Prevalence, Pathophysiology, and Gene–Nutrient Interaction in Metabolic Syndrome

SECTION II Early Life Nutrition and Metabolic Syndrome in Children and Adolescents

SECTION III   Demographic Determinants and Lifestyle Changes in Metabolic Syndrome

SECTION IV   Specific Conditions Related to Metabolic Syndrome

SECTION V   Effects of Dietary Components in Metabolic Syndrome

SECTION VI Dietary Patterns in Metabolic Syndrome

Preface

Metabolic syndrome (MetS) comprises pathological conditions that include insulin resistance, arterial hypertension, visceral adiposity, and dyslipidemia, which favor the development of cardiovascular diseases (CVDs). Existing evidence suggests that MetS, as well as obesity and diabetes mellitus type 2, are rising in developed and in developing countries. Although obesity and insulin resistance constitute the leading causes of MetS, many other pathophysiological mechanisms, such as pro-inflammatory adipokines, hyperuricemia, nitric oxide, and oxidative stress, may contribute to the potential cardiovascular risk factors related to the syndrome. On the other hand, increases in anti-inflammatory adipokine (adiponectin) and antioxidant mechanisms could protect from some CVDs. Nutritional intervention through different dietary patterns and individualized dietary components has been attempted to attenuate the detrimental or increase the beneficial mechanisms in order to decrease the potential risk of the clinical features of MetS. The Mediterranean diet and Dietary Approach to Stop Hypertension are the main standard diets utilized, whereas many foods may also contribute to the prevention and treatment of MetS, such as olive oil, soy-based products, fish oil, green tea, nuts, whole grains, and berries. This book focuses on the continuing efforts to understand the pathophysiology underlying MetS and the development of strategies to prevent and treat these conditions through nutrition intervention.

Isaias Dichi
Andréa Name Colado Simão
Londrina, Brazil

Editors

Dr. Isaias Dichi graduated in medicine and specialized in internal medicine. He earned his master's degree, in 1993, and PhD, in 1997, in physiopathology in internal medicine, nutrition and metabolism, from São Paulo State University (UNESP-Botucatu). Dr. Dichi is currently a professor of internal medicine and clinical nutrition at the State University of Londrina, Paraná, Brazil. He works in the following research areas: physiopathology and diet therapy for metabolic syndrome with fish oil n-3 fatty acids, olive oil, soy, berries, and probiotics; physiopathology and diet therapy for other inflammatory diseases, such as inflammatory bowel disease, rheumatoid disease, and systemic erythematosus lupus with fish oil n-3 fatty acids, olive oil, and probiotics; prevention and treatment of iron deficiency and iron-deficiency anemia; and nutrition and metabolism in chronic diseases. Medical education and film interpretation are his other areas of interest. He was director of the Health Sciences Center of the University of Londrina during 2006–2010.

Dr. Andréa Name Colado Simão graduated in pharmacy and biochemistry in 1997 and earned her MS in experimental pathology in 2004 and PhD in health sciences in 2008. Dr. Simão is currently a professor of clinical immunology at the State University of Londrina, Paraná, Brazil. She has accomplished nutritional intervention with fish oil, olive oil, soy, cranberry, and probiotics in metabolic syndrome. Dr. Simão has also been studying the effects of oxidative stress on many chronic diseases, such as metabolic syndrome, systemic lupus erythematosus, rheumatoid arthritis, psoriasis, multiple sclerosis, hepatitis C, HIV, and breast cancer.

Contributors

Lucilene Rezende Anastácio
Minas Gerais Federal University
Minas Gerais, Brazil
and
Nutrition Department
Itaúna University
Itaúna, Brazil

Catherine J. Andersen
Department of Nutritional Sciences
University of Connecticut
Storrs, Connecticut

Fabiola Malaga Barreto
Department of Food Science Post Graduation
    Program
State University of Londrina
Londrina, Brazil

Arpita Basu
Department of Nutritional Sciences
Oklahoma State University
Stillwater, Oklahoma

Maria Fernanda Giovanetti Biagioni
Internal Medicine Department
Botucatu Medical School
Sao Paulo State University
São Paulo, Brazil

Christopher N. Blesso
Department of Nutritional Sciences
University of Connecticut
Storrs, Connecticut
and
Department of Pathology–Lipid Sciences
Wake Forest University
Winston-Salem, North Carolina

Rachel Clare Brown
Department of Human Nutrition
University of Otago
Dunedin, New Zealand

Philip C. Calder
Faculty of Medicine
Human Development and Health Academic
    Unit
University of Southampton
and
Southampton General Hospital
Southampton, United Kingdom

Adrian James Cameron
World Health Organization (WHO)
    Collaborating Centre for Obesity Prevention
Deakin University
Geelong, Victoria, Australia

Roberta Soares Lara Cassani
Itu Nutrition Institute
and
Laboratory of Investigation in Metabolism and
    Diabetes
State University of Campinas
UNICAMP
Campinas, Brazil

**Alexandra Wynne-Ankaret Hamilton
Chisholm**
Department of Human Nutrition
University of Otago
Dunedin, New Zealand

Maria Isabel Toulson Davison Correia
Department of Surgery
Alfa Institute of Gastroenterology
and
University Hospital
and
Minas Gerais Federal University
Minas Gerais, Brazil

Rui Curi
Department of Physiology and Biophysics
Institute of Biomedical Sciences
University of São Paulo
São Paulo, Brazil

Angelica Dante
Department of Life, Health and Environmental
   Sciences
University of L'Aquila
L'Aquila, Italy

Lucia Helena da Silva Miglioranza
Food Science and Technology Department
State University of Londrina
Londrina, Brazil

Giovambattista Desideri
Department of Life, Health and Environmental
   Sciences
University of L'Aquila
L'Aquila, Italy

Emmanuel James Diamantopoulos
Department of Internal Medicine
and
Unit of Vascular Medicine
Evangelismos State General Hospital
Athens, Greece

Isaias Dichi
Department of Internal Medicine
University of Londrina
Londrina, Brazil

Stefania Di Agostino
Department of Life, Health and Environmental
   Sciences
University of L'Aquila
L'Aquila, Italy

Leandro Arthur Diehl
Department of Internal Medicine
Health Sciences Center
State University of Londrina
Londrina, Brazil

Paolo Di Giosia
Department of Life, Health and Environmental
   Science
University of L'Aquila
L'Aquila, Italy

Fernanda Aparecida Domenici
Laboratory of Molecular Biology and
   Nutrigenomics
Department of Internal Medicine
University of São Paulo
Ribeirao Preto, Brazil

Fotios Drakopanagiotakis
Department of Internal Medicine
and
Unit of Vascular Medicine
Evangelismos State General Hospital
Athens, Greece

Anthony Fardet
Unité de Nutrition Humaine
Université d'Auvergne
and
Clermont-Ferrand & Clermont Université
Clermont-Ferrand, France

Elis Carolina de Souza Fatel
Department of Nutrition
Federal University of Southern Border
Realeza, Paraná, Brazil

William Feng
Department of Chemical Biology
Ernest Mario School of Pharmacy
Rutgers, The State University of New Jersey
Piscataway, New Jersey

Maria Luz Fernandez
Department of Nutritional Sciences
University of Connecticut
Storrs, Connecticut

Claudio Ferri
Department of Life, Health and Environmental
   Sciences
University of L'Aquila
L'Aquila, Italy

Jarlei Fiamoncini
Department of Physiology and Biophysics
Institute of Biomedical Sciences
University of São Paulo
São Paulo, Brazil

Evanthia Gouveri
Department of Internal Medicine
and
Unit of Vascular Medicine
Evangelismos State General Hospital
Athens, Greece

Paulo Cezar Casado Graça
Philadelphia Institute of Londrina
UNIFIL
Londrina, Brazil

Davide Grassi
Department of Life, Health and Environmental
    Sciences
University of L'Aquila
L'Aquila, Italy

Sandro Massao Hirabara
Department of Physiology and Biophysics
Institute of Biomedical Sciences
University of São Paulo
and
Institute of Physical Activity Sciences and
    Sports
Cruzeiro do Sul University
São Paulo, Brazil

Jungil Hong
Department of Food Science & Technology
College of Natural Science
Seoul Women's University
Seoul, South Korea

Tatiana Mayumi Veiga Iriyoda
Department of Internal Medicine
State University of Londrina
Londrina, Brazil

Ana Paula Kallaur
Health Sciences Center
State University of Londrina
and
Department of Clinical Analysis
University North of Paraná
Londrina, Brazil

Mauricio da Silva Krause
School of Biomolecular and Biomedical
    Science
Conway Institute of Biomolecular and
    Biomedical Research
University College Dublin
Dublin, Ireland

Jacqueline Isaura Alvarez Leite
Department of Biochemistry and Immunology
and
Alpha Institute of Gastroenterology
Minas Gerais Federal University
Minas Gerais, Brazil

Cristiane Maria Mártires de Lima
Division of Medical Nutrition
School of Medicine of Ribeirão Preto
University of São Paulo
Ribeirão Preto, Brazil

Marcell Alysson Batisti Lozovoy
Department of Clinical Analysis
University North of Paraná
and
Department of Pathology, Clinical Analysis,
    and Toxicology
University of Londrina
Londrina, Brazil

Timothy J. Lyons
Centre for Experimental Medicine
Queen's University of Belfast
Northern Ireland, United Kingdom

Francesca Mai
Department of Life, Health and Environmental
    Sciences
University of L'Aquila
L'Aquila, Italy

Suzana Mantovani
Clinical Dietitian and Consultant to Medical
    Nutrition
Zürich, Switzerland

Júlio Sérgio Marchini
Division of Medical Nutrition
School of Medicine of Ribeirão Preto
University of São Paulo
Ribeirão Preto, Brazil

Guilherme Figueiredo Marquezine
Department of Clinical Medicine
Health Sciences Center
State University of Londrina
Londrina, Brazil

Letizia Martella
Department of Life, Health and Environmental
    Sciences
University of L'Aquila
L'Aquila, Italy

Gláucia Maria Ferreira da Silva Mazeto
Internal Medicine Department
Botucatu Medical School
Sao Paulo State University
Unesp
São Paulo, Brazil

Adriana Lúcia Mendes
Internal Medicine Department
Botucatu Medical School
Sao Paulo State University
Unesp
São Paulo, Brazil

Édison Miglioranza
Clinical Immunology and Molecular Diagnosis
    Laboratories
Health Sciences Center
State University of Londrina
Londrina, Brazil

Hitomi Okubo
MRC Lifecourse Epidemiology Unit
University of Southampton
Southampton General Hospital
Southampton, United Kingdom

Sérgio Alberto Rupp de Paiva
Internal Medicine Department
Botucatu Medical School
Sao Paulo State University
Unesp
São Paulo, Brazil

Sílvia Justina Papini
Internal Medicine Department
Botucatu Medical School
Sao Paulo State University
Unesp
São Paulo, Brazil

Federica Patrizi
Department of Life, Health and Environmental
    Sciences
University of L'Aquila
L'Aquila, Italy

Javier Sanchez Perona
Department of Food and Health
Instituto de la Grasa
Spanish Council for Scientific Research
Sevilla, Spain

Edna Maria Vissoci Reiche
Clinical Immunology and Molecular Diagnosis
    Laboratories
Department of Pathology, Clinical Analysis,
    and Toxicology
Health Sciences Center
State University of Londrina
Londrina, Brazil

Fernando Vissoci Reiche
Specialist in Clinical Cardiology and
    Echocardiopraphy
Heart Institute of Londrina
Londrina, Brazil

Siân Robinson
MRC Lifecourse Epidemiology Unit
University of Southampton
Southampton General Hospital
Southampton, United Kingdom

Leticia Prates Roma
Institute of Biomedical Sciences
University of São Paulo
São Paulo, Brazil

Talita Romanatto
Department of Physiology and Biophysics
Institute of Biomedical Sciences
University of São Paulo
São Paulo, Brazil

Flávia Troncon Rosa
Department of Nutrition
Philadelphia Institute of Londrina and Health
    Sciences Center
State University of Londrina
Londrina, Brazil

Roberta Deh Souza Santos
Department of Structural and Functional
    Biology
Institute of Biology
State University of Campinas
Campinas, Brazil

Bruna Miglioranza Scavuzzi
Department of Health Sciences
State University of Londrina
Londrina, Brazil

Jose Henrique da Silvah
Division of Medical Nutrition
School of Medicine of Ribeirão Preto
University of São Paulo
Ribeirão Preto, Brazil

Andréa Name Colado Simão
Department of Pathology, Clinical Analysis,
    and Toxicology
University of Londrina
Londrina, Brazil

Vivian Marques Miguel Suen
School of Medicine of Ribeirão Preto
University of São Paulo
Ribeirão Preto, Brazil

Hilton Kenji Takahashi
Institute of Clinical and Experimental Research
Catholic University of Louvain
Louvain-la-Neuve, Belgium

Siew Ling Tey
Department of Human Nutrition
University of Otago
Dunedin, New Zealand

Hélio Vannucchi
School of Medicine of Ribeirao Preto
and
Laboratory of Molecular Biology and
    Nutrigenomics
Department of Internal Medicine
School of Medicine of Ribeirao Preto
University of Sao Paulo
Ribeirao Preto, Brazil

Chung S. Yang
Department of Chemical Biology
Ernest Mario School of Pharmacy
Rutgers, The State University of New Jersey
New Jersey, Piscataway

Section I

Prevalence, Pathophysiology, and Gene–Nutrient Interaction in Metabolic Syndrome

1 Metabolic Syndrome Measurement and Worldwide Prevalence

Adrian James Cameron

CONTENTS

1.1 METABOLIC SYNDROME IN WORLDWIDE CONTEXT

The global prevalence of first obesity, then metabolic syndrome (MetS) and diabetes, have been on the rise since at least the middle of the twentieth century. The new millennium has seen a continuation of this trend. The threat to individuals, national health care systems and health budgets from the MetS and its common consequence, type 2 diabetes, has seen diabetes become only the second disease after AIDS to be the subject of a United Nations resolution. Diabetes is now one of the most common noncommunicable diseases globally, and the fourth or fifth leading cause of death in most developed countries (International Diabetes Federation 2012). Over one-third of a billion people were estimated to have diabetes in 2011 (90% type 2 diabetes), with projections suggesting that by 2030 this number will exceed 500 million (International Diabetes Federation 2012). A frequently unappreciated statistic is that some 80% of those living with diabetes are living in low- and middle-income countries. This is despite a "Western lifestyle" often being blamed for its development.

Considerable evidence now exists linking the MetS and diabetes with an increased risk of cardiovascular diseases (CVDs). Various estimates suggest that between one-half and two-thirds of deaths among people with diabetes are due to cardiovascular causes such as ischemic heart disease and stroke (Barr et al. 2007, Grundy et al. 1999, Morrish et al. 2001). Compared to those without diabetes, the risk of coronary artery disease, stroke, and peripheral arterial disease is two to four times higher in the diabetic population, more particularly among women. Similarly, risk for CVDs is elevated in those with the MetS (Ford 2005).

1.2 WHAT IS THE METABOLIC SYNDROME?

The MetS is observed as a clustering of abnormalities related to increased risk of both type 2 diabetes and CVDs. One or both of insulin resistance and visceral adiposity are thought to precede (Cameron et al. 2008) and be the root cause of these abnormalities that include hyperglycemia, elevated blood pressure, and dyslipidemia (elevated triglyceride levels and reduced levels of high-density lipoprotein cholesterol [HDL-C]). A range of other clinical features including elevated inflammatory markers, a prothrombotic state, polycystic ovarian syndrome, and others have also been linked to the MetS. Clinical definitions of the MetS have been designed specifically to identify those demonstrating the characteristic clustering of risk factors with prevention of the development of type 2 diabetes and CVD being the goal.

1.2.1 INSULIN RESISTANCE SYNDROME OR METABOLIC SYNDROME?

The relationship between insulin resistance and the MetS has been the cause of a general misunderstanding of the purpose of the MetS. The terms MetS and insulin resistance syndrome have often been used interchangeably, but the different names are a reflection of different underlying concepts and different goals (Reaven 2004). Insulin resistance, which manifests as a reduction in insulin-mediated glucose disposal, has been recognized to be a precursor of hyperglycemia and diabetes since the 1930s (Himsworth 1936). We now know that considerable variation exists in the insulin-mediated ability to dispose of glucose within the population (Yeni-Komshian et al. 2000). Most insulin-resistant people are able to compensate with the production of extra insulin by the pancreatic beta cells. In fact, individuals exhibiting otherwise normal glucose levels but hyperinsulinemia are not uncommon in the population. When the ability to compensate for insulin resistance can no longer be sustained, glucose intolerance and type 2 diabetes are the result.

Research has now shown that the hyperinsulinemia required to maintain normal glucose levels in those with insulin resistance is actually a mixed blessing. In his 1988 Banting lecture (Reaven 1988), Reaven spelled out the negative consequences of insulin resistance, which include an increased risk for glucose intolerance, high plasma triglyceride and low HDL cholesterol concentrations, and hypertension. Since these abnormalities increase the risk of CVD, the most common cause of death in people with diabetes, it was assumed by association that insulin resistance must also have close links with CVD. The "insulin resistance syndrome" was a label given to the numerous physiologic abnormalities and the related clinical outcomes that occur commonly in those with insulin resistance (Reaven 2004). The clinical syndromes associated with insulin resistance include not only type 2 diabetes and CVDs, but also hypertension, polycystic ovary syndrome, nonalcoholic fatty liver disease, sleep apnea, and certain cancers.

The term "MetS" has developed to describe those individuals at increased risk of type 2 diabetes and CVDs due to the metabolic dysfunction apparent in the "insulin resistance syndrome," but without presuming an underlying cause. Prevention of type 2 diabetes and CVD in the clinical scenario were behind the development of a clinical definition of the MetS. Numerous organizations have published modestly differing definitions of the MetS, although thankfully we now have a single, unified definition (Alberti et al. 2009). As clinical constructs, MetS definitions do not need to include all of the abnormalities associated with the dysfunction characteristic of the syndrome, and even include central obesity which is really a cause rather than a consequence of metabolic dysfunction (Cameron et al. 2008).

1.2.2 EVOLUTION OF A DEFINITION FOR THE METABOLIC SYNDROME

Prior to the publication of a harmonized definition of the MetS in 2009 (Alberti et al. 2009) by the International Diabetes Federation (IDF), the American Heart Association (AHA), the U.S. National Heart, Lung, and Blood Institute (NHLBI), the World Heart Federation, the International Association for the Study of Obesity, and the International Atherosclerosis Society, numerous competing definitions existed. The four most widely recognized attempts to define the MetS include proposals by the World Health Organization (WHO) in 1998 (Alberti and Zimmet 1998) (finalized in 1999; World Health Organization 1999); the European Group for the Study of Insulin Resistance (EGIR) also in 1999 (Balkau and Charles 1999); the National Cholesterol Education Program (NCEP) Expert Panel on Detection, Evaluation, and Treatment of High Blood Cholesterol in Adults

(Adult Treatment Panel III) in 2001 (updated in 2005; Grundy et al. 2005); and the IDF in 2006 (Alberti et al. 2006).

The main differences between these definitions were the criteria used to identify obesity (both the cut-points and the measure used), whether individuals with diabetes should be included and how glycemia should be measured, and whether obesity was considered to be an essential component or simply one of several risk factors. Each definition included the same core factors of obesity, hyperglycemia, dyslipidemia, and hypertension, although the WHO definition did also include microalbuminuria (World Health Organization 1999) and the EGIR definition prioritized the measurement of insulin resistance (Balkau and Charles 1999).

By the time that representatives from the organizations responsible for the U.S. NCEP definition and the IDF definition sat down in 2009, these two definitions were in common global use. The only differences between the definitions were related to the structure of the definition and the criteria for obesity cut-points. Regarding structure, both definitions achieved a diagnosis according to the presence of at least three of the five abnormalities, although in the IDF definition obesity was a prerequisite for diagnosis. Regarding cut-points for obesity, waist circumference cut-points for overweight were used in the IDF definition, while cut-points for obesity were used in the U.S. definition. The IDF definition included obesity cut-points according to ethnicity based on growing evidence that some ethnic groups have quite different levels of risk for the same level of waist circumference (Cameron et al. 2010).

The consensus MetS definition has been the global reference for its clinical diagnosis since its publication in 2009 (Alberti et al. 2009). Agreement was reached in this definition that (1) the MetS could be defined according to the presence of any three of five abnormalities, and (2) that obesity could be defined according to obesity cut-points that are most appropriate for an individual (according to either ethnicity or nationality). The criteria for the clinical diagnosis of the MetS according to the consensus definition are seen in Table 1.1, while Table 1.2 outlines the waist circumference thresholds recommended for the classification of abdominal obesity by various organizations according to ethnic group or nationality. In the consensus statement, the specific wording relating to the choice of obesity cut-point used in MetS definitions is that "It is recommended that the IDF cut points (where specific cut-points are provided for Asian, Middle East/Mediterranean, Sub-Saharan African and Ethnic Central and South American populations) be used for non-Europeans and either the IDF or American Heart Association (AHA) and the National Heart, Lung, and Blood Institute (NHLBI) cut points used for people of European origin until more data are available." The consensus document also recognizes that locally, different waist circumference cut-points may be adopted for pragmatic or economic reasons by different health systems or other groups. For these reasons, the definition of the MetS according to the consensus statement will vary between ethnic groups and may also vary within ethnic groups. Within the obesity criteria outlined in the consensus statement (Table 1.2), different cut-points for Asian populations are recommended based on the suggestion of the IDF/WHO (≥90 cm in men, ≥80 cm in women), the Japanese Obesity Society (≥85 cm in men, ≥90 cm in women), and the Co-operative Meta-Analysis Group of the Working Group on Obesity in China (≥85 cm in men, ≥80 cm in women) (Alberti et al. 2009). This variation in suggested cut-points among ethnically similar populations is an example of the uncertainty remaining around the appropriate obesity criterion and highlights the continuing need for more definitive studies.

1.2.3 MetS Prevalence and Choice of Cut-Points for Obesity

Just as the prevalence of the component conditions (overweight, hypertension, hyperglycemia, and dyslipidemia) is critically dependent on the definitions and cut-points used, so is the prevalence of the MetS as a whole. The purpose of prevalence statistics for the MetS is to provide an estimate of the current risk factor burden and the likely burden of CVDs and type 2 diabetes that will result. In addition, prevalence statistics are useful for comparisons between populations or subpopulations,

TABLE 1.1

Criteria for the Clinical Diagnosis of the Metabolic Syndrome

Measure	Categorical Cut-Points
Elevated waist circumference[a]	Population and country-specific definitions[a]
Elevated triglycerides (drug treatment for elevated triglycerides is an alternate indicator[b])	≥150 mg/dL (1.7 mmol/L)
Reduced HDL-C (drug treatment for reduced HDL-C is an alternate indicator[b])	<40 mg/dL (1.0 mmol/L) in males <50 mg/dL (1.3 mmol/L) in females
Elevated blood pressure (antihypertensive drug treatment in a patient with a history of hypertension is an alternate indicator)	Systolic ≥130 and/or diastolic ≥85 mmHg
Elevated fasting glucose[c] (drug treatment of elevated glucose is an alternate indicator)	≥100 mg/dL

Source: Data from Alberti, K.G. et al., *Circulation*, 120(16), 1640, 2009.

HDL-C, high-density lipoprotein cholesterol.

[a] It is recommended that the International Diabetes Federation (IDF) cut-points be used for non-Europeans and either the IDF of American Heart Association (AHA) and the National Heart, Lung, and Blood Institute (NHLBI) cut points used for people of European origin until more data are available (For a list of current recommended waist circumference in different ethnic groups, see Table 1.2).

[b] The most commonly used drugs for elevated triglycerides and reduced HDL-C are fibrates and nicotinic acid. A patient taking one of these drugs can be presumed to have high triglycerides and low HDL-C. High dose ω-3 fatty acids presumes high triglycerides.

[c] Most patients with type 2 diabetes mellitus will have the metabolic syndrome by the proposed criteria.

TABLE 1.2

Recommended Waist Circumference Thresholds for Abdominal Obesity

Population	Organization	Recommended Waist Circumference Threshold for Abdominal Obesity (cm)	
		Men	**Women**
Europe	IDF	≥94	≥80
Caucasian	WHO	≥94 (increased risk)	≥80 (increased risk)
		≥102 (still higher risk)	≥88 (still higher risk)
United States	AHA/NHLBI (ATPIII)[a]	≥102	≥88
Canada	Health Canada	≥102	≥88
European	European Cardiovascular Societies	≥102	≥88
Asian (including Japanese)	IDF	≥90	≥80
Asian	WHO	≥90	≥80
Japanese	Japanese Obesity Society	≥85	≥90
China	Co-operative Task Force	≥85	≥80
Middle East, Mediterranean	IDF	≥94	≥80
Sub-Saharan African	IDF	≥94	≥80
Ethnic Central and South American	IDF	≥90	≥80

Source: Data from Alberti, K.G. et al., *Circulation*, 120(16), 1640, 2009.

IDF, International Diabetes Federation; WHO, World Health Organization.

[a] Recent American Heart Association (AHA) and the National Heart, Lung, and Blood Institute (NHLBI) guidelines for metabolic syndrome (MetS) recognize an increased risk for cardiovascular disease (CVD) and diabetes at waist–circumference thresholds of ≥94 cm in men and ≥80 cm in women and identify these as optional cut-points for individuals or populations with increased insulin resistance.

and for examination of trends over time (Cameron et al. 2009). The existence of four competing definitions of the MetS had previously been an impediment to these aims. The prevalence of the MetS, as well as its component conditions, is entirely dependent on the choice of cut-points to dichotomize the population into those with and without the condition. The practice of dichotomizing continuous variables results in a loss of predictive power, but is necessary for clinical decision making and the creation of diagnostic categories. Calculation of a continuous metabolic risk score that takes advantage of the full spectrum of data available has been suggested; however, such constructs have been recommended only for research purposes (Wijndaele et al. 2006). Considerations in the choice of cut-points include

- Whether cut-points should be related to relationships with a particular adverse outcome
- What that outcome is (or what those outcomes are)
- What percentage of the population is classified
- What statistical technique is most suitable for selecting cut-points
- Whether cut-points should vary by ethnicity
- Whether cut-points in the context of the metabolic syndrome should be the same as when the component is considered as a single risk factor

Given the number of competing priorities, it is not surprising that diagnostic criteria and cut-points are often chosen somewhat arbitrarily. Fortunately, agreement has been achieved on cut-points for all components of the MetS except obesity. Based on differences in their predisposition to the MetS, type 2 diabetes and CVDs at the same level of waist circumference, it is clear that ethnicity-specific obesity cut-points are required (Cameron et al. 2010, Razak et al. 2007, Stevens 2003, Vikram et al. 2003). Unfortunately, little strong evidence exists for appropriate cut-points in different groups. Many of the studies attempting to define cut-points for different populations have used statistical methods based on the Youden Index or receiver operating characteristic (ROC) curve (Cameron et al. 2010). Recently, it has been shown that waist circumference cut-points chosen using the Youden Index are entirely dependent on obesity levels in the population (Cameron et al. 2010). The Youden Index is therefore entirely inappropriate for the selection of obesity cut-points and should not be used for this purpose (Cameron et al. 2010). A clear need exists for cross-sectional and particularly longitudinal data "relating waist circumference to risk for both cardiovascular disease (CVD) and type 2 diabetes" (Alberti et al. 2009). Such studies need to use appropriate statistical techniques (Perkins and Schisterman 2006) so that evidence-based ethnicity-specific obesity cut-points for all populations can be decided upon.

1.3 PREVALENCE IN WORLDWIDE POPULATIONS

The prevalence of the MetS is dictated by multiple attributes of the population, many of which change over time. Genetic predisposition, levels of physical activity and inactivity, population age and sex structure, levels of over- and under-nutrition, and body composition are all important. Regardless of the environmental and underlying genetic influences mediating the prevalence of the MetS, a higher prevalence undoubtedly leads to a greater likelihood of undesirable outcomes such as type 2 diabetes and CVDs.

To assess the prevalence of the MetS using only the most current and up-to-date definition, a literature review was conducted for studies utilizing the consensus MetS definition of Alberti et al. (2009). Two search methods were used. Firstly, among all the citations in Google Scholar of the Alberti consensus definition (n = 1616), those in the English language and with a title that suggested that the prevalence of the MetS may have been reported from a population-based study were selected for further review. Secondly, a search in PubMed was conducted using the following search terms: ("prevalence of the MetS" [Title/Abstract]) OR "MetS prevalence" [Title/Abstract]. Studies were excluded if they were based on a specific clinical population or a narrow age group (i.e., they were not from the general population of adults). Three studies were identified among adolescents or young people that fitted all other inclusion criteria—these studies are reported separately. The most recent publication was chosen if several national reports from a single country existed. As the most recent, revised (2005) definition of the MetS by the United States (U.S.) National Cholesterol Education Program (NCEP) is similar to that of the 2009 consensus definition (with the only distinction being that the consensus definition specified ethnicity-specific waist circumference cut-points, while the NCEP definition had a single waist circumference cut-point for obesity of 102 cm [male] and 88 cm [female]), studies that used the NCEP definition were also reported. Because of this, it is acknowledged that for some populations, the waist circumference cut-points used may not have been appropriate for their ethnicity according to the consensus definition. The original NCEP definition incorporated a cut-point for hyperglycemia of FPG ≥ 6.1 mmol/L (110 mg/dL), whereas in the revised (2005) definition the corresponding figure was FPG ≥ 5.6 mmol/L (100 mg/dL). Due to this difference, studies using the original NCEP definition were excluded. The search for relevant publications was last conducted on April 11, 2013. It should be noted that this search strategy was not intended to result in a comprehensive listing of papers reporting the prevalence of the MetS (for instance, some papers may be in languages other than English and many reports of MetS prevalence may be available in gray literature such as national and regional reports). The strategy was designed, however, to identify a range of studies that can demonstrate the variation in the prevalence of the MetS in countries worldwide.

Table 1.3 shows studies from 19 different countries were identified. Eleven studies (46%) reported the prevalence of the MetS based on the most recent consensus statement. A total of 58% of studies were found to be using waist circumference criteria that were inconsistent with those identified in the consensus statement as most appropriate for their population or ethnic group. The simple explanation for this finding is that the majority of those studies reported the prevalence of the MetS based on the NCEP criteria (which defines waist circumference according to a single set of sex-specific cut-points, regardless of ethnicity). The countries with the highest prevalence of the MetS included Greece (45.7%), India (45.3%), Puerto Rico (43.3%), and Colombia (40.7%). Countries with the lowest prevalence included Peru (18.8%, although the study used cut-points of 102 cm/88 cm for males and females, not consistent with the 2009 consensus definition) (Alberti et al. 2009) and Canada (19.1% or 23.2% depending on the waist circumference cut-point used). The two studies among young adults and the U.S. study in adolescents found comparatively low MetS prevalence figures of 5.3% among 18–30-year-old Lebanese, 1.2% in 18–20-year-old Jamaicans, and 5.8% in 12–19-year-old Americans.

1.4 DISCUSSION

This study represents the first assessment of the prevalence of the MetS worldwide since the publication of a consensus definition in 2009. In comparison with the only similar previous review from 2004 (Cameron et al. 2004), the presence of a single consensus definition makes this review a relatively simple proposition to interpret. Although this review was not exhaustive, the fact that only 24 studies were included here reflects the reality that not all studies of (reasonably) nationally representative populations will include measurement of the 5 MetS components necessary to categorize individuals. More is known of global trends in individual components such as overweight and obesity (Finucane et al. 2011), and diabetes and pre-diabetes (International Diabetes Federation 2012). Nevertheless, the low number of studies is also a testament to the fact that we really know little of the contemporary prevalence of the MetS in most countries. The United States stands out as having good data due to its ongoing national monitoring program (the National Health and Nutrition Examination Survey [NHANES]).

Although comparisons of country prevalence figures are simpler now that a single definition exists, the difference in the use of cut-points for waist circumference in order to identify overweight/obesity remains a source of complexity. Prevalence figures are naturally considerably higher when

TABLE 1.3

Prevalence of the Metabolic Syndrome in 19 countries

Region	City, Country	Study Year	Stated Definition of MetS	Obesity Criteria Used	Survey Population	Age Group, N	Response Rate	Prevalence (%) (95% CI)	Reference
Americas	Latin America, Multiple countries	2008	NCEP-ATPIII, 2005	Waist circumference: >102 cm (male) or >88 cm (female)	Unspecified, M=34%	21–79, n=867	Not reported	San Juan, Puerto Rico=43.3	Marquez-Sandoval et al. (2011)
		2008	NCEP-ATPIII, 2005	Waist circumference: >102 cm (male) or >88 cm (female)	Unspecified, M=34%	18–74, n=1007	Not reported	Talca, Chile=35.5	
		2007	NCEP-ATPIII, 2005	Waist circumference: >102 cm (male) or >88 cm (female)	Convenience, M=54%	22–73, n=155	Not reported	Bucaramanga, Colombia=34.8	
		2007	NCEP-ATPIII, 2005	Waist circumference: >102 cm (male) or >88 cm (female)	Probabilistic, M=54%	20–80, n=1878	Not reported	Arequipa, Peru=18.8	
	Brazil, Federal District	2007	Consensus definition, 2009	Waist circumference: >102 cm (male) or >88 cm (female)	Population based	≥18, n=2130	80%	Total=32.0 (28.9–35.2) M=30.9 (26.1–35.6) F=33.0 (29.5–36.6)	Dutra et al. (2012)
	Peru, San Pedro de Cajas (at 13,000 ft altitude) and Rimac (sea level)	2002–2003	NCEP-ATPIII, 2005	Waist circumference: >102 cm (male) or >88 cm (female)	Population based, M=36%	≥30, n=99 (San Pedro de Cajas) and n=172 (Rimac)	Not reported	San Pedro de Cajas: Total=24.2 (15.7–32.6), M=11.1 (0.8–21.4), F=31.7 (20.2–43.1). Rimac: Total=22.1 (15.9–28.3), M=8.1 (1.3–14.9), F=30.0 (21.5–38.5)	Baracco et al. (2007)
	Colombia, Medellin	2008–2010	Consensus definition, 2009	Waist circumference: >90 cm (male) or >80 cm (female)	Population based, M=30.7%	25–64 years, n=901	Not reported	Total=40.7 (36.4–45.3), M=39.3 (31.0–48.3), F=41.5 (36.5–47.1)	Davila et al. (2013)
	Canada, national	2007–2009	Consensus definition, 2009	Waist circumference: >102 cm (male) or >88 cm (female) Waist circumference: >94 cm (male) or >80 cm (female)	Representative	≥18, n=1800	Not reported	Total=19.1, M=17.8, F=20.5 Total=23.2, M=23.4, F=22.9	Riediger and Clara (2011)
	USA, national	2003–2006	Consensus definition, 2009	Waist circumference: >102 cm (male) or >88 cm (female) Waist circumference: >102 cm (male) or >88 cm (female) for white and African-American and other participants; ≥90 cm (male) and ≥80 cm (female) for Hispanic participants	National, Population based	≥20, n=3461	Not reported	Total=34.3, M=36.1, F=32.4 Total=35.0, M=37.3, F=32.6	Ford et al. (2010)

(Continued)

TABLE 1.3 (*Continued*)
Prevalence of the Metabolic Syndrome in 19 countries

Region	City, Country	Study Year	Stated Definition of MetS	Obesity Criteria Used	Survey Population	Age Group, N	Response Rate	Prevalence (%) (95% CI)	Reference
				Waist circumference: >94 cm (male) or >80 cm (female) for white and African American and other participants; ≥90 cm (male) and ≥80 cm (female) for Hispanic participants				Total = 38.5. M = 41.9. F = 35.0	
Europe	Estonia. national	2008–2009	NCEP-ATPIII, 2005	Waist circumference: >102 cm (male) or >88 cm (female)	Population based	20–74, n = 495	53.20%	Total = 27.9 (24.0–32.1) M = 30.8 (24.8–37.6) F = 25.6 (20.7–31.2)	Eglit et al. (2012)
	Greece. national	2003–2004	Consensus definition, 2009	Waist circumference: >102 cm (male) or >88 cm (female) Waist circumference: >94 cm (male) or >80 cm (female)	Population based	≥18, n = 9669	Not reported	Total = 26.3 Total = 45.7	Athyros et al. (2010)
	Cres Island, Croatia	2007	NCEP-ATPIII, 2005	Waist circumference: >102 cm (male) or >88 cm (female)	General population. sampling unclear	Adult (age group not indicated, median age = 57), n = 385	Not reported	Total = 24.9 M = 33.1 F = 20.5	Kabalin et al. (2012)
	Luxembourg, national	2007–2008	Consensus definition, 2009	Waist circumference: >102 cm (male) or >88 cm (female) Waist circumference: >94 cm (male) or >80 cm (female)	Population based. M = 49%	18–69, n = 1349	32.20%	Total = 24.7 (22.7–26.8), M = 30.8 (27.6–34.0). F = 18.5 (16.1–21.2) Total = 28.0 (25.9–30.2), M = 35.5 (32.2–38.9). F = 20.4 (17.9–23.2)	Alkerwi et al. (2011)
	Spain. Murcia	2003	Consensus definition, 2009	Waist circumference: >102 cm (male) or >88 cm (female) Waist circumference: >94 cm (male) or >80 cm (female)	Population based. M = 46%	≥20, n = 1555	61%	Total = 27.2 (25.2–29.2), M = 28.2 (25.1–31.2), F = 26.3 (23.8–28.9) Total = 33.2 (31.2–35.3), M = 38.9 (35.6–42.2), F = 28.4 (25.8–31.0)	Gavrila et al. (2011)

(Continued)

TABLE 1.3 (*Continued*)
Prevalence of the Metabolic Syndrome in 19 countries

Region	City, Country	Study Year	Stated Definition of MetS	Obesity Criteria Used	Survey Population	Age Group, N	Response Rate	Prevalence (%) (95% CI)	Reference
	Spain, Madrid	2005	NCEP-ATPIII, 2005	Waist circumference: >102 cm (male) or >88 cm (female)	Population based, M=44%	31–70, n=1344	Not reported	Total=24.6 (22.3–26.9); M=28.7 (25.1–32.3); F=20.8 (17.9–23.7)	Martinez et al. (2008)
Asia	India, Chandigarh	Not reported	NCEP-ATPIII, 2005; Consensus definition, 2009	Waist circumference: >102 cm (male) or >88 cm (female); Waist circumference: >90 cm (male) or >80 cm (female)	Population based, M=42%	≥20, n=2225	94.80%	Total=35.8, M=27.7, F=43.2; Total=45.3, M=39.2, F=50.9	Ravikiran et al. (2010)
	India, Berhampur, Orissa	2001	Consensus Definition, 2009	Waist circumference: >90 cm (male) or >80 cm (female)	Population based, M=50%	≥20, n=1178	Not reported	(Age standardized to resident population), Total=33.5; M=24.9; F=42.3	Prasad et al. (2012)
	Malaysia, national	2005–2006	NCEP-ATPIII, 2005	Waist circumference: >90 cm (male) or >80 cm (female)	Population based, M=42%	25–64, n=2366	Not reported	Total=36.1; M=37.2; F=35.3	Tan et al. (2011)
Africa	South Africa, Cape Town, Bellville	2008–2009	Consensus definition, 2009	Waist circumference: >94 cm (male) or >80 cm (female) (implied, not stated explicitly); Waist circumference: >102 cm (male) or >88 cm (female) (implied, not stated explicitly)	Population based, M=19%	≥31, n=563	64.20%	M=35.2, F=68.4; M=26.8, F=62.2	Erasmus et al. (2012)
	Tunisia, Great Tunis	2004–2005	NCEP-ATPIII, 2005	Waist circumference: >102 cm (male) or >88 cm (female)	Population based, M=45%	35–70, n=2712	M=74.8%, F=95.1%	Total=31.2; M=23.9; F=37.3	Altal-Elasmi et al. (2010)

(Continued)

TABLE 1.3 (Continued)
Prevalence of the Metabolic Syndrome in 19 countries

Region	City, Country	Study Year	Stated Definition of MetS	Obesity Criteria Used	Survey Population	Age Group, N	Response Rate	Prevalence (%) (95% CI)	Reference
Middle East	United Arab Emirates—national study		NCEP-ATPIII, 2005	Waist circumference: >102 cm (male) or >88 cm (female)	Population based, M=41.3%	≥20, n=4097	89%	Total=39.6 (38.1–41.1), M=35.1 (32.9–37.4), F=39.6 (38.1–41.1)	Malik and Razig (2008)
	Qatar—national study	2007–2008	NCEP-ATPIII, 2005	Waist circumference: >102 cm (male) or >88 cm (female)	Population based, M=49.3%	≥20, n=1204	80.50%	Total=26.5	Bener et al. (2009)
	Kuwait, national	2008–2009	Consensus definition, 2009	Waist circumference: >102 cm (male) or >88 cm (female) Waist circumference: >90 cm (male) or >80 cm (female)	Population based, M=45%	≥20, n=992	Not reported	Total=36.1, M=34.2, F=37.7 Total=40.9, M=41.7, F=40.1	Al Zenki et al. (2012)
Young adults	Lebanon, Beirut	Not reported	NCEP-ATPIII, 2005	Waist circumference: >102 cm (male) or >88 cm (female)	Random selection of University students, M=53%	18–30, n=381	Not reported	Total=5.3 M=7.0 F=3.3	Chedid et al. (2009)
Young adults	Jamaica, national	2005–2007	Consensus definition, 2009	Waist circumference: >94 cm (male) or >80 cm (female)	Consecutive birth cohort, M=45%	18–20, n=839	57.60%	Total=1.2 (0.5–1.9) M=0.5 (0.2–1.3) F=1.7 (0.5–2.9)	Ferguson et al. (2010)
Adolescents	USA, national	1999–2002	NCEP-ATPIII, 2005	Waist circumference: >102 cm (male) or >88 cm (female)	National, Population based	12–19, n=1826	Not reported	Total=5.8 M=7.0 F=4.5	Cook et al. (2008)

NCEP-ATPIII, National Cholesterol Education Program Adult Treatment Panel III; M, male; F, female.

lower cut-points are preferred. Different study selection criteria and age ranges are additional complications, although an attempt has been made here to only include studies across a broad adult age range. Many countries, from diverse regions of the world, reported a high adult prevalence of the MetS of over 30% and sometimes over 40%. The prevalence of the MetS in Canada was notably lower than all other countries surveyed at around 20% regardless of the waist cut-points used. It is certainly plausible that a considerable survey/publication bias exists in those countries with a high prevalence of the MetS or its constituents are more likely to conduct monitoring surveys than those countries where the prevalence is lower.

Many countries reported prevalence statistics stratified by gender, with interesting patterns present in different areas of the globe. Strikingly, high figures for women were observed in each of India (51% vs. 39% and 42% vs. 25%, women vs. men in the two studies, respectively), South Africa (68% vs. 35%), and Tunisia (37% vs. 24%), as well as Peru (~30% vs. ~10%). The inverse was true (though not as dramatically) in the United States and the majority of European countries with data available (Spain, Luxembourg, Estonia, and Croatia). These opposite trends may reflect cultural differences in the traditional role of women in these societies. The prevalence was similar for both genders in studies from the Middle East; perhaps a surprising finding given the considerably higher obesity prevalence among women in many countries of this region (Wikimedia Foundation, Inc. 2015). Data from urban and rural areas are also likely to differ, with the likelihood of differing trends depending on the level of development of a country. For example, rural people have been found to have higher prevalence in the United States (Trivedi et al. 2013), whereas the opposite has been found in West Africa (Ntandou et al. 2009), China (Zhao et al. 2011), and South Asia (Misra and Khurana 2009). Although focused on adults, this review did find three studies reporting the MetS in younger individuals. The reports from Jamaica and the United States reveal a fivefold difference in prevalence (1.2% vs. 5.8%) despite the Jamaican sample being older. The high prevalence of the MetS in such a young age group (12–19 year olds) and using conservative waist cut-points suggests that the MetS represents a substantial disease burden in U.S. teenagers, the majority of whom are likely to go on to develop type 2 diabetes or CVD later in life.

In conclusion, the presence of a single, unified definition of the MetS now facilitates the monitoring of MetS prevalence both between countries and over time. The stability in the definition of the MetS over the past 4 years is in contrast to the problems created by multiple competing definitions previously. Many countries reported high prevalence figures of over 30% of the adult population, with some countries exceeding 40%. Given the high risk of type 2 diabetes and its complications as well as CVD that the presence of the MetS confers, the figures reported here are alarming and represent a truly global health issue.

REFERENCES

Al Zenki, S., Al Omirah, H., Al Hooti, S. et al. 2012. High prevalence of MetS among Kuwaiti adults—A wake-up call for public health intervention. *Int J Environ Res Public Health* 9(5):1984–1996.

Alberti, K., Zimmet, P. 1998. Definition, diagnosis and classification of diabetes mellitus and its complications. Part 1: Diagnosis and classification of diabetes mellitus. Report of a WHO Consultation. *Diabet Med* 15(7):539–553.

Alberti, K.G., Eckel, R.H., Grundy, S.M. et al. 2009. Harmonizing the metabolic syndrome: A joint interim statement of the International Diabetes Federation Task Force on Epidemiology and Prevention; National Heart, Lung, and Blood Institute; American Heart Association; World Heart Federation; International Atherosclerosis Society; and International Association for the Study of Obesity. *Circulation* 120(16):1640.

Alberti, K.G., Zimmet, P., Shaw, J. 2006. MetS—A new world-wide definition. A consensus statement from the International Diabetes Federation. *Diabet Med* 23(5):469–480.

Alkerwi, A., Donneau, A.F., Sauvageot, N. et al. 2011. Prevalence of the MetS in Luxembourg according to the Joint Interim Statement definition estimated from the ORISCAV-LUX study. *BMC Public Health* 11(1):4.

Allal-Elasmi, M., Haj Taieb, S., Hsairi, M. et al. 2010.The MetS: Prevalence, main characteristics and association with socio-economic status in adults living in Great Tunis. *Diabetes Metab* 36(3):204–208.

Athyros, V.G., Ganotakis, E.S., Tziomalos, K. et al. 2010. Comparison of four definitions of the MetS in a Greek (Mediterranean) population. *Curr Med Res Opin* 26(3):713–719.

Balkau, B., Charles, M.A. 1999. Comment on the provisional report from the WHO consultation. European Group for the Study of Insulin Resistance (EGIR). *Diabet Med* 16(5):442–443.

Baracco, R., Mohanna, S., Seclen, S. 2007. A comparison of the prevalence of MetS and its components in high and low altitude populations in Peru. *Metab Syndr Relat Disord* 5(1):55.

Barr, E.L., Zimmet, P.Z., Welborn, T.A. et al. 2007. Risk of cardiovascular and all-cause mortality in individuals with diabetes mellitus, impaired fasting glucose, and impaired glucose tolerance: The Australian Diabetes, Obesity, and Lifestyle Study (AusDiab). *Circulation* 116(2):151–157.

Bener, A., Zirie, M., Musallam, M. et al. 2009. Prevalence of MetS according to Adult Treatment Panel III and International Diabetes Federation criteria: A population-based study. *Metab Syndr Relat Disord* 7(3):221–229.

Cameron, A.J., Boyko, E.J., Sicree, R.A. et al. 2008. Central obesity as a precursor to the MetS in the AusDiab study and Mauritius. *Obesity* 16(12):2707–2716.

Cameron, A.J., Shaw, J.E., Zimmet, P.Z. 2004. The MetS: Prevalence in worldwide populations. *Endocrin Metab Clin N Am* 33(2):351–376.

Cameron, A.J., Sicree, R.A., Zimmet, P.Z. et al. 2010. Cut-points for waist circumference in Europids and South Asians. *Obesity* (Silver Spring) 18(10):2039–2046.

Cameron, A.J., Zimmet, P.Z., Shaw, J.E. et al. 2009. The MetS: In need of a global mission statement. *Diabet Med* 26(3):306–309.

Chedid, R., Gannage-Yared, M.H., Khalife, S. et al. 2009. Impact of different MetS classifications on the MetS prevalence in a young Middle Eastern population. *Metabolism* 58(6):746–752.

Cook, S., Auinger, P., Li, C. et al. 2008. MetS rates in United States adolescents, from the National Health and Nutrition Examination Survey, 1999–2002. *J Pediatr* 152(2):165–170.

Davila, E.P., Quintero, M.A., Orrego, M.L. et al. 2013. Prevalence and risk factors for MetS in Medellin and surrounding municipalities, Colombia, 2008–2010. *Prev Med* 56(1):30–34.

Dutra, E.S., de Carvalho, K.M., Miyazaki, E. et al. 2012. MetS in central Brazil: Prevalence and correlates in the adult population. *Diabetol Metab Syndr* 4(1):20.

Eglit, T., Rajasalu, T., Lember, M. 2012. MetS in Estonia: Prevalence and associations with insulin resistance. *Int J Endocrinol* 2012:951672.

Erasmus, R.T., Soita, D.J., Hassan, M.S. et al. 2012. High prevalence of diabetes mellitus and MetS in a South African coloured population: Baseline data of a study in Bellville, Cape Town. *S Afr Med J* 102(11 Pt 1):841–844.

Ferguson, T.S., Tulloch-Reid, M.K., Younger, N.O. et al. 2010. Prevalence of the MetS and its components in relation to socioeconomic status among Jamaican young adults: A cross-sectional study. *BMC Public Health* 10:307.

Finucane, M.M., Stevens, G.A., Cowan, M.J. et al. 2011. National, regional, and global trends in body-mass index since 1980: Systematic analysis of health examination surveys and epidemiological studies with 960 country-years and 9.1 million participants. *Lancet* 377(9765):557–567.

Ford, E.S. 2005. Risks for all-cause mortality, cardiovascular disease, and diabetes associated with the MetS: A summary of the evidence. *Diabetes Care* 28(7):1769–1778.

Ford, E.S., Li, C., Zhao, G. 2010. Prevalence and correlates of MetS based on a harmonious definition among adults in the US. *J Diabetes* 2(3):180–193.

Gavrila, D., Salmeron, D., Egea-Caparros, J.M. et al. 2011. Prevalence of MetS in Murcia Region, a southern European Mediterranean area with low cardiovascular risk and high obesity. *BMC Public Health* 11:562.

Grundy, S.M., Benjamin, I.J., Burke, G.L. et al. 1999. Diabetes and cardiovascular disease: A statement for healthcare professionals from the American Heart Association. *Circulation* 100(10):1134–1146.

Grundy, S.M., Cleeman, J.I., Daniels, S.R. et al. 2005. Diagnosis and management of the MetS: An American Heart Association/National Heart, Lung, and Blood Institute Scientific Statement. *Circulation* 25;112(17):e285–e290.

Himsworth, H. 1936. Diabetes mellitus: Its differentiation into insulin-sensitive and insulin insensitive types. *Lancet* 1:117–120.

International Diabetes Federation. 2012. *Diabetes Atlas*, 5th edn. Available from: http://www.idf.org/diabetesatlas/5e/the-global-burden. Accessed January 14, 2013.

Kabalin, M., Sarac, J., Saric, T. et al. 2012. MetS among the inhabitants of the Island of Cres. *Coll Antropol* 36(3):745–754.

Malik, M., Razig, S.A. 2008. The prevalence of the MetS among the multiethnic population of the United Arab Emirates: A report of a national survey. *Metab Syndr Relat Disord* 6(3):177–186.

Marquez-Sandoval, F., Macedo-Ojeda, G., Viramontes-Horner, D. et al. 2011. The prevalence of MetS in Latin America: A systematic review. *Public Health Nutr* 14(10):1702–1713.

Martinez, M.A., Puig, J.G., Mora, M. et al. 2008. MetS: Prevalence, associated factors, and C-reactive protein: The MADRIC (MADrid RIesgo Cardiovascular) Study. *Metabolism* 57(9):1232–1240.

Misra, A., Khurana, L. 2009. The MetS in South Asians: Epidemiology, determinants, and prevention. *Metab Syndr Relat Disord* 7(6):497–514.

Morrish, N.J., Wang, S.L., Stevens, L.K. et al. 2001. Mortality and causes of death in the WHO Multinational Study of Vascular Disease in Diabetes. *Diabetologia* 44(Suppl 2):S14–S21.

Ntandou, G., Delisle, H., Agueh, V. et al. 2009. Abdominal obesity explains the positive rural-urban gradient in the prevalence of the MetS in Benin, West Africa. *Nutr Res* 29(3):180–189.

Perkins, N.J., Schisterman, E.F. 2006. The inconsistency of "optimal" cutpoints obtained using two criteria based on the receiver operating characteristic curve. *Am J Epidemiol* 163(7):670–675.

Prasad, D.S., Kabir, Z., Dash, A.K. et al. 2012. Prevalence and risk factors for MetS in Asian Indians: A community study from urban Eastern India. *J Cardiovasc Dis Res* 3(3):204–211.

Ravikiran, M., Bhansali, A., Ravikumar, P. et al. 2010. Prevalence and risk factors of MetS among Asian Indians: A community survey. *Diabet Res Clin Pract* 89(2):181–188.

Razak, F., Anand, S.S., Shannon, H. et al. 2007. Defining obesity cut points in a multiethnic population. *Circulation* 115(16):2111–2118.

Reaven, G. 1988. Role of insulin resistance in human disease. *Diabetes* 37:1595–1607.

Reaven, G. 2004. The MetS or the insulin resistance syndrome? Different names, different concepts, and different goals. *Endocrinol Metab Clin N Am* 33(2):283–303.

Riediger, N.D., Clara, I. 2011. Prevalence of MetS in the Canadian adult population. *Can Med Assoc J* 183(15):E1127–E1134.

Stevens, J. 2003. Ethnic-specific cutpoints for obesity vs country-specific guidelines for action. *Int J Obes Relat Metab Disord* 27(3):287–288.

Tan, A.K., Dunn, R.A., Yen, S.T. 2011. Ethnic disparities in MetS in Malaysia: An analysis by risk factors. *Metab Syndr Relat Disord* 9(6):441–451.

Trivedi, T., Liu, J., Probst, J.C. et al. 2013. The MetS: Are rural residents at increased risk? *J Rural Health* 29(2):188–197.

Vikram, N.K., Pandey, R.M., Misra, A. et al. 2003. Non-obese (body mass index < 25 kg/m^2) Asian Indians with normal waist circumference have high cardiovascular risk. *Nutrition* 19(6):503–509.

Wijndaele, K., Beunen, G., Duvigneaud, N. et al. 2006. A continuous MetS risk score: Utility for epidemiological analyses. *Diabetes Care* 29(10):2329.

Wikimedia Foundation, Inc. 2015. *Obesity in the Middle East and North Africa*. Available from: http://en.wikipedia.org/wiki/Obesity_in_the_Middle_East_and_North_Africa. (last updated 21st March). Accessed April 27, 2015.

World Health Organization. 1999. Definition, diagnosis and classification of diabetes mellitus and its complications; Part 1: Diagnosis and classification of diabetes mellitus. Geneva, Switzerland: Department of Noncommunicable Disease Surveillance. Report No.: WHO/NCD/NCS/99.2.

Yeni-Komshian, H., Carantoni, M., Abbasi, F. et al. 2000. Relationship between several surrogate estimates of insulin resistance and quantification of insulin-mediated glucose disposal in 490 healthy nondiabetic volunteers. *Diabetes Care* 23(2):171–175.

Zhao, J., Pang, Z.C., Zhang, L. et al. 2011. Prevalence of MetS in rural and urban Chinese population in Qingdao. *J Endocrinol Invest* 34(6):444–448.

2 Pathophysiology of Metabolic Syndrome

Part I—Influence of Adiposity and Insulin Resistance

Jarlei Fiamoncini, Talita Romanatto, Sandro Massao Hirabara, and Rui Curi

CONTENTS

2.1 BIOLOGICAL EFFECTS OF INSULIN

Once in the circulation, insulin triggers several signaling pathways that lead to glucose utilization and reduction of glycemia. This hormone raises glycogen synthesis in skeletal muscle and liver, decreases hepatic glucose output, inhibits lipolysis and induces lipogenesis in adipose tissue, reduces proteolysis, and increases protein synthesis in skeletal muscle. Insulin has also other systemic effects including the modulation of cell proliferation.

The insulin signal is transduced via a plasma membrane heterotetrameric protein with intrinsic tyrosine kinase activity—the insulin receptor (Ballotti et al. 1989, Matschinsky et al. 1998). Once phosphorylated, the insulin receptor induces tyrosine phosphorylation of the insulin receptor substrates (IRS) upon its binding (Ashcroft and Gribble 1999, Pronk et al. 1993). These proteins activate several others, particularly phosphatidyl-inositol (PI) 3-kinase that generates PI-3 phosphate,

PI-3,4-biphosphate, and PI-3,4,5-triphosphate, which then propagate the insulin signal (Nystrom and Quon 1999). The activation of this pathway raises the activity of the protein kinase B (Akt) (Alessi et al. 1996), involved in several insulin effects such as translocation of glucose transporter 4 (Glut4) from intracellular vesicles to the plasma membrane (and thus glucose uptake) (Cheatham et al. 1994), protein synthesis via p70 S6 kinase (p70^{S6K}) activation (Chang and Traugh 1998), glycogen synthesis via glycogen synthase kinase-3 inhibition, and the activity of hormone-sensitive lipase (HSL) (Carlsen et al. 1997).

2.2   INSULIN RESISTANCE

Insulin resistance (IR) is referred when there is an impairment or absence of the effects attributed to this hormone. Usually, this condition is paralleled *in vivo* with high insulin secretion from the β-cells as an attempt to overcome the resistance to the hormone.

In *diabetes mellitus* and obesity, IR is observed in association with an increased concentration of circulating nonesterified fatty acids (NEFA). These metabolites have been implied as causal factors for the development of the IR state. In fact, the prolonged increase in the circulating levels of NEFA leads to a reduction in the action of insulin in skeletal muscle, liver, and adipose tissue (Hunnicutt et al. 1994, Oakes et al. 1997, Randle et al. 1963). The effects of NEFA depend on the kind of fatty acid (FA). Saturated FA like palmitic acid has been associated with IR in adipocytes and skeletal muscle (Hirabara et al. 2007, Montell et al. 2001, Thompson et al. 2000). Several mechanisms have been proposed to explain the effects of NEFA on the onset of IR, as described in the following text.

2.2.1   RANDLE CYCLE

According to this mechanism, when FA availability to the cells is increased, specific metabolites accumulate within the cell leading to a decrease in glucose uptake. In 1963, using rat heart and diaphragm muscle, Randle et al. showed increased intracellular content of glucose and glucose-6-phosphate when the tissues are perfused with fatty acids or ketone bodies paralleled to reduced glucose uptake (Randle et al. 1963). In another study from the same group, it was concluded that in conditions of high concentration of NEFA (diabetes and starvation), the activity of fructose 1,6-bisphosphatase is decreased (Newsholme and Randle 1962). Putting their results together, when FA availability is increased, the increased content of acetyl-CoA and NADH generated by FA β-oxidation inhibits pyruvate dehydrogenase and increases citrate concentration and ATP/ADP ratio. These changes inhibit the activity of phosphofructokinase, impairing the flux of metabolites through the glycolytic pathway. Therefore, there is an accumulation of glucose-6-phosphate, which inhibits hexokinase II, preventing glucose phosphorylation. Since nonphosphorylated glucose is free to exit the cell, this results in inhibition of net transport of glucose. There is a debate on the importance of this mechanism for the development of IR. It has been shown that FA actually leads to a decrease and not an increase of glucose-6-phosphate content before inhibiting glucose transport reference. In spite of that, Randle cycle was observed and credited as a mechanism of IR in prolonged exposure to FA (Massao Hirabara et al. 2003, Roden et al. 1996).

2.2.2   INHIBITION OF INSULIN SIGNALING PATHWAYS

Elevated concentrations of free fatty acids, specially saturated ones, have been shown to inhibit the tyrosine kinase activity of insulin receptor in rat soleus muscle (Massao Hirabara et al. 2003) and activate serine and threonine kinases such as protein kinase C-ε (PKC-ε), PKC-θ, and PKC-δ, leading to IRS phosphorylation in residues that are not compatible with their function as signal transducers (Griffin et al. 1999, Schmitz-Peiffer et al. 1999). Both effects result in decreased transduction of the insulin signal in target cells.

2.2.3 LIPID METABOLITES AND INSULIN RESISTANCE

Several reports have shown the association of ceramides and diacylglycerols with the development of IR. Muscle cells treated with palmitic acid (therefore insulin resistant) show increased concentration of ceramides, and the effects of this fatty acid can be mimicked by using a ceramide analog. Moreover, physical activity decreases ceramide content and improves 2-deoxy-glucose uptake in skeletal muscle (Dobrzyñ and Górski 2002, Schmitz-Peiffer et al. 1999).

2.2.4 MITOCHONDRIAL DYSFUNCTION

Mitochondrial dysfunction has been associated with IR state by several authors. In humans, reduced mitochondrial content and oxidative capacity have been reported in insulin-resistant individuals, including obese and type 2 diabetic subjects (Holloway et al. 2007). Mitochondrial mass is decreased in skeletal muscle cells from insulin-resistant offspring of type 2 diabetic subjects, pointing out for an inherited defect in mitochondrial activity as an early marker for the establishment of IR (Morino et al. 2005). Alterations in the mitochondrial DNA, including mutations, polymorphisms, and epigenetics, can also contribute for the development of IR in conditions such as obesity, diabetes mellitus, and metabolic syndrome (MetS) (Juo et al. 2010).

The contribution of the mitochondrial dysfunction for the establishment of IR is not yet completely understood, but some studies suggest the involvement of signaling pathways activated by lipid metabolites and oxidative stress (Martins et al. 2012). In conditions of normal mitochondrial function, fatty acids are rapidly oxidized with no intracellular lipid accumulation, low reactive oxygen species (ROS) production, and normal insulin sensitivity. However, in conditions of abnormal mitochondrial function, fatty acids are poorly oxidized, resulting in ROS production and fatty acid–derived metabolite accumulation, including free fatty acids, ceramides, diacylglycerol, and triacylglycerol. ROS and lipid metabolites are increased in IR conditions and have been associated to the activation of various serine/threonine kinases, including nuclear factor κB (NFκB), p38 mitogen-activated protein kinase (p38 MAPK), c-Jun NH_2-terminal kinase (JNK), PKC-ζ, and PKC-ϵ (Bloch-Damti et al. 2006, Dey et al. 2005, Schmitz-Peiffer et al. 1997, Tirosh et al. 1999). These proteins contribute to the establishment of the IR state by leading to phosphorylation of serine residues in IRS-1, impairing the insulin-stimulated tyrosine phosphorylation of this protein, resulting in decreased activation of downstream signaling pathways and biological responses to the hormone (Hirabara et al. 2010, Krebs and Roden 2005).

Despite the induction of IR by saturated fatty acids, omega-3 polyunsaturated fatty acids (n-3 PUFA) are related to increased sensitivity to insulin (Chicco et al. 1996, Lombardo and Chicco 2006, Storlien et al. 1987). The mechanisms behind this protective effect of n-3 PUFA seem to involve anti-inflammatory effects and reduction of the content of lipids in the liver and in circulation. These fatty acids activate the transcription factor peroxisome proliferator-activated receptor-alpha (PPARα), inducing peroxisome proliferation in the liver and fatty acid oxidation. As a result, the content of triacylglycerols and other lipid molecules in this organ is reduced (Fiamoncini et al. 2012). It is possible that by lowering the lipid content, these fatty acids prevent the formation of lipid metabolites that can activate inflammatory pathways. n-3 PUFA were also described as the ligands of the G protein–coupled receptor 120 (GPR20), preventing by this way macrophage-induced inflammation (Oh et al. 2010). Short-chain fatty acids were also reported to prevent IR. The immunomodulatory effects of these fatty acids have been credited as one of the mechanisms by which they prevent obesity and related metabolic disorders. Other mechanisms are also involved, and a growing body of evidence is emerging, explaining the protective role of short-chain fatty acids toward IR (Lin et al. 2012, Vinolo et al. 2012).

2.2.5 OBESITY, INSULIN RESISTANCE, AND METABOLIC SYNDROME

Obesity is a multifactorial disease caused by genetic and environmental factors. Its incidence has reached pandemic proportions in recent years. The forecast is very pessimistic. It is estimated that by 2030, 51% of the population will be obese and severe obesity might reach 11% of the population (Finkelstein et al. 2012).

Obesity is associated with high plasma levels of NEFA and peripheral IR that leads to impaired glucose homeostasis (Stumvoll et al. 2005) and MetS. A chronic inflammatory state is also observed in obesity, resulting from the increased production of cytokines from adipose tissue and leucocytes. The inflammation state combined with IR leads to increased lipolysis (McArdle et al. 2013). High plasma levels of NEFA released from adipose tissue and pro-inflammatory cytokines aggravate the IR condition, creating a positive feedback loop.

Hotamisligil et al. (1993) firstly demonstrated the link between obesity and inflammation. These authors reported elevated plasma levels of TNF-α in different models of obesity and that the neutralization of this cytokine ameliorates obesity-induced IR (Hotamisligil et al. 1993). White adipose tissue, primarily thought as a triglyceride storage tissue only, is now recognized as an active secretory organ. The adipose tissue produces several cytokines and hormones called adipokines (namely leptin, adiponectin, TNF-α, IL-1 β, IL-6, MIF, IL-10, and others). Adipose tissue expansion is associated with infiltration of inflammatory cells in obesity that release and propagate pro-inflammatory stimuli, leading to the development of IR. One of the functions of adipose tissue in energy metabolism is to release free fatty acids through lipolysis of triacylglycerols as to provide energetic substrates when low glycemia takes place. This effect is observed in parallel with low plasma levels of insulin, a hormone that prevent lipolysis. In conditions of IR, the counter-regulatory effect of insulin is absent and lipolysis in the adipose tissue increases the circulating levels of NEFA.

The pro-inflammatory adipokines and NEFA derived from adipose tissue have combined effects on the liver: increase gluconeogenesis by preventing the inhibitory effect of insulin on this metabolic pathway, and stimulate lipogenesis (Brown and Goldstein 2008). The increased supply of NEFA and activity of lipogenesis in the liver lead to nonalcoholic fatty liver disease (NAFLD) and increased synthesis and release of very-low-density lipoprotein (VLDL), with effects on atherogenesis (Choi and Ginsberg 2011). Obese subjects have high plasma concentrations of cholesterol, VLDL-triacylglycerols, VLDL-ApoB, and LDL-ApoB, in addition to hyperlipidemia and glucose intolerance (Egusa et al. 1985).

The events described above are the landmarks of the MetS: obesity, inflammation, IR, increased plasma NEFA levels, steatosis, and atherosclerosis (Aballay et al. 2013). Nevertheless, it is difficult to establish a causal relationship among these features (e.g., IR can increase NEFA and high concentrations of circulating NEFA lead to IR).

In addition to atherosclerosis, IR and obesity also lead to the development of hypertension, another feature of the MetS (Chen et al. 2011). Yiannikouris et al. have demonstrated that adipocyte-derived angiotensin II plays an important role in the development of high-fat diet-induced hypertension in mice (Yiannikouris et al. 2012). Another mechanism associated to obesity and hypertension is the activation of the sympathetic nervous system (SNS) observed in this condition as well as in sleep apnea (Sowers 2013). Renal sympathetic denervation reduces systolic and diastolic blood pressure and improves insulin sensitivity in patients with refractory hypertension (Mahfoud et al. 2011, Witkowski et al. 2011). Other mechanisms seem to be involved in the development of hypertension induced by IR such as the effects of inflammatory mediators on vascular relaxation and sodium reabsorption (Sowers 2013).

2.3 HYPOTHALAMIC MECHANISMS OF OBESITY AND INSULIN RESISTANCE

Although not usually classified as a metabolic organ per se, the brain is the site of central regulation of food intake and energy expenditure. The hypothalamus responds to nutrients, insulin released from the pancreas, and leptin secreted from the adipose tissue. Insulin is the second most important adipostatic signal provided to the hypothalamus. Studies since the late 1960s pioneered the investigation concerning the roles of insulin in the central nervous system (Margolis and Altszuler 1967). However, only in the 1990s the functions of insulin in the hypothalamus were described (Carvalheira et al. 2001).

Under physiological conditions, the hypothalamus, acting under the control of peripheral factors, coordinates the perfect coupling between food intake and energy expenditure. As long as the system is fully active, body mass is maintained steady. Insulin inhibits food intake following direct administration into the hypothalamus or adjacent third ventricle, whereas neuron-specific deletion of insulin receptors induces a modest increase of body fat mass (Brüning et al. 2000, Hatfield et al. 1974).

Brain insulin action also influences autonomic function in a variety of ways. For example, injection of insulin directly into the lateral hypothalamus stimulates parasympathetic outflow to the pancreas, whereas injection of insulin in the ventromedial hypothalamus has the opposite effect (Obici et al. 2003). More recent studies suggest that, by increasing hepatic vagal outflow, insulin signaling in the arcuate nucleus enhances liver insulin sensitivity and, in turn, lowers hepatic glucose production (Lam et al. 2005, Sakaguchi et al. 1988). A thermogenic action of insulin was also reported following hypothalamic injection, an effect accompanied by increased firing of sympathetic nerves innervating brown adipose tissue (Sanchez-Alavez et al. 2010).

One of the mechanisms involved in the imbalance between food intake and energy expenditure is the establishment of resistance to the anorexigenic effect of insulin in the CNS (De Souza et al. 2005). To identify the molecular mechanism associated to insulin resistance, several groups have evaluated different models of obesity. The most remarkable findings reveal that, upon diet-induced obesity, the induction of inflammatory activity in the hypothalamus leads to the activation of intracellular signaling pathways promoting a negative cross talk with the insulin signaling pathways, which impairs their physiological anorexigenic activities (Carvalheira et al. 2001, Torsoni et al. 2003).

Currently, four distinct mechanisms are known to play a role in diet- and cytokine-induced resistance to leptin and/or insulin in the hypothalamus of rodents: (1) activation of the serine kinase JNK (De Souza et al. 2005); (2) activation of the serine kinase named I kappa B kinase (IKK) in hypothalamic cells by TNF-α (Zhang et al. 2008) resulting in reduced insulin signaling; (3) stimulation of the suppressor of cytokine signaling (SOCS) expression that provides a negative control for insulin signaling (Bjørbaek et al. 1998, Münzberg et al. 2004); and (4) expression of the tyrosine phosphatase PTP1B that catalyses the dephosphorylation of the insulin receptor (InsR) and insulin receptor substrate (IRS) proteins, turning off the signals generated by insulin (Picardi et al. 2008).

Two distinct neuron subpopulations of the arcuate nucleus of the hypothalamus act as the sensors for the energy stores in the body and coordinate a complex network of neurons that, in due course, control the balance of hunger *versus* satiety, and pro- *versus* antithermogenesis (Flier and Maratos-Flier 1998, Schwartz et al. 2000). These first-order neurons are equipped with receptors and intracellular molecular systems capable of detecting subtle or chronic changes in the concentrations of hormones and nutrients in the bloodstream (Schwartz et al. 2000). The response to these changes is based on the modulation of the firing rate and of neurotransmitter production and release by specific neuron bodies (Horvath 2005). The subpopulations of neurons of the arcuate nucleus are characterized by the neurotransmitters each one produces. One of the subpopulations expresses the orexigenic peptides, neuropeptide Y (NPY) and agouti gene-related protein (AgRP), whereas the other expresses anorexigenic pro-opiomelanocortins (POMC), such as α-melanocyte stimulating hormone (α-MSH), and cocaine- and amphetamine-regulated transcript (CART)

(Horvath 2005, Schwartz et al. 2000). Both subpopulations project to the lateral (LH) and para-ventricular nuclei (PVN) of the hypothalamus, where they control the functions of second-order neurons. In the PVN, two distinct subpopulations of neurons produce the anorexigenic and pro-thermogenic neurotransmitters, thyrotropin-releasing hormone (TRH), and corticotropin-releasing hormone (CRH), whereas in the luteinizing hormone (LH), two other subpopulations produce the predominantly orexigenic neurotransmitter orexin and the predominantly antithermogenic mela-nin-concentrating hormone (MCH) (Cone 2005).

During fasting or when body energy stores are depleted, the expressions of NPY and AgRP are induced, while POMC and CART are inhibited. This coordinated response is dependent on the simultaneous sensing of decreased nutrient availability; reduced levels of the adipostatic hor-mones leptin and insulin; reduced levels of the gut hormones cholecystokinin (CCK), glucagon-like peptide-1 (GLP-1), and gastric inhibitory polypeptide (GIP); and increased levels of the gastric hormone ghrelin (Badman and Flier 2005). Active NPY/AgRPergic neurons send inhibi-tory projections to the PVN, reducing the expressions of TRH and CRH, and stimulatory projec-tions to the LH, boosting the activities of the orexin and MCH expressing neurons. Conversely, following a meal or when body energy stores are replenished, NPY/AgRPergic neurons are inhib-ited and POMC/CARTergic neurons are active. In this context, nutrient availability and the levels of leptin and insulin are increased, as well as the levels of CCK, GLP-1, and GIP. In opposition, the level of ghrelin is reduced. The result is the inhibition of orexin and MCH neurons in the LH and the activation of the CRH and TRH neurons in the PVN (Badman and Flier 2005, Cone 2005, Horvath 2005).

The mechanisms by which second-order neurons effectively control food intake and energy expenditure are under intense investigation. MCH neurons play an important role in the control of energy expenditure. Increased expression of this neurotransmitter restrains animal motility and reduces the expression of the mitochondrial uncoupling protein, UCP1, in brown adipose tissue, leading together to a reduction in energy output (Cone 2005, Pereira-da-Silva et al. 2003). Conversely, the knockout mice for MCH produce a lean phenotype due to a combined effect on feeding and thermogenesis (Qu et al. 1996, Shimada et al. 1998), while the knockout for the main MCH receptor, MCHR1, produces a lean phenotype, predominantly due to increased energy expenditure (Marsh et al. 2002). Orexin has a predominant role in arousal and the control of feed-ing (Chemelli et al. 1999, Farr et al. 2005). In opposition to the neurotransmitters of the LH, the PVN neurotransmitters, TRH and CRH have rather overlapping roles in the control of hunger and thermogenesis (Appel et al. 1991, Schuhler et al. 2007). TRH biosynthesis and release are con-trolled by multiple inputs coming from POMC neurons, leptin direct signals, and other sources such as triiodothyronine (T3) (Fekete and Lechan 2007). Although most studies explore the role of TRH upon the control of thyroid function and, consequently, on thermogenesis, there are plenty of data showing its direct action in the control of feeding (Valassi et al. 2008). Similar to TRH, CRH production is modulated by a number of different inputs, such as signals emanating from the arcuate nucleus and direct actions of leptin, GLP-1, and histamine (Nicholson et al. 2004, Sarkar et al. 2003). The reduction of appetite is the most studied effect of CRH, but several studies point to its pro-thermogenic effects as well (Solinas et al. 2006). Nevertheless, little is known about the mechanisms controlling these phenomena. Some additional pathways of the central nervous sys-tem play modulatory roles in energy balance. The connections of first- and second-order neurons of the hypothalamus with these systems are only beginning to be deciphered (Horvath 2005). The actions of serotonin and norepinephrine to induce satiety and increase energy expenditure have been known for a long time (Leibowitz and Miller 1969, Waldbillig et al. 1981). Even so, these neurotransmitters play rather unspecific and minor regulatory roles in this context, as evidenced by the moderate/severe adverse effects produced by drugs acting through the control of these neurotransmitters and by the limited efficiency of all treatment regimens employing such drugs (Mancini and Halpern 2006).

2.4 ANIMAL MODELS FOR THE STUDY OF METABOLIC SYNDROME, OBESITY AND INSULIN RESISTANCE

Since MetS involves several organs, it is difficult to approach it using single-cell cultured systems and therefore, animal models are widely used in this field. It is rare to find animal models that mimic multifatorial/multisystemic diseases (e.g., specific clinical signs of MetS like central adiposity are not observed in rodents) and there are differences in the cutoff for some biochemical and anthropometric markers on top of species and gender-specific differences.

In spite of that, different animal models can display at least some features of MetS once they are challenged and this makes them valuable to the study of this condition. There are not only several strains of rodents that respond to a dietary challenge but also spontaneous animal models of specific characteristics of metabolic diseases. There are also genetically modified models that develop a phenotype similar to the human MetS.

2.4.1 SPONTANEOUS ANIMAL MODELS OF METABOLIC SYNDROME

In 1949, spontaneous mutant mice that became extremely obese were observed in the Jackson laboratories. It was concluded that it was produced by the mutation of a gene called *ob* (after obese) (Ingalls et al. 1950). These mice are recognizably obese at 6 weeks of age, and when they are 3 months old, they weigh double as their littermates. The *ob* gene was identified and cloned in 1994 (Zhang et al. 1994) and the peptide encoded by this gene isolated, and its effects on the modulation of energy homeostasis were shown in 1995. Considering the lean phenotype given by this peptide, it was called leptin from the Greek "*leptós*," which means "*thin*" (Halaas et al. 1995, Pelleymounter et al. 1995). It was then discovered that leptin is a hormone secreted by the adipose tissue that regulates adipose tissue mass through hypothalamic modulation of energy homeostasis.

The leptin receptor (LEP-R), a single transmembrane domain protein, was firstly cloned by Tartaglia et al. (1995). The mice carrying a point mutation in the leptin receptor are called *db/db* mice and are a model for obesity, diabetes, and dyslipidemia. These mice become obese around 4 weeks of age and display elevated plasma insulin levels as early as 14 days of age and hyperglycemia after 4 weeks (The Jackson Laboratory Database "jaxmice.jax.org/strain/000697.html"). The effects of the mutated *ob* and *db* genes are dependent on the background strain, but normally ob/ob and db/db mice have very similar metabolic profiles. Both display obesity, hyperinsulinemia, hyperglycemia, and elevated cholesterol levels as well as impaired fertility. The obvious difference between these two models is that the ob/ob mice have no circulating leptin, whereas db/db mice have elevated levels of this hormone and do not respond to leptin administration (Kennedy et al. 2010).

2.4.2 AGOUTI YELLOW MICE

The agouti gene "*a*" controls the production of melanin pigments in the skin, defining the coat color of mice. The dominant agouti allele Ay, present in homozygosis, is lethal before the implantation of the blastocyst. Heterozygous mice carrying the dominant agouti allele Ay (Ay/a) develop the yellow mouse syndrome, displaying other than an orange-colored coat, a maturity-onset obesity (Miltenberger et al. 1997).

When expressed in the brain, the agouti protein can bind to the melanocortin 4 receptor (MC4-R), antagonizing the action of the α-MSH, an anorexigenic factor (Yen et al. 1994). Therefore, agouti mice are hyperphagic, obese, and insulin resistant.

2.4.3 DIET-INDUCED MODELS FOR METABOLIC SYNDROME

Diets rich in fat, mono- and disaccharides, or sodium induce some features of the MetS in several murine strains. The severity of the symptoms varies according to gender and strain, and the use of purified diets allow well-controlled feeding experiments and comparisons between different studies. Diets widely used to study MetS are described in the following text.

2.4.3.1   Diets Rich in Cholesterol and Saturated Fat

Some murine strains fed on a diet high in cholesterol and saturated fat display atherosclerotic lesions similar to those observed in humans. The disadvantage of this model is that normally, mice and rats are protected from atherosclerosis due to their antiatherogenic lipoprotein profile. To overcome this limitation, genetically modified mice models were generated so that LDL concentrations are maintained at a high level (Lichtman et al. 1999). LDL receptor or the apolipoprotein E knockout mice, for example, show atherosclerotic lesions once fed diets added with 1% cholesterol for 12 weeks (Teupser et al. 2003). The Golden Syrian hamster is responsive to hypercholesterolemic diets, displaying elevated plasma LDL concentrations when fed on diets containing 0.1% cholesterol (Dietschy et al. 1993).

In addition to dyslipidemia, high-fat diets induce obesity and other features of MetS. The high-fat diet is probably one of the most widely used models to study several characteristics of the MetS. The type as well as the amount of fat used to prepare high-fat diets and the time of treatment can generate different phenotypes. The lack of standardization on the diet preparation makes comparisons between studies difficult. On top of that, the use of nonpurified diets makes the interpretation of certain sets of data almost impossible as these nonpurified diets can significantly vary on their macro- and micronutrient contents. Also, different strains of mice (or different species) respond differently to distinct contents of fat in the diet. When these limitations are considered in the planning of the study, hyperlipidic diets can be valuable tools to induce and study obesity.

2.4.3.2   Diets Rich in Mono- and Disaccharides

Sucrose and particularly its fructose component are associated with elevated circulating triglyceride levels and IR in humans. Typically, chow diet contains around 4% sucrose and 0.5% fructose, but when Wistar or Sprague-Dawley rats are fed on diets containing 65% sucrose, they develop IR and hypertriglyceridemia (Pagliassotti et al. 1996). In hamsters, fructose also induces hypertriglyceridemia and IR. Different mice strains respond differently to sucrose/fructose and, therefore, are not used as a model of hypertriglyceridemia and IR induced by high mono- and disaccharides (Nagata et al. 2004).

2.4.3.3   Diets Rich in Sodium

Hypertension, one of the features associated with MetS, is correlated with high sodium intake in humans. A typical murine-purified diet contains around 1% of sodium, whereas the chow contains 0.4%. The Dahl-salt-sensitive rat develops hypertension after some weeks feeding on a diet containing 4% or 8% of sodium (Ogihara et al. 2002). The same occurs with Sprague-Dawley rats, but in a slower rate. Rats are more popular models for sodium-induced hypertension than mice, since in the last the progression of hypertension can take several months, even on an 8% sodium diet (Yu et al. 2004).

2.4.4   Genetically Modified Mice Models for the Study of Metabolic Syndrome

Mice carrying specific mutations or with some genes knocked out can be created in order to mimic features of MetS. Due to the facility of genome manipulation in mouse, several strains are available and can be used for particular purposes. The adiponectin knockout mouse (adipo$^{-/-}$) is an example and can develop different phenotypes with high concentration of VLDL-TG, IR, and other metabolic deficiencies depending on the diet and time of treatment (Oku et al. 2007). A good review on the topic was written by Kennedy et al. (2010).

In summary, the diversity of animal models gives researchers several possibilities to study MetS or specific features of it. One should always keep in mind that these are murine models to study a human disease and care should be taken when comparing results from animal and human studies. The other big issue is the high variability of phenotypes when a diet model is used in different strains. Sometimes, the comparisons between studies can become difficult and must be done carefully.

2.5 INSULIN RESISTANCE AND PHYSICAL ACTIVITY

It is well established that regular physical activity is an important coadjuvant intervention for preventing and/or treating various syndromes, including obesity, type 2 *diabetes mellitus*, and MetS (Brown et al. 2009, Colberg and Grieco 2009, Misigoj-Durakoviæ and Durakoviæ 2009). Several positive effects have been found by this intervention, for example: (1) improvement of glucose uptake by insulin-independent translocation of glucose transporter-4 (Glut-4) and increased expression of this protein; (2) potentiation of insulin signaling in the post-exercise period; (3) elevation of muscle oxidative capacity, reducing the generation of potentially toxic lipid metabolites to this tissue; (4) favoring expression of genes involved in mitochondrial biogenesis and metabolism, and (5) reduction in inflammation (Goodpaster et al. 2003, McFarlin et al. 2006, Toledo et al. 2007). However, the mechanisms involved are still under investigation.

Regular physical activity improves the IR state not only by increasing glucose uptake and insulin signaling but also by improving the capacity to oxidize fatty acids, reducing the generation and accumulation of lipid derivatives potentially harmful to the cells (Corcoran et al. 2007, Hawley and Lessard 2008, Holloszy 2005). In the liver, regular exercise reduces the expression of phosphoenolpyruvate carboxylase and increases the expression of IRS-2 in diabetic rats (Park et al. 2008), as well as decreases lipid accumulation and IR in obese individuals (Haus et al. 2010, Johnson et al. 2009). In the skeletal muscle of diet-induced obese mice, physical activity reduces IR, S-nitrosylation of proteins involved in insulin signaling, and activation of mammalian target of rapamycin (mTOR) and p38 MAPK (Pauli et al. 2008, Rivas et al. 2009, Vichaiwong et al. 2009). In adipose tissue, regular exercise reduces hypertrophy and hyperplasia in rats submitted to a high-fat diet, increases GLUT-4 expression, and improves insulin sensitivity (Gollisch et al. 2009). In addition, physical activity has anti-inflammatory effects by modulating the expression of specific genes and cytokine production. An increase in plasma concentrations of interleukin-6 (IL-6), IL-1 receptor antagonist (IL-1ra), and IL-10 as well as a decrease in the expression of toll-like receptor-4 (TLR-4) and TNF-α in leucocytes and adipocytes have been observed (McFarlin et al. 2006, Petersen and Pedersen 2005).

The increase in insulin response by physical exercise involves activation of specific signaling pathways, leading to the metabolic effects (such as increased glucose uptake, fatty acid oxidation, and oxygen consumption) and expression of genes related to improved mitochondrial biogenesis, oxidative capacity, insulin signaling, glucose metabolism, and inflammation. During muscle contraction, AMP-activated protein kinase (AMPK) and calcium/calmodulin-dependent protein kinases (CaMKs) are activated (Koulmann and Bigard 2006, Ojuka 2004, Reznick and Shulman 2006). AMPK is a key protein responsible for various effects of physical exercise, including (1) phosphorylation and inhibition of acetyl-CoA carboxylase, reducing the generation of malonyl-CoA, an allosteric inhibitior of carnitine palmitoyl transferase-1 (CPT-1) that favors fatty acid oxidation, (2) increase in the glucose transporter-4 (GLUT-4) translocation to the plasma membrane by an insulin-independent mechanism, resulting in increased glucose uptake, and (3) elevation in the expression of genes related to metabolism and mitochondrial biogenesis, leading to improved oxidative capacity (Kelley and Goodpaster 1999, Ojuka 2004). The CaMKs are involved not only in muscle contraction but also in the increased expression of genes related to mitochondrial biogenesis (Koulmann and Bigard 2006, Reznick and Shulman 2006, Rose et al. 2006).

In summary, regular physical activity is an important intervention against development and for treatment of IR and related disorders, including obesity, type 2 *diabetes mellitus*, and MetS. Further investigations are required to address the understanding of the mechanisms involved in this process and the comprehension of the additive or synergic effects with other pharmacological or nonpharmacological interventions.

2.6 CONCLUDING REMARKS

Obesity and IR are the common ground for most of the MetS features. The expansion of adipose tissue stores as well as the ectopic lipid accumulation leads to an increase of NEFA circulatory concentrations that contributes to the IR establishment.

The accumulation of lipids provides the substrates for the synthesis of several lipid-signaling molecules that activate inflammatory responses, disturbing the insulin signaling pathway. The inhibition of insulin signaling by NEFA or inflammatory mediators increases the concentration of the former, establishing a catastrophic cycle that amplifies itself and makes difficult to distinguish between cause and consequence (Figure 2.1). The effects on tissues responsible for glucose disposal, muscle and liver, seem to be as important as those observed in the CNS and again, what comes first is an open question—is IR firstly established in the CNS or in the periphery? The studies carried out in this area are copious, but it seems that we are only starting to unveil the identity and function of these lipid mediators. With the help of new animal models for the study of metabolism, new approaches are possible, increasing the feasibility of studies to understand the mechanisms behind obesity and MetS. Studies on identification of new lipid-derived molecules using mass spectrometry and nuclear magnetic resonance (NMR) are also contributing to the discovery of new players in this multisystemic syndrome.

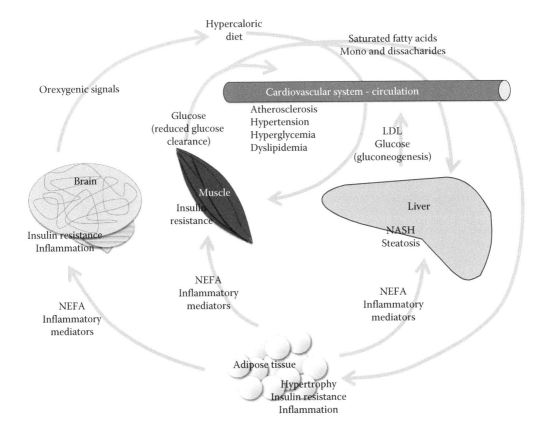

FIGURE 2.1 Role of adiposity, insulin resistance, and inflammation on the pathophysiology of metabolic syndrome. NEFA: nonesterified fatty acids.

REFERENCES

Aballay, L.R., Eynard A.R., Díaz, M.P. et al. 2013. Overweight and obesity: A review of their relationship to metabolic syndrome, cardiovascular disease, and cancer in South America. *Nutrition Reviews* 71:168–179.

Alessi, D.R., Andjelkovic, M., Caudwell, B. et al. 1996. Mechanism of activation of protein kinase B by insulin and IGF-1. *The EMBO Journal* 15:6541–6551.

Appel, N.M., Owens, M.J., Culp, S. et al. 1991. Role for brain corticotropin-releasing factor in the weight-reducing effects of chronic fenfluramine treatment in rats. *Endocrinology* 128:3237–3246.

Ashcroft, F.M. and Gribble, F.M. 1999. ATP-sensitive K+ channels and insulin secretion: Their role in health and disease. *Diabetologia* 42:903–919.

Badman, M.K. and Flier, J.S. 2005. The gut and energy balance: Visceral allies in the obesity wars. *Science* 307:1909–1914.

Ballotti, R., Scimeca, J.C., Kowalski, A., and Van Obberghen, E. 1989. Antiphosphotyrosine antibodies modulate insulin receptor kinase activity and insulin action. *Cellular Signalling* 1:195–204.

Bjørbaek, C., Elmquist, J.K., Daniel Frantz, J., Shoelson S.E., and Flier J.S. 1998. Identification of SOCS-3 as a potential mediator of central leptin resistance. *Molecular Cell* 1:619–625.

Bloch-Damti, A., Potashnik, R., Gual, P. et al. 2006. Differential effects of IRS1 phosphorylated on Ser307 or Ser632 in the induction of insulin resistance by oxidative stress. *Diabetologia* 49:2463–2473.

Brown, M.S. and Goldstein, J.L. 2008. Selective versus total insulin resistance: A pathogenic paradox. *Cell Metabolism* 7:95–96.

Brown, T., Avenell, A., Edmunds, L.D. et al. 2009. Systematic review of long-term lifestyle interventions to prevent weight gain and morbidity in adults. *Obesity Reviews* 10:627–638.

Brüning, J.C., Gautam, D., and Burks, D.J. 2000. Role of brain insulin receptor in control of body weight and reproduction. *Science* 289:2122–2125.

Carlsen, J., Christiansen, K., and Vinten, J. 1997. Insulin stimulated glycogen synthesis in isolated rat hepatocytes: Effect of protein kinase inhibitors. *Cellular Signalling* 9:447–450.

Carvalheira, J.B., Silotob, R.M.P., and Ignacchitti, I. 2001. Insulin modulates leptin-induced STAT3 activation in rat hypothalamus. *FEBS Letters* 500:119–124.

Chang, Y.W. and Traugh, J.A. 1998. Insulin stimulation of phosphorylation of elongation factor 1 (eEF-1) enhances elongation activity. *European Journal of Biochemistry* 251:201–207.

Cheatham, B., Vlahos, C.J., Cheatham, L. et al. 1994. Phosphatidylinositol 3-kinase activation is required for insulin stimulation of pp70 S6 kinase, DNA synthesis, and glucose transporter translocation. *Molecular and Cellular Biology* 14:4902–4911.

Chemelli, R.M., Willie, T., Sintonet, C.M. et al. 1999. Narcolepsy in orexin knockout mice: Molecular genetics of sleep regulation. *Cell* 98:437–451.

Chen, G., McAlister, F.A., Walker, R.L., Hemmelgarn B.R., and Campbell, N.R.C. 2011. Cardiovascular outcomes in framingham participants with diabetes: The importance of blood pressure. *Hypertension* 57:891–897.

Chicco, A., D'Alessandro, M.E., Karabatas, L., Gutman, R., and Lombardo, Y.B. 1996. Effect of moderate levels of dietary fish oil on insulin secretion and sensitivity, and pancreas insulin content in normal rats. *Annals of Nutrition and Metabolism* 40:61–70.

Choi, S.H. and Ginsberg, H.N. 2011. Increased very low density lipoprotein (VLDL) secretion, hepatic steatosis, and insulin resistance. *Trends in Endocrinology and Metabolism: TEM* 22(9):353–363.

Colberg, S.R. and Grieco, C.R. 2009. Exercise in the treatment and prevention of diabetes. *Current Sports Medicine Reports* 8:169–175.

Cone, R.D. 2005. Anatomy and regulation of the central melanocortin system. *Nature Neuroscience* 8:571–578.

Corcoran, M.P., Lamon-Fava, S., and Fielding, R.A. 2007. Skeletal muscle lipid deposition and insulin resistance: Effect of dietary fatty acids and exercise. *The American Journal of Clinical Nutrition* 85:662–677.

De Souza, C.T., Araujo, E.P., Bordin, S. et al. 2005. Consumption of a fat-rich diet activates a proinflammatory response and induces insulin resistance in the hypothalamus. *Endocrinology* 146:4192–4199.

Dey, D., Mukherjee, M., Basu, D. et al. 2005. Inhibition of insulin receptor gene expression and insulin signaling by fatty acid: Interplay of PKC isoforms therein. *Cellular Physiology and Biochemistry* 16:217–228.

Dietschy, J.M., Woollett, L.A., and Spady, D.K. 1993. The interaction of dietary cholesterol and specific fatty acids in the regulation of LDL receptor activity and plasma LDL-cholesterol concentrations. *Annals of the New York Academy of Sciences* 676:11–26.

Dobrzyñ, A. and Górski, J. 2002. Ceramides and sphingomyelins in skeletal muscles of the rat: Content and composition. Effect of prolonged exercise. *American Journal of Physiology: Endocrinology and Metabolism* 282:E277–E285.

Egusa, G., Beltz, W.F., Grundy, S.M., and Howard, B.V. 1985. Influence of obesity on the metabolism of apolipoprotein B in humans. *The Journal of Clinical Investigation* 76:596–603.

Farr, S.A., Banks, W.A., Kumar, V.B., and Morley, J.E. 2005. Orexin-A-induced feeding is dependent on nitric oxide. *Peptides* 26:759–765.

Fekete, C. and Lechan, R.M. 2007. Negative feedback regulation of hypophysiotropic thyrotropin-releasing hormone (TRH) synthesizing neurons: Role of neuronal afferents and type 2 deiodinase. *Frontiers in Neuroendocrinology* 28:97–114.

Fiamoncini, J., Turner, N., Hirabara, S.M. et al. 2013. Enhanced peroxisomal β-oxidation is associated with prevention of obesity and glucose intolerance by fish oil-enriched diets. *Obesity* 21(6):1200–1207.

Finkelstein, E.A., Khavjou, O.A, Thompson, H. et al. 2012. Obesity and severe obesity forecasts through 2030. *American Journal of Preventive Medicine* 42:563–570.

Flier, J.S. and Maratos-Flier, E. 1998. Obesity and the hypothalamus: Novel peptides for new pathways. *Cell* 92:437–440.

Gollisch, K.S.C., Brandauer, J., Jessen, N. et al. 2009. Effects of exercise training on subcutaneous and visceral adipose tissue in normal- and high-fat diet-fed rats. *American Journal of Physiology: Endocrinology and Metabolism* 297:E495–E504.

Goodpaster, B.H., Katsiaras, A., and Kelley, D.E. 2003. Enhanced fat oxidation through physical activity is associated with improvements in insulin sensitivity in obesity. *Diabetes* 52:2191–2197.

Griffin, M.E., Marcucci, M.J., Cline, G.W. et al. 1999. Free fatty acid-induced insulin resistance is associated with activation of protein kinase C theta and alterations in the insulin signaling cascade. *Diabetes* 48:1270–1274.

Halaas, J.L., Gajiwala, K.S., Mafei, M. et al. 1995. Weight-reducing effects of the plasma protein encoded by the obese gene. *Science* 269:543–546.

Hatfield, J.S., Millard, W.J., and Smith, C.J. 1974. Short-term influence of intra-ventromedial hypothalamic administration of insulin on feeding in normal and diabetic rats. *Pharmacology, Biochemistry, and Behavior* 2:223–226.

Haus, J.M., Solomon, T.P.J., Marchetti, C.M., Edmison, J.M., González, F., and Kirwan, J.P. 2010. Free fatty acid-induced hepatic insulin resistance is attenuated following lifestyle intervention in obese individuals with impaired glucose tolerance. *The Journal of Clinical Endocrinology and Metabolism* 95:323–327.

Hawley, J.A. and Lessard, S.J. 2008. Exercise training-induced improvements in insulin action. *Acta Physiologica* 192:127–135.

Hirabara, S., Silveira, L.R., Abdulkader, F., Carvalho, C.R.O., Procópio, J., and Curi, R. 2007. Time-dependent effects of fatty acids on skeletal muscle metabolism. *Journal of Cellular Physiology* 210:7–15.

Hirabara, S.M., Curi, R., and Maechler, P. 2010. Saturated fatty acid-induced insulin resistance is associated with mitochondrial dysfunction in skeletal muscle cells. *Journal of Cellular Physiology* 222:187–194.

Holloszy, J.O. 2005. Exercise-induced increase in muscle insulin sensitivity. *Journal of Applied Physiology* 99:338–343.

Holloway, G.P., Thrush, A.B., Heigenhauser, G.J.F. et al. 2007. Skeletal muscle mitochondrial FAT/CD36 content and palmitate oxidation are not decreased in obese women. *American Journal of Physiology: Endocrinology and Metabolism* 292:E1782–E1789.

Horvath, T.L. 2005. The hardship of obesity: A soft-wired hypothalamus. *Nature Neuroscience* 8:561–565.

Hotamisligil, G.S., Shargill, N.S., and Spiegelman, B.M. 1993. Adipose expression of tumor necrosis factor-alpha: Direct role in obesity-linked insulin resistance. *Science* 259:87–91.

Hunnicutt, J.W., Hardy, R.W., Williford, J., and McDonald, J.M. 1994. Saturated fatty acid-induced insulin resistance in rat adipocytes. *Diabetes* 43:540–545.

Ingalls, A.M., Dickie, M.M., and Snell, G.D. 1950. Obese, a new mutation in the house mouse. *The Journal of Heredity* 41:317–318.

Johnson, N.A., Sachinwalla, T., Walton, D.W. et al. 2009. Aerobic exercise training reduces hepatic and visceral lipids in obese individuals without weight loss. *Hepatology* 50:1105–1112.

Juo, S.-H.H., Lua, M.Y., Bai, R.K. et al. 2010. A common mitochondrial polymorphism 10398A>G is associated metabolic syndrome in a Chinese population. *Mitochondrion* 10:294–299.

Kelley, D.E. and Goodpaster, B.H. 1999. Effects of physical activity on insulin action and glucose tolerance in obesity. *Medicine and Science in Sports and Exercise* 31:S619–S623.

Kennedy, A.J., Ellacott, K.L.J., King, V.L., and Hasty, A.H. 2010. Mouse models of the metabolic syndrome. *Disease Models and Mechanisms* 3:156–166.

Koulmann, N. and Bigard, A.-X. 2006. Interaction between signalling pathways involved in skeletal muscle responses to endurance exercise. *Pflügers Archiv: European Journal of Physiology* 452:125–139.

Krebs, M. and Roden, M. 2005. Molecular mechanisms of lipid-induced insulin resistance in muscle, liver and vasculature. *Diabetes, Obesity and Metabolism* 7:621–632.

Lam, T.K.T., Gutierrez-Juarez, R., Pocai, A., and Rossetti, L. 2005. Regulation of blood glucose by hypothalamic pyruvate metabolism. *Science* 309:943–947.

Leibowitz, S.F. and Miller, N.E. 1969. Unexpected adrenergic effects of chlorpromazine: Eating elicited by injection into rat hypothalamus. *Science* 165:609–611.

Lichtman, A.H., Clinton, S.K., Iiyama, K., Connelly, P.W., Libby, P., and Cybulsky, M.I. 1999. Hyperlipidemia and atherosclerotic lesion development in LDL receptor-deficient mice fed defined semipurified diets with and without cholate. *Arteriosclerosis, Thrombosis, and Vascular Biology* 19:1938–1944.

Lin, H.V., Frassetto, A., Kowalik Jr. E.J. et al. 2012. Butyrate and propionate protect against diet-induced obesity and regulate gut hormones via free fatty acid receptor 3-independent mechanisms. *PloS ONE* 7:e35240.

Lombardo, Y.B. and Chicco, A.G. 2006. Effects of dietary polyunsaturated n-3 fatty acids on dyslipidemia and insulin resistance in rodents and humans. A review. *The Journal of Nutritional Biochemistry* 17:1–13.

Mahfoud, F., Schlaich, M., Kindermann, I. et al. 2011. Effect of renal sympathetic denervation on glucose metabolism in patients with resistant hypertension: A pilot study. *Circulation* 123:1940–1946.

Mancini, M.C. and Halpern, A. 2006. Pharmacological treatment of obesity. *Arquivos Brasileiros de Endocrinologia e Metabologia* 50:377–389.

Margolis, R.U. and Altszuler, N. 1967. Insulin in the cerebrospinal fluid. *Nature* 215:1375–1376.

Marsh, D.J., Weingarth, D.T., Novi, D.E. et al. 2002. Melanin-concentrating hormone 1 receptor-deficient mice are lean, hyperactive, and hyperphagic and have altered metabolism. *Proceedings of the National Academy of Sciences of the United States of America* 99:3240–3245.

Martins, A.R., Nachbar, R.T., Gorjão, R. et al. 2012. Mechanisms underlying skeletal muscle insulin resistance induced by fatty acids: Importance of the mitochondrial function. *Lipids in Health and Disease* 11:30.

Massao Hirabara, S., Carvalho, C.R.O., Mendonça, J.R. et al. 2003. Palmitate acutely raises glycogen synthesis in rat soleus muscle by a mechanism that requires its metabolization (Randle cycle). *FEBS Letters* 541:109–114.

Matschinsky, F.M., Glaser, B., and Magnuson, M.A. 1998. Pancreatic beta-cell glucokinase: Closing the gap between theoretical concepts and experimental realities. *Diabetes* 47:307–315.

McArdle, M.A., Finucane, O.M., Connaughton, R.M., McMorrow, A.M., and Roche, H.M. 2013. Mechanisms of obesity-induced inflammation and insulin resistance: Insights into the emerging role of nutritional strategies. *Frontiers in Endocrinology* 4:52.

McFarlin, B.K., Flynn, M.G., Campbell, W.W. et al. 2006. Physical activity status, but not age, influences inflammatory biomarkers and toll-like receptor 4. *The Journals of Gerontology. Series A, Biological Sciences and Medical Sciences* 61:388–393.

Miltenberger, R.J., Mynatt, R.L., Wilkinson, J.E., and Woychiket R.P. 1997. The role of the agouti gene in the yellow obese syndrome. *The Journal of Nutrition* 127:1902S–1907S.

Misigoj-Durakovięæ, M. and Durakovięæ, Z. 2009. The early prevention of metabolic syndrome by physical exercise. *Collegium Antropologicum* 33:759–764.

Montell, E., Turini, M., Marotta, M. et al. 2001. DAG accumulation from saturated fatty acids desensitizes insulin stimulation of glucose uptake in muscle cells. *American Journal of Physiology: Endocrinology and Metabolism* 280:E229–E237.

Morino, K., Petersen, K.F., Dufouret, S. et al. 2005. Reduced mitochondrial density and increased IRS-1 serine phosphorylation in muscle of insulin-resistant offspring of type 2 diabetic parents. *The Journal of Clinical Investigation* 115:3587–3593.

Münzberg, H., Flier, J.S., and Bjørbaek, C. 2004. Region-specific leptin resistance within the hypothalamus of diet-induced obese mice. *Endocrinology* 145:4880–4889.

Nagata, R., Nishio, Y., Sekine, O. et al. 2004. Single nucleotide polymorphism (-468 Gly to A) at the promoter region of SREBP-1c associates with genetic defect of fructose-induced hepatic lipogenesis [corrected]. *The Journal of Biological Chemistry* 279:29031–29042.

Newsholme, E.A. and Randle, P.J. 1962. Regulation of glucose uptake by muscle. 6. Fructose 1,6-diphosphatase activity of rat heart and rat diaphragm. *The Biochemical Journal* 83:387–392.

Nicholson, R.C., King, B.R., and Smith, R. 2004. Complex regulatory interactions control CRH gene expression. *Frontiers in Bioscience* 9:32–39.

Nystrom, F.H. and Quon, M.J. 1999. Insulin signalling: Metabolic pathways and mechanisms for specificity. *Cellular Signalling* 11:563–574.

Oakes, N.D., Cooney, G.J., Camilleri, S., Chisholm, D.J., and Kraegen, E.W. 1997. Mechanisms of liver and muscle insulin resistance induced by chronic high-fat feeding. *Diabetes* 46:1768–1774.

Obici, S., Feng, Z., Arduini, A., Conti, R., and Rossetti, L. 2003. Inhibition of hypothalamic carnitine palmitoyltransferase-1 decreases food intake and glucose production. *Nature Medicine* 9:756–761.

Ogihara, T., Asano, T., and Ando, K. 2002. High-salt diet enhances insulin signaling and induces insulin resistance in Dahl salt-sensitive rats. *Hypertension* 40:83–89.

Oh, D.Y., Talukdar, S., Bae, E.J. et al. 2010. GPR120 is an omega-3 fatty acid receptor mediating potent anti-inflammatory and insulin-sensitizing effects. *Cell* 142:687–698.

Ojuka, E.O. 2004. Role of calcium and AMP kinase in the regulation of mitochondrial biogenesis and GLUT4 levels in muscle. *The Proceedings of the Nutrition Society* 63:275–278.

Oku, H., Matsuuraa, F., Koseki, M. et al. 2007. Adiponectin deficiency suppresses ABCA1 expression and ApoA-I synthesis in the liver. *FEBS Letters* 581:5029–5033.

Pagliassotti, M.J., Prach, P., Koppenhafer, T.A., and Pan, D. 1996. Changes in insulin action, triglycerides, and lipid composition during sucrose feeding in rats. *The American Journal of Physiology* 271:R1319–R1326.

Park, S., Hong, S.M., and Sung, S.R. 2008. Exendin-4 and exercise promotes beta-cell function and mass through IRS2 induction in islets of diabetic rats. *Life Sciences* 82:503–511.

Pauli, J.R., Ropelle, E.R., Cintra, D. et al. 2008. Acute physical exercise reverses S-nitrosation of the insulin receptor, insulin receptor substrate 1 and protein kinase B/Akt in diet-induced obese Wistar rats. *The Journal of Physiology* 586:659–671.

Pelleymounter, M.A., Culen, M.J., Baker, B. et al. 1995. Effects of the obese gene product on body weight regulation in ob/ob mice. *Science* (*New York*) 269:540–543.

Pereira-da-Silva, M., Torsoni, M.A., Nourani, H.V. et al. 2003. Hypothalamic melanin-concentrating hormone is induced by cold exposure and participates in the control of energy expenditure in rats. *Endocrinology* 144:4831–4840.

Petersen, A.M.W. and Pedersen, B.K. 2005. The anti-inflammatory effect of exercise. *Journal of Applied Physiology* (Bethesda, MD: 1985) 98:1154–1162.

Picardi, P.K., Calegari, V.C., Prada, P.O. et al. 2008. Reduction of hypothalamic protein tyrosine phosphatase improves insulin and leptin resistance in diet-induced obese rats. *Endocrinology* 149: 3870–3880.

Pronk, G.J., McGlade, J., Pelicci, G., Pawson, T., and Bos, J.L. 1993. Insulin-induced phosphorylation of the 46- and 52-kDa Shc proteins. *The Journal of Biological Chemistry* 268:5748–5753.

Qu, D., Ludwig, D., Gammeltoft, S. et al. 1996. A role for melanin-concentrating hormone in the central regulation of feeding behaviour. *Nature* 380:243–247.

Randle, P.J., Garland, P.B., Hales, C.N., and Newsholme, E.A. 1963. The glucose fatty-acid cycle. Its role in insulin sensitivity and the metabolic disturbances of diabetes mellitus. *Lancet* 1:785–789.

Reznick, R.M. and Shulman, G.I. 2006. The role of AMP-activated protein kinase in mitochondrial biogenesis. *The Journal of Physiology* 574:33–39.

Rivas, D.A., Yaspelkis, B.B., Hawley, J.A., and Lessard, S.J. 2009. Lipid-induced mTOR activation in rat skeletal muscle reversed by exercise and 5′-aminoimidazole-4-carboxamide-1-beta-D-ribofuranoside. *The Journal of Endocrinology* 202:441–451.

Roden, M., Price, T.B., Perseghin, G. et al. 1996. Mechanism of free fatty acid-induced insulin resistance in humans. *The Journal of Clinical Investigation* 97:2859–2865.

Rose, A.J., Kiens, B., and Richter, E.A. 2006. Ca2+-calmodulin-dependent protein kinase expression and signalling in skeletal muscle during exercise. *The Journal of Physiology* 574:889–903.

Sakaguchi, T., Takahashi, M., and Bray, G.A. 1988. Diurnal changes in sympathetic activity. Relation to food intake and to insulin injected into the ventromedial or suprachiasmatic nucleus. *The Journal of Clinical Investigation* 82:282–286.

Sanchez-Alavez, M., Tabarean, I.V., Osborn, O. et al. 2010. Insulin causes hyperthermia by direct inhibition of warm-sensitive neurons. *Diabetes* 59:43–50.

Sarkar, S., Feketeb, C., Légrádia, G., and Lechan, R.M. 2003. Glucagon like peptide-1 (7–36) amide (GLP-1) nerve terminals densely innervate corticotropin-releasing hormone neurons in the hypothalamic paraventricular nucleus. *Brain Research* 985:163–168.

Schmitz-Peiffer, C., Browne, C.L., Oakes, N.D. et al. 1997. Alterations in the expression and cellular localization of protein kinase C isozymes epsilon and theta are associated with insulin resistance in skeletal muscle of the high-fat-fed rat. *Diabetes* 46:169–178.

Schmitz-Peiffer, C., Craig, D.L., and Biden, T.J. 1999. Ceramide generation is sufficient to account for the inhibition of the insulin-stimulated PKB pathway in C2C12 skeletal muscle cells pretreated with palmitate. *The Journal of Biological Chemistry* 274:24202–24210.

Schuhler, S., Warner, A., Finney, N., Bennett, G.W., Ebling, F.J.P., and Brameld, J.M. 2007. Thyrotrophin-releasing hormone decreases feeding and increases body temperature, activity and oxygen consumption in Siberian hamsters. *Journal of Neuroendocrinology* 19:239–249.

Schwartz, M.W., Woods, S.C., Porte Jr. D., Seeley, R.J., and Baskin, D.G. 2000. Central nervous system control of food intake. *Nature* 404:661–671.

Shimada, M., Tritos, N.A., Lowell, B.B., Flier, J.S., and Maratos-Flier, E. 1998. Mice lacking melanin-concentrating hormone are hypophagic and lean. *Nature* 396:670–674.

Solinas, G., Summermatter, S., Mainieri, D. et al. 2006. Corticotropin-releasing hormone directly stimulates thermogenesis in skeletal muscle possibly through substrate cycling between de novo lipogenesis and lipid oxidation. *Endocrinology* 147:31–38.

Sowers, J.R. 2013. Diabetes mellitus and vascular disease. *Hypertension* 61:943–947.

Storlien, L.H., Kraegen, E.W., Chrisholm, D.J., Ford, G.L., Bruce, D.G., and Pascoe, W.S. 1987. Fish oil prevents insulin resistance induced by high-fat feeding in rats. *Science (New York)* 237:885–888.

Stumvoll, M., Goldstein, B.J., and van Haeften, T.W. 2005. Type 2 diabetes: Principles of pathogenesis and therapy. *Lancet* 365:1333–1346.

Tartaglia, L.A., Dembski, M., Weng, X. et al. 1995. Identification and expression cloning of a leptin receptor, OB-R. *Cell* 83:1263–1271.

Teupser, D., Persky, A.D., and Breslow, J.L. 2003. Induction of atherosclerosis by low-fat, semisynthetic diets in LDL receptor-deficient C57BL/6J and FVB/NJ mice: Comparison of lesions of the aortic root, brachiocephalic artery, and whole aorta (en face measurement). *Arteriosclerosis, Thrombosis, and Vascular Biology* 23:1907–1913.

Thompson, A.L., Lim-Fraser, M.Y.C., Kraegen, E., and Cooney, G. 2000. Effects of individual fatty acids on glucose uptake and glycogen synthesis in soleus muscle in vitro. *American Journal of Physiology: Endocrinology and Metabolism* 279:E577–E584.

Tirosh, A., Potashnik, R., Bashan, N., and Rudich, A. 1999. Oxidative stress disrupts insulin-induced cellular redistribution of insulin receptor substrate-1 and phosphatidylinositol 3-kinase in 3T3-L1 adipocytes. A putative cellular mechanism for impaired protein kinase B activation and GLUT4 translocation. *The Journal of Biological Chemistry* 274:10595–10602.

Toledo, F.G.S., Menshikova, E.V., Ritov, V.B. et al. 2007. Effects of physical activity and weight loss on skeletal muscle mitochondria and relationship with glucose control in type 2 diabetes. *Diabetes* 56:2142–2147.

Torsoni, M.A., Carvalheira, J.B., Pereira-da-Silva, M., Carvalho-Filho, M.A., Saad, M.J.A., and Velloso, L.A. 2003. Molecular and functional resistance to insulin in hypothalamus of rats exposed to cold. *American Journal of Physiology: Endocrinology and Metabolism* 285:E216–E223.

Valassi, E., Scacchi, M., and Cavagnini, F. 2008. Neuroendocrine control of food intake. *Nutrition, Metabolism, and Cardiovascular Diseases* 18:158–168.

Vichaiwong, K., Henriksen, E.J., Toskulkao, C., Prasannarong, M., Bupha-Intr, T., and Saengsirisuwan, V. 2009. Attenuation of oxidant-induced muscle insulin resistance and p38 MAPK by exercise training. *Free Radical Biology and Medicine* 47:593–599.

Vinolo, M.A.R., Rodrigues, H.G., Festuccia, W.T. et al. 2012. Tributyrin attenuates obesity-associated inflammation and insulin resistance in high-fat-fed mice. *American Journal of Physiology: Endocrinology and Metabolism* 303:272–282.

Waldbillig, R.J., Bartness, T.J., and Stanley, B.G. 1981. Increased food intake, body weight, and adiposity in rats after regional neurochemical depletion of serotonin. *Journal of Comparative and Physiological Psychology* 95:391–405.

Witkowski, A., Prejbisz, A., Florczak, E. et al. 2011. Effects of renal sympathetic denervation on blood pressure, sleep apnea course, and glycemic control in patients with resistant hypertension and sleep apnea. *Hypertension* 58:559–565.

Yen, T.T., Gill, A.M., Frigeri, L.G., Barsh, G.S., and Wolff, G.L. 1994. Obesity, diabetes, and neoplasia in yellow A(vy)/- mice: Ectopic expression of the agouti gene. *The FASEB Journal: Official Publication of the Federation of American Societies for Experimental Biology* 8:479–488.

Yiannikouris, F., Gupte, M., Putnam, K. et al. 2012. Adipocyte deficiency of angiotensinogen prevents obesity-induced hypertension in male mice. *Hypertension* 60:1524–1530.

Yu, Q., Larson, D.F., Slayback, D., Lundeen, T.F., Baxter, J.H., and Watson, R.R. 2004. Characterization of high-salt and high-fat diets on cardiac and vascular function in mice. *Cardiovascular Toxicology* 4:37–46.

Zhang, X., Zhang, G., Zhang, H., Karin, M., Bai, H., and Cai, D. 2008. Hypothalamic IKKbeta/NF-kappaB and ER stress link overnutrition to energy imbalance and obesity. *Cell* 135:61–73.

Zhang, Y., Proenca, R., Maffei, M., Barone, M., Leopold, L., and Friedman, J.M. 1994. Positional cloning of the mouse obese gene and its human homologue. *Nature* 372:425–432.

3 Pathophysiology of Metabolic Syndrome

Part II—Influence of Inflammatory Status and Oxidative Stress

*Hilton Kenji Takahashi, Leticia Prates Roma,
and Mauricio da Silva Krause*

CONTENTS

3.1 INTRODUCTION

The World Health Organization (WHO) states that overweight and obesity are the fifth leading risk for global deaths (James 2008). At least 2.8 million adults die each year as a result of being overweight or obese. The metabolic syndrome (MetS) is a cluster of obesity-related metabolic derangements such as insulin resistance, hypertension, hyperglycemia, and dyslipidemia, which predispose the development of type 2 diabetes, cardiovascular disease (CVD), and mortality (Reaven 2008). Subjects with MetS have three times risk of suffering a heart attack or stroke, twice of dying from such an event, and fivefold greater risk of developing type 2 diabetes when compared to normal subjects (Stern et al. 2004). Beyond these factors, many other path physiologic features have been identified in patients with MetS, such as chronic systemic inflammation, which has its origin in the links between the adipose tissue and the immune system, and increased oxidative stress, which is known to contribute to the progression of this disease.

Adipose tissue can influence and communicate with many other organs, including the brain, heart, vasculature, liver, and muscle through the production of various secretory factors known as adipokines. Adipokines have both pro- and anti-inflammatory activities, and the balance between the different factors is crucial for determining homeostasis throughout the body based on nutritional status. When adipocyte dysfunction occurs as a result of adipose tissue expansion (which may be due to overnutrition or physical inactivity, for example), dysregulation of adipokine production can have local or systemic effects on inflammation responses, thereby contributing to the initiation and progression of obesity-induced metabolic and cardiovascular complications. Such inflammatory condition in combination with an increased surplus of metabolic substrates also triggers an oxidative stress event, which has an important role on the development and extent of MetS complications. Among anti-inflammatory adipokines, adiponectin has been subject of intense investigation (Ouchi et al. 2003a, Berg and Scherer 2005). Low plasma levels of adiponectin have been reported to be associated with obesity-linked development of insulin resistance, type 2 diabetes, and CVD. Several experimental studies suggest that adiponectin can exhibit insulin-sensitizing, fat-burning, and anti-inflammatory properties as well as modulatory effect on oxidative stress in several tissues, thereby thwarting simultaneously several facets of MetS.

3.2 OBESITY AND INFLAMMATION

Obesity—in particular, excess visceral adiposity—is strongly associated with insulin resistance, hypertension, and dyslipidemia, which contribute to high rates of mortality and morbidity. This association was first described by Vague in 1956, who suggested that abdominal obesity may predispose to diabetes and CVD (Vague 1956). Since then, accumulating evidences indicate that a state of chronic inflammation has a crucial role in the pathogenesis of obesity-related metabolic dysfunction (Hotamisligil 2006, Shoelson et al. 2006). Indeed, clinical and epidemiological studies have described a clear connection between the development of low-grade inflammatory responses and metabolic diseases, particularly in the context of obesity and type 2 diabetes. Duncan and Schmidt (2006), Takamoshi et al. (2003) reported a positive correlation between body mass and peripheral leukocyte counts. Since then, a large number of studies showed a correlation between the excessive adipose mass (as occurs in obese individuals) and increased levels of pro-inflammatory marker C-reactive protein (CRP) in the blood. Increased levels of CRP, and its inducer interleukin-6 (IL-6), are predictive of the development of type 2 diabetes and CVD in various populations (Visser et al. 1999, Lowe 2001, Pradhan et al. 2001), and therefore, Ridker et al. (2004) proposed the inclusion of CRP as a component of MetS. In addition, interventions aimed at causing weight loss lead to reduction in the levels of pro-inflammatory proteins, including CRP and IL-6 (Esposito et al. 2003). Although this correlation is based on the higher circulating levels of inflammatory markers, the inflammation itself originates locally in adipose tissue as a consequence of excessive fat deposition, and later reaches the systemic circulation.

3.2.1 INFLAMMATORY RESPONSE

Inflammation is a coordinated physiological response of the organism to harmful stimuli such as infection or tissue injury aiming at the restoration of impaired homeostasis. This response requires the coordinated action of many cell types such as leukocytes (macrophages, lymphocytes, granulocytes), connective tissue cells (fibroblasts), smooth muscle cells, mesangial cells, and mediators, as cytokines (interleukines, hemlines) and growth factors (Lawrence and Gilroy 2007). The normal acute inflammatory response involves the delivery of plasma components and leukocytes to the site of insult and is initiated by tissue-resident macrophages and mast cells, in the case of innate response to infection, leading to a production of different types of inflammatory mediators (chemokines, cytokines, vasoactive amines, eicosanoids, and products of proteolytic cascades) (Medzhitov 2008). The stimulated endothelium allows extravasation of neutrophils and soluble components to the tissue, where they become activated releasing toxic agents and proteolytic enzymes to the extracellular milieu (Serhan 2007). If successful, the injurious agent is eliminated and inflammation resolution and tissue repair follow. This is achieved by switching the lipid mediators from pro-inflammatory (e.g., prostaglandins) to anti-inflammatory and pro-resolution ones (lipoxins, resolvins, and protectins) and by the action of tissue-resident and newly recruited macrophages (Serhan 2007). The whole process is associated with an increased basal metabolic rate and represents the focused and rapid response of the immune system to a site of injury or infection. However, if the neutralization and removal of the noxious stimuli or even if the clearance of apoptotic inflammatory cells from the inflamed tissue fail, the inflammatory process persists and a state of chronic inflammation or autoimmunity may arise (Lawrence and Gilroy 2007).

3.2.2 Nature of Metabolic-Induced Inflammation

The inflammatory state that accompanies MetS does not completely fit into the definition of inflammation, in that it is not accompanied by infection and no massive tissue injury seems to have taken place. Furthermore, the dimension of the inflammatory activation is not large and so it is often called low-grade inflammation. Williamson (1901) observed that salicylates could improve insulin sensitivity and glucose responsiveness in type 2 diabetes. This observation raised the first hypothesis that metabolic disorders could be associated with low-grade chronic inflammation. Multiple large population-based epidemiological studies demonstrated that abnormal levels of inflammatory molecules such as tumor necrosis factor-α (TNF-α), plasminogen activator inhibitor type 1 (PAI-1), and CRP are elevated in metabolic disorders such as obesity, MetS, type 2 diabetes, and CVD, suggesting that metabolic inflammation could be a mediator rather than a bystander marker of these diseases (Festa et al. 2002, Freeman et al. 2002, Hanley et al. 2004).

Adipose tissue mainly comprises of adipocytes, although other cell types contribute to its growth and function, including pre-adipocytes, lymphocytes, macrophages, fibroblasts, and vascular cells, and it can respond rapidly and dynamically to alterations in nutrient excess through adipocyte hypertrophy and hyperplasia (Halberg et al. 2008). Moreover, white adipocytes have been suggested to share embryonic origin, the mesoderm, with immune cells, while characterization of adipose tissue–resident lymphocytes led to the notion that this tissue was an ancestral immune organ (Caspar-Bauguil et al. 2005). More recently, immature hematopoietic cells have been found in adipose tissue; hence it has been proposed as a site for formation and maturation of immune cell precursors (Poglio et al. 2010).

Under conditions of positive energy balance, the adipose tissue stores dietary triglycerides into lipid droplets, until these are hydrolyzed through lipolysis, releasing free fatty acids (FFA) when required by the body energy demands. Adipocytes confer to the adipose tissue an excellent buffering capacity as these cells can expand in situations of caloric abundance and return to its initial state during periods of fasting or negative energy balance. The overloading intake of food leads to a chronic lipid storage, which induces the hypertrophy of mature fat cells and the hyperplasia of adipocyte precursors (Arner et al. 2010). However, if chronic positive calorie balance exceeds these storing mechanisms, a spillover of FFA undergoes into circulation inducing their accumulation to other metabolic tissues such as heart, liver, skeletal muscle, and pancreas (Bays et al. 2007), resulting in adverse clinical outcomes as insulin resistance, insulinopenia, and CVD (Raz et al. 2005, Jensen 2006). The release of FFA also contributes to the dyslipidemia found in MetS as hypertriglyceridemia and to increased proportion of low-density lipoprotein particles (Yu and Ginsberg 2005).

In obesity, the progressive adipocyte enlargement is followed by a reduction of blood supply with consequent hypoxia. It has been proposed that hypoxia could be an inciting etiology of adipocyte necrosis and macrophage infiltration (Trayhurn et al. 2008). Experimental observations from macrophages cultured in hypoxic conditions revealed an increased expression of inflammatory genes such as TNF-α and IL-6 (Ye 2009, Yin et al. 2009).

In normal adipose tissue, macrophages are located around dead adipocytes. One of their functions is to help on the clearance of the necrotic fragments, which contribute for the triggering of the inflammatory response (Cinti et al. 2005). Moreover, macrophages are also required for the formation of new blood vessels at the site of inflammation and ischemic areas (Cursiefen et al. 2004, Khmelewski et al. 2004). However, histological studies of adipose tissue in obese individuals and in animal models of obesity have shown an infiltration by a large number of macrophages, which appeared as crown-shaped aggregates, similar to those observed in other known inflammatory conditions, such as rheumatoid arthritis, and grew larger with increasing degrees of obesity (Weisberg et al. 2003).

The accumulation of macrophages in adipose tissue has been shown to be proportional to adiposity in both humans and mice models, and sustained weight loss results in a reduction in the number of adipose tissue macrophages that is accompanied by a decrease in the pro-inflammatory profiles of obese individuals (Cancello et al. 2005). There is also a preferential infiltration of macrophages into visceral over subcutaneous adipose tissue (Harman-Boehm et al. 2007). The origin of the macrophage infiltration is still under debate, but a study regarding bone marrow cell transplantation in irradiated mice showed that the macrophages that infiltrated the adipose tissue were derived from bone marrow (Weisberg et al. 2003). This finding led to the concept that macrophage aggregates could partially explain the obesity-related inflammatory state, since increased levels of TNF-α, IL-6, and resistin are produced by activated macrophages, which may directly contribute to the insulin resistance mechanisms in adipose tissue (Xu et al. 2003b, Trayhurn and Wood 2005). In support of this hypothesis, two different phenotypes for adipose tissue–resident macrophages were described: one that acts as pro-inflammatory, known as M1, and another that acts as anti-inflammatory, the M2. Interestingly, obesity has been associated with a switch from the M2 to the M1 phenotype, that is, to a more pro-inflammatory profile (Lumeng et al. 2007). Furthermore, the absence of the M2 phenotype has been associated with a higher susceptibility to obesity, inflammation, and insulin resistance (Odegaard et al. 2007). Not only macrophages but also other cell types such as mast cells and natural killer T cells are known to increase in obese adipose tissue compared with lean tissue and may contribute to the inflammatory milieu and metabolic pathophysiology (Liu et al. 2009, Ohmura et al. 2010). Moreover, it has been demonstrated that immature fat cells can transdifferentiate into macrophages (Charriere et al. 2003). However, the enhanced macrophage infiltration explains in part but not completely the increased production of inflammatory mediators.

Until early 1990s, adipose tissue was considered as a passive energy store for the body (triglyceride storage and FFA release in response to changing energy demands) also functioning as heat insulation and mechanical cushioning. This view changed dramatically after the discovery that adipose tissue also functions as an active endocrine organ through the secretion of several cytokines collectively referred as adipokines. Hotamisligil et al. (1993) demonstrated that TNF-α is produced not only by immunocompetent cells but also by adipocytes. Zhang et al. (1994) discovered another adipokine, leptin. This discovery provided a breakthrough in the understanding of adipose tissue functions, since leptin was demonstrated to be a hormonal link between adipose tissue and food intake. To date, more than 50 bioactive adipokines have been discovered. Among these, and in addition to leptin and TNF-α, IL-6, IL-1β, resistin, PAI-1, acylation stimulating protein (ASP), monocyte chemoattractant protein (MCP-1), and adiponectin should be mentioned (Kershaw and Flier 2004). These observations allowed understanding the links between the adipose tissue, inflammation, and other pathological manifestations of the MetS.

The ability of adipocytes to secrete adipokines reinforced the condition of adipose tissue as a mediator of inflammation and innate immunity. Like macrophages, adipocytes are sensitive to infectious disease agents and cytokine-mediated inflammation. In response to these signals, adipocytes have been shown to induce expression and secretion of TNF-α, IL-6, PAI-1, and MCP-1 among other acute phase mediators of inflammation, contributing significantly to systemic inflammation.

Moreover, these mediators can induce a specific type of insulin resistance, known as stress-induced diabetes or diabetes of injury, as seen in the cases of sepsis, acute myocardial infarction, and trauma. This can be interpreted as an evolutionary adaptive mechanism of glucose supply for cells that uses them exclusively as neurons and phagocytic cells. Although these short-term compensatory and adaptive measures are kept in a delicate control, the disruption of the systemic metabolic function can be detrimental (Van den Berghe et al. 2001, Dellinger et al. 2008). In the other way, adipocytes also secrete anti-inflammatory adipokines such as the secreted frizzled-related protein 5 (SFRP5), visceral adipose tissue–derived serene protease inhibitor (Vaspin), ometin-1, apelin, and adiponectin. These adipokines enhance the insulin-induced glucose uptake in adipocytes and other tissues such as muscle, liver, and kidneys, and suppress the expression of pro-inflammatory adipokines such as TNF-α, leptin, and resistin. The levels of pro/anti-inflammatory adipokine secretion are tightly controlled.

In obesity and chronic metabolic-related disorders, the inflammation response and insulin resistance, in contrast to the trauma/infection conditions, cannot be triggered and sustained by inflammatory mediators alone. Instead, the chronic excess of nutrients such as glucose and lipids are considered the triggers of the inflammatory signaling. They activate c-jun N-terminal kinase (JNK), inhibitor of k kinase (IKK), or protein kinase R (PKR) pathways, which in turn activate the transcription factor activated protein 1 (AP-1), nuclear factor-kappa B (NF-κB), and interferon regulatory factor (IRF), resulting in increased expression of pro-inflammatory cytokines in adipose tissue (Nakamura et al. 2010, Solinas and Karin 2010). In models of healthy and lean animals, fasting/feeding cycles induce a low level of inflammatory response in metabolic cells, which is resolved when nutrients are metabolized. During high-fat diet or excess feeding in obesity, response to food become more intense and frequent, and resolution of the inflammatory response becomes less efficient, raising the baseline of inflammation in adipose tissue (Gregor and Hotamisligil 2011). The inflammatory response by adipocytes induces the activation of the endothelial cells through upregulation of adhesion molecules synthesis such as the intracellular adhesion molecule 1 (ICAM-1) and vascular cell adhesion molecule 1 (VCAM-1) and an increase in vascular permeability. The overexpression of these adhesion molecules and MCP-1 by adipocytes induces the recruitment of circulating monocytes and macrophages to adipose tissue, therefore amplifying the inflammation even further (Kanda et al. 2006). The persistent activation of the inflammatory pathway by nutrients further disrupts metabolic functions, as insulin sensitivity, leading to more stress and inflammation in a vicious cycle. This link between inflammatory mediators and insulin resistance in obesity and type 2 diabetes was demonstrated by Uysal et al. (1997) using tumor necrosis factor receptor (TNFR) knockout mice. They observed that the absence of TNFRs protects these mice from obesity-induced insulin resistance.

The elevation of the plasmatic FFA levels in obesity due to the blunted capacity of insulin to inhibit lipolysis followed by excessive intake of dietary lipids (Cnop 2008) can trigger the metabolic inflammatory response through the toll-like receptor 4 (TLR4). The TLR4 is normally expressed in macrophages, myeloid dendritic cells (DCs), mast cells, and B-lymphocytes, and is responsible to activate the innate immune response. The TLR4 binds to the lipopolysaccharide of gram-negative bacterial cell walls, activating the inflammatory pathway through JNK and NF-κB signaling pathways. Saturated fatty acids can mimic this response binding directly to this receptor. Several studies have shown that TLR4 is overexpressed in the adipose tissue of both humans and animal models, which induced the expression of inflammatory cytokines in the presence of saturated fatty acids (Shi et al. 2006, Bes-Houtmann et al. 2007, Vitseva et al. 2008). It was also described that TNF-α can induce lipolysis and inhibit the activity of the nuclear receptor peroxisome proliferator-activated receptor gamma (PPAR-γ or PPARG), which is essential to adipogenesis and maintenance of adipocyte gene expression and function, allowing these cells to make and store lipids and thus maintain insulin sensitivity (Feingold et al. 1992, Guilherme et al. 2008). Therefore, it has been suggested that a paracrine loop between adipocytes and macrophages establishes a vicious circle that aggravates the inflammatory changes in adipose tissue involving fatty acids and TNF-α. Enlarged adipocytes release saturated fatty acids in excess that activate macrophages through TLR4 signaling. As a result, macrophages secrete TNF-α, which in turn acts on TNFR1 and induces inflammatory changes in hypertrophied adipocytes through activation of NF-κB as well as enhanced fatty acid release (Furuhashi et al. 2008).

3.3 ADIPONECTIN

Adiponectin is a hormone secreted exclusively by adipocytes under normal conditions. It is a key mediator of systemic insulin sensitivity and glucose homeostasis. These effects are achieved by a diverse set of effects on several important targets, including the liver, pancreas, cardiac myocytes, and the immune system and even the adipose tissue itself. The main metabolic effects of adiponectin are to suppress hepatic glucose output while suppressing inflammatory responses in many other cell types, including macrophages. In fact, administration of adiponectin to diabetic mice models has been shown to reduce hyperglycemia by improving insulin sensitivity, and in obese mice, it increases fatty acid oxidation and reduces the plasmatic levels of glucose, FFA, and triglycerides.

3.3.1 ADIPONECTIN STRUCTURE

Adiponectin is a 30 kDa protein, a member of the complement 1q (C1q) superfamily, and shares homology with collagens VIII and X, and complement factor C1q. This adipokine has a globular C-terminal domain and a collagenous N-terminal domain, which allows it to form multimer complexes prior to secretion. A cysteine residue in the collagenous portion is a critical mediator of higher-order complexes, which may represent the most bioactive form of this protein (Berg et al. 2002). In human plasma, adiponectin exists as low-molecular-weight (LMW) trimers, middle-molecular-weight (MMW) hexamers of ~180 kDA, and high-molecular-weight (HMW) multimers (12-mers, 15-mers, 18-mers) higher than 300 kDa (Waki et al. 2003).

The adiponectin gene is located on chromosome 3, locus 3q27, a region recently mapped as a susceptibility locus for type 2 diabetes and adiposity (Wu et al. 2002). The gene transcription is regulated by several transcription factors including C/EBP-a, C/EBP-b, SREBP, PPAR-γ, and SP-1, which are required for basal and induced adiponectin transcription (Barth et al. 2002, Iwaki et al. 2003, Seo et al. 2004, Qiao et al. 2005).

Ten relatively common single-nucleotide polymorphisms (SNPs) were identified in the adiponectin gene, with slight variability among ethnic groups. Two of them are associated with an increased risk for type 2 diabetes. SNP 276 in intron 2 (G vs. T) and SNP 45 in exon 2 (T vs. G) were associated with lower plasma adiponectin levels, higher insulin resistance index, and increased risk of type 2 diabetes. Both SNPs correlated with obesity in a Caucasian population (Vasseur et al. 2002). In French Caucasians, two other SNPs, in the promoter region of the adiponectin gene, SNP 11377 and 11391, were significantly associated with hypoadiponectinemia and type 2 diabetes (Vasseur et al. 2005). In spite of these associations clearly demonstrated between the SNPs and hypoadiponectinemia in different populations, their relations with other phenotypes of the MetS remain conflicting (Heid et al. 2006).

In addition to the relatively common SNPs, eight mutations in the adiponectin gene have been reported, some of which are significantly related to diabetes and hypoadiponectinemia (Hara et al. 2002). Arg112Cys and Ile164Thr mutants did not assemble into trimers, which caused impaired secretion from the cell and hypoadiponectinemia. The Gly84Arg and Gly90Ser mutants led to impaired higher multimerization, which was clinically associated with diabetes (Waki et al. 2003).

Although most adiponectin exists in the plasma as full-length adiponectin, it was reported that a small amount of globular adiponectin (~1% of total adiponectin), generated by proteolytic cleavage, was detected in human plasma (Fruebis et al. 2001). It is speculated that the cleavage of adiponectin takes place locally and that the cleaved product is abundant in such regions, in spite of its low systemic concentration (Waki et al. 2005). Even if the globular domain is commonly considered as the receptor-binding/effector domain, it was shown that the amino-terminal region of adiponectin is a physiologically functional domain as well and that a novel receptor, which recognizes this region, may exist in some types of cells (Ujiie et al. 2006).

Adiponectin circulates at a high concentration (approximately 10 μg/mL, ranging from 2 to 30 μg/mL), which is 10^3 higher than that of major hormones (e.g., leptin, insulin, and cortisone) and 10^6 higher than that of most inflammatory cytokines (e.g., TNF-α and IL-6) (Shimada et al. 2004). Circulating levels of adiponectin are tightly controlled and remain relatively constant, despite the rapid turnover of the circulating pool within a few hours (5–6 h) (Trujillo and Scherer 2005). In healthy humans, adiponectin secretion follows a circadian rhythm, with a significant decline at night and a nadir in the early morning (Gavrila et al. 2003).

Although adiponectin is secreted by adipose tissue, clinical studies reported lower adiponectin levels in obese compared with lean individuals. According to Arita's study, the mean plasma adiponectin level was ~4 μg/mL in a group of obese patients compared with a mean level of 9 μg/mL in normal subjects (Arita et al. 1999). Plasmatic levels of adiponectin are also decreased in patients with type 2 diabetes or coronary artery disease compared with healthy individuals. This decrease is significantly more pronounced in patients who suffer from both pathologies.

3.3.2 ADIPONECTIN REGULATION

Adipose expression and secretion of adiponectin is regulated by numerous hormonal and environmental factors. Adiponectin regulation has been intensively studied but remains highly controversial in some aspects.

3.3.3 NUTRITIONAL REGULATION

The issue of possible acute FFA-induced regulation of adiponectin is still unclear and deserves further investigation. A study demonstrated a rapid and slight increase in plasma adiponectin after FFA infusion in humans (Staiger et al. 2002). However, treatment with a transient plasma FFA-reducing drug, acipimox, led to ambiguous results: either no effect on plasma adiponectin or an acute proportional downregulation (Staiger et al. 2002). Besides, intake of diets rich in n-3 polyunsaturated fatty acids led to elevated systemic concentrations of adiponectin, independent of food intake or adiposity, and could explain the antidiabetic effects of such diets to some extent (Flachs et al. 2006).

Fasting, feeding, or glycemia would be of minor influence on adiponectin expression and levels. Apart from one study resulting in a slight and transient increase in plasma adiponectin after a meal (Calvani et al. 2004), other studies did not show any modifications (Kmiec et al. 2005). Likewise, small caloric-restriction-induced weight loss is inefficient in stimulating adiponectin levels (Garaulet et al. 2004, Xydakis et al. 2004), contrary to more important weight reductions leading to a significant reduction in fat mass.

3.3.4 FAT MASS AND DISTRIBUTION OF FAT MASS

There seems to be a clear relationship between adiponectin and fat mass in humans. Adiponectin expression is decreased in obesity. Accordingly, plasma adiponectin levels are negatively correlated with body mass index (BMI) and even more with fat mass (Kern et al. 2003). Although the adiponectin gene is upregulated during the differentiation process of normal adipocytes, it has been demonstrated that there is a downregulation of its expression in differentiated hypertrophic adipocytes, suggesting feedback inhibition during the development of obesity (Nadler et al. 2000). Conversely, malnourished patients with anorexia nervosa have markedly higher adiponectin levels relative to age- and gender-matched controls (Delporte et al. 2003). However, when adipocyte function is dramatically altered due to a loss on adipose mass, as in lipodystrophies, the occurrence of hypoadiponectinemia is observed (Haque et al. 2002, Mynarcik et al. 2002).

In addition to associations with body mass, adiponectin expression levels depend on body fat distribution. Intra-abdominal fat is more negatively correlated with adiponectin levels than subcutaneous fat (Cnop et al. 2003). In addition, *ex vivo* analysis of adipose tissue in lean and obese patients or mice showed higher adiponectin protein and mRNA levels in omental versus subcutaneous adipose tissue (Motoshima et al. 2002).

Adiponectin actions are mainly mediated by adiponectin receptor 1 (AdipoR1) and 2 (AdipoR2). AdipoR1 is ubiquitously expressed, but most abundantly in skeletal muscle, whereas AdipoR2 is predominantly expressed in liver. Both receptors are related, although distantly, to G protein-coupled receptor family. These two receptors are predicted to have seven transmembrane domains but are functionally distinct from the other receptors because they exhibit an inverted topology with an intracellular N-terminus and extracellular C-terminus (Yamauchi et al. 2003).

AdipoR1 has high affinity for globular adiponectin and very low affinity for full-length adiponectin, whereas AdipoR2 has an intermediate affinity for both forms of this adipokine. This observation, together with the localization of both receptors, is consistent with the fact that full-length adiponectin has a greater effect on hepatic metabolic signaling, whereas both forms, and particularly the globular form, elicit metabolic effects in skeletal muscle.

3.3.5   BIOEFFECTS OF ADIPONECTIN

Numerous reports from experimental models demonstrated that adiponectin protects against obesity-linked metabolic dysfunction. Adiponectin administration to a diabetic mice model has been shown to reduce hyperglycemia by enhancing insulin activity (Berg and Scherer 2005), and when given to obese mice, it increases fatty acid oxidation in muscle tissue and reduces plasma levels of glucose, FFA, and triglycerides (Fruebis et al. 2001). In line with these observations, adiponectin-deficient mice develop exacerbated diet-induced insulin resistance (Maeda et al. 2002, Nawrocki et al. 2006), whereas transgene-mediated overexpression of adiponectin in ob/ob mice improves glucose metabolism independently of weight loss (Kim et al. 2007).

The beneficial effects of adiponectin on insulin sensitivity seem to be mediated in part by its ability to activate AMP-activated protein kinase (AMPK) in skeletal muscle and liver, because AMPK activation leads to an increase in fatty acid oxidation and glucose uptake in muscle tissue, and inhibition of gluconeogenesis in liver (Tomas et al. 2002, Yamauchi et al. 2002). Adiponectin is thought to mediate AMPK activation through interactions with AdipoR1 and 2. Accordingly, AdipoR2 deficiency results in reduced adiponectin-induced AMPK activation, increased glucose production, and impaired insulin resistance, whereas AdipoR2 deficiency causes decreased activity of PPAR-α signaling pathways and enhanced insulin resistance (Yamauchi et al. 2007). The disruption of both receptors abolishes adiponectin binding and actions, leading to exacerbation of glucose intolerance.

Adipocytes are known to express AdipoR1 and 2 (Rasmussen et al. 2006), suggesting that adiponectin is able to act locally in an autocrine and paracrine fashion to influence adipose tissue function. One of the most striking effects of adiponectin on adipose tissue is seen in the transgenic ob/ob mouse overexpressing adiponectin. In this model, the transgene mouse displays greater adiposity than the ob/ob mouse, with the excess weight accounted for by a greater subcutaneous fat mass (while intra-abdominal and hepatic fat matched that in wild-type mice) (Kim et al. 2007). Histological examination has shown that the expanded adipose tissue consists of a larger number of adipocytes with a significantly lower average cell size compared with the lipid-engorged adipocytes seen on the ob/ob background. Furthermore, mRNA levels of several key genes involved in lipid metabolism, including peroxisome proliferator-activated receptor gamma 2 (PPARG2) and proliferator-activated receptor gamma, coactivator 1 alpha (PGC1a), are upregulated in the white adipose tissue of these mice, suggesting a generalized improvement in lipid metabolism (Kim et al. 2007, Asterholm and Scherer 2010).

Concurrently, overexpression of adiponectin leads to decreased infiltration of macrophages into adipose tissue (Kim et al. 2007) and this adipokine acts locally to suppress the release of a number of pro-inflammatory cytokines (i.e., TNF-α, IL-6) from adipocytes and surrounding stromal vascular cells (Ajuwon and Spurlock 2005, Dietze-Schroeder et al. 2005, Ohashi et al. 2010). These findings demonstrate the complex interplay between local and systemic inflammation.

3.3.6 Adiponectin and Inflammation

Unquestionably, adiponectin exerts important effects on local inflammation in adipose tissue. However, there are significant anti-inflammatory properties of adiponectin that extend beyond this microenvironment. Insofar, these effects are relevant as systemic inflammation may promote insulin resistance. Plasma adiponectin levels are negatively correlated with CRP levels in obese or diabetic patients, and low adiponectin levels are associated with higher CRP levels in nondiabetic or healthy subjects (Ouchi et al. 2003a,b). Transgenic overexpression of adiponectin in ob/ob mice leads to morbid obesity, but there is marked improvement in glucose metabolism, accompanied by a reduction in macrophage numbers in adipose tissue and decreased expression of TNF-α in fat pads (Kim et al. 2007). Similarly, the acute administration of adiponectin to ob/ob mice improves fatty liver disease through suppression of TNF-α production (Xu et al. 2003a). Therefore, it seems that the ability of adiponectin to suppress pro-inflammatory cytokine production may be an important feature in its ability to reverse metabolic dysfunction.

Accumulating evidence suggests that adiponectin-mediated modulation of macrophage function and phenotype contributes to its role in controlling inflammation (Ouchi et al. 2011). Adiponectin suppresses the growth and proliferation of bone marrow–derived granulocyte and macrophage progenitors while not affecting other hematopoietic cell lines (Yokota et al. 2000). In addition, inflammatory functions in macrophages are affected: phagocytic activity is inhibited in human macrophages incubated with adiponectin (Yokota et al. 2000), as is the release of pro-inflammatory cytokines (Yokota et al. 2000, Wulster-Radcliffe et al. 2004). Lipopolysaccharide-stimulated TNF-α and IL-6 release from macrophages is inhibited through decreased NF-κB translocation into the nucleus (Wulster-Radcliffe et al. 2004, Ajuwon and Spurlock 2005) as well as production of the anti-inflammatory cytokine IL-10 is increased (Kumada et al. 2004, Wolf et al. 2004, Ohashi et al. 2010). Conversely, peritoneal macrophages and adipose tissue stromal vascular fraction cells of adiponectin-null mice display an increased expression of pro-inflammatory M1-type markers, with higher levels of TNF-α, MCP-1, and IL-6 production than wild-type mice (Ohashi et al. 2010). The increases in these cytokines can be reversed by exogenous administration of recombinant adiponectin, which also promotes the polarization of macrophages toward an M2 phenotype (Ohashi et al. 2010).

Adiponectin influences macrophage function in a diverse array of tissues, not only in adipose tissue but also in peritoneal, alveolar (Ohashi et al. 2010), and hepatic macrophages (Mandal et al. 2011); all of them display M2 polarization under the influence of adiponectin. In the context of atherogenesis, adiponectin inhibits macrophage transformation into lipid-laden foam cells (Ouchi et al. 2001, Tian et al. 2009). Ectopic production of adiponectin by macrophages in transgenic mice leads to improved systemic insulin sensitivity after high-fat diet feeding and protection from atherosclerosis when crossed with Low-Density Lipoprotein (LDL)-deficient mice (Luo et al. 2010).

These data highlight the place of adiponectin at the intersection of systemic immune responses and metabolic disease.

3.4 METABOLIC TISSUE DYSFUNCTION, SYSTEMIC INFLAMMATION, AND OXIDATIVE STRESS

Yudkin et al. (1999) demonstrated the relationship between adiposity and increased circulating levels of IL-6, TNF-α, and CRP in human subjects. Similarly other studies have also demonstrated the association of abdominal fat (Lapice et al. 2009) and total body fat (Hermsdorff et al. 2011) with acute-phase marker levels, supporting the observation that a low-level chronic inflammatory state is related with insulin resistance and endothelial dysfunction, thus linking obesity and CVD. Indeed, Pischon et al. (2008) conducted a large study in Europe demonstrating that increases in both BMI and abdominal adiposity are strong predictors of mortality risk.

The increased levels of circulating IL-6 and TNF-α derived from adipose tissue demonstrated to have a role in hepatic insulin resistance. IL-6 is known to induce the hepatic release of CRP, but it also impairs insulin sensitivity through the increased expression of suppressor of cytokine signaling 3 (SOCS-3) protein, which binds and inhibits the insulin receptor (Sabio et al. 2008). TNF-α was identified to activate JNK pathway, thereby inducing a serine instead of a tyrosine phosphorylation of the insulin receptor substrate 1 (IRS-1) (Sabio et al. 2008). Both cytokines thus contribute to the inhibition of the downstream insulin signaling.

CRP is mostly produced by hepatocytes under transcriptional control by IL-6. Ouchi et al. (2003b) have shown that the adipose tissue also secretes CRP and its expression is correlated with adiposity. CRP binds to autologous ligands such as plasma lipoproteins, damaged cell membranes, phospholipids, and apoptotic cells and extrinsic ligands such as components of bacteria, fungi, and parasites (Pepys and Hirschfield 2003). When bounded to these ligands, CRP is recognized by C1q and activates the complement pathway (Thompson et al. 1999). Marked increases in CRP occur with inflammation, infection, trauma, and tissue necrosis and malignant neoplasia. Thus, this protein is used as acute-phase marker. Several studies associated high levels of CRP with risk of CVD and the severity of atherosclerosis. It has been demonstrated that CRP can bind to oxidized LDL and to partly degraded LDL as found in atheromatous plaque, promoting the complement activation and thus inflammation in the plaques (Bhakdi et al. 1999). It was also verified that CRP can impair insulin signaling in vascular endothelial cells (Xu et al. 2007) and myotubes (D'Alessandris et al. 2007).

Patients with MetS also exhibit a procoagulant state as evidenced by increased levels of circulating PAI-1. The presence of endothelial dysfunction and dyslipidemia triggers platelet aggregability increasing the risk of a thrombotic event (Nieuwdorp et al. 2005) and the increased deposition of platelets and fibrinous products, which contributes to atherogenesis (De Pergola and Pannacciulli 2002). Furthermore, CRP can also induce the expression of PAI-1 and decrease tissue plasminogen activator (tPA) in endothelial cells (Devaraj et al. 2003).

Regarding the effect of pro-inflammatory adipokines due to excessive visceral fat, the hypertrophied adipocytes are also characterized by a hyperlipolytic state conferred by insulin resistance (Mittelman et al. 2002). As a consequence, the lipid overflow from adipose tissue is deposited at undesirable storage sites such as liver, heart, and skeletal muscle through a process called ectopic fat deposition (Sethi and Vidal-Puig 2007, Britton and Fox 2011).

In the liver, the excessive lipid influx can alter its metabolism impairing insulin-stimulated glycogen synthesis and suppressing hepatic gluconeogenesis. The lipid accumulation in the liver parallels with weight gain and adiposity, which induces the development of hepatic steatosis. In fact, steatosis induces a subacute inflammatory response in liver similar to that seen with lipid accumulation in adipocytes with activation of resident macrophages, the Kupffer cells, and lymphocytes, contributing to insulin resistance through activation of the NF-kB inflammatory pathway (Boden et al. 2005, Cai et al. 2005). The increased accumulation of lipid and the transport of pro-inflammatory adipokines carried through the portal circulation contribute to the development of insulin resistance in the liver and amplify the inflammatory status of the organ with increased expression of inflammatory cytokines IL-6, TNF-a, and CPR, augmenting the systemic inflammation seen in patients with MetS (Wouters et al. 2008).

MetS has also been associated with an increased risk of CVD such as myocardial infarction, stroke, and coronary microvascular dysfunction. The Bogalusa Heart Study evaluated normotensive, prehypertensive, and hypertensive adults and showed that the early natural history of hypertension was characterized by excess adiposity and increased blood pressure beginning in childhood and also by unfavorable changes in risk variables of MetS occurring through young adulthood

(Nguyen et al. 2008). Fat depots surround both heart and blood vessels. The epicardial adipose tissue is located along the large coronary arteries and on the surface of the ventricles and the apex of the heart, whereas perivascular adipose tissue surrounds the arteries (Nguyen et al. 2008). Therefore, factors secreted from these fat depots can directly modulate the function of the heart and the vasculature (Karastergiou et al. 2010). The majority of adipokines released from adipose tissue, including TNF-α, leptin, PAI-1, MCP-1, and resistin, exert deleterious effects on the cardiovascular system. In obesity, the expansion of adipose tissues leads to overproduction of these pro-inflammatory adipokines, thereby contributing to the pathogenesis of CVD.

3.4.1 MetS and Oxidative Stress

Recent evidences suggest that reactive oxygen species (ROS) may be a novel component of the MetS. Initial observations pointed out that accumulation of ROS due to chronic elevation of glucose and FFA can decrease glucose uptake in muscles and adipose tissue, induce insulin resistance, and impair insulin secretion by pancreatic islets (impaired insulin secretion by pancreatic islets) (Evans et al. 2003, Szypowska and Burgering 2011). Moreover, an increase in ROS production and their deleterious effects, such as hypertension and atherosclerosis by directly affecting vascular wall cells, was observed in both animal models of obesity and human obese patients (Roberts et al. 2006, Vincent and Taylor 2006). Interestingly, ROS levels can be decreased with weight loss as other proinflammatory markers, ameliorating the effects of MetS (Vincent and Taylor 2006).

3.4.1.1 Oxidative Stress

The formation of ROS (which also includes reactive nitrogen species [RNS]) is a well-established physiological event in aerobic metabolism that convenes enzymic and nonenzymic resources, known as antioxidant defenses, to remove these oxidizing species. An imbalance between oxidants and antioxidants, the two terms of the equation that defines *oxidative stress*, and the consequent damage to cell molecules constitute the basic tenet of several pathophysiological states, such as neurodegenerative, cancer, endothelial dysfunction, hypertension, and atherosclerotic CVD, diabetes, and aging.

3.4.1.2 Reactive Oxygen Species

ROS, for example, superoxide anion (O_2^-) and hydrogen peroxide (H_2O_2), are natural by-products of the aerobic metabolism and even their basal levels have important roles in cell signaling and homeostasis. For example, controlled ROS production in pancreatic β-cells are necessary for glucose-stimulated insulin secretion (Newsholme et al. 2012), maintenance of myocardial proper function (Zhang et al. 2012), and adipocyte differentiation (Lee et al. 2009, Kanda et al. 2011). The half-life and reactivity of these various species are very different, which is an indication of the different biological functions of these molecules (Droge 2002).

Formation of $O_2^{\bullet-}$ can be considered the initial step for the subsequent formation of other ROS. It is generated by the single electron reduction of molecular oxygen (O_2). A well-known source of electrons for reduction of molecular oxygen is the mitochondrion. The increase in superoxide formation in the electron transport chain is associated with a high (inner) mitochondrial membrane potential. This causes a decrease in the electron flow through the respiratory chain (NADH, flavins, ubiquinone) and low rate of respiration, leading to elevated oxygen concentration within mitochondria and increasing the probability of superoxide formation by the retained electrons at various sites in the mitochondrial respiratory chain (Murphy 2009).

Another site, the enzyme complex NADPH oxidase (NOX), is able to transfer electrons from NADPH to molecular oxygen to generate $O_2^{\bullet-}$. NOX activation is widely associated with efficient killing of pathogens by phagocytes, such as macrophages, monocytes, DCs, and neutrophils, that form ROS from NOX within the phagosomal membrane (Bylund et al. 2010). NOX-derived ROS have also been shown in other tissues stimulating mitogenic signaling and proliferation

(Arnold et al. 2001). In the cardiovascular system, for example, NOX-derived ROS can induce cardiac remodeling through proliferation of vascular smooth cells and fibroblasts. Moreover, ROS, through the regulation of hypoxia-inducible factor 1 (HIF-1), are also important in O_2 sensing, which is essential for maintaining normal O_2 homeostasis (Goyal et al. 2004). NOX is also expressed in pancreatic β-cells where their function is related to regulation of insulin secretion and cell integrity (Oliveira et al. 2003, Uchizono et al. 2006).

In addition to mitochondria and NADPH oxidases, additional cellular sources of ROS production include a host of other intracellular enzymes such as xanthine oxidase, cyclooxygenases, cytochrome P450 enzymes, lipoxygenases, and other organelles as the endoplasmic reticulum and peroxysomes that produce oxidants as part of their normal function (Finkel 2011).

$O_2^{\cdot-}$, by comparison to other free radicals, is a poorly reactive species and can exist in solution for considerable time (and thus diffuse) before reacting with specific intracellular targets (to yield other highly reactive species) or with specific clusters of iron–sulfur in target proteins (Benov 2001). Being a charged species, superoxide cannot freely cross biological membranes, but may do so via anion channels; its fate in cells and tissues is mostly determined by the activity of various site-specific enzymes (extracellular, cytoplasmic, and mitochondrial) as well as by the activity of superoxide dismutase (SOD) family, which converts superoxide into molecular oxygen and H_2O_2 (Weisiger and Fridovich 1973). H_2O_2 is an even less reactive species; however, due to its small size and uncharged nature, it can diffuse across membranes through aquaporins and mediate oxidative events far from its site of production (Kirkinezos and Moraes 2001, Dalla Sega et al. 2014). Despite their low reactivity, some proteins contain specific cysteine residues that are prone to oxidation by H_2O_2, which are critical to hydrogen peroxide–based signaling systems. H_2O_2 is the substrate for the majority of the antioxidant systems in the cell, such as glutathione and catalase, which convert it into H_2O and O_2. These systems are required to minimize the reaction controlling the conversion of H_2O_2 to $HO^{\cdot}$, a highly reactive species, through the Fenton reaction in the presence of free transition metals as Fe^{2+} and Cu^+ (Murphy 2009). $HO^{\cdot-}$ has a very short half-life, but it virtually reacts with any molecule in its proximity such as DNA, membrane lipids, proteins, and carbohydrates. Because of no known scavenger, most of cellular oxidative damages attributed to H_2O_2 is derived from $HO^{\cdot}$ reactivity, which can only be minimized by diminishing the availability of H_2O_2 itself and free transition metals.

RNS are by definition $NO^{\cdot}$-derived species. $NO^{\cdot}$ is a signal transducing radical and endogenously synthesized from L-arginine, O_2, and NADPH in the presence of the enzyme nitric oxide synthase in macrophages, endothelial cells, neutrophils, hepatocytes, neurone, and many other cells. Among its important actions are relaxation of smooth muscles of blood vessels (vasodilatation), neurotransmitter, platelets activation, and aggregation. It is a highly reactive radical and diffuses freely across cell membranes. $NO^{\cdot}$ chemically combines with $O_2^{\cdot-}$ in a diffusion-controlled reaction, resulting in the formation of peroxynitrite ($ONOO^-$). Interestingly, this reaction depletes the bioactivity of NO, thus limiting its action. For example, the regulation of vascular tone by modulation of vasodilatation has been associated with decreased NO bioavailability through quenching by $O_2^{\cdot-}$ to form $ONOO^{\cdot-}$ (Kajiya et al. 2007). $ONOO^-$ itself is very reactive species, which can directly react with various biological targets such as lipids and proteins, and with transition metals present in macromolecules such as hemoglobin and cytochrome, by oxidizing ferrous heme to corresponding ferric form.

3.4.1.3 Oxidative Stress Definition

ROS levels are kept in a tight balance, but their concentration can be dramatically increased under some pathophysiological conditions, and this may result in alteration of metabolic pathway activity and/or alterations in the structure of cellular membranes, DNA, or proteins, inducing cell dysfunction and ultimately cell death (Limon-Pacheco and Gonsebatt 2009).

Oxidative stress is currently viewed as an imbalance between pro- and antioxidants in favor of the former, which implicates a loss of redox signaling. It can be triggered by excessive ROS production as well as by low antioxidant enzyme activities. Excessive levels of ROS not only directly damage cells by oxidizing DNA, protein, and lipids but also indirectly damage cells by activating a variety of stress-sensitive intracellular signaling pathways such as NF-kB, p38 MAPK, JNK/SAPK, hexosamine, and others (Kaneto et al. 2001, Evans et al. 2002, Henriksen et al. 2011). Activation of these pathways results in the increased expression of numerous gene products that may cause cellular damage and play a major role in the etiology of late complications such as type 2 diabetes and aging (Evans et al. 2002). As a general rule, the maintenance of the physiological redox state is dictated by balance between the production of ROS (essential for physiological signaling) and the antioxidant defenses. If this balance is disrupted, for example, by an uncontrolled rise in ROS synthesis or by a decline in antioxidant defenses, the cell is now in a condition of oxidative stress (Evans et al. 2002, Singh et al. 2009).

3.4.1.4 Overnutrition and Oxidative Stress

As mentioned before, ROS generation is a natural by-product of the aerobic metabolism. In mitochondria that are actively making ATP, the rate of $O_2^{\bullet-}$ production is low, the electron carriers are relatively oxidized, and the respiration rate is high. However, the high surplus of metabolic fuel, such as glucose and lipids, stimulates the oxidation of these metabolites. In a scenario of low demand of ATP such as lack of physical activity, it will favor a low respiration rate and mitochondrial generation of $O_2^{\bullet-}$. It has been proposed that elevated ROS from mitochondrial respiratory chain can act as a feedback signal under conditions of excess nutrient supply and low ATP demand, slowing the oxidation of substrate and stimulating the storage of fat, thus decreasing ROS production (James et al. 2012). However, the generation of ROS during chronic overnutrition does not decrease; instead, it is augmented reflecting into accumulated oxidative damages. Another explanation comes from the fact that NADPH oxidase can be activated by nutrients such as fatty acids. Elevated levels of fatty acids in accumulated fat may thus activate NADPH oxidase and induce/aggravate the production of ROS in obese condition (Han et al. 2010, 2012).

3.4.1.5 MetS-Related Complications and Oxidative Stress

Although chronic low-level inflammation status is one of the hallmarks of the obesity-related complications, a large body of evidences support the concept that oxidative stress may have an important role on MetS manifestation, such as atherosclerosis, endothelial dysfunctions, hypertension, and diabetes (Keaney et al. 2003, Hutcheson and Rocic 2012, Whaley-Connell and Sowers 2012). Rather than a consequence, the increase in oxidative stress markers in MetS patients could be an early event of these chronic components related to MetS.

Furukawa et al. (2004), using a nondiabetic obese mice model, have shown that an increase of fat increased ROS in adipose tissue and it was associated with an augmented expression of NADPH oxidase and decreased expression of the antioxidant enzymes SOD and catalase. Interestingly, ROS production was selectively increased in accumulated fat but not in muscle, liver, and aorta. Another important observation of this study was the increase of the marker of lipid peroxidation malondialdehyde (MDA) in adipose tissue. Plasma analysis has shown an increase of circulating H_2O_2 and MDA, which suggests that obesity *per se* can induce a systemic oxidative stress and may alter the function of remote organs. Independent *in vitro* studies using either primary or permanent adipocyte culture have found that exposure to high glucose and/or fatty acids concentrations can reduce insulin sensitivity and increase ROS levels (Rudich et al. 1998, Talior et al. 2003, Lin et al. 2005, Soares et al. 2005). Increased ROS production can also trigger an inflammatory response through increased secretion of TNF-α, IL-6, PAI-1, and decrease secretion of so-called anti-inflammatory adipokines, such as adiponectin, apelin, and Sfrp5 (Furukawa et al. 2004, Lin et al. 2005). Moreover, direct actions of pro-inflammatory cytokines on adipocytes can also induce ROS generation, and therefore, it may amplify the inflammatory signal (Hahn et al. 2014).

3.4.1.5.1 Insulin Resistance and Oxidative Stress

An important feature of obesity is the recruitment and activation of macrophage in the adipose tissue. Because macrophages are known to produce and export high quantity of ROS, this may also be associated with increased generation of the ROS pool in this tissue. In fact, it is known that ROS can induce the expression of MCP-1 (Lo et al. 2005, Sun et al. 2009, Quan et al. 2011). With the augmented expression of NADPH oxidase in adipocytes by ROS from the tissue microenvironment and the generation of further ROS from the surrounding, this process may lead to further infiltration of macrophages and amplification of the inflammation status. Therefore, a vicious cycle that augments ROS via macrophages is also an important feature of oxidative stress in adipose tissue inflammation. It has also recently been demonstrated that products of lipid peroxidation such as trans-4-hydroxy-2-nonenal (4HNE) are elevated in adipose tissue of obese mice, and it can activate macrophages inducing the release of pro-inflammatory cytokines as TNF-α, which in turn induces higher levels of fasting glucose and a moderate glucose intolerance (Frohnert et al. 2014).

It is well studied that the excess of metabolic substrates, such as glucose and fatty acids, and systemic chronic inflammation have a driven role in the pathogenesis of obesity-related insulin resistance (Reaven 1988), and more recently, it has been reported that oxidative stress is likely an important component. In a study using cultured adipocytes, it was observed that treatment with TNF-α induces insulin resistance within a few days. Interestingly increased ROS levels preceded the development of insulin resistance, which was almost completely abolished with the use of anti-oxidant n-acetylcysteine (NAC) (Houstis et al. 2006). Other groups have reported that oxidative stress induced by H_2O_2 generation decreased insulin-stimulated glucose transport and GLUT4 translocation in both adipocytes and skeletal muscle cell lines (Tirosh et al. 1999, Maddux et al. 2001). Although several studies pointed out that hyperglycemia can induce oxidative stress, it is unlikely that it can trigger insulin resistance *per se* since high glucose levels are only seen after the onset of insulin resistance itself. One common feature of insulin resistance is a decrease in mitochondrial activity due to the ectopic fat accumulation in insulin-responsive tissues, such as skeletal muscle, liver, and adipose tissue. The changes observed included decreased mitochondrial oxidative activity and ATP synthesis, a condition that favors the generation of ROS (Petersen et al. 2004, Petersen and Shulman 2006). Therefore, the excessive uptake of fatty acids by peripheral tissue due to obesity-related elevations of fatty acids (spilled over from the adipose tissue) and together with pro-inflammatory adipokines can induce an excessive generation of ROS contributing to the triggering of insulin resistance in the liver and skeletal muscle rather than glucose (Aronis et al. 2005, Utzschneider and Kahn 2006, Qatanani and Lazar 2007, McArdle et al. 2013). In the liver, exacerbation of oxidative stress also induces important hepatocellular damages, such as lipid peroxidation and DNA fragmentation, activation of Kupffer cells with consequent upregulation of the expression of pro-inflammatory mediator and further ROS generation, overproduction of pro-inflammatory cytokines by the liver itself, and severe oxidation of biomolecules such as cytochrome P450 with loss of their functions (Videla 2009). In the skeletal muscle, in addition to the exacerbated impaired fatty acid oxidation and its accumulation and a response to pro-inflammatory adipokines, oxidative stress inhibits glycogen accumulation and decreases expression of insulin receptors and GLUT4 translocation inhibition (Maddux et al. 2001, Bonnard et al. 2008). With the loss of insulin response, its effect on vascular system is also lost. Insulin can activate endothelial NO synthase and thus stimulate NO synthesis and vasodilatation of skeletal muscle vasculature allowing tissue perfusion for substrate and other hormone delivery (Clark et al. 1995). Therefore, oxidative stress in skeletal muscle also diminishes NO availability contributing to the development of tissue insulin resistance.

3.4.1.5.2 Pancreatic β-Cell and Oxidative Stress

During obesity, there is an increasing demand for insulin to maintain proper glucose homeostasis toward an increasing energetic supply for the body. As a consequence, an increase in β-cell mass and activity is observed in order to secrete more insulin. However, due to the continuous insulin demand and chronic exposure to substrates and inflammatory cytokines, a progressive failure in β-cell function and survival is observed (Eizirik et al. 1994). Pancreatic β-cells are known to express low quantities of the classical antioxidant enzymes SOD, catalase, and glutathione peroxidase when compared to other tissues such as liver and skeletal muscle. Therefore, these cells are much more prone to oxidative damages (Lenzen et al. 1996). Many studies have reported that β-cell dysfunction in obesity-related complications is derived from the combination of chronic exposure to hyperglycemia and FFA (Jacqueminet et al. 2000, Poitout et al. 2010, Van Raalte and Diamant 2011). Moreover, these effects seem to be related with the induction of oxidative stress, which in turn can also activate other cellular stress pathways through activation of NF-kB inducing pro-apoptotic events in the β-cell (Weir et al. 2001, Laybutt et al. 2002).

3.4.1.5.3 Endothelium and Oxidative Stress

Endothelial dysfunction can be defined as a reduction in the availability of vasodilator mediators, in particular NO, and the increase of vasoconstrictors. NO decrease can be associated with an inhibition of expression/activity of the endothelial NO synthase or excessive inactivation of NOS by ROS. Oxidative stress in the endothelium is strongly associated with the development of CVD (Madamanchi et al. 2005). Regarding MetS, most of endothelial abnormalities are more evident with the development of insulin resistance, being influenced by the effects of hyperglycemia, hyperlipidemia, inflammatory adipokines, and the decreased insulin availability. Although it is unclear which of these factors mostly influence endothelial dysfunction, oxidative stress is considered a link that triggers the damage caused by them (Madamanchi et al. 2005, Cozma et al. 2009, Frey et al. 2009). Oxidative stress itself also potentially activates harmful mechanisms, which contribute to CVD. ROS can increase adhesion molecules and oxidation of LDL, which are key factors for the development of atherosclerosis (Vogiatzi et al. 2009, Parthasarathy et al. 2010), and upregulate endothelin-1, which induces vasoconstriction (Ruef et al. 2001, Callera et al. 2006) and oxidative injuries in vasculature structure (Harrison and Ohara 1995, Engin et al. 2012).

3.4.1.5.4 Systemic Oxidative Stress

There is a consensus that the adipose tissue has a central role on the development of MetS. Adipose tissue is known to secrete several inflammatory adipokines and FFA that are targeted to many other tissues such as liver and skeletal muscle, where it will unleash several modifications on cellular function such as decreased uptake of glucose, increased lipid deposit, exacerbation of ROS generation, and triggering of oxidative stress. Moreover, adipose tissue is the major source of the plasma ROS leading to the elevation of systemic oxidative stress (Furukawa et al. 2004). It was verified in several studies, using either human patients or animal models, that an increase in plasma levels of ROS in obese subjects correlates with a decrease in the concentration of plasmatic antioxidant enzymes such as extracellular SOD, catalase, and glutathione peroxidase (Beltowski et al. 2000, Melissas et al. 2006, Sfar et al. 2013). A study comparing the effect of acute hyperglycemia in normal and nondiabetic obese patients demonstrated that during an oral glucose tolerance test (OGTT), plasma glucose from the obese group was higher than in control group, and this increase was followed by a significant increase of plasmatic levels of H_2O_2 (Qin et al. 2012). In addition, the increase in hyperlipidemic diet intake itself contributes to generation of ROS since these lipids are prone to be oxidized, releasing lipid peroxide adducts, thus increasing the oxidative stress status in obesity (de Burgos et al. 1992, Beltowski et al. 2000, Olusi 2002, Udilova et al. 2003, Sies et al. 2005). Taken together, these studies strongly suggest that an increase in plasmatic ROS levels might be a predictor of the development of obesity-related pathologies and of the MetS itself.

Recent clinical studies have focused on the use of oxidative stress biomarkers in epidemiological studies regarding MetS. Growing evidences show a positive correlation with these markers with obesity and insulin resistance. Urakawa et al. (2003) observed that plasma 8-epi prostaglandin F2 alpha (8-epi-PGF2a) levels, a product derived from lipid peroxidation, is increased in obese subjects and these values were significantly correlated with BMI. Moreover, a significant negative correlation was found between 8-epi-PGF2a and insulin response, indicating a relationship between insulin resistance and oxidative stress. Park et al. (2009) observed a positive association between adiposity and the plasmatic level of F2-isoprostane (F2Isop), another lipid peroxide marker. In the same study, it was also observed that together with oxLDL, F2Isop was positively correlated with insulin resistance as assessed by the homeostasis model assessment (HOMA) of insulin resistance. Interestingly, F2Isop correlation with insulin resistance was only considered positive when it was corrected by the BMI, indicating that this marker might be closely related with the oxidative stress effects derived from obesity. Other studies have also observed that urinary levels of 8-epi-PGF2a were elevated in obese subjects (Keaney et al. 2003, Furukawa et al. 2004, Meigs et al. 2007).

An interesting study from Yubero-Serrano et al. (2013) has demonstrated a relationship between the number of MetS components and the degree of oxidative stress in patients with MetS. The components selected for the study were waist circumference >102 cm (men) or >88 cm (women); fasting glucose 5.5–7.0 mmol^{-1}; triglycerides >1.5 mmol^{-1}; HDL <1.0 mmol^{-1} (men) or <1.3 mmol^{-1} (women); and blood pressure >130/85 mmHg or treatment of previously diagnosed hypertension. As expected, MetS subjects with more MetS components showed a higher oxidative stress level. A significant positive correlation was established with the number of components of MetS and the activity of SOD and glutathione peroxidase and lipid peroxide levels. It was found that SOD activity could be the most relevant oxidative stress marker in MetS patients and could also be used as a predictive tool to determine the degree of underlying oxidative stress in MetS. Interestingly, a tendency for a negative correlation decrease with NO bioavailability and the number of MetS parameters was also observed, which was most evident in patients with four or five components of MetS, indicating that it could be used to predict the incidental development of CVD events.

3.4.1.5.5 *Adiponectin and Oxidative Stress*

As previously described, adiponectin exerts insulin-sensitizing effects in liver and skeletal muscle and suppress inflammatory events, and recently its antioxidant effects have been studied intensively. However, the mechanisms of how adiponectin decreases oxidative stress remain unclear. *In vitro* experiments suggest a decrease in NADPH oxidase activity through activation of AMPK and generation of cAMP (Motoshima et al. 2004, Kim et al. 2010, Lu et al. 2012). Moreover, adiponectin can induce NO synthesis, by upregulation of NO synthase expression ameliorating endothelial function, and could also act as an antioxidant by quenching $O_2^{\cdot-}$ and generating peroxynitrite (Motoshima et al. 2004, Hui et al. 2012, Yuan et al. 2012).

Although adipokines expression is tightly controlled in the normal adipose tissue, in obesity the expression of inflammatory adipokines is favored and a drastic decrease in anti-inflammatory adipokines such as adiponectin is observed. Several studies have shown a very significant correlation between decreased levels of plasma adiponectin and the development of obesity and its derived complications (Nakanishi et al. 2005, Osei et al. 2005, Zhu et al. 2008, Chen et al. 2012, Gustafsson et al. 2013). Besides the increase in systemic oxidative stress markers and its relationship with the development of insulin resistance and other obesity-related complications, recent clinical studies report that the decrease in plasma adiponectin levels could also correlate with the extent of systemic oxidative stress. Independent studies pointed out a significant correlation between increased urinary level of 8-iso prostaglandin F2α (8-Iso-PGF2α) and decreased plasma concentration of adiponectin in subjects with obesity, insulin resistance, and diabetes mellitus when compared to normal subjects (Furukawa et al. 2004, Nakanishi et al. 2005, Fujita et al. 2006). Chen et al. (2012) have shown that in patients with MetS a significant decrease in plasma antioxidant enzymes positively correlated with decreased levels of adiponectin, and as expected, a positive correlation was found between inflammatory markers and oxidative stress status. Furthermore, in their study a concentration of adiponectin below 7.90 μg/mL was associated with a greater risk of MetS development.

The association between adiponectin and oxidative stress is more evident when therapeutic approaches are employed in order to increase its plasmatic levels. Furukawa et al. (2004) have demonstrated that the use of NADPH oxidase inhibitor, apocynin, in obese mice led to an increase in adiponectin expression and decreased TNF-α expression, which were accompanied by the suppression of oxidative stress in adipose tissue. Weight loss either by caloric restriction diet or by surgery, with reduction in the BMI and fat mass, have also shown to increase adiponectin levels (Kopp et al. 2005, Swarbrick et al. 2006, Ding et al. 2012). Interestingly, physical exercise itself does not influence adiponectin concentration independently of weight loss (Hulver et al. 2002). Del Ben et al. (2012) have conducted a study where a dietary intervention with moderately low-calorie diet (600 calories/day) was given to MetS patients. The loss of more than 5% of initial weight significantly reduced urinary 8-Iso-PGF2a and increased plasma concentrations of adiponectin and antioxidants. These findings suggest that such increase was likely due to reduced consumption of molecules with antioxidant property secondary to oxidative stress lowering.

3.5   CONCLUDING REMARKS

Although adipose tissue inflammation is considered the initiator of the obesity-derived complications, increased generation of ROS and induction of oxidative stress have emerged as a link between these two phenomena. Increased ROS generation can induce oxidative stress in the tissues influenced by the alterations of adipose tissue such as in liver and skeletal muscle or act systemically. It is still unclear whether oxidative stress is a cause or a consequence of fat inflammation, but it is clear that strategies that target the improvement of antioxidant defenses ameliorate MetS complications. Such improvement is also followed by an increase in adiponectin levels, which also confer antioxidant and anti-inflammatory properties. Moreover, increase in adiponectin levels improves insulin response.

Therefore, apart from the adoption of a healthier life style, studies focusing on the improvement of endogenous antioxidant defenses could be used as a promising treatment of MetS.

REFERENCES

Ajuwon, K.M. and Spurlock, M.E. 2005. Adiponectin inhibits LPS-induced NF-kappaB activation and IL-6 production and increases PPARgamma2 expression in adipocytes. *Am J Physiol Regul Integr Comp Physiol* 288: R1220–R1225.

Arita, Y., Kihara, S., Ouchi, N. et al. 1999. Paradoxical decrease of an adipose-specific protein, adiponectin, in obesity. *Biochem Biophys Res Commun* 257: 79–83.

Arner, E., Westermark, P.O., Spalding, K.L. et al. 2010. Adipocyte turnover: Relevance to human adipose tissue morphology. *Diabetes* 59: 105–109.

Arnold, R.S., Shi, J., Murad, E. et al. 2001. Hydrogen peroxide mediates the cell growth and transformation caused by the mitogenic oxidase Nox1. *Proc Natl Acad Sci USA* 98: 5550–5555.

Aronis, A., Madar, Z., and Tirosh, O. 2005. Mechanism underlying oxidative stress-mediated lipotoxicity: Exposure of J774.2 macrophages to triacylglycerols facilitates mitochondrial reactive oxygen species production and cellular necrosis. *Free Radic Biol Med* 38: 1221–1230.

Asterholm, I.W. and Scherer, P.E. 2010. Enhanced metabolic flexibility associated with elevated adiponectin levels. *Am J Pathol* 176: 1364–1376.

Barth, N., Langmann, T., Scholmerich, J., Schmitz, G., and Schaffler, A. 2002. Identification of regulatory elements in the human adipose most abundant gene transcript-1 (apM-1) promoter: Role of SP1/SP3 and TNF-alpha as regulatory pathways. *Diabetologia* 45: 1425–1433.

Bays, H.E., Chapman, R.H., Grandy, S., and Group, S.I. 2007. The relationship of body mass index to diabetes mellitus, hypertension and dyslipidaemia: Comparison of data from two national surveys. *Int J Clin Pract* 61: 737–747.

Beltowski, J., Wojcicka, G., Gorny, D., and Marciniak, A. 2000. The effect of dietary-induced obesity on lipid peroxidation, antioxidant enzymes and total plasma antioxidant capacity. *J Physiol Pharmacol* 51: 883–896.

Benov, L. 2001. How superoxide radical damages the cell. *Protoplasma* 217: 33–36.

Berg, A.H., Combs, T.P., and Scherer, P.E. 2002. ACRP30/adiponectin: An adipokine regulating glucose and lipid metabolism. *Trends Endocrinol Metab* 13: 84–89.

Berg, A.H. and Scherer, P.E. 2005. Adipose tissue, inflammation, and cardiovascular disease. *Circ Res* 96: 939–949.

Bes-Houtmann, S., Roche, R., Hoareau, L. et al. 2007. Presence of functional TLR2 and TLR4 on human adipocytes. *Histochem Cell Biol* 127: 131–137.

Bhakdi, S., Torzewski, M., Klouche, M., and Hemmes, M. 1999. Complement and atherogenesis: Binding of CRP to degraded, nonoxidized LDL enhances complement activation. *Arterioscler Thromb Vasc Biol* 19: 2348–2354.

Boden, G., She, P., Mozzoli, M. et al. 2005. Free fatty acids produce insulin resistance and activate the proinflammatory nuclear factor-kappaB pathway in rat liver. *Diabetes* 54: 3458–3465.

Bonnard, C., Durand, A., Payroll, S. et al. 2008. Mitochondrial dysfunction results from oxidative stress in the skeletal muscle of diet-induced insulin-resistant mice. *J Clin Invest* 118: 789–800.

Britton, K.A. and Fox, C.S. 2011. Ectopic fat depots and cardiovascular disease. *Circulation* 124: e837–e841.

Bylund, J., Brown, K.L., Movitz, C., Dahlgren, C., and Karlsson, A. 2010. Intracellular generation of superoxide by the phagocyte NADPH oxidase: How, where, and what for? *Free Radic Biol Med* 49: 1834–1845.

Cai, D., Yuan, M., Frantz, D.F. et al. 2005. Local and systemic insulin resistance resulting from hepatic activation of IKK-beta and NF-kappaB. *Nat Med* 11: 183–190.

Callera, G.E., Tostes, R.C., Yogi, A., Montezano, A.C., and Touyz, R.M. 2006. Endothelin-1-induced oxidative stress in DOCA-salt hypertension involves NADPH-oxidase-independent mechanisms. *Clin Sci (Lond)* 110: 243–253.

Calvani, M., Scarfone, A., Granato, L. et al. 2004. Restoration of adiponectin pulsatility in severely obese subjects after weight loss. *Diabetes* 53: 939–947.

Cancello, R., Henegar, C., Viguerie, N. et al. 2005. Reduction of macrophage infiltration and chemoattractant gene expression changes in white adipose tissue of morbidly obese subjects after surgery-induced weight loss. *Diabetes* 54: 2277–2286.

Caspar-Bauguil, S., Cousin, B., Galinier, A. et al. 2005. Adipose tissues as an ancestral immune organ: Site-specific change in obesity. *FEBS Lett* 579: 3487–3492.

Charriere, G., Cousin, B., Arnaud, E. et al. 2003. Preadipocyte conversion to macrophage. Evidence of plasticity. *J Biol Chem* 278: 9850–9855.

Chen, S.J., Yen, C.H., Huang, Y.C. et al. 2012. Relationships between inflammation, adiponectin, and oxidative stress in metabolic syndrome. *PLoS One* 7: e45693.

Cinti, S., Mitchell, G., Barbatelli, G. et al. 2005. Adipocyte death defines macrophage localization and function in adipose tissue of obese mice and humans. *J Lipid Res* 46: 2347–2355.

Clark, M.G., Colquhoun, E.Q., Rattigan, S. et al. 1995. Vascular and endocrine control of muscle metabolism. *Am J Physiol* 268: E797–E812.

Cnop, M. 2008. Fatty acids and glucolipotoxicity in the pathogenesis of type 2 diabetes. *Biochem Soc Trans* 36: 348–352.

Cnop, M., Havel, P.J., Utzschneider, K.M. et al. 2003. Relationship of adiponectin to body fat distribution, insulin sensitivity and plasma lipoproteins: Evidence for independent roles of age and sex. *Diabetologia* 46: 459–469.

Cozma, A., Orasan, O., Sampelean, D. et al. 2009. Endothelial dysfunction in metabolic syndrome. *Rom J Intern Med* 47: 133–140.

Cursiefen, C., Chen, L., Borges, L.P. et al. 2004. VEGF-A stimulates lymphangiogenesis and hemangiogenesis in inflammatory neovascularization via macrophage recruitment. *J Clin Invest* 113: 1040–1050.

D'Alessandris, C., Lauro, R., Presta, I., and Sesti, G. 2007. C-reactive protein induces phosphorylation of insulin receptor substrate-1 on Ser307 and Ser 612 in L6 myocytes, thereby impairing the insulin signalling pathway that promotes glucose transport. *Diabetologia* 50: 840–849.

Dalla Sega, F.V., Zambonin, L., Fiorentini, D. et al. 2014. Specific aquaporins facilitate Nox-produced hydrogen peroxide transport through plasma membrane in leukaemia cells. *Biochim Biophys Acta* 1843: 806–814.

de Burgos, A.M., Wartanowicz, M., and Ziemlanski, S. 1992. Blood vitamin and lipid levels in overweight and obese women. *Eur J Clin Nutr* 46: 803–808.

De Pergola, G. and Pannacciulli, N. 2002. Coagulation and fibrinolysis abnormalities in obesity. *J Endocrinol Invest* 25: 899–904.

Del Ben, M., Angelico, F., Cangemi, R. et al. 2012. Moderate weight loss decreases oxidative stress and increases antioxidant status in patients with metabolic syndrome. *ISRN Obes* 2012: 960427.

Dellinger, R.P., Levy, M.M., Carlet, J.M. et al. 2008. Surviving sepsis campaign: International guidelines for management of severe sepsis and septic shock: 2008. *Crit Care Med* 36: 296–327.

Delporte, M.L., Brichard, S.M., Hermans, M.P., Beguin, C., and Lambert, M. 2003. Hyperadiponectinaemia in anorexia nervosa. *Clin Endocrinol (Oxf)* 58: 22–29.

Devaraj, S., Xu, D.Y., and Jialal, I. 2003. C-reactive protein increases plasminogen activator inhibitor-1 expression and activity in human aortic endothelial cells: Implications for the metabolic syndrome and atherothrombosis. *Circulation* 107: 398–404.

Dietze-Schroeder, D., Sell, H., Uhlig, M., Koenen, M., and Eckel, J. 2005. Autocrine action of adiponectin on human fat cells prevents the release of insulin resistance-inducing factors. *Diabetes* 54: 2003–2011.

Ding, Q., Ash, C., Mracek, T., Merry, B., and Bing, C. 2012. Caloric restriction increases adiponectin expression by adipose tissue and prevents the inhibitory effect of insulin on circulating adiponectin in rats. *J Nutr Biochem* 23: 867–874.

Duncan, B.B., and Schmidt, M. I. 2006. The epidemiology of low-grade chronic systemic inflammation and type 2 diabetes. *Diabetes technology & therapeutics* 8: 7–17.

Droge, W. 2002. Free radicals in the physiological control of cell function. *Physiol Rev* 82: 47–95.

Eizirik, D.L., Sandler, S., Welsh, N. et al. 1994. Cytokines suppress human islet function irrespective of their effects on nitric oxide generation. *J Clin Invest* 93: 1968–1974.

Engin, A.B., Sepici-Dincel, A., Gonul, II, and Engin, A. 2012. Oxidative stress-induced endothelial cell damage in thyroidectomized rat. *Exp Toxicol Pathol* 64: 481–485.

Esposito, K., Pontillo, A., Di Palo, C. et al. 2003. Effect of weight loss and lifestyle changes on vascular inflammatory markers in obese women: A randomized trial. *JAMA* 289: 1799–1804.

Evans, J.L., Goldfine, I.D., Maddux, B.A., and Grodsky, G.M. 2002. Oxidative stress and stress-activated signalling pathways: A unifying hypothesis of type 2 diabetes. *Endocr Rev* 23: 599–622.

Evans, J.L., Goldfine, I.D., Maddux, B.A., and Grodsky, G.M. 2003. Are oxidative stress-activated signalling pathways mediators of insulin resistance and beta-cell dysfunction? *Diabetes* 52: 1–8.

Feingold, K.R., Doerrler, W., Dinarello, C.A., Fiers, W., and Grunfeld, C. 1992. Stimulation of lipolysis in cultured fat cells by tumor necrosis factor, interleukin-1, and the interferons is blocked by inhibition of prostaglandin synthesis. *Endocrinology* 130: 10–16.

Festa, A., D'Agostino Jr., R., Tracy, R.P., and Haffner, S.M. 2002. Elevated levels of acute-phase proteins and plasminogen activator inhibitor-1 predict the development of type 2 diabetes: The insulin resistance atherosclerosis study. *Diabetes* 51: 1131–1137.

Finkel, T. 2011. Signal transduction by reactive oxygen species. *J Cell Biol* 194(1): 7–15.

Flachs, P., Mohamed-Ali, V., Horakova, O. et al. 2006. Polyunsaturated fatty acids of marine origin induce adiponectin in mice fed a high-fat diet. *Diabetologia* 49: 394–397.

Freeman, D.J., Norrie, J., Caslake, M.J. et al. 2002. C-reactive protein is an independent predictor of risk for the development of diabetes in the West of Scotland Coronary Prevention Study. *Diabetes* 51: 1596–1600.

Frey, R.S., Ushio-Fukai, M., and Malik, A.B. 2009. NADPH oxidase-dependent signalling in endothelial cells: Role in physiology and pathophysiology. *Antioxid Redox Signal* 11: 791–810.

Frohnert, B.I., Long, E.K., Hahn, W.S., and Bernlohr, D.A. 2014. Glutathionylated lipid aldehydes are products of adipocyte oxidative stress and activators of macrophage inflammation. *Diabetes* 63: 89–100.

Fruebis, J., Tsao, T.S., Javorschi, S. et al. 2001. Proteolytic cleavage product of 30-kDa adipocyte complement-related protein increases fatty acid oxidation in muscle and causes weight loss in mice. *Proc Natl Acad Sci USA* 98: 2005–2010.

Fujita, K., Nishizawa, H., Funahashi, T., Shimomura, I., and Shimabukuro, M. 2006. Systemic oxidative stress is associated with visceral fat accumulation and the metabolic syndrome. *Circ J* 70: 1437–1442.

Furuhashi, M., Fucho, R., Gorgun, C.Z. et al. 2008. Adipocyte/macrophage fatty acid-binding proteins contribute to metabolic deterioration through actions in both macrophages and adipocytes in mice. *J Clin Invest* 118: 2640–2650.

Furukawa, S., Fujita, T., Shimabukuro, M. et al. 2004. Increased oxidative stress in obesity and its impact on metabolic syndrome. *J Clin Invest* 114: 1752–1761.

Garaulet, M., Viguerie, N., Porubsky, S. et al. 2004. Adiponectin gene expression and plasma values in obese women during very-low-calorie diet. Relationship with cardiovascular risk factors and insulin resistance. *J Clin Endocrinol Metab* 89: 756–760.

Gavrila, A., Peng, C.K., Chan, J.L. et al. 2003. Diurnal and ultradian dynamics of serum adiponectin in healthy men: Comparison with leptin, circulating soluble leptin receptor, and cortisol patterns. *J Clin Endocrinol Metab* 88: 2838–2843.

Goyal, P., Weissmann, N., Grimminger, F. et al. 2004. Upregulation of NAD(P)H oxidase 1 in hypoxia activates hypoxia-inducible factor 1 via increase in reactive oxygen species. *Free Radic Biol Med* 36: 1279–1288.

Gregor, M.F. and Hotamisligil, G.S. 2011. Inflammatory mechanisms in obesity. *Annu Rev Immunol* 29: 415–445.

Guilherme, A., Virbasius, J.V., Puri, V., and Czech, M.P. 2008. Adipocyte dysfunctions linking obesity to insulin resistance and type 2 diabetes. *Nat Rev Mol Cell Biol* 9: 367–377.

Gustafsson, S., Lind, L., Soderberg, S. et al. 2013. Oxidative stress and inflammatory markers in relation to circulating levels of adiponectin. *Obesity* (Silver Spring) 21: 1467–1473.

Hahn, W.S., Kuzmicic, J., Burrill, J.S. et al. 2014. Proinflammatory cytokines differentially regulate adipocyte mitochondrial metabolism, oxidative stress, and dynamics. *Am J Physiol Endocrinol Metab* 306: E1033–E1045.

Halberg, N., Wernstedt-Asterholm, I., and Scherer, P.E. 2008. The adipocyte as an endocrine cell. *Endocrinol Metab Clin N Am* 37: 753–768, x–xi.

Han, C.Y., Kargi, A.Y., Omer, M. et al. 2010. Differential effect of saturated and unsaturated free fatty acids on the generation of monocyte adhesion and chemotactic factors by adipocytes: Dissociation of adipocyte hypertrophy from inflammation. *Diabetes* 59: 386–396.

Han, C.Y., Umemoto, T., Omer, M. et al. 2012. NADPH oxidase-derived reactive oxygen species increases expression of monocyte chemotactic factor genes in cultured adipocytes. *J Biol Chem* 287: 10379–10393.

Hanley, A.J., Festa, A., D'Agostino Jr., R.B. et al. 2004. Metabolic and inflammation variable clusters and prediction of type 2 diabetes: Factor analysis using directly measured insulin sensitivity. *Diabetes* 53: 1773–1781.

Haque, W.A., Shimomura, I., Matsuzawa, Y., and Garg, A. 2002. Serum adiponectin and leptin levels in patients with lipodystrophies. *J Clin Endocrinol Metab* 87: 2395.

Hara, K., Boutin, P., Mori, Y. et al. 2002. Genetic variation in the gene encoding adiponectin is associated with an increased risk of type 2 diabetes in the Japanese population. *Diabetes* 51: 536–540.

Harman-Boehm, I., Bluher, M., Redel, H. et al. 2007. Macrophage infiltration into omental versus subcutaneous fat across different populations: Effect of regional adiposity and the comorbidities of obesity. *J Clin Endocrinol Metab* 92: 2240–2247.

Harrison, D.G. and Ohara, Y. 1995. Physiologic consequences of increased vascular oxidant stresses in hypercholesterolemia and atherosclerosis: Implications for impaired vasomotion. *Am J Cardiol* 75: 75B–81B.

Heid, I.M., Wagner, S.A., Gohlke, H. et al. 2006. Genetic architecture of the APM1 gene and its influence on adiponectin plasma levels and parameters of the metabolic syndrome in 1,727 healthy Caucasians. *Diabetes* 55: 375–384.

Henriksen, E.J., Diamond-Stanic, M.K., and Marchionne, E.M. 2011. Oxidative stress and the etiology of insulin resistance and type 2 diabetes. *Free Radic Biol Med* 51: 993–999.

Hermsdorff, H.H., Zulet, M.A., Puchau, B., and Martinez, J.A. 2011. Central adiposity rather than total adiposity measurements are specifically involved in the inflammatory status from healthy young adults. *Inflammation* 34: 161–170.

Hotamisligil, G.S. 2006. Inflammation and metabolic disorders. *Nature* 444: 860–867.

Hotamisligil, G.S., Shargill, N.S., and Spiegelman, B.M. 1993. Adipose expression of tumor necrosis factor-alpha: Direct role in obesity-linked insulin resistance. *Science* 259: 87–91.

Houstis, N., Rosen, E.D., and Lander, E.S. 2006. Reactive oxygen species have a causal role in multiple forms of insulin resistance. *Nature* 440: 944–948.

Hui, X., Lam, K.S., Vanhoutte, P.M., and Xu, A. 2012. Adiponectin and cardiovascular health: An update. *Br J Pharmacol* 165: 574–590.

Hulver, M.W., Zheng, D., Tanner, C.J. et al. 2002. Adiponectin is not altered with exercise training despite enhanced insulin action. *Am J Physiol Endocrinol Metab* 283: E861–E865.

Hutcheson, R. and Rocic, P. 2012. The metabolic syndrome, oxidative stress, environment, and cardiovascular disease: The great exploration. *Exp Diabetes Res* 2012: 271028.

Iwaki, M., Matsuda, M., Maeda, N. et al. 2003. Induction of adiponectin, a fat-derived antidiabetic and anti-atherogenic factor, by nuclear receptors. *Diabetes* 52: 1655–1663.

Jacqueminet, S., Briaud, I., Rouault, C., Reach, G., and Poitout, V. 2000. Inhibition of insulin gene expression by long-term exposure of pancreatic beta cells to palmitate is dependent on the presence of a stimulatory glucose concentration. *Metabolism* 49: 532–536.

James, A.M., Collins, Y., Logan, A., and Murphy, M.P. 2012. Mitochondrial oxidative stress and the metabolic syndrome. *Trends Endocrinol Metab* 23: 429–434.

James, W.P. 2008. WHO recognition of the global obesity epidemic. *Int J Obes* (*Lond*) 32(Suppl 7): S120–S126.

Jensen, M.D. 2006. Is visceral fat involved in the pathogenesis of the metabolic syndrome? Human model. *Obesity* (Silver Spring) 14(Suppl 1): 20S–24S.

Kajiya, M., Hirota, M., Inai, Y. et al. 2007. Impaired NO-mediated vasodilation with increased superoxide but robust EDHF function in right ventricular arterial microvessels of pulmonary hypertensive rats. *Am J Physiol Heart Circ Physiol* 292: H2737–H2744.

Kanda, H., Tateya, S., Tamori, Y. et al. 2006. MCP-1 contributes to macrophage infiltration into adipose tissue, insulin resistance, and hepatic steatosis in obesity. *J Clin Invest* 116: 1494–1505.

Kanda, Y., Hinata, T., Kang, S.W., and Watanabe, Y. 2011. Reactive oxygen species mediate adipocyte differentiation in mesenchymal stem cells. *Life Sci* 89: 250–258.

Kaneto, H., Xu, G., Song, K.H. et al. 2001. Activation of the hexosamine pathway leads to deterioration of pancreatic beta-cell function through the induction of oxidative stress. *J Biol Chem* 276: 31099–31104.

Karastergiou, K., Evans, I., Ogston, N. et al. 2010. Epicardial adipokines in obesity and coronary artery disease induce atherogenic changes in monocytes and endothelial cells. *Arterioscler Thromb Vasc Biol* 30: 1340–1346.

Keaney Jr., J.F., Larson, M.G., Vasan, R.S. et al. 2003. Obesity and systemic oxidative stress: Clinical correlates of oxidative stress in the Framingham Study. *Arterioscler Thromb Vasc Biol* 23: 434–439.

Kern, P.A., Di Gregorio, G.B., Lu, T., Rassouli, N., and Ranganathan, G. 2003. Adiponectin expression from human adipose tissue: Relation to obesity, insulin resistance, and tumor necrosis factor-alpha expression. *Diabetes* 52: 1779–1785.

Kershaw, E.E. and Flier, J.S. 2004. Adipose tissue as an endocrine organ. *J Clin Endocrinol Metab* 89: 2548–2556.

Khmelewski, E., Becker, A., Meinertz, T., and Ito, W.D. 2004. Tissue resident cells play a dominant role in arteriogenesis and concomitant macrophage accumulation. *Circ Res* 95: E56–E64.

Kim, J.E., Song, S.E, Kim, Y.W. et al. 2010. Adiponectin inhibits palmitate-induced apoptosis through suppression of reactive oxygen species in endothelial cells: Involvement of cAMP/protein kinase A and AMP-activated protein kinase. *J Endocrinol* 207: 35–44.

Kim, J.Y., van de Wall, E., Laplante, M. et al. 2007. Obesity-associated improvements in metabolic profile through expansion of adipose tissue. *J Clin Invest* 117: 2621–2637.

Kirkinezos, I.G. and Moraes, C.T. 2001. Reactive oxygen species and mitochondrial diseases. *Semin Cell Dev Biol* 12: 449–457.

Kmiec, Z., Pokrywka, L., Kotlarz, G. et al. 2005. Effects of fasting and refeeding on serum leptin, adiponectin and free fatty acid concentrations in young and old male rats. *Gerontology* 51: 357–362.

Kopp, H.P., Krzyzanowska, K., Mohlig, M. et al. 2005. Effects of marked weight loss on plasma levels of adiponectin, markers of chronic subclinical inflammation and insulin resistance in morbidly obese women. *Int J Obes (Lond)* 29: 766–771.

Kumada, M., Kihara, S., Ouchi, N. et al. 2004. Adiponectin specifically increased tissue inhibitor of metalloproteinase-1 through interleukin-10 expression in human macrophages. *Circulation* 109: 2046–2049.

Lapice, E., Maione, S., Patti, L. et al. 2009. Abdominal adiposity is associated with elevated C-reactive protein independent of BMI in healthy nonobese people. *Diabetes Care* 32: 1734–1736.

Lawrence, T. and Gilroy, D.W. 2007. Chronic inflammation: A failure of resolution? *Int J Exp Pathol* 88: 85–94.

Laybutt, D.R., Kaneto, H., Hasenkamp, W. et al. 2002. Increased expression of antioxidant and antiapoptotic genes in islets that may contribute to beta-cell survival during chronic hyperglycemia. *Diabetes* 51: 413–423.

Lee, H., Lee, Y.J., Choi, H., Ko, E.H., and Kim, J.W. 2009. Reactive oxygen species facilitate adipocyte differentiation by accelerating mitotic clonal expansion. *J Biol Chem* 284: 10601–10609.

Lenzen, S., Drinkgern, J., and Tiedge, M. 1996. Low antioxidant enzyme gene expression in pancreatic islets compared with various other mouse tissues. *Free Radic Biol Med* 20: 463–466.

Limon-Pacheco, J. and Gonsebatt, M.E. 2009. The role of antioxidants and antioxidant-related enzymes in protective responses to environmentally induced oxidative stress. *Mutat Res* 674: 137–147.

Lin, Y., Berg, A.H., Iyengar, P. et al. 2005. The hyperglycemia-induced inflammatory response in adipocytes: The role of reactive oxygen species. *J Biol Chem* 280: 4617–4626.

Liu, J., Divoux, A., Sun, J. et al. 2009. Genetic deficiency and pharmacological stabilization of mast cells reduce diet-induced obesity and diabetes in mice. *Nat Med* 15: 940–945.

Lo, I.C., Shih, J.M., and Jiang, M.J. 2005. Reactive oxygen species and ERK 1/2 mediate monocyte chemotactic protein-1-stimulated smooth muscle cell migration. *J Biomed Sci* 12: 377–388.

Lowe, G.D. 2001. The relationship between infection, inflammation, and cardiovascular disease: An overview. *Ann Periodontol* 6: 1–8.

Lu, J.P., Hou, Z.F., Duivenvoorden, W.C. et al. 2012. Adiponectin inhibits oxidative stress in human prostate carcinoma cells. *Prostate Cancer Prostatic Dis* 15: 28–35.

Lumeng, C.N., Bodzin, J.L., and Saltiel, A.R. 2007. Obesity induces a phenotypic switch in adipose tissue macrophage polarization. *J Clin Invest* 117: 175–184.

Luo, N., Liu, J., Chung, B.H. et al. 2010. Macrophage adiponectin expression improves insulin sensitivity and protects against inflammation and atherosclerosis. *Diabetes* 59: 791–799.

Madamanchi, N.R., Vendrov, A., and Runge, M.S. 2005. Oxidative stress and vascular disease. *Arterioscler Thromb Vasc Biol* 25: 29–38.

Maddux, B.A., See, W., Lawrence Jr., J.C. et al. 2001. Protection against oxidative stress-induced insulin resistance in rat L6 muscle cells by micromolar concentrations of alpha-lipoic acid. *Diabetes* 50: 404–410.

Maeda, N., Shimomura, I., Kishida, K. et al. 2002. Diet-induced insulin resistance in mice lacking adiponectin/ACRP30. *Nat Med* 8: 731–737.

Mandal, P., Pratt, B.T., Barnes, M., McMullen, M.R., and Nagy, L.E. 2011. Molecular mechanism for adiponectin-dependent M2 macrophage polarization: Link between the metabolic and innate immune activity of full-length adiponectin. *J Biol Chem* 286: 13460–13469.

McArdle, M.A., Finucane, O.M., Connaughton, R.M., McMorrow, A.M., and Roche, H.M. 2013. Mechanisms of obesity-induced inflammation and insulin resistance: Insights into the emerging role of nutritional strategies. *Front Endocrinol (Lausanne)* 4: 52.

Medzhitov, R. 2008. Origin and physiological roles of inflammation. *Nature* 454: 428–435.

Meigs, J.B., Larson, M.G., Fox, C.S. et al. 2007. Association of oxidative stress, insulin resistance, and diabetes risk phenotypes: The Framingham Offspring Study. *Diabetes Care* 30: 2529–2535.

Melissas, J., Malliaraki, N., Papadakis, J.A. et al. 2006. Plasma antioxidant capacity in morbidly obese patients before and after weight loss. *Obes Surg* 16: 314–320.

Mittelman, S.D., Van Citters, G.W., Kirkman, E.L., and Bergman, R.N. 2002. Extreme insulin resistance of the central adipose depot in vivo. *Diabetes* 51: 755–761.

Motoshima, H., Wu, X., Sinha, M.K. et al. 2002. Differential regulation of adiponectin secretion from cultured human omental and subcutaneous adipocytes: Effects of insulin and rosiglitazone. *J Clin Endocrinol Metab* 87: 5662–5667.

Motoshima, H., Wu, X., Mahadev, K., and Goldstein, B.J. 2004. Adiponectin suppresses proliferation and superoxide generation and enhances eNOS activity in endothelial cells treated with oxidized LDL. *Biochem Biophys Res Commun* 315: 264–271.

Murphy, M.P. 2009. How mitochondria produce reactive oxygen species. *Biochem J* 417: 1–13.

Mynarcik, D.C., Combs, T., McNurlan, M.A. et al. 2002. Adiponectin and leptin levels in HIV-infected subjects with insulin resistance and body fat redistribution. *J Acquir Immune Defic Syndr* 31: 514–520.

Nadler, S.T., Stoehr, J.P., Schueler, K.L. et al. 2000. The expression of adipogenic genes is decreased in obesity and diabetes mellitus. *Proc Natl Acad Sci USA* 97: 11371–11376.

Nakamura, T., Furuhashi, M., Li, P. et al. 2010. Double-stranded RNA-dependent protein kinase links pathogen sensing with stress and metabolic homeostasis. *Cell* 140: 338–348.

Nakanishi, S., Yamane, K., Kamei, N. et al. 2005. A protective effect of adiponectin against oxidative stress in Japanese Americans: The association between adiponectin or leptin and urinary isoprostane. *Metabolism* 54: 194–199.

Nawrocki, A.R., Rajala, M.W., Tomas, E. et al. 2006. Mice lacking adiponectin show decreased hepatic insulin sensitivity and reduced responsiveness to peroxisome proliferator-activated receptor gamma agonists. *J Biol Chem* 281: 2654–2660.

Newsholme, P., Rebelato, E., Abdulkader, F. et al. 2012. Reactive oxygen and nitrogen species generation, antioxidant defenses, and beta-cell function: A critical role for amino acids. *J Endocrinol* 214: 11–20.

Nguyen, Q.M., Srinivasan, S.R., Xu, J.H., Chen, W., and Berenson, G.S. 2008. Changes in risk variables of metabolic syndrome since childhood in pre-diabetic and type 2 diabetic subjects: The Bogalusa Heart Study. *Diabetes Care* 31: 2044–2049.

Nieuwdorp, M., Stroes, E.S., Meijers, J.C., and Buller, H. 2005. Hypercoagulability in the metabolic syndrome. *Curr Opin Pharmacol* 5: 155–159.

Odegaard, J.I., Ricardo-Gonzalez, R.R., Goforth, M.H. et al. 2007. Macrophage-specific PPARgamma controls alternative activation and improves insulin resistance. *Nature* 447: 1116–1120.

Ohashi, K., Parker, J.L., Ouchi, N. et al. 2010. Adiponectin promotes macrophage polarization toward an anti-inflammatory phenotype. *J Biol Chem* 285: 6153–6160.

Ohmura, K., Ishimori, N., Ohmura, Y. et al. 2010. Natural killer T cells are involved in adipose tissues inflammation and glucose intolerance in diet-induced obese mice. *Arterioscler Thromb Vasc Biol* 30: 193–199.

Oliveira, H.R., Verlengia, R., Carvalho, C.R. et al. 2003. Pancreatic beta-cells express phagocyte-like NAD(P) H oxidase. *Diabetes* 52: 1457–1463.

Olusi, S.O. 2002. Obesity is an independent risk factor for plasma lipid peroxidation and depletion of erythrocyte cytoprotective enzymes in humans. *Int J Obes Relat Metab Disord* 26: 1159–1164.

Osei, K., Gaillard, T., and Schuster, D. 2005. Plasma adiponectin levels in high risk African-Americans with normal glucose tolerance, impaired glucose tolerance, and type 2 diabetes. *Obes Res* 13: 179–185.

Ouchi, N., Kihara, S., Arita, Y. et al. 2001. Adipocyte-derived plasma protein, adiponectin, suppresses lipid accumulation and class A scavenger receptor expression in human monocyte-derived macrophages. *Circulation* 103: 1057–1063.

Ouchi, N., Kihara, S., Funahashi, T., Matsuzawa, Y., and Walsh, K. 2003a. Obesity adiponectin and vascular inflammatory disease. *Curr Opin Lipidol* 14: 561–566.

Ouchi, N., Kihara, S., Funahashi, T. et al. 2003b. Reciprocal association of C-reactive protein with adiponectin in blood stream and adipose tissue. *Circulation* 107: 671–674.

Ouchi, N., Parker, J.L., Lugus, J.J., and Walsh, K. 2011. Adipokines in inflammation and metabolic disease. *Nat Rev Immunol* 11(2): 85–97.

Park, K., Gross, M., Lee, D.H. et al. 2009. Oxidative stress and insulin resistance: The coronary artery risk development in young adults study. *Diabetes Care* 32: 1302–1307.

Parthasarathy, S., Raghavamenon, A., Garelnabi, M.O., and Santanam, N. 2010. Oxidized low-density lipoprotein. *Methods Mol Biol* 610: 403–417.

Pepys, M.B. and Hirschfield, G.M. 2003. C-reactive protein: A critical update. *J Clin Invest* 111: 1805–1812.

Petersen, K.F. and Shulman, G.I. 2006. Etiology of insulin resistance. *Am J Med* 119: S10–S16.

Petersen, K.F., Dufour, S., Befroy, D., Garcia, R., and Shulman, G.I. 2004. Impaired mitochondrial activity in the insulin-resistant offspring of patients with type 2 diabetes. *N Engl J Med* 350: 664–671.

Pischon, T., Boeing, H., Hoffmann, K. et al. 2008. General and abdominal adiposity and risk of death in Europe. *N Engl J Med* 359: 2105–2120.

Poglio, S., De Toni-Costes, F., Arnaud, E. et al. 2010. Adipose tissue as a dedicated reservoir of functional mast cell progenitors. *Stem Cells* 28: 2065–2072.

Pradhan, A.D., Manson, J.E., Rifai, N., Buring, J.E. and Ridker, P.M. 2001. C-reactive protein, interleukin 6, and risk of developing type 2 diabetes mellitus. *Jama* 286: 327–334.

Poitout, V., Amyot, J., Semache, M. et al. 2010. Glucolipotoxicity of the pancreatic beta cell. *Biochim Biophys Acta* 1801: 289–298.

Qatanani, M. and Lazar, M.A. 2007. Mechanisms of obesity-associated insulin resistance: Many choices on the menu. *Genes Dev* 21: 1443–1455.

Qiao, L., Maclean, P.S., Schaack, J. et al. 2005. C/EBPalpha regulates human adiponectin gene transcription through an intronic enhancer. *Diabetes* 54: 1744–1754.

Qin, C.M., Wang, R., Yin, F.Z. et al. 2012. The change in one-hour postload plasma glucose levels, and an analysis of its related factors in abdominally obese Han Chinese men with normal glucose tolerance. *J Diabetes Compl* 26: 536–539.

Quan, Y., Jiang, C.T., Xue, B., Zhu, S.G., and Wang, X. 2011. High glucose stimulates TNFalpha and MCP-1 expression in rat microglia via ROS and NF-kappaB pathways. *Acta Pharmacol Sinica* 32: 188–193.

Rasmussen, M.S., Lihn, A.S., Pedersen, S.B. et al. 2006. Adiponectin receptors in human adipose tissue: Effects of obesity, weight loss, and fat depots. *Obesity* (Silver Spring) 14: 28–35.

Raz, I., Eldor, R., Cernea, S., and Shafrir, E. 2005. Diabetes: Insulin resistance and derangements in lipid metabolism. Cure through intervention in fat transport and storage. *Diabetes Metab Res Rev* 21: 3–14.

Reaven, G.M. 2008. Insulin resistance: the link between obesity and cardiovascular disease. *Endocrinology and metabolism clinics of North America* 37: 581–601, vii-viii.

Reaven, G.M. 1988. Banting lecture 1988. Role of insulin resistance in human disease. *Diabetes* 37: 1595–1607.

Ridker, P.M., Wilson, P.W., and Grundy, S.M. 2004. Should C-reactive protein be added to metabolic syndrome and to assessment of global cardiovascular risk? *Circulation* 109: 2818–2825.

Roberts, C.K., Barnard, R.J., Sindhu, R.K. et al. 2006. Oxidative stress and dysregulation of NAD(P)H oxidase and antioxidant enzymes in diet-induced metabolic syndrome. *Metabolism* 55: 928–934.

Rudich, A., Tirosh, A., Potashnik, R. et al. 1998. Prolonged oxidative stress impairs insulin-induced GLUT4 translocation in 3T3-L1 adipocytes. *Diabetes* 47: 1562–1569.

Ruef, J., Moser, M., Kubler, W., and Bode, C. 2001. Induction of endothelin-1 expression by oxidative stress in vascular smooth muscle cells. *Cardiovasc Pathol* 10: 311–315.

Sabio, G., Das, M., Mora, A. et al. 2008. A stress signalling pathway in adipose tissue regulates hepatic insulin resistance. *Science* 322: 1539–1543.

Seo, J.B., Moon, H.M., Noh, M.J. et al. 2004. Adipocyte determination- and differentiation-dependent factor 1/sterol regulatory element-binding protein 1c regulates mouse adiponectin expression. *J Biol Chem* 279: 22108–22117.

Serhan, C.N. 2007. Resolution phase of inflammation: Novel endogenous anti-inflammatory and proresolving lipid mediators and pathways. *Annu Rev Immunol* 25: 101–137.

Sethi, J.K. and Vidal-Puig, A.J. 2007. Thematic review series: Adipocyte biology. Adipose tissue function and plasticity orchestrate nutritional adaptation. *J Lipid Res* 48: 1253–1262.

Sfar, S., Boussoffara, R., Sfar, M.T., and Kerkeni, A. 2013. Antioxidant enzymes activities in obese Tunisian children. *Nutr J* 12: 18.

Shi, H., Kokoeva, M.V., Inouye, K. et al. 2006. TLR4 links innate immunity and fatty acid-induced insulin resistance. *J Clin Invest* 116: 3015–3025.

Shimada, K., Miyazaki, T., and Daida, H. 2004. Adiponectin and atherosclerotic disease. *Clin Chim Acta* 344: 1–12.

Shoelson, S.E., Lee, J., and Goldfine, A.B. 2006. Inflammation and insulin resistance. *J Clin Invest* 116: 1793–1801.

Sies, H., Stahl, W., and Sevanian, A. 2005. Nutritional, dietary and postprandial oxidative stress. *J Nutr* 135: 969–972.

Singh, P.P., Mahadi, F., Roy, A., and Sharma, P. 2009. Reactive oxygen species, reactive nitrogen species and antioxidants in etiopathogenesis of diabetes mellitus type-2. *Indian J Clin Biochem* 24: 324–342.

Soares, A.F., Guichardant, M., Cozzone, D. et al. 2005. Effects of oxidative stress on adiponectin secretion and lactate production in 3T3-L1 adipocytes. *Free Radic Biol Med* 38: 882–889.

Solinas, G. and Karin, M. 2010. JNK1 and IKKbeta: Molecular links between obesity and metabolic dysfunction. *FASEB J* 24: 2596–2611.

Staiger, H., Tschritter, O., Kausch, C. et al. 2002. Human serum adiponectin levels are not under short-term negative control by free fatty acids in vivo. *Horm Metab Res* 34: 601–603.

Stern, M.P., Williams, K., Gonzalez-Villalpando, C., Hunt, K.J., and Haffner, S.M. 2004. Does the metabolic syndrome improve identification of individuals at risk of type 2 diabetes and/or cardiovascular disease? *Diabetes Care* 27: 2676–2681.

Sun, J., Xu, Y., Dai, Z., and Sun, Y. 2009. Intermittent high glucose stimulate MCP-l, IL-18, and PAI-1, but inhibit adiponectin expression and secretion in adipocytes dependent of ROS. *Cell Biochem Biophys* 55: 173–180.

Swarbrick, M.M., Austrheim-Smith, I.T., Stanhope, K.L. et al. 2006. Circulating concentrations of high-molecular-weight adiponectin are increased following Roux-en-Y gastric bypass surgery. *Diabetologia* 49: 2552–2558.

Szypowska, A.A. and Burgering, B.M. 2011. The peroxide dilemma: Opposing and mediating insulin action. *Antioxid Redox Signal* 15: 219–232.

Talior, I., Yarkoni, M., Bashan, N., and Eldar-Finkelman, H. 2003. Increased glucose uptake promotes oxidative stress and PKC-delta activation in adipocytes of obese, insulin-resistant mice. *Am J Physiol Endocrinol Metab* 285: E295–E302.

Thompson, D., Pepys, M.B., and Wood, S.P. 1999. The physiological structure of human C-reactive protein and its complex with phosphocholine. *Structure* 7: 169–177.

Tirosh, A., Potashnik, R., Bashan, N. and Rudich, A. 1999. Oxidative stress disrupts insulin-induced cellular redistribution of insulin receptor substrate-1 and phosphatidylinositol 3-kinase in 3T3-L1 adipocytes. A putative cellular mechanism for impaired protein kinase B activation and GLUT4 translocation. *The Journal of biological chemistry* 274: 10595–10602.

Tian, L., Luo, N., Klein, R.L. et al. 2009. Adiponectin reduces lipid accumulation in macrophage foam cells. *Atherosclerosis* 202: 152–161.

Tamakoshi, K., Yatsuya, H., Kondo, T., Hori, Y., Ishikawa, M., Zhang, H., Murata, C., Otsuka, R., Zhu, S. and Toyoshima, H. 2003. The metabolic syndrome is associated with elevated circulating C-reactive protein in healthy reference range, a systemic low-grade inflammatory state. *International journal of obesity and related metabolic disorders: journal of the International Association for the Study of Obesity* 27: 443–449.

Tomas, E., Tsao, T.S., Saha, A.K. et al. 2002. Enhanced muscle fat oxidation and glucose transport by ACRP30 globular domain: Acetyl-CoA carboxylase inhibition and AMP-activated protein kinase activation. *Proc Natl Acad Sci USA* 99: 16309–16313.

Trayhurn, P. and Wood, I.S. 2005. Signalling role of adipose tissue: Adipokines and inflammation in obesity. *Biochem Soc Trans* 33: 1078–1081.

Trayhurn, P., Wang, B., and Wood, I.S. 2008. Hypoxia in adipose tissue: A basis for the dysregulation of tissue function in obesity? *Br J Nutr* 100: 227–235.

Trujillo, M.E. and Scherer, P.E. 2005. Adiponectin—Journey from an adipocyte secretory protein to biomarker of the metabolic syndrome. *J Intern Med* 257: 167–175.

Uchizono, Y., Takeya, R., Iwase, M. et al. 2006. Expression of isoforms of NADPH oxidase components in rat pancreatic islets. *Life Sci* 80: 133–139.

Udilova, N., Jurek, D., Marian, B. et al. 2003. Induction of lipid peroxidation in biomembranes by dietary oil components. *Food Chem Toxicol* 41: 1481–1489.

Ujiie, H., Oritani, K., Kato, H. et al. 2006. Identification of amino-terminal region of adiponectin as a physiologically functional domain. *J Cell Biochem* 98: 194–207.

Urakawa, H., Katsuki, A., Sumida, Y. et al. 2003. Oxidative stress is associated with adiposity and insulin resistance in men. *J Clin Endocrinol Metab* 88: 4673–4676.

Utzschneider, K.M. and Kahn, S.E. 2006. Review: The role of insulin resistance in nonalcoholic fatty liver disease. *J Clin Endocrinol Metab* 91: 4753–4761.

Uysal, K.T., Wiesbrock, S.M., Marino, M.W., and Hotamisligil, G.S. 1997. Protection from obesity-induced insulin resistance in mice lacking TNF-alpha function. *Nature* 389: 610–614.

Vague, J. 1956. The degree of masculine differentiation of obesities: A factor determining predisposition to diabetes, atherosclerosis, gout, and uric calculous disease. *Am J Clin Nutr* 4: 20–34.

Van den Berghe, G., Wouters, P., Weekers, F. et al. 2001. Intensive insulin therapy in critically ill patients. *N Engl J Med* 345: 1359–1367.

Van Raalte, D.H. and Diamant, M. 2011. Glucolipotoxicity and beta cells in type 2 diabetes mellitus: Target for durable therapy? *Diabetes Res Clin Pract* 93(Suppl 1): S37–S46.

Vasseur, F., Helbecque, N., Dina, C. et al. 2002. Single-nucleotide polymorphism haplotypes in the both proximal promoter and exon 3 of the APM1 gene modulate adipocyte-secreted adiponectin hormone levels and contribute to the genetic risk for type 2 diabetes in French Caucasians. *Hum Mol Genet* 11: 2607–2614.

Vasseur, F., Helbecque, N., Lobbens, S. et al. 2005. Hypoadiponectinaemia and high risk of type 2 diabetes are associated with adiponectin-encoding (ACDC) gene promoter variants in morbid obesity: Evidence for a role of ACDC in diabesity. *Diabetologia* 48: 892–899.

Videla, L.A. 2009. Oxidative stress signalling underlying liver disease and hepatoprotective mechanisms. *World J Hepatol* 1: 72–78.

Vincent, H.K. and Taylor, A.G. 2006. Biomarkers and potential mechanisms of obesity-induced oxidant stress in humans. *Int J Obes (Lond)* 30: 400–418.

Visser, M., Bouter, L.M., McQuillan, L.M., Wener, M.H., and Harris, T.B. 1999. Elevated C-reactive protein levels in overweight and obese adults. *JAMA* 282: 2131–2135.

Vitseva, O.I., Tanriverdi, K., Tchkonia, T.T. et al. 2008. Inducible toll-like receptor and NF-kappaB regulatory pathway expression in human adipose tissue. *Obesity* (Silver Spring) 16: 932–937.

Vogiatzi, G., Tousoulis, D., and Stefanadis, C. 2009. The role of oxidative stress in atherosclerosis. *Hellenic J Cardiol* 50: 402–409.

Waki, H., Yamauchi, T., Kamon, J. et al. 2003. Impaired multimerization of human adiponectin mutants associated with diabetes. Molecular structure and multimer formation of adiponectin. *J Biol Chem* 278: 40352–40363.

Waki, H., Yamauchi, T., Kamon, J. et al. 2005. Generation of globular fragment of adiponectin by leukocyte elastase secreted by monocytic cell line THP-1. *Endocrinology* 146: 790–796.

Weir, G.C., Laybutt, D.R., Kaneto, H., Bonner-Weir, S., and Sharma, A. 2001. Beta-cell adaptation and decompensation during the progression of diabetes. *Diabetes* 50 Suppl 1: S154–S159.

Weisberg, S.P., McCann, D., Desai, M. et al. 2003. Obesity is associated with macrophage accumulation in adipose tissue. *J Clin Invest* 112: 1796–1808.

Weisiger, R.A. and Fridovich, I. 1973. Superoxide dismutase. Organelle specificity. *J Biol Chem* 248: 3582–3592.

Whaley-Connell, A. and Sowers, J.R. 2012. Oxidative stress in the cardiorenal metabolic syndrome. *Curr Hypertens Rep* 14: 360–365.

Williamson, R.T. 1901. On the treatment of glycosuria and diabetes mellitus with sodium salicylate. *Br Med J* 1: 760–762.

Wolf, A.M., Wolf, D., Rumpold, H., Enrich, B., and Tilg, H. 2004. Adiponectin induces the anti-inflammatory cytokines IL-10 and IL-1RA in human leukocytes. *Biochem Biophys Res Commun* 323: 630–635.

Wouters, K., van Gorp, P.J., Bieghs, V. et al. 2008. Dietary cholesterol, rather than liver steatosis, leads to hepatic inflammation in hyperlipidemic mouse models of nonalcoholic steatohepatitis. *Hepatology* 48: 474–486.

Wu, X., Cooper, R.S., Borecki, I. et al. 2002. A combined analysis of genome wide linkage scans for body mass index from the National Heart, Lung, and Blood Institute Family Blood Pressure Program. *Am J Hum Genet* 70: 1247–1256.

Wulster-Radcliffe, M.C., Ajuwon, K.M., Wang, J., Christian, J.A., and Spurlock, M.E. 2004. Adiponectin differentially regulates cytokines in porcine macrophages. *Biochem Biophys Res Commun* 316: 924–929.

Xu, A., Wang, Y., Keshaw, H. et al. 2003a. The fat-derived hormone adiponectin alleviates alcoholic and nonalcoholic fatty liver diseases in mice. *J Clin Invest* 112: 91–100.

Xu, H., Barnes, G.T., Yang, Q. et al. 2003b. Chronic inflammation in fat plays a crucial role in the development of obesity-related insulin resistance. *J Clin Invest* 112: 1821–1830.

Xu, J.W., Morita, I., Ikeda, K., Miki, T., and Yamori, Y. 2007. C-reactive protein suppresses insulin signalling in endothelial cells: Role of spleen tyrosine kinase. *Mol Endocrinol* 21: 564–573.

Xydakis, A.M., Case, C.C., Jones, P.H. et al. 2004. Adiponectin, inflammation, and the expression of the metabolic syndrome in obese individuals: The impact of rapid weight loss through caloric restriction. *J Clin Endocrinol Metab* 89: 2697–2703.

Yamauchi, T., Kamon, J., Minokoshi, Y. et al. 2002. Adiponectin stimulates glucose utilization and fatty-acid oxidation by activating AMP-activated protein kinase. *Nat Med* 8: 1288–1295.

Yamauchi, T., Kamon, J., Ito, Y. et al. 2003. Cloning of adiponectin receptors that mediate antidiabetic metabolic effects. *Nature* 423: 762–769.

Yamauchi, T., Nio, Y., Maki, T. et al. 2007. Targeted disruption of AdipoR1 and AdipoR2 causes abrogation of adiponectin binding and metabolic actions. *Nat Med* 13: 332–339.

Ye, J. 2009. Emerging role of adipose tissue hypoxia in obesity and insulin resistance. *Int J Obes* (*Lond*) 33: 54–66.

Yin, J., Gao, Z., He, Q. et al. 2009. Role of hypoxia in obesity-induced disorders of glucose and lipid metabolism in adipose tissue. *Am J Physiol Endocrinol Metab* 296: E333–E342.

Yokota, T., Oritani, K., Takahashi, I. et al. 2000. Adiponectin, a new member of the family of soluble defense collagens, negatively regulates the growth of myelomonocytic progenitors and the functions of macrophages. *Blood* 96: 1723–1732.

Yu, Y.H. and Ginsberg, H.N. 2005. Adipocyte signalling and lipid homeostasis: Sequelae of insulin-resistant adipose tissue. *Circ Res* 96: 1042–1052.

Yuan, F., Li, Y.N., Liu, Y.H. et al. 2012. Adiponectin inhibits the generation of reactive oxygen species induced by high glucose and promotes endothelial NO synthase formation in human mesangial cells. *Mol Med Rep* 6: 449–453.

Yubero-Serrano, E.M., Delgado-Lista, J., Pena-Orihuela, P. et al. 2013. Oxidative stress is associated with the number of components of metabolic syndrome: LIPGENE study. *Exp Mol Med* 45: e28.

Yudkin, J.S., Stehouwer, C.D., Emeis, J.J., and Coppack, S.W. 1999. C-reactive protein in healthy subjects: Associations with obesity, insulin resistance, and endothelial dysfunction: A potential role for cytokines originating from adipose tissue? *Arterioscler Thromb Vasc Biol* 19: 972–978.

Zhang, Y., Proenca, R., Maffei, M. et al. 1994. Positional cloning of the mouse obese gene and its human homologue. *Nature* 372: 425–432.

Zhang, Y., Tocchetti, C.G., Krieg, T., and Moens, A.L. 2012. Oxidative and nitrosative stress in the maintenance of myocardial function. *Free Radic Biol Med* 53: 1531–1540.

Zhu, W., Cheng, K.K., Vanhoutte, P.M., Lam, K.S., and Xu, A. 2008. Vascular effects of adiponectin: Molecular mechanisms and potential therapeutic intervention. *Clin Sci* (*Lond*) 114: 361–374.

4 Vitamin D in Metabolic Syndrome

Adriana Lúcia Mendes, Maria Fernanda Giovanetti Biagioni,
Sérgio Alberto Rupp de Paiva, and
Gláucia Maria Ferreira da Silva Mazeto

CONTENTS

4.1   INTRODUCTION

The metabolic syndrome (MS) is a complex disorder characterized by simultaneous occurrence of metabolic abnormalities, including high blood pressure (HBP), central adiposity, dyslipidemia (high serum LDL-cholesterol and triglycerides and low serum HDL-cholesterol) and insulin resistance (WHO 1999, Muredach et al. 2003). These conditions are highly prevalent in Western societies and are associated with a fivefold risk of developing type 2 diabetes mellitus (DM2) and a two- to threefold risk of developing cardiovascular diseases (CVD). Today, these diseases are considered some of the main health problems of the twenty-first century (Zimmet and Alberti 2006). MS is also associated with other comorbidities, such as thrombophilia, proinflammatory state (Sutherland et al. 2004), nonalcoholic fatty liver disease (Kotronen et al. 2007), and reproductive disorders (Ehrmann et al. 2006, Corona et al. 2007).

MS causes and mechanisms may be diverse and reflect the interaction of genetic environmental aspects (Laaksonen et al. 2002, Cornier et al 2008). In this context, there has been growing interest on the possible involvement of vitamin D in MS genesis, especially considering the relationship of this vitamin with energy expenditure (Teegarden et al. 2008) and insulin resistance (Pittas et al. 2007), in addition to its anti-inflammatory and immune-modulating effects (Holick 2005).

4.2   VITAMIN D

Vitamin D, a steroid hormone, is considered a vitamin since it is also obtained from food. In foods, it is found in the form of ergocalciferol (vitamin D2), produced by plants and fungi, and cholecalciferol (vitamin D3) (Miller and Portalle 1999).

Although scarce, dietary sources of vitamin D, such as egg yolk, liver, butter, and milk, are essential for meeting the recommended daily requirement (Ladhani et al. 2004). In addition to the foods fortified with vitamin D, dietary sources include liver oil from fish such as tuna, halibut and especially

TABLE 4.1
Amount of Dietary Vitamin D (Cholecalciferol) in 100 g of Food

Food	Cooking Unit/Grams	Amount of Vitamin D (IU)
Fish liver oil	1 table spoon (10 g)	1000
Sardine oil	1 table spoon (10 g)	33.2
Raw Atlantic herring	100 g	1628
Salmon	100 g	763
Skimmed milk (1% fat)	1 cup (240 mL)	124.8
Whole milk (3.25% fat)	1 cup (240 mL)	96
Oat breakfast cereal	1 portion (30 g)	42.9
Raw chicken egg	1 medium unit	17.5
Mushroom	100 g	21
Salted butter	1 tablespoon (32 g)	17.9
Parmesan cheese	100 g	28

Source: U.S. Department of Agriculture, Agricultural Research Service, USDA national nutrient database for standard reference, Release 25, Nutrient data laboratory home page, http://www.ars.usda.gov/ba/bhnrc/ndl, 2012. (Accessed Apr 22, 2015.)

cod, and fish such as salmon, mackerel, sardine, eel, and herring (Calvo and Whiting 2006, U.S. Department of Agriculture 2012). Table 4.1 shows the main natural dietary sources of vitamin D.

In humans, cholecalciferol can also be synthesized in the skin from 7-dehydrocholesterol when the skin is exposed to solar ultraviolet-B radiation, forming pre-vitamin D (Holick 2005). Roughly, 80%–90% of the body vitamin D stems from skin synthesis and the remainder from the diet (Table 4.1) (Holick 1999).

In order to perform its functions, vitamin D needs to be transformed into its active metabolite, a process that requires two successive hydroxylations (FAO/WHO 2002). The first phase of

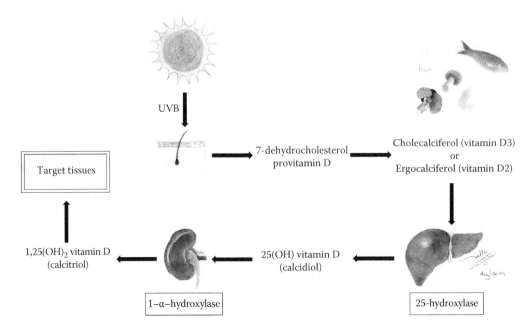

FIGURE 4.1 Representative scheme of vitamin D metabolism.

this process occurs in the liver, promoted by the enzyme 25-hydroxylase on carbon 25, forming 25-hydroxyvitamin D_3 [25 (OH)D_3], or calcifediol, the most abundant metabolite of vitamin D present in the blood, and whose measure is an indicator of its level in the body (Premaor and Furlanetto 2006). The second hydroxylation occurs mainly in the proximal tubules of the kidneys promoted by the enzyme 1 α-hydroxylase on carbon 1, forming 1,25-dihydroxyvitamin D [1,25(OH)$_2D_3$], the active metabolite known as calcitriol (Holick 1999, 2005, Miller and Portalle 1999). Figure 4.1 shows the processes involved in vitamin D activation. Once in the circulation, 1,25(OH)$_2D_3$ will act on all body tissues with calcitriol receptors (Holick 2004).

4.3 VITAMIN D SUFFICIENCY

An individual's vitamin D status is given by the plasma level of calcifediol. Determination of 1,25(OH)$_2D_3$ is not indicated because of its extremely short half-life and difficulty associated with estimating its serum level (Mosekilde 2005). Some authors suggest that adequate vitamin D status is that capable of maintaining the parathyroid hormone (PTH) in the normal range, given that vitamin D deficiency increases PTH, stimulating bone resorption, and increasing renal calcium absorption. Studies have reported a balance between calcium absorption and appropriate PTH levels when serum 25(OH)D_3 is close to 20 ng/mL (Chapuy et al. 1997, Tangpricha et al. 2002, Vieth et al. 2003).

According to recent Endocrine Society guidelines, vitamin D deficiency is defined by serum 25(OH)D_3 below 20 ng/mL and insufficiency by serum 25(OH)D_3 between 21 and 29 ng/mL (Table 4.2) (Holick et al. 2011).

4.4 EPIDEMIOLOGY

Currently, vitamin D deficiency or insufficiency is considered a world health problem because of the implication of this condition on the development of various diseases (Kimball et al. 2008).

Data published in many recent studies done worldwide indicate that vitamin D and calcium deficiencies are highly prevalent in the general population (30%–80%) and affect both genders and different age groups (Su and Zemel 2008).

The National Health and Nutrition Examination Survey—2003–2006 (NHANES) assessed the prevalence of vitamin D deficiency and its correlates in the American population and found a prevalence of vitamin D deficiency of 41.6%, that is, levels of 25(OH)D_3 below 20 ng/mL. Additionally, deficiency was more common in obese and hypercholesterolemic individuals (Zhao et al. 2010). Indeed, some population subgroups are at greater risk for vitamin D deficiency, especially the elderly. It is estimated that anything from 20% to 100% of the elderly American, Canadian, and European population may be vitamin D deficient (Holick et al. 2011).

TABLE 4.2
Individual Vitamin D Status according to Serum 25(OH)D_3

25(OH)D_3 (ng/mL)	Vitamin D Status
<20	Deficiency
21–29	Insufficiency
30–100	Sufficiency
>100	Excess
>150	Poisoning

Sources: Data from Grant, W.B. and Holick, M.F., *Altern. Med. Rev.*, 10(2), 94, 2005; Holick, M.F. et al., *J. Clin. Endocrinol. Metab.*, 96(7), 1911, 2011.

Despite the more favorable latitudes found in Brazil, high prevalence of vitamin D deficiency and insufficiency have been reported, especially in the elderly and during winter (Maeda et al. 2010), but they have also been seen in younger and healthy populations (Preamaor and Furnaletto 2006). Depending on the studied group, vitamin D deficiency rates may come close to 80% (Preamaor and Furnaletto 2006, Saraiva et al. 2007, Unger et al. 2010, Peters et al. 2012).

The causes of vitamin D deficiency or insufficiency may be numerous, among them little sun exposure and obesity (Schuch et al. 2009). The percentages of individuals with inadequate vitamin D intake range from 85.4% to 99.0% (Peters et al. 2009, Pinheiro et al. 2009, IBGE 2010). Moreover, since vitamin D is fat soluble, its absorption is promoted by consumption of high-fat foods absorbed in the jejunum-ileum portion of the gastrointestinal tract. Thus, deficiency may also stem from consuming low-fat meals, in addition to the much studied malabsorptive component (Ruiz-Tovar et al. 2012).

4.5 VITAMIN D TARGETS

Calcitriol has many targets, such as brain, pancreatic, gastric, intestinal, skin and gonadal tissues, and immune cells (Holick 2004), among others. However, the main function of vitamin D is to maintain the intra- and extracellular calcium levels within a physiologically acceptable range. This is possible because of the bond between $1,25(OH)2D_3$ and its intranuclear receptor (VDR). VDR is widely distributed not restricted to classical vitamin D target tissues, which explains the various actions of this vitamin (Holick 2004). In the nucleus, vitamin D bonds to specific DNA sequences, called vitamin D response elements (VDRE) (Barsony and Prufer 2002), resulting in the transcription of a messenger ribonucleic acid (mRNA) that regulates the translation of many proteins, including the vitamin D–dependent calcium-binding protein (CaBP) responsible for the transcellular transport of calcium in the intestine. VDR clearly controls essential genes associated with bone metabolism, oxidative stress, chronic diseases, and inflammation (Haussler et al. 2008, 2013). Yet, recently Wang and DeLuca (2011) showed the inexistence of VDR in skeletal and heart muscles, suggesting that vitamin D acts on these targets in an indirect or nongenomic manner.

4.6 ROLE OF VITAMIN D ON THE METABOLIC SYNDROME

Studies on the action of vitamin D on metabolic processes and its clinical repercussions date from the seventeenth century (Bouillon et al. 2008). The vast amount of data on vitamin D deficiency/ insufficiency published globally has aroused great interest in research centers, which frequently identify repercussions of such deficiency not only on bone metabolism, but also on vital cellular processes, such as cellular differentiation and proliferation, and on insulin secretion, immune system, and various noncommunicable chronic diseases (Zemel 2003, Peterlick and Cross 2005, Bouillon et al. 2008, Heaney et al. 2008, James 2008, Kimball et al. 2008, Prentice et al. 2008, Kahn et al. 2011, Skaaby et al. 2012). As a matter of fact, recent studies suggest that low vitamin D levels may be associated with greater risk of cardiovascular and metabolic diseases, including DM2 (Knekt et al. 2008, Kahn et al. 2011) and CVD (Dobnig et al. 2008, Giovannucci et al. 2008, Wang et al. 2008, Skaaby et al. 2012).

Vitamin D is strongly associated with individual risk factors for MS, with inverse association with the presence of this syndrome (Chiu et al. 2004, Ford 2005, Pinelli et al. 2010, Yin et al. 2012). Some authors reported an approximate threefold increase in the prevalence of MS in individuals with hypovitaminosis D (Ford 2005). On the other hand, adequate vitamin D levels reduce vulnerability to MS by 54% (Chiu et al. 2004). Nevertheless, some studies have associated other vitamin D–related elements, not its deficiency, with MS. In this sense, PTH levels in obese men and women (Reis et al. 2007, Hjelmesaeth et al. 2009) and calcium levels (Liu et al. 2005) have been associated with the syndrome. Hence, the relationship of MS and its associated factors with vitamin D deficiency is not very clear.

Considering the individual risk factors for MS, the Women's Health Initiative Calcium/ Vitamin D Supplementation Study (WHI CaD Study) assessed menopausal women and found that serum $25(OH)D_3$ was inversely associated with serum triglyceride levels, triglyceride/ HDL-cholesterol ratio, excess weight, and MS. These associations were not dependent on demographic characteristics or on the traditional risk factors for cardiovascular and metabolic diseases (Jackson et al. 2006).

A recent review found that vitamin D deficiency can promote changes in insulin secretion, glucose intolerance, and DM2 (Pittas et al. 2010). Accordingly, $1,25(OH)_2D_3$ acts on the pancreas, increasing insulin production (Holick et al. 2004). This action could occur directly, by VDR activation, or indirectly, by calcemic hormones and inflammatory cytokines (Thorand et al. 2011). Some cross-sectional studies indicate that hypovitaminosis D is associated with higher serum levels of inflammatory markers, such as interleukin-6 (IL-6), tumor necrosis factor-alpha (TNF-α), and C-reactive protein (CRP) in healthy and obese individuals (Dobnig et al. 2008, Peterson and Heffernan 2008, Ngo et al. 2010, Jablonski et al. 2011). Moreover, its indirect effect may be mediated by the intra- and extracellular calcium flow in pancreatic β-cells induced by higher PTH and $1,25(OH)_2D_3$ levels (Zemel 2003). In this context, calcium is essential for insulin action on fat and muscle tissues. Literature data show that changes in the calcium levels of these tissues may increase peripheral insulin resistance, that is, vitamin D and/or calcium levels are inversely associated with insulin resistance (Chiu et al. 2004, Liu et al. 2005, Pittas et al. 2007).

Studies have shown that obese individuals have low serum $25(OH)D_3$ and high serum PTH (Arunabh et al. 2003, Snidjer et al. 2005). In addition to less sun exposure because of seclusion, these findings might be mainly related to the high percentage of body fat in obese individuals, which reduces vitamin D bioavailability and causes a cascade of reactions that begins in the hypothalamus and results in high sensation of hunger and low-energy expenditure (Schuch et al. 2009). This situation also generates a disproportional increase in intracellular calcium levels, preventing catecholamine-induced lipolysis, and increasing fatty acid synthase expression, thereby contributing to fat tissue synthesis (Su and Zemel 2008). Indeed, there seems to be a link between adequate vitamin D status and high-energy expenditure (Teegarden et al. 2008).

Studies have shown a positive association between vitamin D deficiency and high cardiovascular risk, and possibly HBP (Li et al. 2002, Giovannucci et al. 2008, Kendrick et al. 2009).

Some previously known mechanisms may explain such association. First, $1,25(OH)_2D_3$ helps to regulate the renin–angiotensin axis since hypovitaminosis D directly suppresses the expression of the renin gene (Xiang et al. 2005) and may thereby increase blood pressure (Li et al. 2002). Second, smooth muscle and endothelial cells have vitamin D receptors and can convert $25(OH)D_3$ into $1,25(OH)_2D_3$ (Zehnder et al. 2002, Somjen et al. 2005). Finally, secondary hyperparathyroidism caused by vitamin D deficiency promotes myocyte hypertrophy and vascular remodeling. Studies suggest that PTH has a proinflammatory effect, stimulating smooth muscle cells to release cytokines. Vitamin D deficiency and/or high PTH levels also promote calcification of heart structures, compromising cardiovascular function (Anderson et al. 2010, 2011).

Considering the various MS aspects, Bolland et al. (2011) found a correlation between serum $25(OH)D_3$ and blood glucose, fasting insulin, serum lipids, and adiposity, and concluded that high serum levels of this vitamin are inversely associated with diabetes, dyslipidemia, obesity, and MS. Moreover, they concluded that for each unit vitamin D level increase, there is a 3.57-fold decrease in metabolic risk (Bolland et al. 2011). This finding is in agreement with those of other authors who reported that adults with hypovitaminosis D seem to be at higher risk of insulin resistance and MS because of pancreatic beta-cell dysfunction and higher rate of DM2 (Snidjer et al. 2005). A study done with 542 Arab Americans of both genders found a negative correlation between serum vitamin D and homeostasis model assessment of insulin resistance (HOMA-IR), hypertriglyceridemia, and glycated hemoglobin (A1c) in men and a positive correlation between serum vitamin D and HDL-cholesterol (Pinelli et al. 2010). Chacko et al. (2011) found an inverse association between serum vitamin D and body fat, serum triglycerides, triglyceride/HDL ratio, and MS prevalence.

No significant associations were found between serum vitamin D and LDL-cholesterol, HDL-cholesterol, insulin, glucose, HOMA-IR, or homeostasis model assessment of beta-cell function (HOMA-β) (Chacko et al. 2011).

4.7   METABOLIC SYNDROME RESPONSE TO VITAMIN D SUPPLEMENTATION

The role of vitamin D supplementation on SM and/or its main associated factors still requires further elucidation. A study done with mouse preadipocytes found an association between 25(OH)D$_3$ level and adipogenesis inhibition (Wood 2008). Another study with postmenopausal women taking 1000 mg of calcium and 400 IU of cholecalciferol per day found that they gained less weight than the unsupplemented group (Caan et al. 2007). After 1 year of supplementation with high dosages of vitamin D, Beilfuss and colleagues (2012) found a reduction in serum IL-6 but insulin resistance and serum TNF-α remained the same.

Studies that assessed the efficiency of vitamin D supplementation suggest an improvement in insulin secretion (Orwoll et al. 1994, Chiu et al. 2004). According to Borissova and colleagues (2003), an increase in serum 25(OH)D$_3$ from 10 to 30 ng/mL may improve insulin sensitivity by 60%. Intervention studies suggest that supplementations with dosages equal to or higher than 800 IU of 25(OH)D$_3$ and/or calcium seem to be particularly important for preventing the development of DM2 in individuals with DM2-related risk factors (Pittas et al. 2006).

4.8   FINAL CONSIDERATIONS

The consequences of vitamin D deficiency are a global public health problem. In addition to the effects of vitamin D on bone metabolism, knowledge is needed on the nonclassical hypovitaminosis D-related aspects, such as its effects on the immune and cardiovascular systems and on insulin sensitivity, and its anti-inflammatory properties. Such knowledge will allow the development of recommendations for correcting vitamin D inadequacies related to MS genesis and/or progression.

REFERENCES

Anderson, J.L., May, H.T., Horne, B.D. et al. 2010. Relation of vitamin D deficiency to cardiovascular risk factors, disease status, and incident events in a general healthcare population. *Am J Cardiol* 106(7):963–968.

Anderson, J.L., Vanwoerkom, R.C., Horne, B.D. et al. 2011. Parathyroid hormone, vitamin D, renal dysfunction, and cardiovascular disease: Dependent or independent risk factors? *Am Heart J* 162(2):331–339.

Arunabh, S., Pollack, S., Yeh, J., Aloia, J.F. 2003. Body fat content and 25-hydroxivitamin D levels in health women. *J Clin Endocrinol Metab* 88(1):157–161.

Barsony, J., Prufer, K. 2002. Vitamin D receptor and retinoid X receptor interactions in motion. *Vitam Horm* 65:345–376.

Beilfuss, J., Berg, V., Sneve, M., Jorde, R., Kamycheva, E. 2012. Effects of a 1-year supplementation with cholecalciferol on interleukin-6, tumor necrosis factor-alpha and insulin resistance in overweight and obese subjects. *Cytokine* 60(3):870–874.

Bolland, M.J., Grey, A., Avenell, A., Gamble, G.D., Reid, I.R. 2011. Calcium supplements with or without vitamin D and risk of cardiovascular events. *BMJ* 342:d2040.

Borissova, A.M., Tankova, T., Kirilov, G., Dakovska, L., Kovacheva, R. 2003. The effect of vitamin D3 on insulin secretion and peripheral insulin sensitivity in type 2 diabetic patients. *Int J Clin Pract* 57:258–261.

Bouillon, R., Carmeliet, G., Verlinden, L. et al. 2008. Vitamin D and human health: Lessons from vitamin D receptor null mice. *Endocr Rev* 29(6):726–776.

Caan, B., Neuhouser, M., Aragaki, A. et al. 2007. Calcium plus vitamin D supplementation and risk of postmenopausal weight gain. *Arch Intern Med* 167(9):893–902.

Calvo, M.S., Whiting, S.J. 2006. Public Health Strategies to overcome barriers to optimal vitamin D status in population with special needs. *J Nutr* 136:1135–1139.

Chacko, S.A., Song, Y., Manson, J.E., Horn, L.V., Eaton, C., Martin, L.W. 2011. Serum 25-hydroxyvitamin D concentrations in relation to cardiometabolic risk factors and metabolic syndrome in postmenopausal women. *Am J Clin Nutr* 94:209–217.

Chapuy, M.C., Preziosi, P., Maamer, M. et al. 1997. Prevalence of vitamin D insufficiency in an adult normal population. *Osteoporos Int* 7(5):439–443.

Chiu, K.C., Chu, A., Go, V.L., Saad, M.F. 2004. Hypovitaminosis D is associated with insulin resistance and beta cell dysfunction. *Am J Clin Nutr* 79:820–825.

Cornier, M.A., Dabelea, D., Hernandez, T.L. et al. 2008. The metabolic syndrome. *Endocr Rev* 29:777–822.

Corona, G., Mannucci, E., Petrone, L. et al. 2007. NCEPATPIII: Defined metabolic syndrome, type 2 diabetes mellitus, and prevalence of hypogonadism in male patients with sexual dysfunction. *J Sex Med* 4:1038–1045.

Dobnig, H., Pilz, S., Scharnagl, H. et al. 2008. All-cause and cardiovascular mortality. *Arch Intern Med* 168:1340–1349.

Ehrmann, D.A., Liljenquist, D.R., Kasza, K. et al. 2006. Prevalence and predictors of the metabolic syndrome in women with polycystic ovary syndrome. *J Clin Endocrinol Metab* 91:48–53.

FAO/WHO. 2002. Human vitamin and mineral requirements. Disponível em. http://www.fao.org/es/ESN/Vitrni/vitrni.html. Accessed November 25, 2011.

Ford, E.S. 2005. Prevalence of the metabolic syndrome defined by the International Diabetes Federation among adults in the U.S. *Diabetes Care* 28:2745–2749.

Giovannucci, E., Liu, Y., Hollis, B.W., Rimm, E.B. 2008. 25-Hydroxyvitamin D and risk of myocardial infarction in men: A prospective study. *Arch Intern Med* 168:1174–1180.

Grant, W.B., Holick, M.F. 2005. Benefits and requirements of vitamin D for optimal health: A review. *Altern Med Rev* 10(2):94–111.

Haussler, M.R., Haussler, C.A., Bartik, L. et al. 2008. Vitamin D receptor: Molecular signaling and actions of nutritional ligands in disease prevention. *Nutr Rev* 66:S98–S112.

Haussler, M.R., Whitfield, G.K., Kaneko, I. et al. 2013. Molecular mechanisms of vitamin D action. *Calcif Tissue Int* 92(2):77–98.

Heaney, R.P., Armas, L.A.G., Shary, J.R. et al. 2008. 25-Hydroxilation of vitamin D3: Relation to circulating vitamin D3 under various input conditions. *Am J Clin Nutr* 87(6):1738–1742.

Hjelmesaeth, J., HofsØ, D., Aasheim, E.T. et al. 2009. Parathyroid hormone, but not vitamin D, is associated with the metabolic syndrome in morbidly obese women and men: A cross-sectional study. *Cardiovasc Diabetol* 8:7.

Holick, M.F. 1999. Evolutions biologic function, and recommended dietary allowances for vitamin D. In: Holick, M.F. (ed.) *Vitamin D: Physiology, Molecular Biology, and Clinical Applications*, 1st edn. Humana Press: Totowa, NJ, pp. 1–16.

Holick, M.F. 2004. Vitamin D: Importance in the prevention of cancers, type 1 diabetes, heart disease, and osteoporosis. *Am J Clin Nutr* 79:362–371.

Holick, M.F. 2005. The vitamin D epidemic and its health consequences. *J Nutr* 135:2739S–2748S.

Holick, M.F., Bischoff-Ferrari, H.A., Gordon, C.M. et al. 2011. Endocrine Society. Evaluation, treatment, and prevention of vitamin D deficiency: An endocrine society clinical practice guideline. *J Clin Endocrinol Metab* 96(7):1911–1930.

Jablonski, K.L., Chonchol, M., Pierce, G.L., Walker, A.E., Seals, D.R. 2011. 25-Hydroxyvitamin D deficiency is associated with inflammation-linked vascular endothelial dysfunction in middle-aged and older adults. *Hypertension* 57:63–69.

Jackson, R.D., LaCroix, A.Z., Gass, M. et al. 2006. Calcium plus vitamin D supplementation and the risk of fractures. *N Engl J Med* 354:669–683.

James, W.P. 2008. 22nd Marabou symposium: The changing faces of vitamin D. *Nut Rev* 66(5):286–290.

Kahn, L.S., Satchidanand, N., Kopparapu, A., Goh, W., Yale, S., Fox, C.H. 2011. High prevalence of undetected vitamin D deficiency in an urban minority primary care practice. *J Natl Med Assoc* 103(5):407–411.

Kendrick, J., Targher, G., Smits, G., Chonchol, M. 2009. 25-Hydroxyvitamin D deficiency is independently associated with cardiovascular disease in the Third National Health and Nutrition Examination Survey. *Atherosclerosis* 205(1):255–260.

Kimball, S., Fuleihan, G.H., Vieth, R. 2008. Vitamin D: A growing perspective. *Crit Rev Clin Lab Sci* 45(4):339–414.

Knekt, P., Laaksonen, M., Mattila, C. et al. 2008. Serum vitamin D and subsequent occurrence of type 2 diabetes. *Epidemiology* 19:666–671.

Kotronen, A., Westerbacka, J., Bergholm, R. et al. 2007. Liver fat in the metabolic syndrome. *J Clin Endocrinol Metab* 92:3490–3497.

Laaksonen, D.E., Lakka, H.M., Niskanen, L. et al. 2002. Metabolic syndrome and development of diabetes mellitus: Application and validation of recently suggested definitions of the metabolic syndrome in a prospective cohort study. *AM J Epidemiol* 156(11):1070–7.

Ladhani, S., Srinivasan, L., Buchanan, C., Allgrove, J. 2004. Presentation of vitamin D deficiency. *Arch Dis Child* 89:781–784.

Li, Y., Kong, J., Wei, M. et al. 2002. 1,25-Dihydroxyvitamin D3 is a negative endocrine regulator of the renin-angiotensin system. *J Clin Invest* 110:229–238.

Liu, S., Song, Y., Ford, E. et al. 2005. Dietary calcium, vitamin D, and the prevalence of metabolic syndrome in middle-aged and older U.S. women. *Diabetes Care* 28:2926–2932.

Maeda, S.S., Kunii, I.S., Hayashi, L.F., Lazaretti-Castro, M. 2010. Increases in summer serum 25-hydroxyvitamin D (25OHD) concentrations in elderly subjects in São Paulo, Brazil vary with age, gender and ethnicity. *BMC Endocr Disord* 10:12.

Miller, W.L., Portalle, A.A. 1999. Genetic disorders of vitamin D biosynthesis. *Pediatr Endocrinol* 28(4):825–840.

Mosekilde, L. 2005. Vitamin D and the elderly. *Clin Endocrinol* 62(3):265–281.

Muredach, P., Reilly, M.P., Rader, D.J. 2003. The metabolic syndrome: More than a sum of its parts? *Circulation* 108:1546–1551.

Ngo, D.T., Sverdlov, A.L., McNeil, J.J., Horowitz, J.D. 2010. Does vitamin D modulate asymmetric dimethylarginine and C-reactive protein concentrations? *Am J Med* 123:335–341.

Orwoll, E., Riddle, M., Prince, M. 1994. Effects of vitamin D on insulin and glucagon secretion in non-insulin-dependent diabetes mellitus. *Am J Clin Nutr* 59:1083–1087.

Peterlick, M., Cross, H.S. 2005. Vitamin D and calcium deficits predispose for multiple chronic diseases. *Eur J Clin Invest* 35(5):290–304.

Peters, B.S.E., dos Santos, L.C., Fisberg, M., Wood, R.J., Martini, L.A. 2009. Prevalence of vitamin D insufficiency in Brazilian adolescents. *Ann Nutr Metab* 54:15–21.

Peterson, C.A., Heffernan, M.E. 2008. Serum tumor necrosis factor-alpha concentrations are negatively correlated with serum 25(OH) D concentrations in healthy women. *J. Inflamm* (*Lond*) 5:10.

Pinelli, N.R., Jaber, L.A., Brown, M.B., Herman, W.H. 2010. Serum 25-hydroxy vitamin D and insulin resistance, metabolic syndrome, and glucose intolerance among Arab Americans. *Diabetes Care* 33(6):1373–1375.

Pinheiro, M.M., Schuch, N.J., Genaro, P.S. et al. 2009. Nutrient intakes related to osteoporotic fractures in men and women: The Brazilian Osteoporosis Study (BRAZOS). *Nutr J* 8:6.

Pittas, A.G., Chung, M., Trikalinos, T. et al. 2010. Systematic review: Vitamin D and cardiometabolic outcomes. *Ann Intern Med* 152:307–314.

Pittas, A.G., Dawson-Hughes, B., Li, M. et al. 2006. Vitamin D and calcium intake in relation to type 2 diabetes in women. *Diabetes Care* 29:650–656.

Pittas, A.G., Lau, J., Hu, F.B., Dawson-Hughes, B. 2007. The role of vitamin D and calcium in type 2 diabetes. A systematic review and metanalysis. *J Clin Endocrinol Metab* 92:2017–2029.

Premaor, M.O., Furlanetto, T.W. 2006. Hipovitaminose D em adultos: Entendendo melhor a apresentação de uma velha doença. *Arq Bras Endocrinol Metab* 50(1):25–37.

Prentice, A., Goldberg, G., Schoenmakers, I. 2008. Vitamin D across the lifescycle: Physiology and biomarkers. *Am J Clin Nutr* 88(2):500S–506S.

Reis, J., von Mühlen, D., Kritz-Silverstein, D., Wingard, D., Barrett-Connor, E. 2007. Vitamin D, parathyroid hormone levels, and the prevalence of metabolic syndrome in community-dwelling older adults. *Diabetes Care* 30:1549–1555.

Ruiz-Tovar, J., Oller, I., Tomas, A. et al. 2012. Mid-term effects of sleeve gastrectomy on calcium metabolism parameters, vitamin D and parathormone (PTH) in morbid obese women. *Obes Surg* 22(5):797–801.

Saraiva, G.L., Cendoroglo, M.S., Ramos, L.R. et al. 2007. Prevalence of vitamin D deficiency, insufficiency and secondary hyperparathyroidism in the elderly inpatients and living in the community of the city of São Paulo, Brazil. *Arq Bras Endocrinol Metab* 51(3):437–442.

Schuch, N.J., Garcia, V.C., Matini, L.A. 2009. Vitamina D e doenças endocrinometabólicas. *Arq Bras Endocrinol Metab* 53:625–633.

Skaaby, T., Husemoen, L.L., Pisinger, C. et al. 2012. Vitamin D status and changes in cardiovascular risk factors: A prospective study of a general population. *Cardiology* 123(1):62–70.

Snidjer, M.B., van Dam, R.M., Visser, M. 2005. Adiposity in relation to vitamin D status and parathyroid hormone levels: A population-based study in older men and women. *J Clin Endocrinol Metab* 90:4119–4123.

Somjen, D., Weisman, Y., Kohen, F. et al. 2005. 25-Hydroxyvitamin D3-1alpha-hydroxylase is expressed in human vascular smooth muscle cells and is upregulated by parathyroid hormone and estrogenic compounds. *Circulation* 111(13):1666–1671.

Su, X., Zemel, M.B. 2008. 1Alpha, 25-dihydroxyvitamin D and corticosteroid regulate adipocyte nuclear vitamin D receptor. *Int J Obes (Lond)* 32(8):1305–1311.

Sutherland, J.P., McKinley, B., Eckel, R.H. 2004. The metabolic syndrome and inflammation. *Metab Syndr Relat Disord* 2(2):82–104.

Tangpricha, V., Pearce, E.N., Chen, T.C., Holick, M.F. 2002. Vitamin D insufficiency among free-living healthy young adults. *Am J Med* 112(8):659–662.

Teegarden, D., White, K.M., Lyle, R.M. et al. 2008.Calcium and dairy product modulation of lipid utilization and energy expenditure. *Obesity* 16:1566–1572.

Thorand, B., Zierer, A., Huth, C. et al. 2011. Effect of serum 25-hydroxivitamin D on risk for type 2 diabetes may be partially mediated by subclinical inflammationn: Results from the MONICA/RORA Ausburg study. *Diabetes Care* 34:2320–2322.

Unger, M.D., Cuppari, L., Titan, S.M. et al. 2010. Vitamin D status in a sunny country: Where has the sun gone? *Clin Nutr* 29(6):784–788.

U.S. Department of Agriculture, Agricultural Research Service. 2012. USDA national nutrient database for standard reference, Release 25. Nutrient data laboratory home page. http://www.ars.usda.gov/ba/bhnrc/ndl. Accessed April 22, 2015.

Vieth, R., Ladak, Y., Walsh, P.G. 2003. Age-related changes in the 25-hydroxyvitamin D versus parathyroid hormone relationship suggest a different reason why older adults require more vitamin D. *J Clin Endocrinol Metab* 88(1):185–191.

Wang, T.J., Peencina, M.J., Booth, S.L. et al. 2008. Vitamin D deficiency and risk cardiovascular Disease. *Circulation* 117:503–511.

Wang, Y., DeLuca, H.F. 2011. Is the vitamin d receptor found in muscle? *Endocrinology* 152(2):354–363.

Wood, R.J. 2008. Vitamin D and adipogenesis: New molecular insights. *Nutr Rev* 66(1):40–46.

World Health Organization. 1999. Definition diagnosis and classification of diabetes mellitus and its complications. Report of a WHO Consultation. Part 1: Diagnosis and classification of diabetes mellitus. World Health Organization: Geneva, Switzerland.

Xiang, W., Kong, J., Chen, S. et al. 2005. Cardiac hypertrophy in vitamin D receptor knockout mice: Role of the systemic and cardiac renin-angiotensin systems. *Am J Physiol Endocrinol Metab* 288(1):E125–E132.

Yin, X., Sun, Q., Zhang, X. et al. 2012. Serum 25(OH)D is inversely associated with metabolic syndrome risk profile among urban middle-aged Chinese population. *Nutr J* 11:68.

Zehnder, D., Bland, R., Chana, R.S. et al. 2002. Synthesis of 1,25-dihydroxyvitamin D(3) by human endothelial cells is regulated by inflammatory cytokines: A novel autocrine determinant of vascular cell adhesion. *J Am Soc Nephrol* 13(3):621–629.

Zemel, M.B. 2003. Mechanisms of dairy modulation of adiposity. *J Nutr* 133:252S–256S.

Zhao, G., Ford, E.S., Li, C. 2010. Association of serum concentrations of 25-hydroxyvitamin D and parathyroid hormone with surrogate markers of insulin resistance among U.S. adults without physician-diagnosed diabetes: NHANES, 2003–2006. *Diabetes Care* 33:344–347.

Zimmet, P., Alberti, G. 2006. The IDF definition: Why we need a global consensus. *Diabetes Voice* 51:12–15. http://www.idf.org/sites/default/files/attachments/article_409_en.pdf. Accessed April 22, 2015.

5 Genetic Polymorphisms and Gene–Nutrient Interaction in Metabolic Syndrome

Edna Maria Vissoci Reiche, Ana Paula Kallaur,
Fernando Vissoci Reiche, and Paulo Cezar Casado Graça

CONTENTS

5.1   INTRODUCTION

Metabolic syndrome (MetS) is a complex disorder characterized by central obesity, insulin resistance, dyslipidemia with raised triacylglycerols, and reduced high-density lipoprotein cholesterol (HDL-C), hypertension, and inflammation (Moller and Kaufman, 2005). While details differ between numerous definitions, all agree on the essential components, such as obesity, insulin resistance/glucose intolerance, dyslipidemia, and hypertension (NCEP ATP III, 2002). MetS is a high-prevalence condition, affecting almost a quarter of the global adult population, increasing among men and women of all ages and ethnicities and correlating with the global epidemic of obesity and type 2 diabetes mellitus (T2DM) (Ford et al., 2010). MetS is associated with severe health complications, such as an increased risk of T2DM and cardiovascular disease (CVD). Interactions between genetic and environmental factors, such as diet and lifestyle, particularly over-nutrition and sedentary behavior, promote the progression and pathogenesis of these polygenic diet-related diseases (Phillips, 2013). Heritability rates of 25%–40% are attributed for body mass index fat (Vogler et al., 1995), and 10%–30% for MetS (Henneman et al., 2008; Bellia et al., 2009), indicating that these conditions are partly heritable.

MetS is defined by the presence of three or more of the following criteria: central obesity, high blood pressure, hypertriacylglycerolemia, low HDL-C, and/or altered fasting glucose (NCEP ATP III, 2002). The etiology of MetS may be due to a combination of genetic and environmental factors, mainly dietary and physical activity (Figure 5.1). The concept of environmental factors is complex and is associated with the lifestyle habits, such as smoking, consumption of drugs, toxic exposition, and educational and socioeconomic levels. However, food is an environmental factor that deserves attention since the individual is permanently exposed.

Obesity, one of MetS criteria, is a complex disease resulting from a chronic and long-term positive energy balance in which both genetic and environmental factors are involved. Weight reduction methods are mainly focused on dietary changes and increased physical activities. However, responses to nutritional intervention programs show a wide range of interindividual variation, which is importantly influenced by genetic determinants. Subjects carrying several obesity-related genetic variants show differences in response to calorie-restriction programs. Furthermore, there is evidence indicating that dietary compounds not only fuel the body but also participate in the modulation of gene expression. Thus, the expression pattern and nutritional regulation of several obesity-related genes have been studied, as well as those that are differentially expressed by caloric restriction (Abete et al., 2012). In the area of obesity, *leptin* (*LEP*) and *leptin receptor* (*LEPR*) gene mutations have emerged as leading candidates toward predicting the risk of obesity (Li et al., 1999; Chagnon et al., 2000).

CVD is one of the healthy complications of MetS and is becoming the leading cause of morbidity and mortality worldwide. CVD is a complex multifactorial disease influenced by genetic and environmental factors, such as diet. Whole genomic and candidate gene association studies are two main approaches used in the cardiovascular genetics to identify disease-causing genes and to show the influence of genotype on the responsiveness to dietary factors or nutrients that may reduce CVD risk (Engler, 2009).

MetS is not only a risk factor for CVD, but often both of them have the same shared susceptibility genes, as several genetic variants have shown a predisposition to both diseases. Due to the spread of robust genome-wide association studies (GWAS), the number of candidate genes in MetS and CVD susceptibility increases very rapidly. Genes influencing lipid metabolism exert effects on the circulating triacylglycerol levels. As the elevated levels of triacylglycerols can be associated

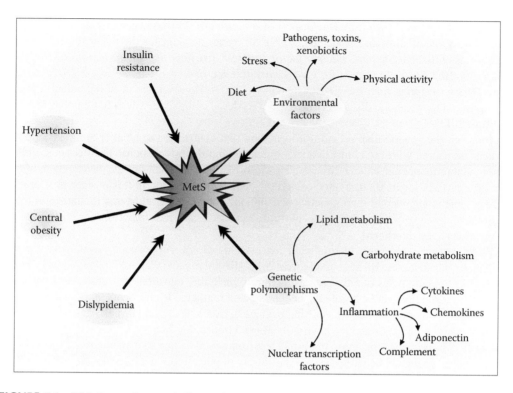

FIGURE 5.1 Risk factors for metabolic syndrome (MetS). Cardiometabolic risk determinants (including dyslipidemia, central obesity, hypertension, and insulin resistance), environmental factors (diet, stress, pathogens, toxins, xenobiotics, physical activity), and common genetic polymorphisms (variations in genes encoding for key molecules of lipid and carbohydrate metabolism, inflammation, and nuclear transcription factors) that are associated with the development of MetS.

with disease phenotypes, some of these genetic variants can have susceptibility features in both MetS and CVD (Krisfali et al., 2010).

Some gene–nutrient interactions are associated with MetS and CVD. Soy ingestion, where the most abundant active compounds are genistein and daidzein, reduces the genes expression related with the development of CVD, and consequently, MetS. Diets rich in omega-3 polyunsaturated fatty acids (n-3 PUFAs), such as α-linolenic acid (ALA), eicosapentaenoic acid (EPA), and docosahexaenoic acid (DHA), are associated with decreased incidence and severity of CVD. At least some of the beneficial effects of these dietary fatty acids are mediated by metabolites such as prostaglandins, leukotrienes, thromboxanes, and resolvins.

The effects of n-3 PUFAs often differ from those of other fatty acids with very similar structures, such as arachidonic acid (n-6 PUFAS) and their corresponding metabolites. Specific receptors exist for fatty acids or their metabolites that are able to regulate gene expression and coordinately affect metabolic or signaling pathways associated with CVD. The four nuclear receptor (NR) subfamilies that respond to dietary and endogenous ligands and have implications for MetS are peroxisome proliferator-activated receptors (PPARs), retinoid X receptors (RXR), liver X receptors (LXR), and the farnesoid X receptor (FXR) (Vanden Heuvel, 2009).

The Human Genome Project concluded in 2003 was crucial to supply the tools and information about genetics aspects of innumerous allelic variants that are associated with susceptibility and resistance for several monogenic and complex diseases. Monogenic disorders account for up to 5% of all cases of obesity and diabetes. Mutations in a number of genes including *LEP*, *LEPR*, *pro-opimelanocortin* (*POMC*), and *melacortin-4 receptor* (*MC4R*) have been associated with monogenic obesity (Andreasen and Andersen, 2009). Six genes account for the majority of the monogenic forms of diabetes: *hepatic nuclear factor 1α* (*HNF-1α*), *hepatic nuclear factor 4α* (*HNF-4α*), *hepatic nuclear factor 1β* (*HNF-1β*), *glucokinase* (*GCK*), *insulin promoter factor 1* (*IPF-1*), and *neuro D1 transcription factor* (*NEURODI*) (Gloyn, 2003). However, for most individuals, genetic predisposition to metabolic diseases, which are considered complex diseases, has a polygenic basis (Phillips, 2013).

Moreover, the genetic map provides information that contributes to identify some genetic biomarkers associated with the clinical course, outcome, and therapy response of infectious, inflammatory, autoimmune, and cancer diseases. This information contributes to the development of new therapy approaches, which takes into account the genetic host factors. In this postgenomic era, the study of genetic factors and their genetic contribution to the disease addresses fundamental issues in our understanding of the pathogenesis of the disease and opens new opportunities for therapeutic interventions to be developed.

GWAS carried out by large international consortia are discovering genetic variants that contribute to metabolic diseases (Billings and Florez, 2010; Hirschhom and Gajdos, 2011). Genomes evolve in response to many types of environmental stimuli, including nutrition. Therefore, the expression of genetic information can be highly dependent on, and regulated by, nutrients, micronutrients, and phytochemicals found in food. The shifting balance between health and disease states involves the complex interplay of genes and the environment, which includes diet.

Nutrition is probably the most important environmental factor that modulates expression of genes involved in metabolic pathways and the variety of phenotypes associated with obesity, MetS, and T2DM (Phillips, 2013). Dietary and plasma fatty acid composition may alter the risk of MetS and are the major environmental factors associated with the syndrome (Groop, 2000; Vessby, 2003; Roche et al., 2005; Phillips et al., 2006).

Until recently, nutrition research has been directed toward nutrient deficiencies and impaired health; however, one current aim of nutrition is improving health through personalization of diet. The concept that food compounds can affect physiological functions by interacting and modulating molecular mechanisms has revolutionized the field of nutrition (Steven and Sieber, 1994). In association with environmental factors, nutrients interact with the human genome at molecular, cellular, and systemic levels, modulating gene expression and endocrine and immune systems functions.

It is widely known that the effect of dietary changes on plasma biomarker concentrations differs significantly between individuals. There is increasing evidence that supports the concept that this variability in response is an intrinsic characteristic of the individual, rather than being the result of different dietary compliances with experimental protocols (Perez-Martinez et al., 2012).

5.2 NUTRIGENETICS AND NUTRIGENOMICS

Polymorphisms in genes coding for key molecules of several physiological pathways, such as lipid and carbohydrate metabolism, inflammatory response, systemic coagulation, blood pressure regulation, and cell adhesion have been implicated in the pathophysiology of several nontransmitted chronic diseases, such as atherosclerosis, diabetes mellitus, dyslipidemia, stroke, and MetS. The knowledge about communication between genes and food compounds, such as nutrients and bioactive compounds, enables the emergence of two sciences, named nutrigenetics and nutrigenomics (Steven and Sieber, 1994).

Nutrigenetics refers the effects of genetic variant in the diet and disease interaction, with the identification of genes responsible for different responses to diet while nutrigenomics refers the studies of how the constituents of the diet interact with genes and their products and how they alter phenotype. Bioactive food compounds can interact with genes affecting transcription factors, protein expression, and metabolic production (Garcia-Cañas et al., 2010). Biologically active molecules can modulate the gene expression and can affect health and disease (endpoints) (Figure 5.2).

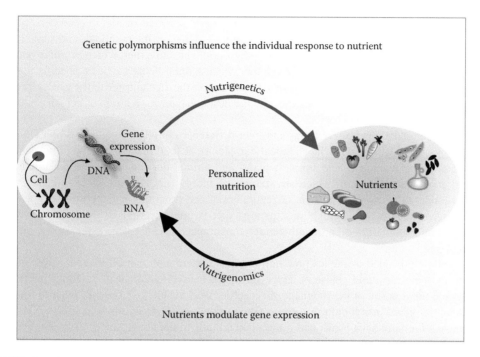

FIGURE 5.2 Concepts o f nutrigenetics and nutrigenomics. Nutrigenetics studies the effect of genetic variation in the disease–nutrient interaction with the aim to generate dietary recommendations, considering the risk and benefits of specific diet or dietary compounds for the individual, taken into account the genetic profile. Nutrigenomics studies the influence of nutrients in the gene expression, and the response of gene expression after the consumption of nutrients.

The classical example of nutrigenetics is the accumulation of phenylalanine in the blood, responsible for brain damage in patients with phenylketunuria (PKU), which is an autosomal recessive metabolic genetic disorder characterized by homozygous or compound heterozygous mutations in the *hepatic enzyme* phenylalanine hydroxylase (*PAH*) gene, rendering it nonfunctional. The *PAH* gene is located on the long arm of the chromosome 12 (12q22-q24.1) and includes about 90,000 base pairs in 13 exons. More than 500 mutations in the *PAH* gene have been identified in people with PKU. Most of these mutations change single amino acids in phenylalanine hydroxylase. For example, the most common mutation in many populations replaces the amino acid arginine (Arg) with the amino acid tryptophan (Trp) at position 408 (Arg408Trp or R408W) (Woo et al., 1983). PAH deficiency causes a spectrum of disorders, including classic PKU and a less severe accumulation of phenylalanine (hyperphenylalaninemia). For this reason, the newborns carriers of this genetic disease are immediately submitted to a special diet, poor in phenylalanine. In the past, this disease was not diagnosed using genetic tests; however, this disease and the dietary prescription fit in the nutrigenetics concept.

Nutrigenomics studies suggest that all the solutions to improve quality of life are in the diet with the ability to interfere in the gene expression in each individual. The genome in each individual is single; so, each individual may have a personalized diet and each nutrient could be prescribed, actually, as a medicine. However, for this statement may become reality, it is necessary to understand how the bioactive compounds of the nutrients interact with the genome. The aim of the nutrigenomic science is to identify the genes that, if activated, can trigger the processes that result in the development of several diseases. With this information, it will be possible to avoid or delete these mechanisms by the simple approach of eating the nutrients that act directly in the gene control.

The biological singularity is responsible for the variety of effects of diet in each person. There exists considerable interindividual variation in response to dietary interventions, and some of them may benefit certain individuals or population subgroups. The same diet, which presents beneficial effects to a person, can be ineffective to another. Each human being carries a specific gene that regulates how the body will burn the calories. In addition to the diet adjusted to the genetic profile of each individual, nutrigenomics studies indicate the best behavior for a group of persons, according to the dietary lifestyle of each region.

Human subpopulations present intra- and inter-differences in allele frequencies and DNA haplotype blocks, and together with the chemical complexity of food make the study of nutrient–gene interactions highly complex. The simplest plant- and animal-derived foods contain hundreds of chemical constituents, some of which are sources of energy (e.g., glucose or certain fatty acids), while others serve as essential nutrient or regulators of cell functions (e.g., certain fatty acids and phytoestrogens such as genistein). Consequently, diet is often overlooked as an important variable in experimental design even though dietary constituents can alter gene expression and/or gene structure.

Two well-documented examples how nutrient–gene interaction can affect gene expression are provided by hyperforin and genistein. Hyperforin, the active ingredient in St. John's wort, binds to the ligand binding site of the pregnane X receptor (Watkins et al., 2003) and induces transcription of reporter genes in cell culture systems (Rebbeck et al., 2004; Tirona et al., 2004). Genistein, an isoflavone found in soya beans and other plants, binds to the active site of estrogen receptor β (Pike et al., 1999) and induces estrogen-specific gene expression in uteri of rats fed genistein-supplemented food (Nacif et al., 2002). Previous reviews discuss these and other molecular processes directly affected by nutrients and show how nutrient–gene interactions affect health (Kaput and Rodrigues, 2004).

The risk for developmental and degenerative diseases increases with DNA damage, which in turn is dependent on nutritional status. The optimal concentration of micronutrients for preventions of genome damage is dependent on genetic polymorphisms that alter the function of genes involved directly or indirectly in the uptake and metabolism of micronutrients required for DNA repair, DNA replication, and chromosomal stability. Multiple micronutrients and their interactions with the inherited and/or acquired genome determine DNA damage and genome instability rates. The challenge is to identify for each individual the combination of micronutrients and their doses, named nutriome that optimizes genome instability, including telomere integrity and functionality and DNA repair. Using nutrient array systems with high-content analysis diagnosis of DNA, cell death and cell growth, it is possible to define, on an individual basis, the optimal nutriome for DNA damage prevention and cancer growth control (Fenech, 2014).

Currently, it has been recognized the increasing ability to optimize nutrition and maintain a state of good health through longer periods of life. The new field of nutrigenomics with focuses on the interaction between bioactive dietary components and the genome recognizes that current nutritional guidelines may be ideal for only a relatively small proportion of the population.

There is good evidence that nutrition has significant influences on the expression of genes, and, likewise, genetic variation can have a significant effect on food intake, metabolic response to food, individual nutrient requirements, food safety, and the efficacy of disease-protective dietary factors. For example, a significant number of human studies in various areas are increasing the evidence for interactions between genetic variants in several genes and the metabolic response to diet, including the risk of obesity. The control of food intake is profoundly affected by polymorphisms either in genes encoding taste receptors or in genes encoding a number of peripheral signaling peptides such as insulin, leptin, ghrelin, cholecystokinin, and corresponding receptors. Total dietary intake and the satiety value of various foods will profoundly influence the effects of these genes. Identifying the key genetic variants that are likely to influence the health of an individual provides an approach to understanding and, ultimately, to optimizing nutrition at the population or individual level with the potential of preventing, delaying, or reducing the symptoms of chronic diseases (Fergusson, 2006).

Genetic variation and numerous environmental influences put the study of these interactions beyond the scope and expertise of any researcher, institute, or program. Resolving experimental design issues that originate from complexities of gene–environmental interactions will probably require pooling of information from several population groups (Kaput et al., 2005).

In the last years, two well-designed studies have been conducted to evaluate how gene–diet interactions influence susceptibility to MetS. The first was known as the Genetic of Lipid Lowering Drugs and Diet Network (GOLDN) study, including 1200 individuals recruited from two genetically homogeneous and predominantly white racial areas (Mineapolis and Salt Lake City, USA) (GOLDN, 2008). The second study is the Diet, Genomics, and the Metabolic Syndrome: an Integrated Nutrition, Agrofood, Social, and Economic Analysis (LIPGENE). LIPGENE is a large European, multicenter project including 486 individuals with MetS from eight countries (Ireland, the United Kingdom, Norway, France, the Netherlands, Spain, Poland, and Sweden (Shaw et al., 2009)).

Diet–gene interactions are complex and are likely to require large populations for adequate statistical power. Moreover, nutritional genomics requires systems biology approaches, necessary for analyzing gene–environmental interactions, but it also requires discipline-specific expertise and is expensive. The methods and technical skills range from genotyping, nutritional epidemiology, microarray analysis, proteomics, metabolomics, bioinformatics, pathology, and diverse clinical assessments, in models ranging from cell culture to experimental animals and human populations. Significant number of investigators is developing nutrigenomics programs in various countries, and each of them will probably face similar problems in developing and adapting cutting-edge technologies for high-dimensional research efforts. The strategic and technical knowledge challenges of nutritional genomics justify the sharing of resources and knowledge to avoid duplication in developing experimental tools, software programs, and computational models (Kaput et al., 2005).

The study of these complex interactions requires the development of advanced analytical approaches combined with bioinformatics. Thus, to carry out these studies, the "omic" technologies such as transcriptomics, proteomics, and metabolomics approaches are employed together with an adequate integration of the information they provide (Garcia-Cañas et al., 2010). These approaches include analysis of mRNA, proteins, and metabolites.

Traditional methods for identification of genetic variations of single-nucleotide polymorphisms (SNPs) may involve consideration of individual variants, using methodologies such as restriction fragment length polymorphism (RFLP) or quantitative real-time PCR assays. Other methods for the studies of diet–gene interactions are the microarrays. Expression profiling using microarrays offers a powerful tool to gain a comprehensive view of biological systems by measuring the expression of thousands of genes simultaneously (Garosi et al., 2005).

The current biological molecular approaches allow the identification of more than 500,000 polymorphisms per person. However, only some of them seem to have functional effect. In epigenetic events, polymorphisms are responsible for modifying the phenotype and even for the functions of genes, resulting in metabolic changes such as increase or decrease in dietary intake requirements. The challenge is to understand how this interaction works on the balance between health and disease. The knowledge of the genetic variants that are associated with these changes may contribute to the development of functional foods taking into account the genetic host factors.

Several gene–nutrient interactions are linked with the benefit or risk for diseases; however, the situation is highly complex and it is necessary the information on polymorphisms in many genes and how they interact with different nutrients before conclusion about what is good for an individual and what is not.

The number of studies investigating gene–nutrient interactions related to MetS continues to grow, and has potential for reducing the risk of disease at the level of the individual genotype. Given the importance of understanding the interaction between nutrient and gene, the purpose of the present chapter is to review the literature about the main advances in nutrigenetics and nutrigenomics regarding the gene–nutrient interactions associated with the development of MetS.

5.3 GENETIC POLYMORPHISMS

Currently, it is known that the human genome has 30,000–35,000 genes distributed among the 23 pairs of chromosome, a smaller number than was previously supposed. Protected inside the nucleus, there are 23 pairs of chromosome, each one with the complementary DNA double strand, composed by 3 billion of 4 types of chemical substances named nitrogenous bases. The pair of nitrogenous bases consists of a purine linked to a pyrimidine as follows: adenine (A)–thymine (T) and guanine (G)–cytosine (C) in DNA, and A–uracil (U) and G–C in RNA. The different combinations of these four molecules determinate the genetic code of each individual. The gene is the DNA unity that contains information for one specific inherited characteristic for the code to a specific protein synthesis.

The sequencing of the human genome laid the foundation for one of the most significant scientific contributions to humankind—an evidence-based understanding that while human individuals are genetically similar, each retains a unique genetic identity underlying the wide array of biochemical, physiological, and morphological phenotypes in human populations. Ancestral groups share about 86%–90% of genetic variations in our species. One of the discoveries of the Human Genome Project was the identification of the difference in the genetic sequence that results in a wide variation in the individual's response against environmental factors, such as diet (Jorde and Wooding, 2004).

Genetic variations that occur at a frequency of more than 1% in a study population are named as genetic polymorphisms. Polymorphism arises as result of mutation and the type of mutation that created them refers to different polymorphisms. The simplest type of polymorphism results from a single base mutation, which substitutes one nucleotide for another. The polymorphism at the site harboring such changes has been termed a SNP. For example, two sequenced DNA fragments from different individuals, CCTTGCCTA to CCTTGCTTA, contain a difference in a single nucleotide. The C nucleotide was changed to T nucleotide, creating two alleles.

Other polymorphisms are created by insertions or deletions (*indels*) of one or more base pairs, repeats of a large number of nucleotides (variable number of tandem repeats [VNTR] or minisatellite), and repeats of a small number of nucleotides (short tandem repeat [STR] or microsatellite). Despite success in identifying genetic contributors to common metabolic phenotypes, only part of the heritable component of these traits has been explained. VNTR is likely to be responsible for some of the unexplained variation. As observed with SNPs, it is probable that both rare and common VNTRs contribute to susceptibility to metabolic diseases. Recent efforts to map VNTRs in control populations have defined their size, frequency, and distribution. Many of the identified VNTRs overlap genes with important functions in metabolic pathways. The overlap of VNTRs that were found in control datasets with functional candidate genes or genes with previous evidence of association with MetS presents an important subset for future VNTRs association studies (Lanktree and Hegele, 2008).

SNPs are the most common type of sequence variation in the human genome. The 10–30 million SNPs in humans represent 90% of all sequence variations (Collins et al., 1998). Many of these SNPs have no known function, but many others alter the expression of critical genes involved in metabolism. In the exonic region of a gene, which encodes for a protein, an SNP can lead to substitution of an amino acid in protein; this causes a change in protein structure and can result in loss or gain of function. In the regulatory region of a gene that contains the switches (transcription factor binding sites) that turn the gene on or off, an SNP can change gene expression and thereby alter the amount of protein available to perform its function in metabolism. Such SNPs often decrease the amount of functional protein because they inhibit gene expression, but some SNPs can increase gene expression if they result in a defective region of the gene that normally acts inhibiting gene expression. When SNPs occur in genes critical for metabolism, they create metabolic inefficiencies that can influence requirements for, and responses to, a nutrient (Zeisel, 2012).

SNPs are the key factors in human genetic variation and provide a molecular basis for phenotypic differences between individuals. The knowledge and identification of these SNPs associated with the individual response to diet integrate the nutrigenetics (Fogg-Johnson and Kaput, 2003). The effect of a polymorphism depends on its interactions with environmental factors that predispose patients to dyslipidemia, such as being overweight, physical inactivity, or smoking (Freeman et al., 1994; Vohl et al., 1999).

Most SNPs are not responsible for a disease state. However, they can be located near a gene associated with a certain disease and, for this reason, may serve as biological markers for pinpointing a disease on the human genome map. Application of association study can detect differences between the SNP patterns of two groups (control-disease), thereby indicating which pattern is most likely associated with the disease-causing gene. Using SNPs to study the genetics of diet or drug response will help in the creation of "personalized" nutrition or "personalized" medicine, respectively.

5.4 PATHWAYS OF GENE–NUTRIENT INTERACTION IN METABOLIC SYNDROME

Genes are turned on and off based on the metabolic signals received by the nucleus from internal and external factors. Nutrients are among the most influent environmental stimuli that modulate the expression of genes encoding the proteins of energy metabolism, cell differentiation, and cell growth. The expression of genes is highly dependent on, and regulated by, nutrients, micronutrients, and phytochemicals found in food (Kaput et al., 2005).

Nutrients can affect gene expression directly or indirectly. At the cellular levels, nutrients may (1) act directly as ligands for transcription factor receptors; (2) be metabolized by metabolic pathways, causing changes in the concentrations of substrates or intermediates involved in gene regulation or cell signaling; and (3) alter signal transduction pathways and signaling (Kaput et al., 2004). Nutrients and their metabolites bind to several receptors in the NR superfamily of transcription factors to activate them and influence a variety of specific genes and cellular functions.

The NRs are some of the sensors of dietary lipids. Members of the NR superfamily act as intracellular transcription factors that directly regulate gene expression in response to lipophilic molecules. To date, more than 300 NRs have been cloned and several of them respond to dietary lipids, including the fatty receptors PPAR, LXR, RXR, *HNF-4α*, and FXR. Most NRs regulate gene expression predominantly in the same fashion. When a ligand binds to its cognate receptor, a conformational change occurs leading to the activation that alters the protein–protein interfaces of the molecule. As a result, the activated receptor interacts with an NR response element within the regulatory region of a target gene; upon recruitment of various transcriptional coactivators and subsequent RNA polymerase II, initiation of transcription of the target gene occurs. The dietary and intermediary metabolites activate these NRs and genes regulated by them affecting a wide variety of functions, including fatty acid metabolism, reproductive development, and detoxification of foreign substances (Vanden Heuvel, 2009) (Figure 5.3).

Recent findings revealed that polyphenols could interact with cellular signaling cascades regulating the activity of transcription factors and consequently affecting the expression of genes. Moreover, polyphenols have been shown to affect the expression of microRNAs (miRNA) (Milenkovic et al., 2013). miRNAs are short (22 nucleotides) double-stranded regulatory noncoding RNAs and have emerged as critical regulators of gene expression at the posttranscriptional level (Ambros, 2004; Bartel, 2009). The expression of miRNAs can be affected by different external stimuli including nutrients such as vitamins, lipids, and phytochemicals. Over 100 miRNAs, involved in the control of different cellular processes such as inflammation or apoptosis, were identified as modulated by polyphenols. The majority of studies were carried out in vitro using different cell lines and few of them were performed in animals (Milenkovic et al., 2013).

To date, thousands of miRNAs have been discovered, and it is thought that these small molecules may regulate >60% of all gene transcripts (Friedman et al., 2009). Specifically, miR-33a/b and

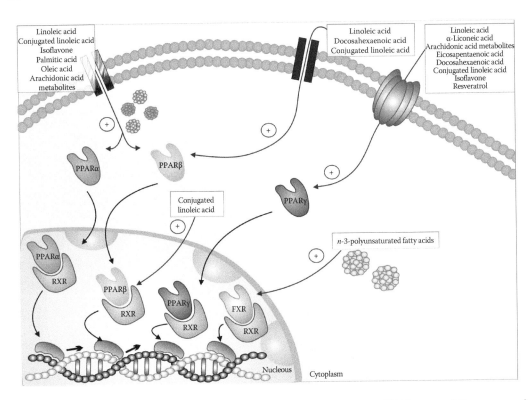

FIGURE 5.3 Gene–nutrient interactions by activation of nuclear receptors (NRs), some of the sensors of dietary lipids. Members of the NRs superfamily, such as peroxisome proliferator–activated receptor (PPAR), retinoid X receptors (RXR), and the farnesoid X receptor (FXR) act as intracellular transcription factors that directly regulate gene expression in response to lipophilic molecules. The natural PPAR alpha (PPARα) ligands in human serum are palmitic acid, oleic acid, linoleic acid, arachidonic acid, n-3 polyunsaturated fatty acid, and α-linoleic acid. The natural PPAR gamma (PPARγ) ligands are fatty acids and eicosanoid derivatives, such as the fatty acids linoleic acid, α-linoleic acid, arachidonic acid, and eicosapentaenoic acid. The natural PPAR beta (PPARβ) ligands are n-3 polyunsaturated fatty acids and conjugated linoleic acid. The RXR ligands are docosatetraenoic acid and fatty acids (unsaturated, monosaturated, and polyunsaturated fatty acids). The FXR binds to arachidonic acid, α-linoleic acid, and docosatetraenoic acid.

miR-122 have emerged as key regulators of genes involved in lipid metabolism, insulin signaling, and glucose homeostasis (Fernández-Hernado et al., 2013). The miR-122 is liver specific, plays a critical role in liver homeostasis (Hsu et al., 2012; Tsai et al., 2012), and its inhibition has been associated with the deregulation of genes playing key roles in the control of liver lipid and carbohydrate metabolism. Modulation of miR-33a/b, the foremost liver-related miRNAs, and miR-122 has been proposed to be a promising strategy to treat dyslipidemia and insulin resistance associated with obesity and MetS. Specific polyphenols reduce the levels of these miRNAs (Figure 5.4).

The effect of two grape proanthocyanidin extracts, their fractions and pure polyphenol compounds on miRNA expression depended on the polyphenol chemical structure. Moreover, miR-33a was repressed independently of its host gene *Sterol Regulatory Element-Binding Protein 2* (*SREBP2*). Therefore, the ability of resveratrol (3,5,4′-trihydroxy-*trans*-stilbene, a plant polyphenol that is naturally occurring in grapes, red wine, and peanuts), and11-epigallocattchin-3-gallate (EGCG) to bind miR-33a and miR-122 was measured using nuclear magnetic resonance spectroscopy. Both compounds bound miR-33a and miR-122 differently. The nature of the binding of these compounds to the miRNAs was consistent with their effects on cell miRNA levels. The results suggested that the specific and direct binding of polyphenols to miRNAs emerges as a new posttranscriptional mechanism by which polyphenols could modulate metabolism (Baselga-Escudero et al., 2014).

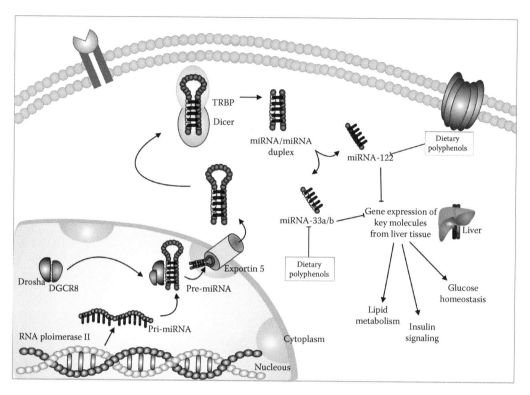

FIGURE 5.4 Gene–polyphenols interactions through the modulation of microRNAs. miRNAs are short double-stranded regulatory noncoding RNAs and have emerged as critical regulators of gene expression at the posttranscriptional level. Specifically, miR-33a/b and miR-122have emerged as key regulators of genes involved in lipid metabolism, insulin signaling, and glucose homeostasis. Specific polyphenols reduce the levels of these miRNAs and the inhibition of these miRNA by the dietary polyphenols has been associated with the deregulation of genes playing key roles in the control of liver lipid and carbohydrate metabolism. Modulation of miR-33a/b and miR-122 has been proposed to be a promising strategy to treat dyslipidemia and insulin resistance associated with obesity and metabolic syndrome.

The nuclear factor κB (NF-κB) is an important transcriptional factor of many genes in both innate and adaptative immune response. NF-κB is an inducible redox-sensitive transcriptional factor responsible for the regulation of complex phenomena, with a pivotal role in controlling cell signaling in the body under certain physiological and pathological conditions. Among other functions, NF-κB controls the expression of genes encoding the pro-inflammatory cytokines, such as cytokines, chemokines, adhesion molecules, inducible enzymes, and growth factors, some of the acute-phase proteins, and immune receptors, all of which play critical roles in controlling most inflammatory processes. This nuclear factor is activated in response to T cell receptor (TCR) signals and is essential for cytokine synthesis. TCR signals lead to serine phosphorylation of IkB by the IkB kinases. The phosphorylation of IkB is followed by attachment of multiple copies of a small protein called ubiquitin. This ubiquitination targets IkB for proteolysis in the cytosolic proteasome, the multienzyme protease complex that degrades many cytosolic proteins. The degraded IkB can no longer bind to NF-κB, which is released and translocated to the nucleus, where it contributes to the transcriptional activation of multiple cytokine genes and cytokine receptor genes.

Since NF-κB represents an important and very attractive therapeutic target to treat many inflammatory diseases, including MetS, most attention has been paid in the last decade to the identification of compounds that selectively interfere with this pathway. A great number of plant-derived substances, including polyphenols, have been evaluated as possible inhibitors of the NF-κB pathway (Nam, 2006).

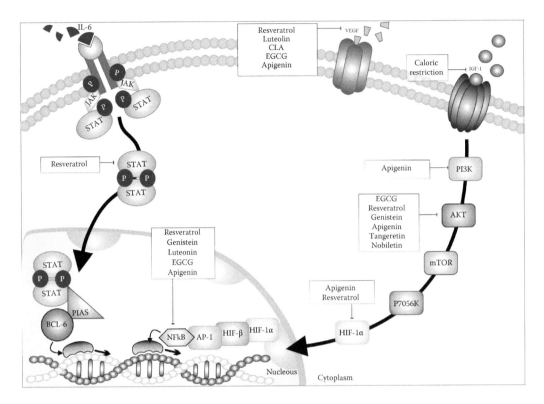

FIGURE 5.5 The gene–polyphenols interactions in the inflammatory response. Among the polyphenolic compounds, apigenin, luteonin, resveratrol, genistein, epigallocatechin-3-gallate (EGCG), epigallocatechin (EGC), epicatechin-3-gallate (ECG), and epicatechin (EC) act inhibiting signaling pathways of the inflammatory response through several mechanisms: (1) hypoxia inducible factor 1-alpha (HIF-1α) protein and the VEGF expression by blocking the phosphatidylinositol 3′-kinase (PI3K)-Akt signaling pathway; (2) by inactivating the nuclear factor κB (NF-κB) through the suppression of p65 phosphorylation; (3) by modulating the MAPK pathway and NF-κB signaling with decrease of the cytokine and chemokine genes expression; and (4) by inhibiting the STAT3 protein and JAK2 phosphorylation, repressing Stat3-regulated Bcl-6, and the lacking of the nuclear translocation of the protein inhibitor of activated STAT3 (PIAS), resulting in an induction of apoptosis.

Resveratrol impairs or delays cardiovascular alterations, cancer, inflammation, metabolic diseases, and aging. In addition to the variety of signaling pathways and the transcriptional networks that resveratrol controls, such as NF-κB, it has been proposed that the protective properties of this polyphenol may arise from its modulation of miRNA (Lançon et al., 2013).

Dietary chemicals can directly affect signal transduction pathways. Hyperforin, polyphenol EGCG, flavonoids (apigenin, luteonin, tangeretin, genistein), polyphenols present in extra-virgin olive oil (EVOO) and virgin olive oil (VOO), other retinoids (vitamin A), resveratrol, and *n*-3 PUFAs and *n*-6 PUFAs are some of the dietary ligands of the NRs and transcriptional factors involved in the gene–nutrient interactions that are discussed in this chapter (Figure 5.5).

5.5 POLYMORPHISMS IN GENES ASSOCIATED WITH LIPID METABOLISM AND REGULATION

Serum lipids have a multifactorial etiology that is determined by a large number of environmental and genetic factors. Genetic and dietary factors influence serum cholesterol concentration, but detailed mechanisms of their interactions are not well known. An increase in dietary cholesterol intake raises serum cholesterol concentrations in some but not in all subjects.

Many polymorphic variants of the genes that regulate lipid metabolism are present in humans, and more than 400 genes are candidate regulators of lipid exchange. Carriers of abnormal alleles exhibit a high risk for obesity and its associated complications, and therefore there is an interest in the association between dyslipidemia, adiposity, and other diseases with different genotypes. Genetic variations of enzymes, receptors, and apolipoproteins (apo), which are essential to low-density lipoprotein cholesterol (LDL-C) metabolism, are partially involved in the regulation of serum LDL-C and total cholesterol. Genes of note include the *apolipoprotein APOA1/C3/A4/A5 cluster, apolipoprotein B (APOB), apolipoprotein E (APOE), cholesterol ester transfer protein (CETP), hepatic and lipoprotein lipases, transcription factor 7–like 2 (TCF7L2), glucokinase regulatory protein (GCRP), fatty acid binding protein, microsomal triglyceride transfer protein, peroxisome proliferator-activated receptor gamma (PPAR-γ), scavenger receptor* class *B type1 (SCARB1)*, and *perilipin (PLIN)* (Phillips, 2013).

5.5.1 *Low-Density Lipoprotein Receptor* Gene Polymorphisms

Hypercholesterolemia can be multifactorial or less frequent monogenic leading to autosomal-dominant hypercholesterolemia (ADH). The first ADH causative gene identified was the *low-density lipoprotein receptor (LDLR)* gene encoding the LDL receptor (LDLR) (Goldstein et al., 1973); the disease was named familial hypercholesterolemia (FH) and its heterozygous prevalence was estimated at 1/500.

LDLR plays a major role in the removal of LDL-C particles from the blood, which, in turn, regulates cholesterol homeostasis. LDLR modulates plasma levels of LDL-C by regulating LDL-C particle uptake by the liver. It also delivers cholesterol to the adrenal gland and gonads for steroid hormone synthesis and to the liver for bile acid synthesis (Brown and Goldstein, 1986). LDLR is responsible for the binding and subsequent cellular uptake of apolipoprotein B- and E-containing lipoproteins (apo B and apo E, respectively).

Located on chromosome 19p13.2, the *LDLR* gene comprises 18 exons and 17 introns and encodes a protein of 839 amino acids (Südhof et al., 1985). More than 1288 different variants in the *LDLR* gene have been reported in FH patients, details of which are given as follows: 55% exonic substitutions, 22% exonic small rearrangements (<100 bp), 11% large rearrangements (>100 bp), 2% promoter variants, 10% intronic variants, and 1 variant in the 3′ untranslated sequence (Usifo et al., 2012). Considering the crucial role of LDLR in cholesterol homeostasis, SNPs in the *LDLR* gene have distinct impact on LDLR structure and function and may contribute to the variation in plasma cholesterol levels in normal and hypercholesterolemic subjects (Brown and Goldstein, 1986; Myant et al., 1991; Gylling et al., 1997; Gudnason et al., 1998; Salazar et al., 1999, 2000a,b,c; DeCastro-Orós et al., 2001). Variations in *LDLR* can interfere to a varying extent with all the different stages of the posttranslational processing, binding, uptake, and subsequent dissociation of the LDL-particle-LDLR complex (Brown and Goldstein, 1986; Gudnason et al., 1998). Individuals who are carriers for such mutations exhibit plasma total cholesterol levels two-fold or more above normal concentration and are at increased risk for developing atherosclerosis and CAD (Brown and Goldstein, 1986).

The polymorphic nature of the *LDLR* gene has been demonstrated by the digestion of the variant alleles of a DNA fragment with restriction enzymes (endonucleases), with the restriction fragment length polymorphism (RFLP) method (Pedersen and Berg, 1988). Some of these polymorphisms are named *Rsa*I (5′ extremity), *Stu*I (exon 2), *Mae*III (exon 4), *Taq*I (intron 4), *Sph*I (intron 6), *Stu*I (exon 8), *Hha*I (exon 11), *Hinc*II (exon 12, C16730T, rs688), *Ava*II (exon 13, T20001C, rs5925), *Msp*I (exon 15), *Pvu*II (intron 15, C>T), *Msp*I and *Nco*I (exon 18), and *Pst*I (3′ extremity), among others (Villéger et al., 2002).

The *Pvu*II polymorphism, located at the intron 15 of the *LDLR* has been considered a genetic marker linked to one of the variations in *LDLR* expression that either structurally alters the receptor activity or alters its function in a regulatory manner (Gudnason et al., 1998). These authors reported an association between the P2 allele with lower levels of plasma lipids than the P1 allele. The *Pvu*II polymorphism may exert an indirect effect on cholesterol metabolism, probably by increasing mRNA stability, activity or increasing the number of LDLR on the cell surface. The intron 15 C/T change is unlikely to be an allelic marker for a functional sequence elsewhere at the gene locus (Gudnason et al., 1998). However, both in vitro functional studies and in silico analysis (Mollaki et al., 2013) could predict whether *LDLR Pvu*II variant exhibits damaging effect at the protein level.

The *LDLR Pvu*II polymorphism has been associated with differences in LDL-C concentration in normo and hypercholesterolemic individuals from different countries (Leitersdorf et al., 1989; Chaves et al., 1996; Gudnason et al., 1998; Salazar et al., 2000a). Individuals carrying the P2P2 genotype exhibited lower LDL-C levels (10%–20%) than those with other genotypes (Gudnason et al., 1998). Among Brazilian population, the P1P1 genotype frequency for the *Pvu*II intron 15 polymorphism (homozygous for the absence of a restriction site) was greater in individuals with high risk for CAD. Moreover, this genotype was strongly associated with high total cholesterol, triacylglycerol, LDL-C, and very-low-density lipoprotein cholesterol (VLDL-C) levels and low HDL-C levels in patients with high risk for CAD. Similarly, the control individuals with the P1P1 genotype presented higher concentrations of total cholesterol and LDL-C compared to those with other genotypes (P1P2 and P2P2 (Salazar et al., 2000a).

5.5.2 *APOLIPOPROTEIN A1* GENE POLYMORPHISMS

The apolipoprotein A-1 (apoA-1) is the major protein component of HDL-C in plasma and exerts a specific role in lipid metabolism. Chylomicrons secreted from the intestinal enterocyte also contain apo A-1, but it is quickly transferred to HDL-C in the bloodstream.

ApoA-1 promotes cholesterol efflux from tissues to the liver for excretion, and it is a cofactor for lecithin cholesterol acyltransferase (LCAT) which is responsible for the formation of most plasma cholesteryl esters. The *APOA1* gene located on chromosome 11 encodes this protein (11q23-q24) that is closely linked with two other *apolipoprotein* genes. Variations in the *APOA1* gene affect, in a different way, the levels of HDL-C. Mutations in the *APOA1* gene cause familial HDL-C deficiency, an inherited condition characterized by low levels of HDL-C and an elevated risk for early-onset CVD, which often occurs before age 50. These mutations lead to an altered apoA-1 protein. Some versions of the altered protein are less able to promote the removal of cholesterol and phospholipids from cells, which decreases the amount of these substances available to form HDL-C. Other versions of the altered protein are less able to stimulate cholesterol esterification, which means cholesterol cannot be integrated into HDL-C particles. Both types of mutation result in low HDL-C levels.

A specific SNP in the promoter of the *APOA1* gene, named -75G/A, has been extensively studied in relation to apoA-1 and HDL-C levels (Juo et al., 1999). Interactions with dietary factors could modulate the effect of this genetic SNP. Carriers of the A allele for this SNP showed an increase in HDL-C concentrations with increased intake of PUFAs. Whereas those homozygous for the more common G allele showed a predictable lowering of HDL-C levels with increased intake of PUFAs (Ordovas, 2004). The influence of gender has also been demonstrated in this specific interaction. In women carrier of the A allele, higher PUFAs intake were associated with higher HDL-C concentrations, whereas the opposite effect was observed in GG women in the Framingham Study. PUFAs intake had no significant effect on either HDL-C or ApoA-1 concentrations in men (Ordovas et al., 2002b). The basis of Apo heterogeneity is related to a copy number variation in one of its protein domains, kringle IV type 2 (KIV$_2$), which exists in 5–50 identically repeated copies.

Previously, all the scientists believed that all the persons that adopted a diet rich in PUFAs omega-3 (*n*-3) and omega-6 (*n*-6) would be able to increase the HDL-C levels and, consequently, to reduce the risk for CVD. Nowadays, the scientists know that is not simple. Some women with specific variation in the *APOA1* gene can present an opposite response with the consumption of these nutrients, with a decrease in the HDL-C levels.

Increased PUFAs intake reduces both LDL-C and HDL-C. However, recent work suggests that the response to PUFAs depends on genotype. The -75G/A *APOA1* SNP influenced the postprandial LDL-C response to a monounsaturated (MUFA) diet. After consumption of a high MUFA diet, carriers of the A allele showed significant increases in LDL-C concentrations, which were not noted in GG individuals (Lopez-Miranda et al., 1994).

Approximately, 75% of individuals are homozygous GG for the -75G/A *APOA1* SNP and, in these individuals, increased PUFAs intake is associated with decreased HDL-C. However, in heterozygous GA or homozygotes AA, increased PUFAs intake has the opposite effect, increasing HDL-C. This strongly suggests that there is an interaction between diet and genotype in determining the benefit or risk of increased PUFAs intake. A specific population group might benefit from a high PUFAs diet. As a single factor, an SNP may have no observable effect on metabolism or phenotype, but it may have under different nutritional conditions (Hesketh et al., 2006).

In addition, the postprandial LDL-C response to dietary fat is influenced by the presence of the *347Ser* variant of the *APOA4* gene. Thus, carriers of the *347Ser* allele presented a greater decrease in LDL-C levels when they were switched from the saturated fatty acid (SFA) to the National Cholesterol Education Program (NCEP) type 1 diet than those with the homozygous *347Thr* allele (Jansen et al., 1997). It has been demonstrated that the presence of *APOA1* and *APOA4* SNPs can even influence the effects of dietary fat on LDL particle size and oxidation in healthy young adults (Gomez et al., 2010).

5.5.3 *APOLIPOPROTEIN B* GENE POLYMORPHISMS

Apolipoprotein B (ApoB) is an essential protein for the formation of chylomicrons in the small intestine and for the secretion of VLDL-C in the liver. This is the major protein in human LDL-C and VLDL-C and it is synthesized in the liver and intestine. This protein is essential for the assembly, secretion, and metabolism of lipoprotein particles and for the removal of LDL-C from the circulation by LDLR on cell surfaces (Brown and Goldstein, 1986; Young, 1990).

APOB gene is located on chromosome 2p23-p24 and several mutations and SNPs are associated with either variation in plasma lipid concentrations (Forti et al., 2003) or with CAD and myocardial infarction (Wu et al., 1994; Turner et al., 1995; Gardemann et al., 1998). Structural and genetic alterations in *apoB* gene are associated with defective binding to LDLR and lead to hypercholesterolemia (Avogaro et al., 1980; Levy, 1981; Lewis, 1983).

The SNPs in *apoB* include the *Xba*I at exon 26 (C7673T, rs693), *Eco*RI at exon 29 (G12669A, rs1042031), *Msp*I at exon 26 (rs676210), an indel at exon 1 within the signal peptide (rs17240441), and a hypervariable region at the 3′ end (3′HVR) (Ludwig and McCarthy, 1990; Tai et al., 1998). These SNPs are associated with variability in serum cholesterol levels and coronary atherosclerosis (Berg, 1986; Hansen et al., 1997; Stepanov et al., 1998; Guzmán et al., 2000). The indel, *Msp*I (rs676210), *Xba*I (rs693), and 3′HVR polymorphisms may be associated with variations in lipid levels, CAD, and myocardial infarction (Berg, 1986; Hegele et al., 1986; Law et al., 1986; Talmud et al., 1987; Peacock et al., 1992), but these findings are controversial (Myant et al., 1989; Glisić et al., 1997).

The *Xba*I polymorphism in exon 26 of the *apoB* gene is associated with increased total cholesterol, altered postprandial lipoprotein metabolism, and increased CAD (Genest et al., 1990; Ukkola et al., 1993; Lopez-Miranda et al., 1997). The *Eco*RI polymorphism in exon 29 is associated with variations in total cholesterol and triacylglycerol levels, obesity, and CAD (Paulweber et al., 1990; Peacock et al., 1992; Pouliot et al., 1994; Stepanov et al., 1998). Furthermore, the signal peptide indel polymorphism is associated with increased serum triacylglycerol, total cholesterol, and LDL-C levels (Bohn et al., 1994; Hong et al., 1997).

5.5.4 *APOLIPOPROTEIN E* GENE POLYMORPHISMS

The apoE protein is incorporated in the structure of HDL-C, VLDL-C, chylomicrons, and lipo-lytic degradation products (i.e., the remnants of chylomicrons and intermediate density lipopro-tein cholesterol [IDL-C]). ApoE is important for the catabolism of triacylglycerol-rich lipoproteins and reverse cholesterol transport in various tissues (Forti et al., 2003), which involves its binding to LDLR and the apoE hepatic receptor, the activation of enzymes including hepatic lipase, and hepatic production of VLDL-C (Shore and Shore, 1973; Ginsberg, 1998). The LDLR in the liver can clear both LDL- and apoE-containing lipoproteins but the LRP-mediated clearance of remnants is absolutely dependent on apoE (Linton et al., 1998). Moreover, apoE influences enteral cholesterol absorption, immunoregulation, and neurobiological events such as neuronal repair, remodeling, and protection (Mahley and Huang, 1999; Schwanke et al., 2002).

This apolipoprotein presents three major isoforms (APOE2, APOE3, and APOE4) that modulate lipid levels and these isoforms differ in their affinity for binding to apoE receptor and LDLR, and to other lipoprotein particles (Moreno et al., 2004).

APOE gene is located at the long arm of chromosome 19 and encodes a protein of 299 amino acids (Forti et al., 2003). A common polymorphism, named *Hha*I (T112C, rs429358 and C158T, rs7412), is located in exon 4 and generates three alleles (ε2, ε3, and ε4); these alleles determine the six genotypes (ε2/ε2, ε2/ε3, ε2/ε4, ε3/ε3, ε3/ε4, and ε4/ε4) (Shore and Shore, 1973; Forti et al., 1997; Mahley and Huang, 1999; Schwanke et al., 2002). The allele frequencies differ significantly between ethnic groups (Hallman et al., 1991; Gerdes et al., 1992), but ε3 is the most common allele in several populations (Eichner et al., 2002). The *APOE* polymorphisms modify the protein struc-ture and function (Schwanke et al., 2002) and ApoE isoforms interact differently with lipoprotein receptors, altering their metabolism and consequently the plasma level of the circulating lipids (Siest et al., 1995).

In industrialized societies, individuals carrying the ε4 allele exhibit high serum levels of total cholesterol and LDL-C, while individuals carrying the ε3 allele exhibit intermediate levels and those carrying the ε2 allele present the lowest levels (Davignon et al., 1988). Associations between the ε4 allele and increased total cholesterol and LDL-C levels and between the ε2 allele and low lev-els of these lipids have been documented in many studies, independently of ethnic group (Hallman et al., 1991).

The affinity for the receptor depends on the polymorphism *Hha*I (exon 4) in *APOE* gene. Studies have shown that ε4 allele is associated with CHD due to the increases in LDL-C levels (Davignon et al., 1988; Salazar et al., 2000b; Pedro-Bolet et al., 2001). Salazar et al. (2000b) also showed that the ε4/ε4 genotype was associated with CHD and higher levels of total cholesterol, triacylglycerol, and LDL-C when compared to controls. Compared with individuals with the commonest ε3/ε3 genotype, ε2 carriers exhibited a 20% lower risk for CHD and ε4 carrier had higher risk. Indeed, individuals with the ε2/ε2 genotype had about 31% lower mean LDL-C concentrations than those with the ε4/ε4 genotype.

However, not everyone with the ε4 allele develops CHD, which suggests that other genetic or environmental factors could influence the final phenotype. It has been demonstrated that *APOE* gene promoter -219G/T polymorphism increases LDL-C concentrations and susceptibility to oxi-dation in response to a diet rich in SFA. Carriers of the T allele showed higher concentrations of apoB and LDL-C after SFA diet compared with GG carriers. In carriers of the T allele, decreases in LDL-C and apoB were significantly higher when they changed from the saturated to the high-carbohydrate diet compared with GG individuals (Moreno et al., 2004). This particular SNP could explain individual differences in response to a diet. It has been demonstrated that the same -219G/T polymorphism determines insulin sensitivity in response to dietary fat in healthy young adults with *APO*ε3/ε3 genotype (Moreno et al., 2005).

Intervention studies demonstrated clear evidence that *APOE* locus could interact with dietary SFA, increasing LDL-C concentrations and increasing CVD risk, which appears more evident in ε4 carriers. However, we need to be cautious before drawing general conclusions, given that studies varied widely in the number and type of population, and in the composition and duration of the dietary interventions (Garcia-Rios et al., 2012).

Other illustration of this interaction is the SNP (2219G/T) in the promoter of the *APOE* gene that exerts little effect on fasting triacylglycerol levels but does influence postprandial triacylglycerol clearance; similarly, following fish oil supplementation, postprandial triacylglycerol levels were lowered more in the apoE2 subgroup for a specific SNP within the *APOE* coding region (Hesketh et al., 2006).

5.5.5 *APOE5* Gene Polymorphism and Postprandial State

A common SNP in the *APOE5* gene (-1131T/C) has been clearly related with higher triacylglycerols concentration among those carrying the C allele. With this SNP, it is possible to understand how gene–diet interaction can modulate the effect of a genetic polymorphism (Lai et al., 2006; Park et al., 2010; Sánches-Moreno et al., 2011). In the Framingham study, the consistent association was demonstrated between the -1131T/C and fasting triacylglycerols concentrations. A significant interaction was demonstrated between this SNP and PUFAs intake. The -1131C allele was associated with an increase in fasting triacylglycerols and in remnant-like particle triacylglycerol concentrations only in individuals consuming >6% of energy from PUFAs.

The postprandial period is considered the physiological state in human metabolism, where the assessment of the postprandial lipemic response is the best way to identify disturbances in lipid metabolism (Perez-Martines et al., 2011c). Accumulating evidence points to a role for postprandial lipemia in the pathogenesis of metabolic diseases such as obesity, CVD, and MetS (Le and Walter, 2007; Stalenhoef and de Graaf, 2008). The postprandial state following a fatty meal, especially when the meal is rich in SFA, induces physiological postprandial hypertriacylglycerolemia that may play a pivotal role in the control of atherogenesis. Regarding genetic component, multiple lipid candidate genes have been investigated in order to explain the wide variability in postprandial response.

Several genetic association studies have underscored the *APOE5* as a major gene that is involved in the postprandial lipoprotein metabolism. The *APOE5* gene promoter SNP -1131T/C was evaluated in 51 healthy *APOEε3/ε3* male volunteers who underwent a vitamin A fat-load test consisting of 1 g of fat/kg body weight and 60,000 IU of vitamin A. The healthy men carrying the -1131 C allele presented higher postprandial triacylglycerol levels and markedly higher postprandial responses in both large and small triacylglycerol-rich lipoprotein.

5.5.6 *Peroxisome Proliferator-Activated Receptor Gamma* Gene Polymorphisms

Other gene–diet interactions that influence HDL-C metabolism involving the *PPAR-γ* gene have been demonstrated (Memisoglu et al., 2003; Robitaille et al., 2003). The peroxisome proliferator-activated receptors (PPARs) regulate the expression of several genes related to the carbohydrate and lipid metabolism. PPARs exist as three subtypes (α, β, and γ) that vary in expression, ligand recognition, and biological function. PPARα was the first transcription factor identified as a potential fatty acid receptor and regulates fatty acid transport, fatty acid binding proteins, fatty acyl-coenzyme A (CoA) synthesis, microsomal, peroxisomal, and mitochondrial fatty acid oxidation, ketogenesis, and fatty acid desaturation.

Natural PPARα ligands in human serum include palmitic acid, oleic acid, linoleic and arachidonic acid (AA). Notably, PPARα is the only PPAR subtype that binds to a wide range of SFAs (Vanden Heuvel et al., 2006). VLDL and LDL contain PPARα ligands (Chawla et al., 2003; Ziouzenkova et al., 2003). Activation of PPARα is seen when lipoprotein lipase (LPL) is added to VLDL, showing that the endogenous ligands are probably fatty acids or their metabolites esterified into triacylglycerols (Figure 5.3).

PPARγ is expressed in many tissues, including adipose, muscle, vascular cells, macrophages, and epithelial cells of the mammary gland, prostate, and colon (Spiegelman, 1998). Activated PPARγ induces LPL and fatty acid transporters (CD36), enhances adipocyte differentiation, and inhibits cytokine and cyclooxygenase-2 (COX-2) expression, perhaps by modulating nuclear factor-κB function. Clinically relevant antidiabetic agents such as pioglitazone and rosiglitazone are potent PPARγ agonists (Kd in low nanomolar range). A number of fatty acids and eicosanoid derivatives bind and activate PPARγ in the micromolar range (Krey et al., 1997). Unlike the PPARα subtype, PPARγ has a clear preference for PUFAs (Vanden Heuvel et al., 2006). The fatty acids linoleic acid, ALA, arachidonic acid, and EPA bind PPARγ within the range of concentrations of free fatty acids found in human serum. Although fatty acids are not particularly efficacious activators of PPARγ, intracellular conversion of fatty acids to eicosanoids through 15-lipoxygenase greatly increased PPARγ-mediated transactivation (Willson and Wahli, 1997) (Figure 5.3).

The PPAR-γ is expressed mainly in the adipocyte tissue and is a NR that regulates specific genes of adipocytes and contributes to the adipocyte differentiation. The PPAR-γ modulates the expression of genes that are involved in the entry of lipids into the cells, the triacylglycerols synthesis, the fatty acids oxidation, and the extracellular metabolism of cholesterol. Several polymorphisms have been described in the *PPAR-γ* gene, such as those located in the codons 12, 113, 318, 425, 477, and 495. These include a very rare gain-of-function mutation (Pro115Gln) associated with obesity but not insulin resistance (Ristow et al., 1998), two loss-of-function mutations (Val290Met and Pro467Leu) reported in three individuals with severe insulin resistance but normal body weight (Barroso et al., 1999), the silent CAC478CAT mutation (Deeb et al., 1998), and the highly prevalent SNP of the codon 12 of the *PPAR-γ*, which results in a proline for alanine substitution (Pro12Ala) (Yen et al., 1997).

The Pro12Ala SNP has been widely studied and the total fat intake has been shown to be correlated with plasma HDL-C concentrations. It is the result of a CCA-to-GCA missense mutation in codon 12 of exon B of the *PPAR-γ* gene. This exon encodes the NH_2-terminal residue that defines the adipocyte-specific PPAR-γ2 isoform (Yen et al., 1997).

Variation in the *PPAR-γ* gene alters the risk for adiposity in adults, with evidence of interaction with diet. The Pro12Ala SNP of the *PPAR-γ2 locus* modulates the relationship between energy intake and body weight in T2DM patients (Vaccaro et al., 2007). This study provides evidence of a differential susceptibility to fat accumulation, and, hence, weight gain, in response to habitual high energy intake for Ala carriers compared with Pro/Pro homozygotes. Among Pro12Pro homozygotes, total fat intake was inversely correlated with HDL-C concentrations (Memisoglu et al., 2003). However, among 12Ala variant allele carriers, the intake of total fat was directly correlated with HDL-C concentrations. Although PPAR-γ is a critical transcriptional regulator of adipogenesis, it has also been proposed to be a mediator of physiological responses to lipids as it promotes the HDL-induced cholesterol efflux in adipocytes (Zhao et al., 2008).

The Pro12Ala phenotype was associated with T2DM and obesity in male individuals. Carriers of the Ala12 exhibit lower risk to T2DM, higher loss of weight when are treated with metformin or when they change lifestyle when compared with carriers of the Pro12. The homeostasis model assessment of insulin resistance (HOMA-IR) was lower among the Ala12Ala than the Pro12Pro subjects (Stumvoll and Häring, 2002). The adiposity in children is also influenced by the Pro12Ala polymorphism in a sex-specific and age-dependent manner and there is evidence of an age-dependent gene–diet (SFA, TF) interaction, suggesting that the type of fat intake modifies the effect of the Pro12 allele on obesity-related measures (Dedoussis et al., 2011).

5.5.7 PROPROTEIN CONVERTASE SUBTILISIN/KEXIN TYPE 9 GENE POLYMORPHISMS

Another protein related to dyslipidemia is proprotein convertase subtilisin/kexin type 9 (PCSK9). The *PCSK9* gene is located on chromosome 1 (1p32), has 12 exons, and encodes a 692 amino acid protein. There are several mutations in *PCSK9*, including c.G1120T (p.Asp374Tyr), c.T381A (p.Ser127Arg), c.T646A (p.Phe216Leu), c.A654T (p.Arg218Ser), R46L (rs11591147), and rs11206510. Mutations in *PCSK9* cause ADH (Abifadel et al., 2003). The overexpression of PCSK9 cells accelerates the degradation of cell-surface LDLR through a nonproteasomal mechanism in a postendoplasmic reticulum compartment and leads to increased total cholesterol and LDL-C (Benjannet et al., 2004; Maxwell et al., 2005).

5.5.8 CHOLESTERYL ESTER TRANSFER PROTEIN GENE POLYMORPHISMS

Cholesteryl ester transfer protein (CETP) is an enzyme with a key role in HDL-C metabolism. CETP promotes the exchange of triacylglycerol and cholesterol between lipoproteins, and it transfers cholesteryl esters from HDL-C to other lipoproteins for subsequent absorption of cholesterol by hepatocytes. Cholesteryl esters are transferred to LDL-C and VLDL-C in exchange for triacylglycerol (Yen et al., 1989; Tall, 1995; Barter, 2002). By increasing the amount of cholesteryl esters in LDL-C and VLDL-C, CETP increases the atherogenicity of these lipoproteins. High plasma CETP concentration is associated with reduced HDL-C, a strong and independent risk factor for atherosclerosis (McPherson et al., 1991; Tall, 1993).

The *CETP* gene is located on chromosome 16 and contains 16 exons (Angelon et al., 1990; Callen et al., 1992). The protein is expressed primarily in the liver, spleen, and adipose tissue, but low levels have been detected in the small intestine, adrenal glands, heart, kidney, and skeletal muscle (Ordovas et al., 2000). CETP-deficient patients exhibit elevated plasma HDL-C levels and low plasma LDL-C levels (Inazu et al., 1994).

The *Taq*IB (rs708272) polymorphism affects lipid transfer activity and HDL-C. *Taq*IB (rs708272) is one of the best studied polymorphisms in *CETP*; it consists of a silent guanine-to-adenine nucleotide substitution in intron1. The less common allele, B2, is associated with decreased CETP activity, and in normolipemic individuals, this allele is associated with an increase in HDL-C due to decreased CETP activity (Drayna and Lawn, 1987; Kondo et al., 1989; Freeman et al., 1994; Hannuksela et al., 1994).

5.5.9 LIPOPROTEIN LIPASE GENE POLYMORPHISMS

LPL is linked to the vascular endothelium and plays a crucial role in plasma lipoprotein processing. LPL catalyzes triacylglycerol hydrolysis, which is the limiting step in the removal of triacylglycerol-rich lipoproteins such as chylomicrons, VLDL-C, and LDL-C from the circulation (Eckel, 1989). LPL acts as a ligand for LDLR-related protein and for the uptake of VLDL-C and LDL-C (Mulder et al., 1993).

The *LPL* gene is located on chromosome 8 (8p22) and is composed of 10 exons (Deeb and Peng, 1989; Oka et al., 1990). The known polymorphisms result in three functional variants: D9N (G28A, rs1801177), S291N (A1127G, rs268), and serine447-Stop (S447X) or *Mnl*I (rs328), and two SNPs located on introns; *Hind*III at intron 8 (T381G, rs320) and *Pvu*II at intron 6 (rs285). Generally, these variants are associated with increased triacylglycerols, but the S447X mutation, which truncates the last two amino acids of the polypeptide chain, decreases triacylglycerols (Hokanson, 1999; Wittrup et al., 1999; Razzaghi et al., 2000). Two genetic variations at the *LPL* gene (rs328 and rs1059611) influence plasma lipid concentrations, mainly triacylglycerol rich-lipoprotein, and interact with plasma *n*-6 PUFAs to modulate lipid metabolism. The comprehension of these gene–nutrient interactions could help the understanding of the pathogenesis of MetS (Garcia-Rios et al., 2011; Povel et al., 2011).

A study investigated whether the association of *LPL Hind*III (H1/H1) and S447X SNPs explained the interindividual variability observed during the postprandial state (López-Miranda et al., 2004). Fifty healthy apo ε3 male volunteers underwent a vitamin A fat-load test consisting of 1 g of fat/kg body weight and 60,000 IU of vitamin A. The fatty meal consisted of two cups of whole milk, eggs, bread, bacon, cream, walnuts, and butter, which was consumed within 20 min. The meal provided

1 g fat and 7 mg cholesterol/kg body weight and contained 60% fat, 15% protein, and 25% carbohydrates. After meal, individuals were not allowed to consume any calorie-containing food for 11 h. Blood samples were drawn before the meal, every hour until the 6th hour, and every 2 h and 30 min until the 11th hour. The results showed that carriers of the H1 allele (H1S447 and H1X447 genotypes) presented a lower postprandial lipemic response than carriers of the H2S447 genotype (homozygotes for the H2 allele of the *LPLHind*III SNP and S447 allele). This result is significant since the modifications observed in postprandial lipoprotein metabolism might be involved in the increased prevalence of CAD observed in homozygous individuals for the H2 allele of the *LPL Hind*III SNP (Mattu et al., 1994).

5.5.10 *Hepatic Lipase* Gene Polymorphisms

Variability in the *LIPC* gene, which encodes a key enzyme involved in reverse cholesterol transport, is also associated with interactions between intake of fat and concentrations of HDL-C. This gene codifies an enzyme that can process HDL-C when this molecule is enriched in triacylglycerols. Indeed, this enzyme can convert the phospholipid-rich HDL2 into HDL3. Other example of gene–nutrient interaction that influences the plasma parameter of lipid metabolism, such as HDL-C levels that are affected by the level of dietary fat, is the *-514C/T* SNP in the promoter of the *LIPC* gene. The T allele is associated with decreased plasma hepatic lipase activity and increased HDL-C, but TT subjects may have impaired adaptation to higher animal-fat diets that could result in higher cardiovascular risk (Hesketh et al., 2006). Moreover, -514 C/T SNP in *LIPC* gene interacted with dietary fat in determining HDL-C levels and subclasses of HDL-C in which the T allele was associated with significantly greater HDL-C concentrations and large HDL-C size only in subjects consuming <30% of energy from fat (Ordovas et al., 2002a).

Similarly, it has been shown that the dietary AA intake influences the atherogenic effect of allelic variation in the *5-lipoxygenase* gene. The 5-lipoxygenase promoter normally contains five tandem Sp1 binding sites but individuals with variation in the number of these sites show increased atherosclerosis and this effect was enhanced by dietary arachidonic acid but lowered by dietary *n*-3 PUFAs intake. Again, this illustrates that nutritional status influences benefit–risk assessment of specific nutrients and genotypes.

5.5.11 *Period 2* Gene Polymorphisms

The *Period 2* (*PER2*) gene, a circadian clock gene, is a member of the *Period* family of genes and is expressed in a circadian pattern in the suprachiasmatic nucleus, the primary circadian pacemaker in the mammalian brain. Genes in this family encode components of the circadian rhythms of locomotor activity, metabolism, and behavior.

Variants of *PER2* gene have been linked to MetS. Garcia-Rios et al. (2012) investigated whether SNPs in the *PER2* locus (rs934945 and rs2304672) interact with various classes of plasma fatty acids to modulate plasma lipid metabolism in 381 participants with MetS in the European LIPGENE study. The rs2304672 SNP interacted with plasma total SFA concentrations to affect fasting plasma triacylglycerols, triacylglycerol-rich lipoprotein, total cholesterol, apoC-II, apoB, and apoB-48 concentrations. Carriers of the minor allele, with the genotypes GC + GG when received the highest SFA concentration exhibited a higher plasma triacylglycerol levels and higher triacylglycerol-rich lipoprotein than those carrying the CC genotype.

Moreover, individuals carrying the minor G allele for rs2304672 SNP and with a higher SFA concentration exhibited higher plasma concentrations of apo C-II, apo C-III, and apoB-48 compared with the carriers of the CC genotype. These results demonstrated that the rs2304672 polymorphism in the *PER2* gene locus may influence lipid metabolism by interacting with the plasma total SFA concentration in individuals with MetS and the understanding of these gene–nutrient interactions could help to provide a better knowledge of the pathogenesis in MetS (Garcia-Rios et al., 2012).

5.5.12 Gene–Nutrient Interaction Studies in LDL-C

A heterogeneity in LDL-C concentrations and LDL-C size is observed among different individuals, probably as result of a combination of gene and nutrient interactions. Several studies were carried out in order to evaluate the gene interactions in LDL-C levels. Carriers of the T allele of the SNP rs405509 on the *APOE* gene showed higher concentrations of apoB and LDL-C after SFA diet compared with GG carriers (Moreno et al., 2004). Carriers of the minor allele of the SNP re1800206 on the *PPARγ* gene presented higher fasting total cholesterol LDL-C and apoB after a single fat load composed of 60% calories as fat, 15% as protein, and 25% as carbohydrates (Tanaka et al., 2007).

Other study showed that carriers of the A allele of the SNP rs670 on the *APOA1* gene presented a significant increase in LDL-C after a high MUFA diet, compared with GG carriers (Lopes-Miranda et al., 1994). Carriers of the *347Ser* allele of the SNP rs675 in the *APOA4* gene presented a greater decrease in LDL-C when were switched from the saturated to the NCEP type 1 diet compared with *347Thr* homozygous (Jansen et al., 1997).

5.5.13 Gene–Nutrient Interaction Studies in HDL-C

PUFAs intake modulates the effects of the SNP rs670 on the *ApoA1* gene on HDL-C concentrations in a sex-specific manner. In female carriers of the A allele, higher PUFAs intake were associated with higher HDL-C levels. The opposite effect was observed in GG women carriers. These interactions were not demonstrated in men (Ordovas 2004).

Other study evaluated the SNPs rs361525 and rs1800629 on the *TNF*-α gene and the results showed that PUFAs intake was positively associated with HDL-C levels in carriers of the *-238A* allele, but negatively in those with the *-238*GG genotype. However, the intake of PUFAs was inversely associated with HDL-C in carriers of the *-308A* allele, but not in those with the *-308*GG genotype (Fontaine-Bisson et al., 2007).

5.5.14 Gene–Nutrient Interaction Studies in Triacylglycerols

PUFAs interact with the L162V SNP (rs1800206) in the *PPARα* gene affecting the plasma triacylglycerols and apolipoprotein C-III concentrations in the Framingham Heart Study. The 162V allele was associated with a greater triacylglycerol and apoC-III levels only in individuals consuming a low-PUFAs diet (Tai et al., 2005).

The SNP rs662799 on the *APOA5* gene also interacted with diet. The -1131C allele was associated with an increase in fasting triacylglycerols and in remnant-like particle triacylglycerol concentrations only in individuals consuming >6% of energy from PUFAs (Lai et al., 2006).

Carriers of the minor allele at the rs1799983 in *NOS3* gene have plasma triacylglycerols concentrations, which are more responsive to *n*-3 PUFAs (Ferguson et al., 2010a).

5.5.15 Gene–Diet Interactions after Acute Ingestion of Olive Oil

An increasing amount of data indicate that fatty acids and polyphenols, present in EVOO, modulate the expression of key atherosclerotic-related genes in vascular (macrophages, endothelial and smooth muscle cells) and peripheral blood mononuclear cells (PBMCs), toward a less-atherogenic gene profile. These compounds exert an effect after acute ingestion of the oil and during the postprandial state and may provide protection during several stages of atherosclerosis.

All evidence for the impact of olive oil on gene expression is derived from research using animal or human cells in culture. Recent *in vitro* studies have shown that sustained consumption of VOO influences PBMCs gene expression upregulating the expression of genes associated with DNA repair proteins, such as the excision repair cross complementation group (ERCC-) and the X-ray repair complementing defective repair Chinese hamster cells 5 (XRCC-5). VOO consumption also upregulated aldehyde dehydrogenase 1 family, member A1 (*ALDH1A1*) and *lipoic acid synthetase* (*LIAS*) gene expression. *ALDH1A1* is a gene encoding a protein that protects cells from the oxidative stress induced by lipid peroxidation; the LIAS protein plays an important role in α-(+)-lipoic acid (LA) synthesis. LA is an important antioxidant that has been shown to inhibit atherosclerosis in mouse models of human atherosclerosis due to its anti-inflammatory, antihypertriacylglycerolemic, and weight-reducing effects. Moreover, apoptosis-related genes, such as *baculoviral IAP repeat containing protein* (*BICR-1*) and TNF (ligand) superfamily, member 10 (*TNSF-10*) were also upregulated. BIRC-1 inhibits apoptosis while TNSF-10 promotes macrophages and lymphocytes apoptosis (Khymenets et al., 2009).

VOO ingestion modified the expression of the following genes: (1) upregulated the *O-linked N-acetylglucosamine transferase* (*OGT*) gene; (2) *ubiquitin specific peptidase 48* (*USP-48*); (3) *peroxisome proliferator-activated receptor-binding protein* (*PPARBP*); (4) *disintegrin and metalloproteinase domain 17* (*ADAM-17*); (5) prevented an increase in *cyclo-oxygenase-2* (*COX-2*) gene expression and decreased *monocyte chemotactic protein 1* (*MCP-1*) gene expression (Llorente-Cortés et al., 2010); (6) prevented *low-density lipoprotein receptor-related protein-1* (*LRP-1*) overexpression in high cardiovascular risk population; and (7) increased the expression of genes involved in intracellular process of thrombosis, such as the *tissue factor pathway inhibitory* (*FFPI*) (Ortega et al., 2012).

The olive oil polyphenols play a significant role in the downregulation of pro-atherogenic genes in human PBMCs after 3 months of a dietary intervention with a traditional Mediterranean diet (TMD) + VOO and TMD + washed virgin olive oil (WVOO) that has the same characteristics as VOO, except for the lower polyphenol content. The dietary intervention decreased the expression of genes related to inflammation, such as *interferon gamma* (*IFN-γ*), *Rho G1Pase activating protein-13* (*ARHGAP-15*), *interleukin 7 receptor* (*IL-7R*), and oxidative stress-related genes, such as *adrenergic β-2 receptor surface* (*ADRB2*) (Konstantinidou et al., 2010; Ortega et al., 2012).

5.6 POLYMORPHISMS IN GENES ASSOCIATED WITH CARBOHYDRATE METABOLISM

Although many SNPs have been linked to certain MetS features, there are few studies analyzing the influence of SNPs on carbohydrate metabolism in MetS. Carbohydrate metabolism is an important target, given its key implications in chronic diseases, such as T2DM and longevity (Delgado-Lista et al., 2014).

Several individual gene variants of the carbohydrate metabolism have been associated with MetS. The *CEBPA*, *GCKR*, *Calpain-10*, or transcription factor 7-like 2 (*TCF7L2*) loci were associated with different MetS-related traits, such as impaired β-cell function or insulin resistance, especially under certain dietary conditions (Delgado-Lista et al., 2011a, 2013; Perez-Martinez et al., 2011a,b). GWAS identified more than 50 *loci* relevant to obesity and diabetes, and the most important T2DM susceptibility gene known so far, *TCF7L2* rs7903146 SNP. *TCF7L2* polymorphisms have also been associated with MetS components such as dyslipidemia and waist circumference (Melzer et al., 2006).

Some GWAS were focused on associations with the prevalence of MetS or clinical criteria (Kraja et al., 2011; Kristiansson et al., 2012). A review pooled all available data regarding carbohydrate metabolism in patients with MetS and identified *TCF7L2, FTO, ADCY5, FADS1, GLIS3, IGF1,* and *PPARγ* as candidate genes (Phillips et al., 2009; Phillips, 2013), whereas another GWAS identified other genes such as *GCKR, ETFB,* and *TMX2* as potential candidates (Kristiansson et al., 2012).

Nine hundred and four SNPs selected on biological plausibility were evaluated for the influence on eight fasting and dynamic markers of carbohydrate metabolism, by performance of an intravenous glucose tolerance test (Delgado-Lista et al., 2014). Fasting and postprandial samples of 450 patients with MetS from the LIPGENE study were included. From 382 initial gene–phenotype associations between SNPs and any phenotype variables, 61 (16% of the preselected variables) remained significant after bootstrapping. Top SNPs affecting glucose metabolism variables were as follows: fasting glucose, rs26125 (*PPARγ-C1B*); fasting insulin, rs4759277 (*LRP1*); C-peptide, rs4759277 (*LRP1*); homeostasis assessment of insulin resistance, rs4759277 (*LRP1*); quantitative insulin sensitivity check index, rs184003 (*AGER*); sensitivity index, rs7301876 (*ABCC9*); acute insulin response to glucose, rs290481 (*TCF7L2*); and disposition index, rs12691 (*CEBPA*).

The *PPARγ-1C* rs26125 variable ranked as the top SNP influencing fasting glucose. Carriers of the rare A allele had lower glucose compared with the homozygotes for the common allele. The protein encoded by this gene is a key regulator of several transcription factors and NRs and is involved in metabolic processes such as nonoxidative glucose metabolism or regulation of energy expenditure (Handshin and Spiegelman, 2006; Franks et al., 2014). The SNP in the *LRP1* rs4759277 was the top SNP influencing three glucose metabolism variables, such as fasting insulin, C-peptide, and HOMA-IR. The LRP1 expression decreased in visceral fat of obese persons (Clemente-Postigo et al., 2011), and recent data suggest that LRP1 participates in the translocation of GLT4 glucose transporters from intracellular membranes to cell surface to internalize glucose (Bogan, 2012).

The *AGER* (advanced glycosylation end-products receptors) or *RAGE* gene SNP (rs184003) ranked as the top SNP influencing the quantitative insulin sensitivity check index (QUICKI). *AGER* has been implicated in several functions and has been linked to inflammation, oxidative stress, and endothelial dysfunction in T2DM (Delgado-Lista et al., 2014).

5.6.1 *CALPAIN10* GENE POLYMORPHISMS

Calpain10 (CAPN10) is an important molecule in β-cell and acts as a fuel sensor and determinant of insulin exocytosis, with actions at the mitochondria and plasma membrane, respectively. Genetic and functional data indicate that CAPN10 plays an important role in insulin resistance and intermediate phenotypes, including those associated with adipocytes (Saez et al., 2008). *CAPN10* gene is located at the long arm of the chromosome 2 (2q37) and encodes a ubiquitously expressed member of the calpain-like cysteine protease family. Some *CAPN10* SNPs act as a regulator of CAPN10 expression (Shaw et al., 2009).

The *CAPN10* gene has been associated with several components of MetS, such as elevated plasma cholesterol levels (Wu et al., 2005), hypertriacylglycerolemia (Carlsson et al., 2004), body mass index (Shima et al., 2003), and hypertension (Garant et al., 2002). The rs2953171 *CAPN10* genetic polymorphism influences insulin sensitivity by interacting with plasma SFA levels in MetS individuals (Perez-Martinez et al., 2011b). Subjects with low plasma SFA levels and carriers of the GG genotype presented lower fasting insulin concentrations and HOMA-IR and higher glucose effectiveness compared with those carrying the minor A allele (GA and AA genotypes). In contrast, the carriers of GG genotype with the highest levels of plasma SFA presented higher fasting insulin and HOMA-IR and lower glucose effectiveness, compared with those with the A allele.

5.6.2 *GLUCOKINASE REGULATORY PROTEIN* GENE POLYMORPHISMS

Glucokinase (GK), a key enzyme that regulates glucose homeostasis, converts glucose to glucose-6-phosphate in pancreatic β-cells, liver hepatocytes, specific hypothalamic neurons, and gut enterocytes. In hepatocytes, GK regulates glucose uptake and glycogen synthesis, suppresses glucose production, and is subject to the endogenous inhibitor GK regulatory protein (GKRP). During fasting, GKRP binds, inactivates, and sequesters GK in the nucleus, which removes GK from the gluconeogenic process and prevents a futile cycle of glucose phosphorylation. Compounds that directly hyperactivate GK (GK activators) lower blood glucose levels and are being clinically evaluated as potential therapeutics for the treatment of T2DM. In liver and pancreatic islet cells, GCKR acts as a glucose sensor responsible for glucose phosphorylation in the first step of glycolysis. The overexpression of GCKR in the liver of experimental model increased GK activity leading to the lowered blood glucose and increased triacylglycerol concentrations (O'Doherty et al., 1999).

The *GCKR* gene is located in the short arm of the chromosome 2 (2p23.3) and SNPs are associated with plasma triacylglycerols and insulin concentrations. The minor T allele of the rs780094 SNP, or rs1260326, a variant in high-linkage disequilibrium, was associated with decreased fasting glucose, increased serum triacylglycerols, and C-reactive protein levels (Orho-Melander et al., 2008; Perez-Martinez et al., 2009). Carriers of the CC genotype and with *n*-3 PUFAs levels below the population median presented higher fasting insulin concentrations, C-peptide levels, and HOMA-IR than those carrying the minor T allele. In contrast, carriers of the CC genotype with the highest levels of plasma *n*-3 PUFAs showed lower fasting insulin concentrations, C-peptide levels, and HOMA-IR, and C-reactive protein, compared to those with the T-allele (Perez-Martinez et al., 2011a). Therefore, the carriers of the GG genotype presented a better genetic profile associated with insulin resistance compared to those with other genotypes of the rs780094 SNP in the *GCKR*.

5.6.3 *UNCOUPLING PROTEIN 1* GENE POLYMORPHISMS

The *uncoupling protein 1* (*UCP1*) gene is located on chromosome 4 (4q28-q31) and presents six exons. This gene encodes the UCP1 that is exclusively expressed in mitochondria of brown adipocytes where it uncouples respiration from ATP synthesis, dissipating the proton gradient as heat. The UCP1 enzyme plays important roles in metabolic and energy balance and regulation, cold- and diet-induced thermogenesis, and in decreasing the reduction of reactive oxygen species (ROS) by mitochondria, important mechanisms associated with the pathogenesis of obesity and T2DM (Dalgaard and Pedersen, 2001; Azzu and Brand, 2010). For this reason, a number of genetic studies have been investigated the association between the *UCP1* genetic variants with obesity and T2DM. Particular attention was paid to -3826 A/G (rs1800592), -1766 A/G, and -112A/C polymorphisms in the promoter region of the *UCP1* gene. Other SNP evaluated are Ala64Thr in the exon 2 and Met299Leu SNP in the exon 5 of the *UCP1* gene. While some studies showed an association of one or more of these SNPs with obesity, T2DM, body fat accumulation, body mass index, or other characteristic of MetS, other studies failed to demonstrate these associations (see the review by Brondani et al., 2012).

The effects of the -3826 A/G (rs1800592) polymorphism are more evident. The -3826G allele has been associated with reduced *UCP1* mRNA expression in intraperitoneal adipose tissue of obese individuals (Esterbauer et al., 1998), with reduced HDL-C levels (Sale et al., 2007), increased triacylglycerols (Matsushita et al., 2003), LDL-C levels, and increased systolic and/or diastolic blood pressure (Oh et al., 2004). An association between the -3826G allele and T2DM, insulin resistance or increased insulin or glucose levels was also reported (Heilbronn et al., 2000). Moreover, the -3826A/-112A/Met229 UCP1 haplotype was associated with increased risk for T2DM in Indian individuals (Vimaleswaran et al., 2010).

5.6.4 *PHOSPHOENOLPYRUVATE CARBOXYKINASE* GENE POLYMORPHISMS

The cytosolic phosphoenolpyruvate carboxykinase (PEPCK-C) enzyme is the main control point for the regulation of gluconeogenesis. The cytosolic enzyme encoded by the *PCK1* gene, along with guanosine triphosphate (GTP), catalyzes the formation of phosphoenolpyruvate from oxaloacetate, with the release of carbon dioxide and guanosine diphosphate (GDP). The *PCK1* gene is located in the chromosome 20 and its normal expression is under hormonal control, regulated at the transcriptional level by both activators, such as glucagon, and inhibitors, such as insulin. The expression of the *PCK1* gene can also be regulated by glucocorticoids and diet. The *PCK1* gene plays a significant role regulating glucose metabolism, whereas fatty acids are also key metabolic regulators, which interact with transcription factors and influence glucose metabolism. For this reason, the *PCK1* is a potential candidate gene in the pathogenesis of T2DM. The -232C/G SNP (rs2071023) located at the promoter region of the *PCK1* has been associated with an increased risk of T2DM in ethnically different cohorts (Gouni-Berthold et al., 2006; Rees et al., 2009).

Perez-Martinez et al. (2012) demonstrated other example of gene–nutrient interaction associated with MetS. These authors investigated the rs2179706 SNP of the *PCK1* gene in relation to the degree of insulin resistance and plasma fatty acid levels in 443 individuals with MetS, participants in the LIPGENE cohort. These authors also analyzed the *PCK1* gene expression in the adipose tissue of a subgroup of MetS individuals according to the *PCK1* genetic variants. The results showed that rs2179706 SNP interacted with plasma concentration of *n*-3 PUFAs, which were significantly associated with plasma concentrations of fasting insulin, peptide C, and HOMA-IR. Among individuals with *n*-3 PUFAs levels above the population median, carriers of the CC genotype exhibited lower plasma concentrations of fasting insulin and HOMA-IR than those carrying the CC genotype with *n*-3 PUFAs below the median. The carriers of the CC genotype with *n*-3 PUFAs levels above the median showed lower plasma concentrations of peptide C compared to those with the variant T allele. Individuals carrying the variant T allele showed a lower gene *PCK1* expression when compared with those carrying the CC genotype. Taken together, these results demonstrated that the *PCK1* rs2179706 polymorphism interacts with plasma concentration of *n*-3 PUFAs levels modulating insulin resistance in individuals with MetS.

5.7   POLYMORPHISMS IN GENES ASSOCIATED WITH INFLAMMATION

Chronic low-grade inflammation plays a role in the pathogenesis of obesity and insulin resistance (Spranger et al., 2003; Hu et al., 2004), conditions associated with increased risk for MetS, diabetes and CVD. Moreover, the pro-inflammatory status has been considered a key for the pathophysiology of other MetS features. Several SNPs in genes of complement components and proinflammatory cytokines, including *tumor necrosis factor alpha* (*TNF*-α) and *interleukin 6* (*IL-6*), are associated with central obesity, diabetes, and MetS phenotypes (Dalziel et al., 2002; Hamid et al., 2005; Sookoian et al., 2005; Huth et al., 2006; Shen et al., 2008; Phillips et al., 2009).

5.7.1   Complement System Gene Polymorphisms

Complement component C3 (C3), a protein with a central role in the innate immune system, is a novel determinant of MetS. Elevated concentration of C3 has been associated with insulin resistance, diabetes, and MetS. On activation, C3 is converted to its components, including acylation-stimulating protein (ASP), a key player in nonesterified acid (NEFA) transport into adipocytes (Yasruel et al., 1991). C3 has also been positively associated with insulin resistance, obesity, fasting and postprandial triacylglycerol concentrations, hypertension, and CVD (Muscari et al., 2000; Halkes et al., 2001). A significant dose relation between C3 concentrations and the number of MetS components has been reported. After postprandial triacylglycerol, fasting C3 concentrations were the second most important determinant of MetS (van Oostrom et al., 2007).

Epidemiological studies report anti-inflammatory effects of dietary fish, fish oil, and/or long-chain *n*-3 PUFAs (LC *n*-3 PUFAs) intake (Madsen et al., 2001; Lopez-Garcia et al., 2004). However, the findings of intervention trials to confirm the functional effects of dietary PUFAs are mixed (Blok et al., 1997; Mayer-Davis et al., 1997; Lovejoy et al., 2002; Luu et al., 2007; Hartweg et al., 2008), a result that might be due to an interaction between an individual's genetic profile and dietary fat exposure, which affects the risk of MetS (Phillips et al., 2006; Szabo de Edelenyi et al., 2008). The postprandial C3 elevation is related to triacylglycerols and NEFA metabolism (Halkes et al., 2001), and chylomicrons are the strongest stimulators of adipocyte C3 production (Verseyden et al., 2003). PUFASs are ligands of the FXR, a NR that regulates *C3* gene expression (Li et al., 2005).

The potential relation between genetic variations of *C3* and MetS phenotype and whether interaction with PUFAs (a biomarker of dietary) modulates this relation was investigated (Phillips et al., 2009). This was the first case–control study to report association between *C3* polymorphisms and MetS risk and its phenotypes, including dyslipidemia, abdominal obesity, and insulin resistance.

Plasma PUFAs composition and status appeared to modulate these genetic influences. Two SNPs of *C3* gene were associated with MetS: rs11569562 GG homozygotes exhibited decreased MetS risk compared with minor A allele carriers (odds ratio 0.53; 95% confidence interval: 0.35–0.82, $p = 0.0009$), which was augmented by high plasma PUFAs status (odds ratio 0.32; 95% confidence interval: 0.11–0.93, $p = 0.04$). The GG homozygotes had lower C3 concentrations than those AA carriers and showed decreased risk of hypertryglyceridemia compared with A allele carriers, which was further ameliorated by an increase in *n*-3 PUFAs or a decrease in *n*-6 PUFAs. The AA homozygote carriers of the SNP rs2250656 had increased MetS risk relative to minor G allele carriers, which was exacerbated by low *n*-6 PUFAs status. The authors concluded that plasma PUFAs may modulate the susceptibility to MetS that is conferred by C3 polymorphisms, which suggests novel gene–nutrient interactions.

5.7.2 NITRIC OXIDE SYNTHASE GENE POLYMORPHISMS

Another gene–nutrient interaction has been demonstrated between *nitric oxide synthase* (*NOS3*) gene and plasma *n*-3 PUFAs status.

Nitric oxide (NO) is synthesized from the amino acid L-arginine by the enzyme NOS with the concomitant production of L-citrulline. At least three isoforms of NOS have been identified: two constitutive isoforms—neuronal NOS (nNOS) and endothelial NOS (eNOS)—and one inducible isoform (iNOS). NO maintains basal cerebral blood flow (White et al., 1998), reduces both platelet adhesion (Radomski et al., 1987) and aggregation (Radomski et al., 1990), and therefore may exert antithromboembolic effect (Samdani et al., 1997).

NOS3 is a key regulator of redox balance, which is essential in glucose metabolism. Moreover, is an essential enzyme for the regulation of vascular function and blood pressure. *NOS3* SNPs influence vascular reactivity in the set of metabolic stressors, such as an oral fat-load test (Delgado-Lista et al., 2011b), and influence triacylglycerol plasma concentrations (Ferguson et al., 2010a). NOS variants, by reducing the ability of NOS to donate nitric oxide to the cellular metabolic machinery, may impair the function of the β-cells (Delgado-Lista et al., 2014). Carriers of the minor allele for rs1799983 SNP showed higher plasma triacylglycerol concentrations in those with low plasma *n*-3 PUFAs status compared with homozygous individuals for the major allele. Those individuals had a better response to changes in plasma *n*-3 PUFAs after supplementation than major allele homozygotes (Ferguson et al., 2010a). This is of great importance given that those individuals might show greater beneficial effects of *n*-3 PUFAs consumption to reduce plasma triacylglycerol concentrations.

Resveratrol, a polyphenolic phytoalexin found in grapes and wine, has structural similarity to the synthetic estrogen diethylstilbestrol, and has been reported to act as an agonist at the estrogen receptor. Resveratrol can bind to and activate gene transcription by the estrogen receptor subtypes α and β, in estrogen-sensitive tissues and cell lines (Gehm et al., 1997; Henry and Witt, 2002). Resveratrol upregulated *eNOS* mRNA expression in a time- and concentration-dependent manner (up to 2.8-fold). Moreover, eNOS protein expression and eNOS-derived NO production were also increased after long-term incubation with resveratrol. Resveratrol increased the activity of the *eNOS* promoter (3.5 kb fragment) in a concentration-dependent fashion. Resveratrol also stabilized the *eNOS* mRNA. These results underscored the cardiovascular protective effects attributed to resveratrol by stimulating the eNOS expression and activity (Wallerath et al., 2002).

5.7.3 CYTOKINE AND ADIPOKINE GENE POLYMORPHISMS

5.7.3.1 *Tumor Necrosis Factor Alpha* and *Tumor Necrosis Factor Beta* Gene Polymorphisms

Most of the candidate genes that could influence the intensity of the inflammatory response are located on the highly polymorphic region of human chromosome 6, called major histocompatibility complex (MHC). These are genes involved with the antigen recognition pathways and in the expression of proinflammatory cytokines such as TNF-α and TNF-β, named also Lymphotoxin-α (LT-α) (Waterer and Wunderink, 2003).

TNF-α affects insulin signaling, lipid metabolism, adipocyte function (Cawthorn and Sethi, 2008), and plays a central role in various components of MetS (Moller, 2000). In addition, TNF-α acts as a modulator of gene expression in adipocytes and is implicated in the development of insulin resistance (Hotamisligil and Spiegelman, 1994; Jang et al., 2007; Plomgaard et al., 2007) by a variety of mechanisms, including inhibition of insulin receptor signaling, inhibition of glucose transport, and regulating lipid metabolism (Moller, 2000; Cawthorn and Sethi, 2008). TNF-α affects lipid metabolism by inhibiting free fatty acids uptake and lipogenesis and/or by enhancing intracellular lipolysis (Cawthorn and Sethi, 2008).

TNF-α and TNF-β are known to induce inflammation by activating NF-κB nuclear protein upon to biding to TNF receptor and are known to be expressed in atherosclerotic plaques (Bazzoni and Beutler, 1996; Naoum et al., 2006). TNF-α levels may be influenced by age, ethnicity, gender, BMI, circumference waist, and obesity (Hotamisligil et al., 1995; Kern et al., 1995; Olson et al., 2012).

The studies in *TNF* region are of particular interest because *TNF*-α and *TNF*-β genes are tandemly located next to each other within the human leukocyte antigen (HLA) class III genes on the short arm of human chromosome 6, and evolutionary studies suggest a common ancestor for both genes that duplicated during evolution (Zhang et al., 2003).

The interindividual variation in the capacity to produce TNF-α may be caused by differences in either transcription rate, the regulation of mRNA stability, translation efficiency or processing of the mature protein. Polymorphisms in the proteins that regulate this process may cause differences in TNF-α production. Different polymorphisms have been described in the promoter TNF-α gene, such as the SNP at position -308 (TNF-α -308G/A, rs1800629), which consists in a substitution of a G (TNF1 allele, more common) to an A (TNF2 allele, less common). The variant genotype was associated with higher constitutive and inducible levels of *TNF* gene transcription as compared to wild-type genotype (Huizinga et al., 1997).

This SNP has been associated with obesity, insulin resistance, and hypertension. The results of a meta-analysis to assess the association of the TNF-α -308 G/A polymorphism with the components of MetS indicate that individuals who carried the -308A *TNF*-α gene variant are at 23% risk of developing obesity compared with controls and showed significantly higher systolic arterial blood pressure and plasma insulin levels, supporting the hypothesis that the *TNF*-α gene is involved in the pathogenesis of MetS (Sookoian et al., 2005).

Gomez-Delgado et al. (2014) examined whether the consumption of a Mediterranean diet (MedDiet), compared with a low-fat diet, interacts with two SNPs at the *TNF*-α gene (rs1800629, rs1799964) in order to improve triacylglycerols, glycemic control, and inflammation markers. Genotyping, biochemical measurements, dietary intervention, and oral fat load test meal were determined in 507 individuals with MetS. At baseline, 408 carriers of the GG genotype at the rs1800629 SNP showed higher fasting and postprandial triacylglycerols, and high sensitivity C-reactive protein (hsCRP) levels than 99 carriers of the minor A allele, (GA + AA genotypes). After 12 months of MedDiet, baseline differences between genotypes disappeared. The decrease in triacylglycerols and hsCRP was statistically significant in 203 carriers of the GG genotype compared with 48 carriers of the minor A allele. The authors suggested that the rs1800629 at the *TNF*-α gene interacts with MedDiet to influence triacylglycerol metabolism and inflammation status in MetS individuals. These results underscore that a better understanding of the role of gene–diet interactions may be the best strategy for personalized treatment of patients with MetS.

TNF-β is a cytokine produced by T lymphocytes similar to TNF-α and binds to TNF receptors. It is also expressed as a membrane protein, activates endothelial cells and neutrophils, and is thus a mediator of the acute inflammatory response, providing a link between T cell activation and inflammation. These biological effects of TNF-β are the same as those of TNF-α, consistent with their binding to the same receptors. However, because the quantity is much less than the amounts of TNF-α, TNF-β is not readily detected in the circulation. Therefore, TNF-β is usually a locally cytokine and not a mediator of systemic injury (Eigler et al., 1997).

The exon 3 variant of the *TNF-β* gene leads to the substitution at the amino acid position 26 (aspartato to threonine) and correlates with a reduced level of TNF-β production (Messer et al., 1991). The combination of these allelic forms may lead to the different levels of cytokine production in response to various physiological and pathological stimuli and in turn might result in a predisposition to the development of MetS.

An SNP located at position +252 in the first intron of the *TNF-β*, named *Nco*I polymorphism (A252G, rs909253), consists of a G in the allele TNFB1 (allele G) and of an A in the allele TNFB2 (allele A) (Messer et al., 1991). This polymorphism is potentially an influential locus in many inflammatory conditions. The occurrence of the allelic forms of *TNF-β* could undergo intrachromosomal interactions that take place in close proximity to the *TNF-α* promoter in a configuration that potentially underlies selective activation of the *TNF-α* gene (Tsytsykova et al., 2007).

Some of the metabolic markers, such as TC and LDL-cholesterol, were associated with the *TNF-βNco*I polymorphism. An association between the *TNFB2* allele with hyperinsulinemia may contribute to the development of MetS in patients with CAD (Braun et al., 1998). Studies demonstrated an involvement of *TNF-βNco*I polymorphism influencing the levels of VLDL-C and triacylglycerols (Kanková et al., 2002; Asselbergs et al., 2007).

The TNFB2/B2 genotype of the *TNF-βNco*I polymorphism was associated with features of MetS, such as hyperinsulinemia, dyslipidemia, small LDL-C particle, and low adiponectin levels in CAD patients (Jang et al., 2007). The results suggest that the *TNF-βNco*I polymorphism could be already involved in genetic modulation of glucose and lipid homeostasis and regulation of insulin sensitivity in healthy subjects.

The association of the *TNF-βNco*I polymorphism with glucose homeostasis could be probably explained through the proposed effect of this polymorphism on TNF-α or eventually TNF-β levels (Pociot et al., 1993; Wishelow et al., 1996). Kanková et al. (2002) also reported a possible involvement of *TNF-βNco*I polymorphism in the regulation of glucose and lipid homeostasis genetic modulation, and regulation of insulin sensitivity in healthy subjects. The disturbance of this regulation could be a component of several pathogenesis. Japanese men with MetS carrying the TNFB2 variant homozygous genotype significantly presented lower insulin resistance than those carrying the wild-type allele (Hayakawa et al., 2000). A case report showed a Japanese man with diabetes mellitus who developed multiple sclerosis, with markedly decreased secretion of insulin with time. It is possible that changes in immune conditions after the destruction of pancreatic islets or hyperglycemia triggers the onset of multiple sclerosis in men (Katsuki et al., 1998). In contrast, Jang et al. (2007) showed that men with CAD carrying TNFB2/B2 genotype presented increased insulin and HOMA-IR than the other genotypes, showing an association of TNF-β *Nco*I polymorphism and insulin resistance.

5.7.3.2   *IL-6 Gene Polymorphisms*

IL-6 is a major proinflammatory cytokine expressed in several tissues and cell types, including leukocytes, and endothelial and muscle cells. This cytokine can act on many cell types, and like interleukin 1 (IL-1), plays an important role in the systemic inflammatory response. IL-6 plays a key role in the promotion of acute inflammatory response and in the regulation of the production of the acute-phase proteins, such as C-reactive protein (Heinrich et al., 1990), in the activation of endothelial cells (Romano et al., 1997), and in the stimulation of synthesis of fibrinogen and von Willebrand factor. These events result in hypercoagulability status and is likely important in the pathogenesis of vascular inflammation (Yamada et al., 2006).

The *IL-6* gene is located in the short arm of chromosome 7 and the most common SNP is located in its 5′ flanking region (Fishman et al., 1998). The functioning of this gene is implicated in a wide variety of inflammation-associated disease states, including susceptibility to T2DM and glucose disorders (Festa et al., 2001). Both circulating levels of IL-6 and adipose tissue IL-6 content have been correlated with insulin resistance (Bastard et al., 2002) and high IL-6 plasma levels have been found to predict the development of T2DM (Pradhan et al., 2001). The change from G to C at position 174 in the promoter of the *IL-6* gene (-174 G/C SNP) creates a potential site for the transcriptional factor NF-1, considered a repressor of gene expression. The C allele has been associated with reduced gene expression and reduced plasma levels of IL-6 (Fishman et al., 1998; Cardellini et al., 2005). However, the results are conflicting. While some studies demonstrated that individuals with the GG genotype presented higher IL-6 circulation levels under basal condition and in response to inflammatory stimuli (Fishman et al., 1998), other studies failed to demonstrate this effect (Kubaszek et al., 2003).

This -174C/G SNP was also associated with obesity and other comorbidities, such as insulin resistance, MetS, and T2DM (Möhlig et al., 2004; Goyenechea et al., 2007; Stephens et al., 2007). Similarly, the effect of the -174 G/C SNP on insulin resistance and T2DM is conflicting. In a Spanish population, the C/C genotype was associated to increased insulin sensitivity (Fernandez-Real et al., 2000), whereas in a Finnish population subjects carrying the C/C genotype showed lower insulin sensitivity (Kubaszek et al., 2003). Two studies have shown that the G/G genotype was associated with T2DM in Spanish individuals and Pima Indians and in a German Caucasian population (Vozarova et al., 2003; Illig et al., 2004), whereas another study reported that obese German individuals carrying the C/C genotype have increased risk of developing T2DM (Möhlig et al., 2004).

The *IL-6* -174 G/C SNP was also evaluated in two cohorts of individuals, including 275 nondiabetic subjects who underwent a euglycemic-hyperinsulinemic clamp (cohort 1) and 77 patients with morbid obesity who underwent laparoscopic adjustable gastric banding (cohort 2) (Cardellini et al., 2005). In cohort 1, carriers of the -174G/G genotype showed lower insulin sensitivity and higher plasma IL-6 levels in comparison with carriers of the C allele. The -174G/C SNP was independently associated with insulin sensitivity; however, after inclusion of plasma IL-6 concentrations, the polymorphism was excluded from the model explaining insulin sensitivity variability, thus suggesting that the polymorphism was affecting insulin sensitivity by regulating IL-6 plasma levels. Carriers of -174G/G genotype showed increased IL-6 expression compared with subjects carrying the C allele and a significant correlation between adipose *IL-6* mRNA expression and insulin resistance assessed by HOMA-IR was also observed in cohort 2. These results indicate that the -174G/G genotype of the *IL-6* gene may contribute to variations in insulin sensitivity.

The impact of *IL-6* -174 G/C SNP on obesity-related metabolic disorders was evaluated in individuals with excess in body weight (Goyenechea et al., 2007). Subjects carrying the C allele showed higher plasma insulin concentrations and systolic blood pressure than homozygotes for the G allele. A multiple regression analysis showed that the presence of the C allele induced an increase in the HOMA-IR compared with GG subjects. Analyzing the mentioned obesity-related diseases, an enhanced prevalence of presenting high risk of developing these complications was found for the GC and CC genotypes relative to GG, demonstrating that the occurrence of C allele of IL-6 -174 G/C SNP in individuals with excessive body weight is accompanying a higher risk of developing obesity-related metabolic disorders, especially insulin resistance.

The effect of polyphenol-rich cloudy apple juice (CloA) consumption on plasma parameters related to the obesity phenotype and potential effects of interactions between CloA and allelic variants in obesity candidate genes were assessed in obese men (Barth et al., 2012). In a controlled, randomized, and parallel study, 68 non-smoking, nondiabetic men with a body mass index ≥27 kg/m^2) received 750 mL/day CloA (802.5 mg polyphenols) or 750 mL/day control beverage (CB, isocaloric equivalent to CloA) for 4 weeks. Further, study participants were genotyped for SNPs in *PPARγ* (rs1801282), *UCP3* (rs1800849), *IL-6* (rs1800795), *FABP2* (rs1799883), *INSIG2* (rs7566605), and *PGC1* (rs8192678) genes. At the beginning and at the end of intervention, plasma lipids, distinct adipokines and cytokines, as well as anthropometric parameters were determined. The results showed that CloA compared to CB had no significant effect on plasma lipids, plasma adipokine and cytokine levels, body mass index, and waist circumference. However, CloA consumption significantly reduced percent body fat compared to CB. The *IL-6–174* G/C polymorphism showed an interaction with body fat reduction induced by CloA. Solely in carriers of the C/C genotype, but not in G/C or G/G carriers, a significant reduction in body fat after 4 weeks of CloA intervention was detectable. All together, the results indicate that the observed diet–gene interaction might be a first indication for the impact of individual genetic background on CloA-mediated bioactivity on obesity-associated comorbidities.

5.7.3.3 *Adiponectin* Gene Polymorphisms

Adiponectin (ADIPOQ) is the most quantitatively abundant adipokine secreted by adipocytes (Scherer et al., 1995) and sensitizes the body to insulin (Berg et al., 2001; Yamauchi et al., 2002). Concentrations of circulating adiponectin are reduced in obese and T2DM subjects (Arita et al., 1999). Hypoadiponectinemia, caused by interactions of genetic and environmental factors, seems to play an important causal role in insulin resistance, T2DM, and MetS (Weyer et al., 2001; Tschritter et al., 2003; Ryo et al., 2004). It is proposed that this hormone is a key player in the etiology of MetS because it may be an important regulator of insulin sensitivity and inflammation. Functional studies in animal models have shown that adiponectin attenuates insulin resistance by reducing the triacylglycerol content in muscle and liver (Yamauchi et al., 2001).

Several SNPs of the *adiponectin* gene (*ADIPOQ*) gene have been associated with metabolic phenotypes. The *ADIPOQ* is located on the long arm of the chromosome 3 (3q27), which has been reported to be linked to T2DM and MetS (Vasseur et al., 2002). In humans, associations have been found between many genetic polymorphisms in *ADIPOQ*, *ADIPOR1*, and *ADIPOR2* and adiponectin levels, insulin resistance, and MetS phenotypes (Menzaghi et al., 2007; Sheng and Yang, 2008). Polymorphisms in the *ADIPOQ* gene and its receptors, *ADIPOR1* and *ADIPOR2*, may play a role in the pathogenesis and progression of MetS (Vasseur et al., 2006). Moreover, gene–environmental interactions, such as with dietary compounds, may be important in modulating the susceptibility to the development of MetS traits. However, inconsistent results have been reported with the associations of polymorphisms in these genes and metabolic measures that could be due to environmental interactions, particularly dietary factors. Gene–nutrient interactions can modulate the effect of certain polymorphisms in MetS-related trait (Luan et al., 2001). One study conducted in obese females found that there was an interaction between the rs266729 polymorphism of *ADIPOQ* and the percentage of dietary-derived energy from fat with the development of obesity (Santos et al., 2006).

Gene–nutrient interactions were examined in MetS subjects to determine interactions between SNPs in the *ADIPOQ* and its receptors (*ADIPOR2* and *ADIPOR2*) and plasma fatty acid composition and their effects on MetS characteristics (Ferguson et al., 2010b). This dietary intervention study was carried out in 1754 subjects recruited from the LIPGENE. A combination of SNPs previously mentioned in the literature were genotyped, revealing 11 SNPs in three genes: *ADIPOQ* (rs266729, rs822395, rs17366569, rs2241766, and rs1063538), *ADIPOR1* (rs2275737, rs10753929, and rs10920533), and *ADIPOR2* (rs6489323, rs1058322, and rs10848571). Only two SNPs (rs266729 and rs10920533) showed a number of interesting significant associations.

Triacylglycerols, nonesterified fatty acids (NEFA), and waist circumference were significantly different between the genotypes for *ADIPOQ* rs266729 and *ADIPOR1* rs109220533. Minor allele homozygotes for both of these SNPs were identified as having degrees of insulin resistance, as measured by the HOMA-IR, that were highly responsive to differences in plasma SFAs. The SFA-dependent association between *ADIPOR1* rs10920533 and insulin resistance was replicated in cases with MetS.

Two SNPs in genes encoding ADIPOQ (rs266729) and its receptor ADIPOR1 (rs10920533) interact with plasma SFAs to alter insulin sensitivity as measured by HOMA-IR. A reduction in plasma SFAs could be expected to lower insulin resistance in MetS subjects who are minor allele carriers of rs266729 in *ADIPOQ* and rs10920533 in *ADIPOR1*. The genotype at these polymorphisms may play a role in the responsiveness to dietary fatty acid modification and personalized dietary advice to decrease SFA consumption in MetS individuals may be recommended as a possible therapeutic measure to improve insulin sensitivity (Ferguson et al., 2010b).

Goyenechea et al. (2009) investigated whether the *ADIPOQ* gene promoter variant -11391 G/A (rs17300539) could predict the risk of developing traits characterizing MetS and the impact of weight management. The -11391 G/A SNP was genotyped in 180 Spanish volunteers (body mass index of 31.4 ± 3.2 kg/m^2 and with age 35 ± 5 years). Clinical measurements were determined at baseline, following an 8-week low-calorie diet (LCD), and at 32 and 60 weeks. At baseline, the GG genotype was associated with higher HOMA-IR, insulin and triacylglycerol concentrations than other genotypes and was also related with a higher risk of insulin resistance and MetS clinical manifestations. Following the LCD, the increased risk in GG subjects compared with others disappeared. By 32 weeks after dietary therapy (*n* = 84), GG carriers had recovered the risk of metabolic comorbidities and this risk was even more evident after 60 weeks. Altogether, these data show an increased risk of insulin resistance and MetS complications in obese subjects carrying the -11391 GG genotype and the risk was markedly reduced during an energy-restricted diet, but was not sustained. Therefore, carriage of the A allele confers protection from weight regain, and the effect is particularly evident 32–60 weeks after the dietary intervention, when improvement in GG subjects had disappeared.

5.7.4 Gene–Nutrient Interactions in Inflammatory Response

Total plasma PUFA/SFA levels modified the observed additive effects of *IL-6*, *TNF-α*, and *TNF-β* genes (Phillips et al., 2010). When stratified according to median plasma PUFA/SFA levels, MetS risk was fourfold higher in the 3 SNPs risk genotype carriers with the lowest PUFA/SFA levels compared to noncarriers and was thought to be driven by the SFA content, with high SFA levels alone accounting for fivefold increased MetS risk. A low PUFA/SFA ratio also exacerbated their increased risk for several phenotypes such as abdominal obesity, fasting hypertriacylglycerolemia, hypertension, and pro-inflammatory profile. When the risk genotype carriers with the lowest PUFA/SFA levels were compared with their risk genotype carriers with the highest PUFA/SFA levels significant improvements to their metabolic profile were observed. A high PUFA/SFA ratio attenuated genetic predisposition to MetS risk. Risk genotype carriers with the highest PUFA/SFA levels had reduced pro-inflammatory status, lower triacylglycerol levels and HOMA-IR values than risk genotype carriers with the lowest PUFA/SFA levels. Taken together, these results support current guidelines to reduce dietary SFA intake and increase PUFAs consumption.

Phillips et al. (2010) determined the relationship between *TNF-α* rs1800629, *TNF-β* rs915654, and *IL-6* rs1800797 gene polymorphisms with MetS risk and investigated whether plasma fatty acid composition, a biomarker of dietary fat intake, modulated these associations. The study included 1754 individuals from LIPGENE-SU.VI.MAX study of MetS and matched controls. The results showed that *TNF-β* rs915654 minor A allele carriers and *TNF-α* rs1800629 major G allele homozygotes exhibited increased MetS risk compared with those carrying the TT homozygotes and A allele carriers, respectively. The possession of the *IL-6* rs1800797 GG genotype by the *TNF-β* and *TNF-α* risk genotype carriers further increased the risk of MetS, fasting hyperglycemia, high systolic blood pressure, and abdominal obesity. Plasma PUFA to saturated fat ratio exacerbated these effects; subjects in the lowest 50th percentile exhibited even greater risk of MetS, fasting hyperglycemia, high systolic blood pressure, and abdominal obesity. Taken together, the results underscore that *TNF-α* rs1800629, *TNF-β* rs915654, and *IL-6* rs1800797 genotype interactions increased MetS risk, which was further exacerbated by low plasma PUFA to saturated fat exposure, indicating important modulation of genetic risk by dietary fat exposure.

5.7.5 Gene–Flavonoids Interactions in Inflammatory Response

Flavonoids are plant secondary metabolites that are ubiquitous in fruits, vegetables, nuts, seeds, and plants and have been demonstrated to exhibit a broad spectrum of biological activities for human health, including anti-inflammatory properties. Numerous studies have proposed that flavonoids act through a variety of mechanism to prevent and attenuate inflammatory response. A robust review summarizes the most important effects of the flavonoids compounds and the interaction with genes to modulate their expression (Pan et al., 2010) (Figure 5.5).

Among the 2000 polyphenolic compounds, more attention have been paid to the apigenin (flavonoid present in parsley and celery), which is found to inhibit hypoxia-inducible factor 1-alpha (HIF-1α) protein and the vascular endothelial growth factor (VEGF) expression, a signal protein produced by cells that stimulates vasculogenesis and angiogenesis. These effects of apigenin occur by blocking the phosphatidylinositol 3′-kinase (PI3K)-Akt signaling pathway or lipopolysaccharide (LPS)-induced pro-inflammatory cytokines expression by inactivating the NF-κB through the suppression of p65 phosphorylation (Pan et al., 2009). Luteolin is prevalent in thyme and also beets, brussels sprouts, cabbage, and cauliflower and is shown to have great antioxidant activity. Luteolin was found to regulate Mitogen-Activated Protein Kinase (MAPK) pathway and NF-κB signaling that inhibits TNF-α-induced IL-8 production, which is an important inflammatory cytokine (Pan et al., 2010). Luteolin also decreases *TNF-α*, *IL-1*, and *MCP-1* genes expression and increases adiponectin and leptin levels through the enhancement of transcriptional activity of PPARγ in 3T3-L1 adipocytes that might improve obesity-driven insulin resistance (Ding et al., 2010).

Genistein, the major isoflavone abundantly present in soybeans, exerts important anti-inflammatory functions. The treatment with genistein inhibited TNF-α-induced cell adhesion molecules expression, such as CD62E and CD106, and subsequent monocyte adhesion in human endothelial cells; decreased the interaction between monocytes and endothelial cells through the activation of PPARγ that inhibits the monocyte adhesion in culture cells and animal models; inhibited LPS-induced MCP-1 secretion from macrophages and contributed to reduced monocyte migration; inhibited LPS-induced expression of iNOS and nitrotyrosine protein in vascular tissue that prevents hypertension and vascular alterations; inhibited production of proinflammatory molecules such as NO, IL-1β, TNF-α, MCP-1; and increased ADIPOQ levels. All these results indicate that genistein could regulate the inflammatory conditions and improve metabolic parameters (Pan et al., 2010).

Citrus peel is a rich source of polymethoxyflavones, such as tangeretin and nobiletin, and exhibits a broad spectrum of biological activities, such as suppression of IL-1β-induced COX-2 expression through inhibiting activation of MAPK and Akt pathways (Pan et al., 2009). Two new flavones isolated from *Cirsium japonicum* DC pectolinarin and 5,7-dihydroxy-6,4′-dimethoxyflavone were found to reduce high-carbohydrates/high-fat diet-induced diabetes in rat through decreasing plasma glucose and increasing adiponectin levels that may improve glucose and lipid homeostasis (Liao et al., 2010).

The potential for resveratrol to modulate gene expression has been previously reported (Jones et al., 2005). Resveratrol has been shown to bind to and to activate gene transcription by the estrogen receptor subtypes α- and β estrogen-sensitive tissue and cell lines (Wallerath et al., 2002). It is conceivable that changes in gene regulation by this compound contribute to its biological effects. Reports indicate that resveratrol interferes with the MAPK and protein kinase C (PKC) pathways and the signal transducer and activator of transcription 3 (STAT3) signaling. STAT3 is a cytoplasmic protein important for promoting the proliferation, survival, and other biological processes triggered by cytokines and growth factors. An uncontrolled proliferation or failure to undergo cell death is involved in pathogenesis and progression of many human diseases, including CVD. This polyphenol exerts its effect by inhibiting the STAT3 protein and Janus Kinase 2 (JAK2) phosphorylation in several cell lines, repressing Stat3-regulated Bcl-6, and the lacking of the nuclear translocation of the protein inhibitor of activated STAT3 (PIAS). All these effects result in an induction of apoptosis, regulating the uncontrolled proliferation (Kotha et al., 2006) (Figure 5.5).

Green tea has attracted attention for its health benefits due to the catechin compounds, including epigallocatechin-3-gallate (EGCG), epigallocatechin (EGC), epicatechin-3-gallate (ECG), and epicatechin (EC). The potential of green tea in iron-chelating, radical-scavenging, anti-inflammatory and brain-permeable activities increased the consumption of this popular beverage worldwide to prevent cardiovascular, chronic and neurodegenerative diseases (Weinreb et al., 2004; Babu and Liu, 2008). Among the several health benefits, the EGCG has excellent activity against obesity-associated pathogenesis and metabolic disorders. In high fat-diet–induced obesity in animal models, supplementation with dietary EGCG reduced body weight gain and body fat, plasma cholesterol and MCP-1 levels, and decreased lipid accumulation in hepatocytes as well as attenuated insulin resistance (Bose et al., 2008).

5.8 PROBLEMS AND LIMITATIONS OF THE GENETIC ASSOCIATION STUDIES

Genetic variations in populations confound molecular epidemiology studies that seek to analyze gene–disease or nutrient–gene associations. A limited number of results is replicated more than three times (Hirschhorn et al., 2002). Similarly, nonreplicated results associating diet with candidate gene variants are the norm (Loktionov et al., 2000; Loktionov, 2003; Ordovas and Corella, 2004). In addition to population stratification and genetic heterogeneity, other confounders include sample sizes lacking statistical power, inappropriately matched controls, over interpretation of data (Lander and Krunglyak, 1995; Cardon and Bell, 2001), and the influence of other environmental factors. Although there has been a number of GWAS related to nutrigenetics using smaller number of subjects, large-scale dietary intervention studies that demonstrate positive modification of biomarkers in groups with genetic polypmorphisms have been limited. This is understandable considering the cost, management, and significant occurrence of noncompliance problems due to differences in personal dietary habits and cultural factors (Subbiah, 2008).

Although DNA microarray technology is a powerful technique for monitoring changes in gene expression on a global scale in different systems, these assays are complex, and multistep procedures in different laboratories have developed a variety of protocols (Garosi et al., 2005). This approach is associated with a number of technical challenges and potential pitfalls. Firstly, the cost of microarrays continues to drop but is still comparatively high. Secondly, the technical variations between array platforms and analytical procedures that almost inevitably lead to differences in the transcriptional responses observed. Consequently, conflicting data may be produced, important effects may be missed and/or false leads generated. Thirdly, even though production capabilities and the use of microarrays are becoming increasingly well established and widespread, variation still arises due to the overall complexity of the experimental approach. Significant differences exist with regard to fabrication techniques and user protocols. Such differences make the comparison of results across platforms very difficult. All parts of the protocol, such as array production, RNA extraction, cDNA labeling and hybridization, and data analysis techniques, include a multitude of parameters that need to be optimized to reach stable experimental results (Garosi et al., 2005).

A great limitation of the results obtained in experimental studies is the occurrence of the gene–gene interactions, named epistasis that may also alter association of SNP or set of SNP with disease processes. Other problem is the limited understanding of what constitutes an optimal response because we lack key health and disease biomarkers and signatures. At the same time, issues relating to consumer acceptance, privacy protection as well as marketing and distribution of personalized products need to be addressed before personalized nutrition can become commercially viable (De Roos, 2012).

5.9 FUTURE PERSPECTIVES

The nutrition science has been benefited from the concepts of nutrigenetics and nutrigenomics. The nutrigenomics approaches are expected to provide short and long-term advantages to human health in several ways, such as delivering biomarkers for health, delivering early biomarkers for nutrition-related disease disposition, identifying genes and molecular pathways as target for prevention, differentiating dietary responders from nonresponders, and discovering bioactive food components.

The development of functional foods will contribute to the improvement of the quality and benefits of the nutrition for the prevention of multifactorial diseases. Therefore, an interaction between disciplines is required, such as nutrition, biochemistry, immunology, endocrinology, diseases pathogenesis, genetics, molecular epidemiology, molecular biology, and bioinformatics to provide the approaches and an increased understanding of these issues. In addition, better overview of the early phases of the diet-related disease process and the development of potential therapeutic agents by designing new molecules are expected.

The next-generation methods in transcriptomics, proteomics, and metabolomics will continue to improve technically the studies of nutrigenetics and nutrigenomics. These methods have created opportunities for increasing the understanding about the biochemical, molecular, and cellular mechanisms that underlies the beneficial or adverse effects of certain bioactive food compounds. Moreover, these methods will contribute to the identification of genes that are involved in the previous stage of the onset of the disease, therefore, contributing to the identification of molecular biomarkers and the effects of bioactive food compounds on key molecular pathways (Garcia-Cañas et al., 2010).

All individuals do not respond equally or similarly to bioactive components, and interactions at the genetic levels result in variability of response and benefits. Therefore, further research is required to determine the optimal micronutrient combinations and the doses that are required for intervention taking into account the genetic profile of an individual or of groups, based on sex, ethnicity, or specific metabolic imbalance. With this approach, the prescription of personalized diet for health promoting or disease preventing becomes true.

We hope that the availability of high-throughput analytical techniques in clinical laboratories, which can run hundred of SNPs in a day, might eventually lower cost and turnaround times, making possible the research of the metabolic profiling (metabolomics), which can identify variation at the cellular level from a simple peripheral blood sample of individuals with metabolic chronic diseases.

REFERENCES

Abete I, Navas-Carretero S, Marti A, Martinez JA. 2012. Nutrigenetics and nutrigenomics of caloric restriction. *Prog Mol Biol Transl Sci* 108: 323–346.

Abifadel M, Varret M, Rabès J-P et al. 2003. Mutations in PCSK9 cause autosomal dominant hypercholesterolemia. *Nat Genet* 34: 154–156.

Ambros V. 2004. The functions of animal microRNAs. *Nature* 431: 350–355.

Andreasen CH, Andersen G. 2009. Gene–environment interactions and obesity. Further aspects of genome wide association studies. *Nutrition* 25: 998–1003.

Angelon LB, Quinet EM, Gillete TG, Drayna DT, Brown ML, Tall AR. 1990. Organization of the human cholesterylester transfer protein gene. *Biochemistry* 29: 1372–1376.

Arita Y, Kihara S, Ouchi N et al. 1999. Paradoxical decrease of an adipose-specific protein, adiponectin in obesity. *Biochem Biophys Res Commun* 257: 79–83.

Asselbergs FW, Pai JK, Rexrode KM, Hunter DJ, Rim ER. 2007. Effects of Lymphotoxin-α gene and galectin 02 gene polymorphisms on inflammatory biomarkers, cellular adhesion molecules and risk of coronary heart disease. *Clin Sci* 112: 291–298.

Avogaro P, Bon GB, Cazzolato G, Rorai E. 1980. Relationship between apolipoproteins and chemical components of lipoproteins in survivors of myocardial infarction. *Atherosclerosis* 37: 69–76.

Azzu V, Brand MD. 2010. The on–off switches of the mitochondrial uncoupling proteins. *Trends Biochem Sci* 37: 1513–1522.

Babu PV, Liu D. 2008. Green tea catechins and cardiovascular health: An update. *Curr Med Chem* 15: 1840–1850.

Barroso I, Gurnell M, Crowley VE et al. 1999. Dominant negative mutations in human PPAR gamma associated with severe insulin resistance, diabetes mellitus and hypertension. *Nature* 402: 880–883.

Bartel DP. 2009. MicroRNAs: Target recognition and regulatory functions. *Cell* 136: 215–233.

Barter PJ. 2002. Hugh Sinclair Lecture: The regulation and remodeling of HDL by plasma factors. *Atherosclerosis Suppl* 3: 39–47.

Barth SW, Koch TC, Watzl B, Dietrich H, Will F, Bub A. 2012. Moderate effects of apple juice consumption on obesity-related markers in obese men: Impact of diet–gene interaction on body fat content. *Eur J Nutr* 51: 841–850.

Baselga-Escudero L, Blade C, Ribas-Latre A et al. 2014. Resveratrol and EGCG bind directly and distinctively to miR-33a and miR-122 and modulate divergently their levels in hepatic cells. *Nucleic Acids Res* 42: 882–892.

Bastard JP, Maachi M, Tran Van Nhieu J et al. 2002. Adipose tissue IL-6 content correlates with resistance to insulin activation of glucose uptake both in vivo and *in vitro*. *J Clin Endocrinol Metab* 87: 2084–2089.

Bazzoni F, Beutler B. 1996. Tumor necrosis factor ligand and receptor families. *N Engl J Med* 334: 1717–1725.

Bellia A, Giardina E, Lauro D et al. 2009. "The linosa study": Epidemiological and heritability data of the metabolic syndrome in a Caucasian genetic isolate. *Nutr Metab Cardiovasc Dis* 19: 455–461.

Benjannet S, Rhainds D, Essalmani R et al. 2004. NARC-1/PCSK9 and its natural mutants: Zymogen cleavage and effects on the low-density lipoprotein (LDL) receptor and LDL cholesterol. *J Biol Chem* 279: 48865–48875.

Berg AH, Combs TP, Du X, Brownlee M, Scherer PE. 2001. The adipocyte-secreted protein Acrp30 enhances hepatic insulin action. *Nat Med* 7: 947–953.

Berg K. 1986. DNA polymorphism at the apolipoprotein B locus is associated with lipoprotein level. *Clin Genet* 30: 515–520.

Billings LK, Florez JC. 2010. The genetics of type 2 diabetes: What have we learned from GWAS? *Ann N Y Acad Sci* 1212: 59–77.

Blok WL, Deslypere JP, Demacker PN et al. 1997. Pro- and anti-inflammatory cytokines in healthy volunteers fed various doses of fish oil for 1 year. *Eur J Clin Invest* 27: 1003–1008.

Bohn M, Bakken A, Erikssen J, Berg K. 1994. The apolipoprotein B signal peptide insertion/deletion polymorphism is not associated with myocardial infarction in Norway. *Clin Genet* 45: 255–259.

Bogan JS. 2012. Regulation of glucose transporter translocation in health and diabetes. *Annu Rev Biochem* 81: 507–532.

Bose M, Lambert JD, Ju J, Reuhl KR, Shapses SA, Yang CS. 2008. The major green tea polyphenol, (−)-epigallocatechin-3-gallate, inhibits obesity, metabolic syndrome, and fatty liver disease in high-fat-fed mice. *J Nutr* 138: 1677–1683.

Braun J, März W, Winkelmann BR, Donner H, Henning U sadel K, Badenhoop K. 1998. Tumour necrosis factor beta alleles and hyperinsulinaemia in coronary artery disease. *Eur J Clin Invest* 28: 538–542.

Brondani LA, Assmann TS, Duarte GCK, Gross JL, Canani LH, Crispim D. 2012. The role of uncoupling protein 1 (UCP1) on the development of obesity and type 2 diabetes mellitus. *Arq Bras Endocrinol Metab* 56: 215–225.

Brown MS, Goldstein JL. 1986. A receptor-mediated pathway for cholesterol homeostasis. *Science* 232: 34–47.

Callen DF, Hildebrand CE, Reeders S. 1992. Report of the second international workshop on human chromosome 16 mapping. *Cytogenet Cell Genet* 60: 158–167.

Cardellini M, Perego L, D'Adamo M et al. 2005. C-174G polymorphism in the promoter of the interleukin-6 gene is associated with insulin resistance. *Diabetes Care* 28: 2007–2012.

Cardon LR, Bell JI. 2001. Association study designs for complex diseases. *Nat Rev Genet* 2: 91–99.

Carlsson E, Fredriksson J, Groop L, Ridderstrale M. 2004. Variation in the calpain-10 gene is associated with elevated triglyceride levels and reduced adipose tissue messenger ribonucleic acid expression in obese Swedish subjects. *J Clin Endocrinol Metab* 89: 3601–3605.

Cawthorn WP, Sethi JK. 2008. TNFα and adipocyte biology. *FEBS Lett* 582: 117–131.

Chaves FJ, Puig O, García-Sogo M et al. 1996. Seven DNA polymorphisms in the LDL receptor gene: Application to the study of familial hypercholesterolemia in Spain. *Clin Genet* 50: 28–35.

Chawla A, Lee CH, Barak Y et al. 2003. PPAR delta is a very low-density lipoprotein sensor in macrophages. *Proc Natl Acad Sci USA* 100: 1268–1273.

Chagnon YC, WEilmore JH, Borecki LB et al. 2000. Associations between the leptin receptor gene and adiposity in middle ages Caucasian males from the HERITAGE family study. *J Clin Endocrinol Metab* 85: 29–34.

Clemente-Postigo M, Queipo-Ortuno MI, Fernandez-Garcia D, Gomez-Huelgas R, Tinahones FJ, Cardona F. 2011. Adipose tissue gene expression of factors related to lipid processing in obesity. *PLoS One* 6: e24783.

Collins FS, Brooks LD, Chakravarti A. 1998. A DNA polymorphism discovery resource for research on human genetic variation. *Genome Res* 8: 1229–1231.

Dalgaard LT, Pedersen O. 2001. Uncopling proteins: Functional characteristics and role in the pathogenesis of obesity and type II diabetes. *Diabetologia* 44: 946–965.

Dalziel B, Gosby AK, Richman RM, Bryson JM, Caterson ID. 2002. Association of the TNF-alpha-308 G/A promoter polymorphism with insulin resistance in obesity. *Obes Res* 10: 401–407.

Davignon J, Gregg RE, Sing CF. 1988. Apolipoprotein E polymorphisms and atherosclerosis. *Atherosclerosis* 8: 1–21.

DeCastro-Orós I, Pampín S, Bolado-Carrancio A et al. 2001. Functional analysis of LDLR promoter and 5′ UTR mutations in subjects with clinical diagnosis of familial hypercholesterolemia. *Hum Mutat* 32: 868–872.

Dedoussis GV, Manios Y, Kourlaba G et al. 2011. An age-dependent diet-modified effect of the PPARγ Pro12Ala polymorphism in children. *Metabolism* 60: 467–473.

Deeb SS, Peng R. 1989. Structure of the human lipoprotein lipase gene. *Biochemistry* 28: 4131–4135.

Deeb SS, Fajas L, Nemoto M et al. 1998. A Pro12Ala substitution in PPARg2 associated with decreased receptor activity, lower body mass index and improved insulin sensitivity. *Nat Genet* 20: 284–287.

Delgado-Lista J, Garcia-Rios A, Perez-Martinez P et al. 2011b. Gene variations of nitric oxide synthase regulate the effects of a saturated fat rich meal on endothelial function. *Clin Nutr* 30: 234–238.

Delgado-Lista J, Perez-Martinez P, García-Rios A et al. 2011a. Pleiotropic effects of TCF7L2 gene variants and its modulation in the metabolic syndrome: From the LIPGENE study. *Atherosclerosis* 214: 110–116.

Delgado-Lista J, Perez-Martinez P, Garcia-Rios A et al. 2013. A gene variation (rs12691) in the CCAT/enhancer binding protein α modulates glucose metabolism in metabolic syndrome. *Nutr Metab Cardiovasc Dis* 23: 417–423.

Delgado-Lista J, Perez-Martinez P, Solivera J et al. 2014. Top Single Nucleotide polymorphisms affecting carbohydrate metabolism in metabolic syndrome: From the LIPGENE Study. *J Clin Endocrinol Metab* 99: E384–E389.

De Roos B. 2012. Personalised nutrition: Ready for practice? *Proc Nutr Soc* 12: 1–5.

Ding L, Jin D, Chen X. 2010. Luteolin enhances insulin sensitivity via activation of PPARγ transcriptional activity in adipocytes. *J Nutr Biochem* 21: 941–947.

Drayna D, Lawn R. 1987. Multiple RFLPs at the human cholesteryl ester transfer protein (CETP) locus. *Nucleic Acids Res* 15: 4698.

Eckel RH. 1989. Lipoprotein lipase: A multifunctional enzyme relevant to common metabolic diseases. *N Engl J Med* 320: 1060–1068.

Eichner JE, Dunn ST, Perveen G, Thompson DM, Stewart KE, Stroehla BC. 2002. Apolipoprotein E polymorphism and cardiovascular disease: A HuGE review. *Am J Epidemiol* 155: 487–495.

Eigler A, Sinha B, Hartmann G, Endres S. 1997. Taming TNF: Strategies to restrain this proinflammatory cytokine. *Immunol Today* 18: 487–492.

Engler MB. 2009. Nutrigenomics in cardiovascular disease: Implications for the future. *Prog Cardiovasc Nurs* 24: 190–195.

Esterbauer H, Oberkofler H, Liu YM et al. 1998. Uncoupling protein-1 mRNA expression in obese human subjects: The role of sequence variations at the uncoupling protein-1 gene locus. *J Lipid Res* 39: 834–844.

Fenech MF. 2014. Nutriomes and personalized nutrition for DNA damage prevention, telomere integrity maintenance and cancer growth control. *Cancer Treat Res* 159: 427–441.

Ferguson JF, Phillips CM, McMonagle J et al. 2010a. NOS3 gene polymorphisms are associated with risk markers of cardiovascular disease, and interact with omega-3 polyunsaturated fatty acids. Atherosclerosis 211: 539–544.

Ferguson JF, Phillips CM, Tierney AC et al. 2010b. Gene–nutrient interactions in the metabolic syndrome: Single nucleotide polymorphisms in ADIPOQ and ADIPOR1 interact with plasma-saturated fatty acids to modulate insulin resistance. *Am J Clin Nutr* 91: 794–801.

Fergusson LR. 2006. Nutrigenomics: Integrating genomic approaches into nutrition research. *Mol Diagn Ther* 10: 101–108.

Fernández-Hernado C, Ramiréz CM, Goedeke L, Suárez Y. 2013. MicroRNAs in metabolic disease. *Artheroscler Thromb Vasc Biol* l33: 178–185.

Fernandez-Real JM, Broch M, Vendrell J et al. 2000. Interleukin-6 gene polymorphism and insulin sensitivity. *Diabetes* 49: 517–520.

Festa A, D'Agostino R, Tracy RP, Haffner SM. 2001. Elevated levels of acute-phase proteins and plasminogen activator inhibitor-1 predict the development of type 2 diabetes: The Insulin Resistance Athersclerosis Study. *Diabetes* 51: 1131–1137.

Fishman D, Faulds G, Jeffery R et al. 1998. The effect of novel polymorphisms in the interleukin-6 (IL-6) gene on IL-6 transcription and plasma IL-6 levels, and an association with systemic-onset juvenile chronic arthritis. *J Clin Invest* 102: 1369–1376.

Fogg-Johnson N, Kaput J. 2003. Nutrigenomics: An emerging scientific discipline. *Food Technol* 57: 60–67.

Fontaine-Bisson B, Wolever TM, Chiasson JL et al. 2007. Genetic polymorphisms of tumor necrosis factor alpha modify the association between dietary polyunsaturated fatty acids and fasting HDL-cholesterol and apo A-I concentrations. *Am J Clin Nutr* 86: 768–774.

Ford ES, Li C, Zhao G. 2010. Prevalence and correlates of metabolic syndrome based on a harmonious definition among adults in the US. *J Diabetes* 2: 180–193.

Forti N, Fukushima J, Giannini SD. 1997. Perfil lipídico de indivíduos submetidos à cinecoronariografia em diferentes regiões do Brasil. *Arq Bras Cardiol* 68: 333–342.

Forti N, Salazar LA, Diament J, Giannini SD, Hirata M H, Hirata RDC. 2003. Genetic changes and cholesterolemia: Recent Brazilian studies. *Arq Bras Cardiol* 80: 565–571.

Franks PW, Christophi CA, Jablonski KA et al. 2014. Common variation in PPARGC1A/B and progression to diabetes or change in metabolic traits following preventive interventions: The Diabetes Prevention Program. *Diabetologia* 57: 485–490.

Freeman DJ, Griffin BA, Holmes AP et al. 1994. Regulation of plasma HDL cholesterol and subtraction distribution by genetic and environmental factors: Associations between the *Taq*I B RFLP in the CETP gene and smoking and obesity. *Arterioscler Thromb* 14: 336–344.

Friedman RC, Farh KK, Burge CB, Bartel DP. 2009. Most mammalian mRNAs are conserved targets of microRNAs. *Genome Res* 19: 92–105.

Garant M J, Kao WH, Brancati F et al. 2002. SNP43 of CAPN10 and the risk of type 2 diabetes in African-Americans: The Atherosclerosis Risk in Communities Study. *Diabetes* 51: 231–237.

Garcia-Cañas V, Simón C, León C, Cifuentes A. 2010. Advances in nutrigenomics research: Novel and future analytical approaches to investigate the biological activity of natural compounds and food functions. *J Pharm Biomed Anal* 51: 290–304.

Garcia-Rios A, Delgado-Lista J, Perez-Martinez P et al. 2011. Genetic variations at the lipoprotein lipase gene influence plasma lipid concentrations and react with plasma n-6 polyunsaturated fatty acids to modulate lipid metabolism. *Atherosclerosis* 218: 416–422.

Garcia-Rios A, Perez-Martinez P, Delgado-Lista J et al. 2012. A Period 2 genetic variant interacts with plasma SFA to modify plasma lipid concentrations in adults with metabolic syndrome. *J Nutr* 142: 1213–1218.

Gardemann A, Ohly D, Fink M et al. 1998. Association of the insertion/deletion gene polymorphism of the apolipoprotein B signal peptide with myocardial infarction. *Atherosclerosis* 141: 167–175.

Garosi P, De Filippo C, van Erk M, Rocca-Serra P, Sansone S-A, Elliott R. 2005. Defining best practice for microarray analyses in nutrigenomic studies. *Br J Nutr* 93: 425–432.

Gehm BD, McAndrews JM, Chien PY et al. 1997. Resveratrol, a polyphenolic compound found in grapes and wine, is an agonist for the estrogen receptor. *Proc Natl Acad Sci USA* 94: 14138–14143.

Genest Jr JJ, Ordovas JM, McNamara JR et al. 1990. DNA polymorphisms of the apolipoprotein B gene in patients with premature coronary artery disease. *Atherosclerosis* 82: 7–17.

Gerdes LU, Klausen IC, Sihm I, Faergeman O. 1992. Apolipoprotein E polymorphism in a Danish population compared to findings in 45 other study populations around the world. *Genetic Epidemiol* 9: 155–167.

Ginsberg HN. 1998. Lipoprotein physiology. Endocrinology and Metabolism Clinics of North America. 27: 503–519.

Glisić S, Prljić J, Radovanović N, Alavantić D. 1997. Study of apoB gene signal peptide insertion/deletion polymorphism in a healthy Serbian population: No association with serum lipid levels. *Clin Chim Acta* 263: 57–65.

Gloyn AL. 2003. The search for type 2 diabetes genes. *Ageing Res Rev* 2: 111–127.

GOLDN. 2008. Genetics of lipid lowering drugs and diet network. https://dsgweb.wustl.edu/goldn/ [Accessed March 12, 2008].

Goldstein JL, Schrott HG, Hazzard WR, Bierman EL, Motulsky AG. 1973. Hyperlipidemia in coronary heart disease. II. Genetic analysis of lipid levels in 176 families and delineation of a new inherited disorder, combined hyperlipidemia. *J Clin Invest* 52: 1544–1568.

Gomez P, Perez-Martinez P, Mari NC et al. 2010. APOA1 and APOA4 gene polymorphisms influence the effects of dietary fat on LDL particle size and oxidation in healthy young adults. *J Nutr* 140: 773–778.

Gomez-Delgado F, Alcala-Diaz JF, Garcia-Rios A et al. 2014. Polymorphism at the TNF-alpha gene interacts with Mediterranean diet to influence triglyceride metabolism and inflammation status in metabolic syndrome patients: From the CORDIOPREV clinical trial. *Mol Nutr Food Res* 58: 1519–1527.

Gouni-Berthold I, Giannakidou E, Faust M, Berthold HK, Krone W. 2006. Association of the promoter polymorphism -232C/G of the phosphoenolpyruvate carboxykinase gene (PCK1) with type 2 diabetes mellitus. *Diabet Med* 23: 419–425.

Goyenechea E, Collins LJ, Parra D et al. 2009.The -11391 G/A polymorphism of the adiponectin gene promoter is associated with metabolic syndrome traits and the outcome of an energy-restricted diet in obese subjects. *Horm Metab Res* 41: 55–61.

Goyenechea E, Parra D, Martínez JA. 2007. Impact of interleukin 6 -174G>C polymorphism on obesity-related metabolic disorders in people with excess in body weight. *Metab Clin Exp* 56: 1643–1648.

Groop L. 2000. Genetics of the metabolic syndrome. *Br J Nutr* 83(Suppl 1): S39–S48.

Gudnason V, Zhou T, Thormar K et al. 1998. Detection of the low-density lipoprotein receptor gene PvuII polymorphism using the polymerase chain reaction with plasma lipid traits in healthy men and women. *Dis Markers* 13: 209–220.

Guzmán EC, Hirata MH, Quintão EC, Hirata RD. 2000. Association of the apolipoprotein B gene polymorphisms with cholesterol levels and response to fluvastatin in Brazilian individuals with high risk for coronary heart disease. *Clin Chem Lab Med* 38: 731–736.

Gylling H, Kontula K, Koivisto UM, Miettinen HE, Miettinen TA. 1997. Polymorphisms of the genes encoding apoproteins A-I, B, C-III and E and LDL receptor, and cholesterol and LDL metabolism during increase cholesterol intake. Common alleles of the apoprotein E gene show the greatest regulatory impact. *Arterioscler Thromb Vasc Biol* 17: 38–44.

Halkes CJ, van Dijk H, de Jaegere PP et al. 2001. Postprandial increase of complement component 3 in normolipidemic patients with coronary artery disease: Effects of expanded-dose simvastatin. *Arterioscler Thromb Vasc Biol* 21: 1526–1530.

Hallman DM, Boerwinkle E, Saha N et al. 1991. The apolipoprotein E polymorphism: A comparison of allele frequencies and effects in nine populations. *Am J Hum Genet* 49: 338–349.

Hamid YH, Rose CS, Urhammer SA et al. 2005. Variations of the interleukin-6 promoter are associated with features of the metabolic syndrome in Caucasian Danes. *Diabetologia* 48: 251–260.

Handschin C, Spiegelman BM. 2006. Peroxisome proliferator-activated receptor gamma coactivator 1 coactivators, energy homeostasis, and metabolism. *Endocr Rev* 27: 728–735.

Hannuksela ML, Johanna Liinamaa M, Kesaniemi YA, Savolainen MJ. 1994. Relation of polymorphisms in the cholesteryl ester transfer protein gene to transfer protein activity and plasma lipoprotein levels in alcohol drinkers. *Atherosclerosis* 110: 35–44.

Hansen PS, Defesche JC, Kastelein JJ et al. 1997. Phenotypic variation in patients heterozygous for familial defective apolipoprotein B (FDB) in three European countries. *Arterioscler Thromb Vasc Biol* 17: 741–747.

Hartweg J, Perera R, Montori V, Dinneen S, Neil HA, Farmer A. 2008. Omega-3 polyunsaturated fatty acids (PUFA) for type 2 diabetes mellitus. *Cochrane Database Syst Rev* 1: CD003205.

Hayakawa T, Nagai Y, Taniguchi M et al. 2000. Tumor necrosis factor-beta gene NcoI polymorphism decreases insulin in Japanese men. *Metabolism* 48: 1506–1509.

Hegele RA, Huang LS, Herbert PN et al. 1986. Apolipoprotein B-gene DNA polymorphisms associated with myocardial infarction. *N Engl J Med* 315: 1509–1515.

Heilbronn LK, Kind KL, Pancewicz E, Morris AM, Noakes M, Clifton PM. 2000. Association of -3826 G variant in uncoupling protein-1 with increase BMI in overweight Australian women. *Diabetologia* 43: 242–244.

Heinrich PC, Castell JC, Andus T.1990. Interleukin-6 and acute phase response. *Biochem J* 161: 621–636.

Henneman P, Aulchenko YS, Frants RR, van Dijk KW, Oostra BA, van Duijn CM. 2008. Prevalence and heritability of the metabolic syndrome and its individual components in a Dutch isolate: The Erasmus Rucphen Family study. *J Med Genet* 45: 572–577.

Henry LA, Witt DM. 2002. Resveratrol: Phytoestrogen effects on reproductive physiology and behavior in female rats. *Horm Behav* 41: 220–228.

Hesketh J, Wybranska I, Dommels Y et al. 2006. Nutrient–gene interactions in benefit–risk analysis. *Br J Nutr* 95: 1232–1236.

Hirschhom JN, Gajdos ZK. 2011. Genome-wide association studies: Results from the first few years and potential implications for clinical medicine. *Ann Rev Med* 62: 11–24.

Hirschhorn JN, Lohmmueller K, Byrne E, Hirschhorn K. 2002. A comprehensive review of genetic association studies. *Genet Med* 4: 45–61.

Hokanson JE. 1999. Functional variants in the lipoprotein lipase gene and risk of cardiovascular disease. *Curr Opin Lipidol* 10: 393–399.

Hong SH, Lee CC, Kim JQ. 1997. Genetic variation of the apolipoprotein B gene in Korean patients with coronary artery disease. *Mol Cells* 7: 521–525.

Hotamisligil GS, Arner P, Caro JF, Atkinson RL, Spiegelman BM. 1995. Increase adipose tissue expression of tumor necrosis factor-α in human obesity and insulin resistance. *J Clin Invest* 95: 2409–2415.

Hotamisligil GS, Spiegelman BM. 1994. Tumor necrosis factor alpha: A key component of the obesity-diabetes link. *Diabetes* 43: 1271–1278.

Hsu S, Wang B, Kota J et al. 2012. Essential metabolic, anti-inflammatory, and anti-tumorigenic functions of miR-122 in liver. *J Clin Invest* 122: 2871–2883.

Hu FB, Meigs JB, Li TY, Rifai N, Manson JE. 2004. Inflammatory markers and risk of developing type 2 diabetes in women. *Diabetes* 53: 693–700.

Huizinga TW, Westendorp RG, Bollen EL et al. 1997. TNF-alpha promoter polymorphisms, production and susceptibility to multiple sclerosis in different groups of patients. *J Neuroimmunol* 72: 149–153.

Huth C, Heid IM, Vollmert C et al. 2006. IL6 gene promoter polymorphisms and type 2 diabetes: Joint analysis of individual participants' data from 21 studies. *Diabetes* 55: 2915–2921.

Illig T, Bongardt F, Schopfer A et al. 2004. Significant association of the interleukin-6 gene polymorphisms C-174G and A-598G with type 2 diabetes. *J Clin Endocrinol Metab* 89: 5053–5058.

Inazu A, Jiang X-C, Haraki T et al. 1994. Genetic cholesteryl ester transfer protein deficiency caused by two prevalent mutations as a major determinant of increased levels of high-density lipoprotein cholesterol. *J Clin Invest* 94: 1872–1882.

Jang Y, Kim HJ, Koh SJ et al. 2007. Lymphotoxin-α gene 252A>G and metabolic syndrome features in Korean men with coronary artery disease. *Clin Chim Acta* 384: 124–128.

Jansen S, Lopez-Miranda J, Salas J et al. 1997. Effect of 347-serine mutation in apoprotein A-IV on plasma LDL cholesterol response to dietary fat. *Arterioscler Thromb Vasc Biol* 17: 1532–1538.

Jones SB, DePrimo SE, Whitfield ML, Brooks JD. 2005. Resveratrol-induced gene expression profiles in human prostate cancer cells. *Cancer Epidemiol Biomarkers Prev* 14: 596–604.

Jorde LB, Wooding SP. 2004. Genetic classification and "race". *Nat Genet* 36(Suppl 1): S28–S33.

Juo SH, Wysynski DF, Beaty TH, Huang HY, Bailey-Wilson JE. 1999. Mild association between the A/G polymorphism in the promoter of the apolipoprotein A-I gene and apolipoprotein A-I levels: A meta-analysis. *Am J Med Genet* 82: 235–241.

Kanková K, Márová I, Jansen EH, Vasků A, Jurajda M, Vácha J. 2002. Polymorphism Ncol in tumor necrosis factor B is associated with fasting glycemia and lipid parameters in healthy non-obese Caucasian subjects. *Diabetes Metab* 28: 231–237.

Kaput J, JKelin KG, Reyes EJ et al. 2004. Identification of genes contributing to the obese yellow Avy phenotype: Caloric restriction, genotype, diet–genotype interactions. *Physiol Gemomics* 18: 316–324.

Kaput J, Ordovas JM, Ferguson L et al. 2005. The case for strategic international alliances to harness nutritional genomics for public and personal health. *Br J Nutr* 94: 623–632.

Kaput J, Rodrigues RL. 2004. Nutritional genomics: The next frontier in the postgenomic era. *Physiol Gemomics* 16: 166–177.

Katsuki A, Yano Y, Sumida Y et al. 1998. Significant decreased insulin secretion is a diabetic with clinically probable multiple sclerosis. *Intern Med* 37: 865–869.

Kern PAA, Saghizadeh M, Ong JM, Bosch RJ, Deem R, Simsolo RB. 1995. The expression of tumor necrosis factor in human adipose tissue. Regulation by obesity, weight loss, and relationship to lipoprotein lipase. *J Clin Invest* 95: 2111–2119.

Khymenets O, Fitó M, Covas MI et al. 2009. Mononuclear cell transcriptome response after sustained virgin olive oil consumption in humans and exploratory nutrigenomics study. *OMICS* 13: 7–19.

Kondo I, Berg K, Drayna D, Lawn R. 1989. DNA polymorphism at the locus for human cholesteryl ester transfer protein (CETP) is associated with high-density lipoprotein cholesterol and apolipoprotein levels. *Clin Genet* 35: 49–56.

Konstantinidou V, Covas MI, Muñoz-Aguayo D et al. 2010. In vivo nutroigenomic effects of virgin olive oil polyphenols within the frame of the Mediterranean diet: A randomized controlled trial. *FASEB J* 24: 2546–2557.

Kotha A, Sekharam M, Cilenti L et al. 2006. Resveratrol inhibits Src and Stat3 signaling and induces the apoptosis of malignant cells containing activated Stat3 protein. *Mol Cancer Ther* 5: 621–629.

Kraja AT, Vaidya D, Pankow JS et al. 2011. A bivariate genome-wide approach to metabolic syndrome: STAMPEED consortium. *Diabetes* 60: 1329–1339.

Krey G, Braissant O, Kalkhoven E et al. 1997. Fatty acids, eicosanoids, and hypolipidemic agents identified as ligands of peroxisome proliferator-activated receptors by coactivator-dependent receptor ligand assay. *Mol Endocrinol* 11: 779–791.

Krisfali P, Polgár N, Sáfrány E et al. 2010. Triglyceride level affecting shared susceptibility genes in metabolic syndrome and coronary artery disease. *Curr Med Chem* 17: 3533–3541.

Kristiansson K, Perola M, Tikkanen E et al. 2012. Genome-wide screen for metabolic syndrome susceptibility Loci reveals strong lipid gene contribution but no evidence for common genetic basis for clustering of metabolic syndrome traits. *Circ Cardiovasc Genet* 5: 242–249.

Kubaszek A, Pihlajamaki J, Punnonen K, Karhapaa P, Vauhkonen I, Laakso M. 2003. The C-174G promoter polymorphism of the IL-6 gene affects energy expenditure and insulin sensitivity. *Diabetes* 52: 558–561.

Lai CQ, Corella D, Demissie S et al. 2006. Dietary intake of n-6 fatty acids modulates effect of apolipoprotein concentrations, and lipoprotein particle size: The Framingham Heart Study. *Circulation* 113: 2062–2070.

Lançon A, Michaille JJ, Latruffe N. 2013. Effects of dietary phytophenols on the expression of microRNAs involved in mammalian cell homeostasis. *J Sci Food Agric* 93: 3155–3164.

Lander E, Krunglyak L. 1995. Genetic dissection of complex traits: Guidelines for interpreting and reporting results. *Nat Genet* 11: 241–247.

Lanktree M, Hegele RA.2008. Copy number variation in metabolic phenotypes. *Cytogenet Genome Res* 123(1–4): 169–175.

Law A, Wallis SC, Powell LM et al. 1986. Common DNA polymorphism within coding sequence of apolipoprotein B gene associated with altered lipid levels. *Lancet* 1: 1301–1303.

Le NA, Walter MF. 2007. The role of hypertriglyceridemia in atherosclerosis. *Curr Atheroscler Rep* 9: 110–115.

Leitersdorf E, Chakravarti A, Hobbs HH. 1989. Polymorphic DNA haplotypes at the LDL receptor locus. *Am J Hum Genet* 44: 409–421.

Levy RI. 1981. Cholesterol, lipoproteins, apoproteins, and heart disease: Present status and future prospects. *Clin Chem* 27: 653–662.

Lewis B. 1983. The lipoproteins: Predictors, protectors, and pathogens. *Br Med J (Clin Res Ed)* 287: 1161–1164.

Li J, Pircher PC, Schulman IG, Westin SK. 2005. Regulation of complement C3 expression by the bile acid receptor FXR. *J Biol Chem* 280: 7427–7434.

Li WD, Reed DR, Lee JH et al. 1999. Sequence variants in the 5′ flanking region of the leptin gene are associated with obesity in women. *Ann Hum Genet* 63: 227–234.

Linton MF. Hasty AH, Babaev VR, Fazio S. 1998. Hepatic apo E expression is required for remnant lipoprotein clearance in the absence of the low-density lipoprotein receptor. *Journal of Clinical Investigation* 101: 1726–1736.

Liao Z, Chen X, Wu M. 2010. Antidiabetic effect of flavones from *Cirsium japonicum* DC in diabetic rats. *Arch Pharm Res* 33: 353–362.

Llorente-Cortés V, Estruch R, Mena MP et al. 2010. Effect of Mediterranean diet on the expression of pro-atherogenic genes in a population at high cardiovascular risk. *Atherosclerosis* 208: 442–450.

Loktionov A. 2003. Common gene polymorphisms and nutrition: Emerging links with pathogenesis of multi-factorial chronic diseases (review). *J Nutr Biochem* 14: 426–451.

Loktionov A, Scolle S, McKeown N, Binghmam SA. 2000. Gene–nutrition interactions: Dietary behavior associated with high coronary heart disease risk particularly affects serum LDL-cholesterol in apolipoprotein E epsilon4-carrying free-living individuals. *Br J Nutr* 84: 885–890.

Lopez-Garcia E, Schulze MB, Manson JE et al. 2004. Consumption of (*n*–3) fatty acids is related to plasma biomarkers of inflammation and endothelial activation in women. *J Nutr* 134: 1806–1811.

López-Miranda J, Cruz G, Gómez P et al. 2004. The influence of lipoprotein lipase gene variation on post-prandial lipoprotein metabolism. *J Clin Endocrinol Metab* 89: 4721–4728.

Lopez-Miranda J, Ordovas JM, Espino A et al. 1994. Influence of mutation in human apolipoprotein A-1 gene promoter on plasma LDL cholesterol response to dietary fat. *Lancet* 343: 1246–1249.

Lopez-Miranda J, Ordovas JM, Ostos MA et al. 1997. Dietary fat clearance in normal subjects is modulated by genetic variation at the apolipoprotein B gene locus. *Arterioscler Thromb Vasc Biol* 17: 1765–1773.

Lovejoy JC, Smith SR, Champagne CM et al. 2002. Effects of diets enriched in saturated (palmitic), mono-unsaturated (oleic), or trans (elaidic) fatty acids on insulin sensitivity and substrate oxidation in healthy adults. *Diabetes Care* 25: 1283–1288.

Luan J, Browne PO, Harding AH et al. 2001. Evidence for gene–nutrient interaction at the PPAR gamma locus. *Diabetes* 50: 686–689.

Ludwig EH, McCarthy BJ. 1990. Haplotype analysis of the human apolipoprotein B mutation associated with familial defective apolipoprotein B100. *Am J Hum Genet* 47: 712–720.

Luu NT, Madden J, Calder PC et al. 2007. Dietary supplementation with fish oil modifies the ability of human monocytes to induce an inflammatory response. *J Nutr* 137: 2769–2774.

Madsen T, Skou HA, Hansen VE et al. 2001. C-reactive protein, dietary n–3 fatty acids, and the extent of coronary artery disease. *Am J Cardiol* 88: 1139–1142.

Mahley RW, Huang Y. 1999. Apoliprotein E: From atherosclerosis to Alzheimer's disease and beyond. *Curr Opin Lipidol* 10: 207–217.

Matsushita H, Kurabayashi T, Tomita M, Kato N, Tanaka K. 2003. Effects of uncoupling protein 1 and beta-3 adrenergic receptor gene polymorphisms on body size and serum lipid concentrations in Japanese women. *Maturitas* 45: 39–45.

Mattu RK, Needham EW, Morgan R et al. 1994. DNA variants at the LPL gene locus associate with angi-ographically defined severity of atherosclerosis and serum lipoprotein levels in a Welsh population. *Arterioscler Thromb* 14: 1090–1097.

Maxwell KN, Fisher EA, Breslow JL. 2005. Overexpression of PCSK9 accelerates the degradation of the LDLR in a post-endoplasmic reticulum compartment. *Proc Natl Acad Sci USA* 102: 2069–2074.

Mayer-Davis EJ, Monaco JH, Hoen HM et al. 1997. Dietary fat and insulin sensitivity in a triethnic population: The role of obesity. The Insulin Resistance Atherosclerosis Study (IRAS). *Am J Clin Nutr* 65: 79–87.

McPherson R, Mann CJ, Tall AR et al. 1991. Plasma concentrations of cholesteryl ester transfer protein in hyperlipoproteinemia. Relation to cholesteryl ester transfer protein activity and other lipoprotein variables. *Arterioscler Thromb* 11: 797–804.

Melzer D, Murray A, Hurst AJ et al. 2006. Effects of the diabetes linked TCF7L2 polymorphism in a representative older population. *BMC Med* 4: 34.

Memisoglu A, Hu FB, Hankinson SE et al. 2003. Interaction between a peroxisome proliferator-activated receptor gamma gene polymorphism and dietary fat intake in relation to body mass. *Hum Mol Genet* 12: 2923–2929.

Menzaghi C, Trischitta V, Doria A. 2007. Genetic influences of adiponectin on insulin resistance, type 2 diabetes, and cardiovascular disease. *Diabetes* 56: 1198–1209.

Messer G, Spengler U, Jung MC et al. 1991. Polymorphic structure of the tumor necrosis factor (TNF) locus: An Ncol polymorphism in the first intron of the human TNF-beta gene correlates with a variant amino acid in position 26 and a reduced level of TNF-beta production. *J Exp Med* 173: 209–219.

Milenkovic D, Jude B, Morand C. 2013. miRNA as molecular target of polyphenols underlying their biological effects. *Free Radic Biol Med* 64: 40–51.

Mollaki V, Progias P, Drogari E. 2013. Novel LDLR variants in patients with familial hypercholesterolemia: In silico analysis as a tool to predict pathogenic variants in children and their families. *Ann Hum Genet* 77: 426–434.

Moller DE. 2000. Potential role of TNF-α in the pathogenesis of insulin resistance in type 2 diabetes. *Trends Endocrinol Metab* 11: 212–217.

Moller DE, Kaufman KD. 2005. Metabolic syndrome: A clinical and molecular perspective. *Annu Rev Med* 56: 45–62.

Möhlig M, Boeing H, Spranger J et al. 2004. Body mass index and C-174G interleukin-6 promoter polymorphism interact in predicting type 2 diabetes. *J Clin Endocrinol Metab* 89: 1885–1890.

Moreno JA, Perez-Jimenez F, Marin C et al. 2004. Apolipoprotein E gene promoter -219G>T polymorphism increased LDL-cholesterol concentrations and susceptibility to oxidation in response to a diet rich in saturated fat. *Am J Clin Nutr* 80: 1404–1409.

Moreno JA, Pérez-Jimenez F, Marin C, Perez-Martinez P. 2005. The apolipoportein E gene promoter (-219G/T) polymorphism determines insulin sensitivity in response to dietary fat in healthy young adults. *J Nutr* 135: 2535–2540.

Mulder M, Lombardi P, Jansen H, Van Berkel TJC, Frants RR, Havekes LM. 1993. Low-density lipoprotein receptor internalizes low density and very low-density lipoproteins that are bound to heparan sulfate proteoglycans via lipoprotein lipase. *J Biol Chem* 268: 9369–9375.

Muscari A, Massarelli G, Bastagli L et al. 2000. Relationship of serum C3 to fasting insulin, risk factors and previous ischaemic events in middle-aged men. *Eur Heart J* 21: 1081–1090.

Myant NB, Gallagher J, Barbir M, Thompson GR, Wile D, Humphries SE. 1989. Restriction fragment length polymorphisms in the apo B gene in relation to coronary artery disease. *Atherosclerosis* 77: 193–201.

Myant NB, Gallagher JJ, Knight BL et al. 1991. Clinical signs of familial hypercholesterolemia in patients with familial defective apolipoprotein B-100 and normal low-density lipoprotein receptor function. *Arterioscler Thromb Vasc Biol* 11: 691–703.

Nacif JM, Jump ML, Torontali SM et al. 2002. Gene expression profile induced by 17 alpha-ethynyl estradiol, bisphenol A, and genistein in the developing female reproductive system of the rat. *Toxicol Sci* 68: 184–199.

Nam NH. 2006. Naturally occurring NF-kappaB inhibitors. *MiniRev Med Chem* 6: 945–941.

Naoum JJ, Chal H, Lin PH, Lumsden AB, Yao Q, Chen C. 2006. Limphotoxin-α and cardiovascular disease: Clinical association and pathogenic mechanisms. *Med Sci Monit* 12: RA121–RA124.

NCEP ATP III. National Cholesterol Education Program; National Heart, Lung, and Blood Institute; National Institutes of Health. 2002. Third Report of the National Cholesterol Education Program (NCEP) Expert Panel on Detection, Evaluation, and Treatment of High Blood Cholesterol in Adults (Adult Treatment Panel III) final report. *Circulation* 106: 3143–3421.

O'Doherty RM, Lehman DL, Telemaque-Potts S, Newgard CB. 1999. Metabolic impact of glucokinase overexpression in liver: Lowering of blood glucose in fed rats is accompanied by hyperlipidemia. *Diabetes* 48: 2022–2027.

Oh HH, Kim KS, Choi SM, Yang HS, Yoon Y. 2004. The effects of uncoupling protein -1 genotye on lipoprotein cholesterol levels in Korean obese subjects. *Metabolism* 53: 1054–1059.

Oka K, Tkalcevic GT, Nakano T, Tucker H, Ishimura-Oka K, Brown WV. 1990. Structure and polymorphic map of human lipoprotein lipase gene. *Biochim Biophys Acta* 1049: 21–26.

Olson NC, Callas PW, Hanley AJG et al. 2012. Circulating levels of TNF-α are associated with impaired glucose tolerance, increased insulin resistance, and ethnicity: The insulin resistance atherosclerosis study. *J Clin Endocrinol Metab* 97: 1032–1040.

Ordovas JM. 2004. The quest for cardiovascular health in the genomic era: Nutrigenetics and plasma lipoproteins. *Proc Nutr Soc* 63: 145–152.

Ordovas JM, Corella D. 2004. Nutritional genomics. *Annu Rev Genomics Hum Genet* 5: 71–118.

Ordovas JM, Cupples LA, Corella D et al. 2000. Association of cholesteryl ester transfer protein-*Taq*IB polymorphism with variations in lipoprotein subclasses and coronary heart disease risk: The Framingham Study. *Arterioscler Thromb Vasc Biol* 20: 1323–1329.

Ordovas JM, Corella D, Cupples LA et al. 2002b. Polyunsaturated fatty acids modulate the effects of the ApoA1 G-A polymorphism on HDL-cholesterol concentrations in a sex-specific manner: The Framingham Study. *Am J Clin Nutr* 75: 38–46.

Ordovas JM, Corella D, Demissie S et al. 2002a. Dietary fat intake determines the effect of a common polymorphism in the hepatic lipase gene promoter on high-density lipoprotein metabolism: Evidence of a strong dose effect in this gene nutrient interaction in the Framingham Study. *Circulation* 106: 2315–2321.

Orho-Melander M, Melander O, Guiducci C et al. 2008. Common missense variant in the glucokinase regulatory protein gene is associated with increased plasma triglyceride and C-reactive protein but lower fasting glucose concentrations. *Diabetes* 57: 3112–3121.

Ortega A, Varela LM, Bermudez B, Lopez S, Muriana FJG, Abia R. 2012. Nutrigenomics and Atherosclerosis: The postprandial and long-term effects of virgin olive oil ingestion. In: Parthassarathy S (ed.), *Atherogenesis*. Published In Tech: Rijeka, Croatia, pp. 135–160.

Pan MH, Lai CS, Dushenkov S, Ho CT. 2009. Modulation of inflammatory genes by natural dietary bioactive compounds. *Agric Food Chem* 57: 4467–4477.

Pan M-H, Lai C-S, Ho C-T. 2010. Anti-inflammatory activity of natural flavonoids. *Food Funct* 1: 15–31.

Park JKY, Paik JK, Kim OY et al. 2010. Interactions between the APOA5 -1131T.C and the FEN1 10154G>T polymorphisms on n-6 polyunsaturated fatty acids in serum phospholipids and coronary artery disease. *J Lipid Res* 51: 3281–3288.

Paulweber B, Friedl W, Krempler F, Humphries SE, Sandhofer F. 1990. Association of DNA polymorphism at the apolipoprotein B gene locus with coronary heart disease and serum very low-density lipoprotein levels. *Arteriosclerosis* 10: 17–24.

Peacock R, Dunning A, Hamsten A, Tornvall P, Humphries S, Talmud P. 1992. Apolipoprotein B gene polymorphisms, lipoproteins and coronary atherosclerosis: A study of young myocardial infarction survivors and healthy population-based individuals. *Atherosclerosis* 92: 151–164.

Pedersen JC, Berg K. 1988, Normal DNA polymorphism at the low-density lipoprotein receptor (LDLR) locus associated with serum cholesterol level. *Clin Genet* 34: 302–312.

Pedro-Bolet J, Schaeffer EJ, Bakker-Arkema RG et al. 2001. Apolipoprotein E phenotype affects plasma lipid response to atorvastatin in a gender specific manner. *Atherosclerosis* 158: 183–193.

Perez-Martinez P, Corella D, Shen J et al. 2009. Association between glucokinase regulatory protein (GCKR) and apolipoprotein A5 (APOA5) gene polymorphisms and triacylglycerol concentrations in fasting, postprandial, and fenofibrate-treated states. *Am J Clin Nutr* 89: 391–399.

Perez-Martinez P, Delgado-Lista J, Garcia-Rios A et al. 2011a. Glucokinase regulatory protein genetic variant interacts with omega-3 PUFA to influence insulin resistance and inflammation in metabolic syndrome. *PLoS One* 6: e20555.

Perez-Martinez P, Delgado-Lista J, Garcia-Rios A et al. 2011b. Calpain-10 interacts with plasma saturated fatty acid concentrations to influence insulin resistance in individuals with the metabolic syndrome. *Am J Clin Nutr* 93: 1136–1141.

Perez-Martinez P, Garcia-Rios A, Delgado-Lista J, Perez-Jimenez F, Lopez-Miranda J. 2012. Metabolic syndrome: Evidences for a personalized nutrition. *Mol Nutr Food Res* 56: 67–76.

Perez-Martinez P, Garcia-Rios A, Delgado-Lista J, Perez-Jimenez F, Lopez-Miranda J. 2011c. Nutrigenetics of the postprandial lipoprotein metabolism: Evidence from human intervention studies. *Curr Vasc Pharmacol* 9: 287–291.

Phillips CM. 2013. Nutrigenetics and metabolic disease: Current status and implications for personalised nutrition. *Nutrients* 5: 32–57.

Phillips CM, Goumidi L, Bertrais S et al. 2009. Complement component 3 polymorphisms interact with polyunsaturated fatty acids to modulate risk of metabolic syndrome. *Am J Clin Nutr* 90: 1665–1673.

Phillips CM, Goumidi L, Bertrais S et al. 2010. Additive effect of polymorphisms in the IL-6, LTA, and TNF-{alpha} genes and plasma fatty acid level modulate risk for the metabolic syndrome and its components. *J Clin Endocrinol Metab* 95: 1386–1394.

Phillips C, Lopez-Miranda J, Perez-Jimenez F, McManus R, Roche HM. 2006. Genetic and nutrient determinants of the metabolic syndrome. *Curr Opin Cardiol* 21: 185–193.

Pike AC, Brzozowski AM, Hubbard RE et al. 1999. Structure of the ligand-binding domain of oestrogen receptor beta in the presence of a partial agonist and a full antagonist. *EMBO J* 18: 4608–4618.

Plomgaard P, Nielsen AR, Fischer CP et al. 2007. Associations between insulin resistance and TNF-α in plasma, skeletal muscle and adipose tissue in humans with and without type 2 diabetes. *Diabetologia* 50: 2562–2571.

Pociot F, Briant L, Jongencel CV et al. 1993. Association of tumor necrosis factor (TNF) and class II major histocompatibility complex alleles with the secretion of TNF-α and TNF-β by human mononuclear cells: A possible link to insulin-dependent diabetes mellitus. *Eur J Immunol* 23: 224–231.

Pouliot M-C, Despres J-P, Dionne FT et al. 1994. ApoB-100 gene EcoRI polymorphism: Relations to plasma lipoprotein changes associated with abdominal visceral obesity. *Arterioscler Thromb* 14: 527–533.

Povel CM, Boer JM, Reiling E, Feskens EJ. 2011. Genetic variants and the metabolic syndrome: A systematic review. *Obes Rev* 12: 952–967.

Pradhan AD, Manson JE, Rifai N, Buring JE, Ridker PM. 2001. C-reactive protein, interleukin 6, and risk of developing type 2 diabetes mellitus. *JAMA* 286: 327–34.

Radomski MW, Palmer RMJ, Moncada S. 1987. Endogenous nitric oxide inhibits human platelet adhesion to vascular endothelium. *Lancet* 2: 1057–1058.

Radomski MW, Palmer RMJ, Moncada S. 1990. An L-arginine/nitric oxide pathway present in human platelets regulates aggregation. *Proc Natl Acad Sci USA* 87: 5193–5197.

Razzaghi H, Aston CE, Hamman RF, Kamboh MI. 2000. Genetic screening of the lipoprotein lipase gene for mutations associated with high triglyceride/low HDL-cholesterol levels. *Hum Genet* 107: 257–267.

Rebbeck TR, Spitz M, Wu X. 2004. Assessing the functions of genetic variants in candidate gene association studies. *Nat Rev Genet* 5: 589–597.

Rees SD, Britten AC, Bellary S et al. 2009. The promoter polymorphism -232C/G of the PCK1 gene is associated with type 2 diabetes in a UK-resident South Asian population. *BMC Med Genet* 2; 10: 83.

Ristow M, Müller-Wieland D, Pfeiffer A, Krone W, Kahn CR. 1998. Obesity associated with a mutation in a genetic regulator of adipocyte differentiation. *N Engl J Med* 339: 953–959.

Robitaille J, Després JP, Pérusse L, Vohl MC. 2003. The PPAR-gamma P12A polymorphism modulates the relationship between dietary fat intake and components of the metabolic syndrome: Results from the Québec Family Study. *Clin Genet* 63: 109–116.

Roche HM, Phillips C, Gibney MJ. 2005. The metabolic syndrome: The crossroads of diet and genetics. *Proc Nutr Soc* 64: 371–377.

Romano M, Sironi M, Toniatti C et al. 1997. Role of IL-6 and its soluble receptor in induction of chemokines and leukocyte recruitment. *Immunity* 6: 315–325.

Ryo M, Nakamura T, Kihara S et al. 2004. Adiponectin as a biomarker of the metabolic syndrome. *Circ J* 68: 975–981.

Saez ME, Gonzalez-Sanches JL, Ramirez-Lorca R et al. 2008. The CAPN10 gene is associated with insulin resistance phenotypes in the Spanish population. *PLoS One* 3: e2953.

Salazar LA, Cavalli SA, Hirata MH et al. 2000b. Polymorphisms of the low-density lipoprotein receptor gene in Brazilian individuals with heterozygous familial hypercholesterolemia. *Braz J Med Biol Res* 33: 1301–1304.

Salazar LA, Hirata MH, Forti N et al. 2000a. Pvu II intron 15 polymorphism at the LDL receptor gene is associated with differences in serum lipid concentrations in subjects with low and high risk for coronary artery disease from Brazil. *Clin Chim Acta* 293: 75–88.

Salazar LA, Hirata MH, Giannini SD et al. 2000c. Seven DNA polymorphisms at the candidate genes of atherosclerosis in Brazilian woman with angiographically documented coronary artery disease. *Clin Chem Acta* 300: 139–149.

Salazar LA, Hirata MH, Giannini SD et al. 1999. Effects of AvaII and HincII polymorphism of the LDL-receptor gene on serum lipid level of Brazilian individuals with high risk for coronary heart disease. *J Clin Lab Anal* 13: 251–258.

Sale MM, Hsu FC, Palmer ND et al. 2007. The uncoupling protein 1 gene, UCP1, is expressed in mammalian islet cells and associated with acute insulin response to glucose in African American families from the IRAS Family Study. *BMC Endocr Disord* 7: 1.

Samdani AF, Dawson TM, Dawson VL. 1997. Nitric oxide synthase in models of focal ischemia. *Stroke* 28: 1283–1288.

Sánches-Moreno C, Ordovás JM, Smith CE et al. 2011. APOA5 gene variation interacts with dietary fat intake to modulate obesity and circulating triglycerides in a Mediterranean population. *J Nutr* 141: 380–385.

Santos JL, Boutin P, Verdich C et al. 2006. Genotype-by-nutrient interactions assessed in European obese women. A case-only study. *Eur J Nutr* 45: 454–462.

Scherer PE, Williams S, Fogliano M, Baldini G, Lodish HF. 1995. A novel serum protein similar to C1q, produced exclusively in adipocytes. *J Biol Chem* 270: 26746–26749.

Schwanke CHA, Cruz IBM, Leal NF, Scheibe R, Moriguchi Y, Moriguchi EH. 2002. Análise da associação entre polimorfismo do gene da apolipoproteína E e fatores de risco cardiovascular em idosos longevos. *Arq Bras Cardiol* 78: 561–570.

Shaw DI, Tierney AC, McCarthy S et al. 2009. LIPGENE food-exchange model for alteration of dietary fat quantity and quality in free-living participants from eight European countries. *Br J Nutr* 101: 750–759.

Shen J, Arnett DK, Perez-Martinez P. et al. 2008. The effect of IL6–174C/G polymorphism on postprandial triglyceride metabolism in the GOLDN study. *J Lipid Res* 49: 1839–1845.

Sheng T, Yang K. 2008. Adiponectin and its association with insulin resistance and type 2 diabetes. *J Genet Genomics* 35: 321–326.

Shima Y, Nakanishi K, Odawara M, Kobayashi T, Ohta H. 2003. Association of the SNP-19 genotype 22 in the calpain-10 gene with elevated body mass index and hemoglobin A1c levels in Japanese. *Clin Chim Acta* 336: 89–96.

Shore VG, Shore B. 1973. Heterogeneity of human plasma very low-density lipoproteins. Separation of species differing in protein components. *Biochemistry* 12: 502–507.

Siest G, Pillot T, Regis-Bailly A et al. 1995. Apolipoprotein E: An important gene and protein to follow in laboratory medicine. *Clin Chem* 41: 1068–1086.

Sookoian S, Garcia SI, Gianotti TF, Dieuzeide G, Gonzalez CD, Pirola CJ. 2005. The G-308A promoter variant of the tumor necrosis factor-alpha gene is associated with hypertension in adolescents harboring the metabolic syndrome. *Am J Hypertens* 18: 1271–1275.

Sookoian SC, González C, Pirola CJ. 2005. Meta-analysis on the G-308A tumor necrosis factor alpha gene variant and phenotypes associated with the metabolic syndrome. *Obes Res* 13: 2122–2131.

Spiegelman BM. 1998. PPAR-gamma: Adipogenic regulator and thiazolidinedione receptor. *Diabetes* 47: 507–514.

Spranger J, Kroke A, Mohlig M et al. 2003. Inflammatory cytokines and the risk to develop type 2 diabetes: Results of the prospective population-based European Prospective Investigation into Cancer and Nutrition (EPIC)-Potsdam Study. *Diabetes* 52: 812–817.

Stalenhoef AF, de Graaf J. 2008. Association of fasting and nonfasting serum triglycerides with cardiovascular disease and the role of remnant-like lipoproteins and small dense LDL. *Curr Opin Lipidol* 19: 355–361.

Stepanov VA, Puzyrev VP, Karpov RS, Kutmin AI. 1998. Genetic markers in coronary artery disease in a Russian population. *Hum Biol* 70: 47–57.

Stephens JW, Hurel SJ, Lowe GDO, Rumley A, Humphries SE. 2007. Association between plasma IL-6, the IL-6–174G>C variant and the metabolic syndrome in type 2 diabetes mellitus. *Mol Genet Metab* 90: 422–428.

Steven AM, Sieber GM. 1994. Trends in individual fat consumption in the UK 1900–1985. *Br J Nutr* 71: 775–788.

Stumvoll M, Häring H. 2002. The peroxisome proliferator-activated receptor γ2 pro12ala polymorphism. *Diabetes* 51: 2341–2347.

Subbiah MTR. 2008. Understanding the nutrigenomic definitions and concepts at the food-genome junction. *OMICS* 12: 229–235.

Südhof TC, Goldstein JL, Brown MS, Russel DW. 1985. LDL receptor gene: A mosaic of exons shared with different proteins. *Science* 228: 815–822.

Szabo de Edelenyi F, Goumidi L, Bertrais S et al. 2008. Prediction of the metabolic syndrome status based on dietary and genetic parameters, using Random Forest. *Genes Nutr* 3: 173–176.

Tai DY, Pan JP, Lee-Chen GJ. 1998. Identification and haplotype analysis of apolipoprotein B-100 Arg3500 → Trp mutation in hyperlipidemic Chinese. *Clin Chem* 44: 1659–1665.

Tai ES, Corella D, Demissie S et al. 2005. Framingham heart study. Polyunsaturated fatty acids interact with the PPARA-L162V polymorphism to affect plasma triglyceride and apolipoprotein C-III concentrations in the Framingham Heart Study. *J Nutr* 135: 397–403.

Tall A. 1995. Plasma lipid transfer proteins. *Ann Rev Biochem* 64: 235–257.

Tall A. 1993. Plasma cholesteryl ester transfer protein. *J Lipid Res* 34: 1255–1274.

Talmud PJ, Barni N, Kessling AM et al. 1987. Apolipoprotein B gene variants are involved in the determination of serum cholesterol levels: A study in normo- and hyperlipidaemic individuals. *Atherosclerosis* 67: 81–89.

Tanaka T, Ordovas JM, Delgado-Lista J et al. 2007. Peroxisome proliferator-activated receptor alpha polymorphisms and postprandial lipemia in healthy men. *J Lipid Res* 48: 1402–1408.

Tirona RG, Leake BF, Podust LM, Kim RB. 2004. Identification of amino acids in rat pregnane X receptor that determine species-specific activation. *Mol Pharmacol* 65: 36–44.

Tsai WC, Hsu SD, Hsu CS et al. 2012. MicroRNA-122 plays a critical role in liver homeostasis and hepatocarcinogenesis. *J Clin Invest* 122: 2884–2897.

Tschritter O, Frische A, Thamer C et al. 2003. Plasma adiponectin concentrations predict insulin sensitivity of both glucose and lipid metabolism. *Diabetes* 52: 239–243.

Tsytsykova AV, Rajsbaum R, Falvo JV, Ligeiro F, Neely SR, Goldfeld AE. 2007. Activation-dependent intrachromosomal interactions formed by the TNF gene promoter and two distal enhancers. *Proc Natl Acad Sci USA* 104: 16850–16855.

Turner PR, Talmud PJ, Visvikis S, Ehnholm C, Tiret L. 1995. DNA polymorphisms of the apoprotein B gene are associated with altered plasma lipoprotein concentrations but not with perceived risk of cardiovascular disease: European Atherosclerosis Research Study. *Atherosclerosis* 116: 221–234.

Ukkola O, Savolainen MJ, Salmela PI, Von Dickhoff KI, Kesaniemi YA. 1993. Apolipoprotein B gene DNA polymorphisms are associated with macro- and microangiopathy in non-insulin-dependent diabetes mellitus. *Clin Genet* 44: 177–184.

Usifo E, Leigh SE, Whittall RA et al. 2012. Low-density lipoprotein receptor gene familial hypercholesterolemia variant database: Update and pathological assessment. *Ann Hum Genet* 76: 387–401.

Vaccaro O, Lapice E, Monticelli A et al. 2007. Pro12Ala polymorphism of the PPARgamma2 locus modulates the relationship between energy intake and body weight in type 2 diabetic patients. *Diabetes Care* 30: 1156–1161.

Vanden Heuvel JP, Thompson JT, Frame SR, Gillies PJ. 2006. Differential activation of nuclear receptors by perfluorinated fatty acid analogs and natural fatty acids: A comparison of human, mouse, and rat peroxisome proliferator-activated receptor alpha, -beta, and -gamma, liver X receptor-beta, and retinoid X receptor-alpha. *Toxicol Sci* 92: 476–489.

Vanden Heuvel JP. 2009. Cardiovascular disease-related genes and regulation by diet. *Curr Atheroscler Rep* 11: 448–455.

van Oostrom AJ, Alipour A, Plokker TW, Sniderman AD, Cabezas MC. 2007. The metabolic syndrome in relation to complement component 3 and postprandial lipemia in patients from an outpatient lipid clinic and healthy volunteers. *Atherosclerosis* 190: 167–173.

Vasseur F, Helbecque N, Dina C et al. 2002. Single-nucleotide polymorphism haplotypes in the both proximal promoter and exon 3 of the APM1 gene modulate adipocyte-secreted adiponectin hormone levels and contribute to the genetic risk for type 2 diabetes in French Caucasians. *Hum Mol Genet* 11: 2607–2614.

Vasseur F, Meyre D, Froguel P. 2006. Adiponectin, type 2 diabetes and the metabolic syndrome: Lessons from human genetic studies. *Exp Rev Mol Med* 8: 1–12.

Verseyden C, Meijssen S, van Dijk H, Jansen H, Castro Cabezas M. 2003. Effects of atorvastatin on fasting and postprandial complement component 3 response in familial combined hyperlipidemia. *J Lipid Res* 44: 2100–2108.

Vessby B. 2003. Dietary fat, fatty acid composition in plasma and the metabolic syndrome. *Curr Opin Lipidol* 14: 15–19.

Villéger L, Abifadel M, Allard D et al. 2002. The UMD-LDLR database: Additions to the software and 490 new entries to the database. *Hum Mutat* 20: 81–87.

Vimaleswaran KS, Radha V, Ghosh S, Majumder PP, Rao MR, Mohan V. 2010. A haplotype at the UCP1 gene locus contributes to genetic risk for type 2 diabetes in Asian Indians (CURES-72). *Met Syndr Relat Disord* 8: 63–68.

Vogler GP, Sorensen TI, Stunkard AJ, Srinivasan MR, Rao DC. 1995. Influences of genes and shared family environment on adult body mass index assessed in an adoption study by a comprehensive path model. *Int J Obes Relat Metab Disord* 19: 40–45.

Vohl M-C, Lamarche B, Pascot A et al. 1999. Contribution of the cholesteryl ester transfer protein gene TaqIB polymorphism to the reduced plasma HDL-cholesterol levels found in abdominal obese men with the features of the insulin resistance syndrome. *Int J Obes Relat Metab Disord* 23: 918–925.

Vozarova B, Fernandez-Real JM, Knowler WC et al. 2003. The interleukin-6 (−174) G/C promoter polymorphism is associated with type-2 diabetes mellitus in Native Americans and Caucasians. *Hum Genet* 112: 409–413.

Wallerath T, Deckert G, Ternes T et al. 2002. Resveratrol, a polyphenolic phytoalexin present in red wine, enhances expression and activity of endothelial nitric oxide synthase. *Circulation* 106: 1652–1658.

Waterer GW, Wunderink RG. 2003. Science review: Genetic variability in the systematic inflammatory response. *Crit Care* 7: 308–314.

Watkins RE, Maglich JM, Moore LB et al. 2003. A crystal structure of human PXR complex with the St. John's wort compound hyperforin. *Biochemistry* 42: 1430–1438.

Weinreb O, Mandel S, Amit T, Youdim MB. 2004. Neurological mechanisms of green tea polyphenols in Alzheimer's and Parkinson's diseases. *J Nutr Biochem* 15: 506–516.

Weyer C, Funahashi T, Tanaka S et al. 2001. Hypoadiponectinemia in obesity and type 2 diabetes: Close association with insulin resistance and hyperinsulinemia. *J Clin Endocrinol Metab* 86: 1930–1935.

White RP, Deane C, Vallance P, Markus HS. 1998. Nitric oxide synthase inhibition in humans reduces cerebral blood flow but not the hyperemic response to hypercapnia. *Stroke* 29: 467–472.

Willson TM, Wahli W. 1997. Peroxisome proliferator-activated receptor agonists. *Curr Opin Chem Biol* 1: 235–241.

Wishelow CE, Hitman GAA, Raafar I, Bottzzo GF, Sachs JA. 1996. The effect of TNF*β gene polymorphism on TNF-alpha and -beta secretion in patients with insulin dependent diabetes mellitus and healthy controls. *Eur J Immunogenet* 23: 425–435.

Wittrup HH, Tybjarg-Hansen A, Nordestgaard BG. 1999. Lipoprotein lipase mutations, plasma lipids and lipoproteins, and risk of ischemic heart disease: A meta-analysis. *Circulation* 99: 2901–2907.

Woo SL, Lidsky AS, Güttler F, Chandra T, Robson KJ. 1983. Cloned human phenylalanine hydroxylase gene allows prenatal diagnosis and carrier detection of classical phenylketonuria. *Nature* 306: 151–155.

Wu B, Takahashi J, Fu M et al. 2005. Variants of calpain-10 gene and its association with type 2 diabetes mellitus in a Chinese population. *Diabetes Res Clin Pract* 68: 155–61.

Wu JH, Wen MS, Lo SK, Chern MS. 1994. Increased frequency of apolipoprotein B signal peptide sp24/24 in patients with coronary artery disease. General allele survey in the population of Taiwan and comparison with Caucasians. *Clin Genet* 5: 250–254.

Yamada Y, Metoki N, Yoshida H et al. 2006. Genetic risk for ischemic and hemorrhagic stroke. *Arterioscler Thromb Vasc Biol* 26: 1920–1925.

Yamauchi T, Kamon J, Minokoshi Y et al. 2002. Adiponectin stimulates glucose utilization and fatty-acid oxidation by activating AMP-activated protein kinase. *Nat Med* 8: 1288–1295.

Yamauchi T, Kamon J, Waki H et al. 2001. The fat-derived hormone adiponectin reverses insulin resistance associated with both lipoatrophy and obesity. *Nat Med* 7: 941–946.

Yasruel Z, Cianflone K, Sniderman AD, Rosenbloom M, Walsh M, Rodriguez MA. 1991. Effect of acylation stimulating protein on the triacylglycerol synthetic pathway of human adipose tissue. *Lipids* 26: 495–499.

Yen CJ, Beamer BA, Negri C et al. 1997. Molecular scanning of the human peroxisome proliferator activated receptor gamma (hPPAR gamma) gene in diabetic Caucasians: Identification of a Pro12Ala PPAR gamma 2 missense mutation. *Biochem Biophys Res Commun* 241: 270–274.

Yen FT, Deckelbaum RJ, Mann CJ, Marcel YL, Milne RW, Tall AR. 1989. Inhibition of cholesteryl ester transfer protein activity by monoclonal antibody. Effects of cholesteryl ester formation and neutral lipid mass transfer in human plasma. *J Clin Invest* 83: 2018–2024.

Young SG. 1990. Recent progress in understanding apolipoprotein B. *Circulation* 82: 1574–1594.

Zhao SP, Yang J, Li J, Dong SZ, Wu ZH. 2008. Effect of niacin on LXRalpha and PPAR gamma expression and HDL-induced cholesterol efflux in adipocytes of hypercholesterolemic rabbits. *Int J Cardiol* 124: 172–178.

Zeisel HS. 2012. Diet–gene interactions underlie metabolic individuality and influence brain development: Implications for clinical practice derived from studies on choline metabolism. *Ann Nutr Metab* 60 (Suppl. 3): 19–25.

Zhang D-L, Li J-S, Jiang Z-W, Yu B-J, Tang X-M and Zheng H-M. 2003. Association of two polymorphism of tumor necrosis factor gene with acute biliary pancreatitis. *World J Gastroenterol* 9: 824–828.

Ziouzenkova O, Perrey S, Asatryan L et al. 2003. Lipolysis of triglyceride-rich lipoproteins generates PPAR ligands: Evidence for an antiinflammatory role for lipoprotein lipase. *Proc Natl Acad Sci USA* 100: 2730–2735.

Section II

Early Life Nutrition and Metabolic
Syndrome in Children and Adolescents

6 Early Life Nutrition and Metabolic Syndrome

Hitomi Okubo and Siân Robinson

CONTENTS

6.1 INTRODUCTION

Metabolic syndrome (MetS) describes a cluster of risk factors (including central obesity, insulin resistance, glucose intolerance, dyslipidemia, and hypertension) that predispose to type 2 diabetes and cardiovascular disease. Because of the growing prevalence of obesity, which contributes strongly to the risk of MetS, rates are increasing in both developed and developing countries. However, despite its public health importance, the etiology of MetS is still poorly understood.

In the past two decades, there has been growing recognition that the risk of developing cardiovascular disease and other chronic conditions is not just determined by factors acting in adult life, but is also influenced by events much earlier in the lifecourse (Barker et al. 1989, 1993, 2002). There is consistent evidence from epidemiological studies, as well as clinical and experimental findings, to suggest that nutrition and growth in early life play a powerful role in influencing the susceptibility to develop specific degenerative conditions in adulthood. Adopting a lifecourse approach is therefore needed to understand the etiology of adult disease. This chapter focuses specifically on the role of nutrition at critical periods during development in early life, and summarizes the epidemiological evidence regarding its relation with development of MetS.

6.2 EARLY LIFE NUTRITION AND LIFELONG HEALTH

Studies carried out in the 1960s by McCance and Widdowson showed that manipulation of the plane of nutrition in early life had lifelong consequences. Rats raised in small litters, and therefore overfed during a critical period in early postnatal life, grew faster than control rats. They remained larger throughout life, even though normal feeding was established after the period of lactation (McCance 1962). Overfeeding in rats during early postnatal life was subsequently shown to lead to permanent overweight with increased fat deposition, hyperleptinemia, hyperinsulinemia, impaired glucose tolerance, hypertriglyceridemia, and an increased systolic blood pressure in later life (You et al. 1990, Plagemann et al. 1992, 1999). Interestingly, nutritional manipulation after weaning did not have such permanent effects, suggesting that there is a critical period within which variations in postnatal nutrition impact on body composition and later physiological function. This phenomenon linking early nutrition to long-term health was described as *programming* in 1991 by Lucas, and defined as a process whereby a stimulus or insult acting at a critical period of development results in permanent change in the structure and function of the organism (Lucas 1991).

The first evidence of programming in human subjects came from epidemiological studies that linked low birth weight to adverse long-term health effects (Barker et al. 1989). Impaired fetal growth, evidenced by lower birth weight, was shown to be associated with a greater risk of cardiovascular disease, and type 2 diabetes (Barker et al. 1989, Hales et al. 1991, Hales and Barker 1992). These associations, which have now been reproduced in a range of studies across the world, are not explained by differences in gestational age at birth, or by adult lifestyle (Godfrey 2006). This evidence led to the *fetal origins of adult disease* hypothesis, which proposes that environmental factors, such as suboptimal nutrition, *in utero*, trigger metabolic adaptations and program an increased risk of chronic disease in later life. Although the initial hypothesis identified the intrauterine period as being of key importance, it is now clear that there are additional windows of sensitivity, including the period in early postnatal life. In particular, developing organs and physiological systems may be permanently altered in response to the reduced availability of nutrients. These adaptations, while advantageous for short-term survival, may be detrimental to health in later life. Rapidly growing organs are more vulnerable to reduced availability of nutrients, and different organs have different critical periods of development (Roseboom et al. 2006, Rinaudo and Wang 2012). Hence, the timing of the suboptimal nutrition in early life is key in determining the long-term consequences and future risk of disease.

Exploring the factors that affect growth and development in the period from fetal life to infancy may provide new insights into understanding the etiology of MetS and strategies for its prevention. This chapter considers the evidence that links maternal nutrition, fetal growth, and nutrition in infancy/early childhood to the components of MetS in later life.

6.3 MATERNAL NUTRITIONAL FACTORS AND OFFSPRING'S METABOLIC DISEASE

There is now a body of experimental evidence showing that maternal nutritional manipulation in the period extending from conception to lactation can cause permanent changes in body composition and physiology of the offspring (Rinaudo and Wang 2012). Variation in maternal nutrition, in terms of body composition and dietary intake, may affect fetal development both by having direct effects on substrate availability to the fetus as well as indirect effects via changes in placental function and structure (Godfrey 2002).

6.3.1 BEFORE PREGNANCY

Animal models have provided clear evidence to link maternal nutrition before pregnancy to components of the MetS. For example, maternal undernutrition during the period of conception and implantation has been shown to cause hypertension and cardiovascular dysfunction in the offspring (Langley-Evans et al. 1996b, Kwong et al. 2000, Edwards and McMillen 2002, Fernandez-Gonzalez et al. 2004, Gardner et al. 2004). Emerging data from animal studies suggest that overnutrition may also be important—with long-term effects on offspring body composition (Lillycrop and Burdge 2011). In comparison, little is known about maternal influences acting before pregnancy on the risk of MetS in humans. One study has shown an association between prepregnancy maternal obesity and the risk of MetS in children aged 6–11 years (Bony et al. 2005). Using the modified criteria of the National Cholesterol Education Program, children who were born to obese mothers (prepregnancy BMI > 27.3 kg/m²) had a twofold increase in risk of developing MetS (HR = 1.81; 95% CI: 1.03, 3.19; $P = 0.039$) compared with the offspring of mothers whose weight was in the recommended range. A number of studies have examined relationships with individual components of the MetS. The most consistent pattern of association is that high maternal weight before pregnancy is associated with a greater risk of adiposity in the offspring and positively associated with a range of cardiovascular risk factors (Jeffery et al. 2006, Fraser et al. 2010, Tsadok et al. 2011).

Although maternal dietary intake is the key in influencing maternal nutritional status and body composition before pregnancy, there is currently no evidence to link variations in dietary intake in the preconception period to risk of MetS in the offspring.

6.3.2 During Pregnancy

6.3.2.1 Excessive Gestational Weight Gain

To date there have been no studies that have directly addressed the link between gestational weight gain (GWG) and risk of MetS in the offspring, but a number of studies have examined effects on its components. Most commonly, studies have examined associations with offspring adiposity and have reported positive associations with offspring body mass index in childhood (Moreira et al. 2007, Oken et al. 2007, Wrotniak et al. 2008, Dello Russo et al. 2013, Ensenauer et al. 2013), adolescence (Oken et al. 2008), and adulthood (Mamun et al. 2009). Recent studies have shown that exceeding the recommended GWG range, defined by the U.S. Institute of Medicine (IOM) in 2009, has an adverse impact on the risk of childhood overweight and adiposity (Crozier et al. 2010, Ensenauer et al. 2013). However, suboptimal GWG has also been linked to offspring adiposity (Stuebe et al. 2009, Crozier et al. 2010). There is some evidence of associations between excess GWG and clusters of the components of the MetS. For example, according to data from mother-offspring pairs from a U.K. prospective cohort study, women who gained more weight than IOM recommended range during gestation were more likely to have offspring who had greater adiposity, higher levels of systolic blood pressure, C-reactive protein, and interleukin-6 levels and lower high-density lipoprotein cholesterol (HDL-cholesterol) and apoprotein A levels (Fraser et al. 2010). In this study, among children of women who gained insufficient weight (below IOM recommended range), cardiovascular risk factors tended to be similar to those of offspring of women whose weight gain was adequate (Fraser et al. 2010). Further analyses demonstrated that weight gain in early pregnancy (0–14 weeks) was incrementally associated with increased offspring adiposity, but in midpregnancy (14–36 weeks), only high weight gain (>500 g/week) was associated with increased offspring adiposity. GWG from 14 to 36 weeks of gestation was positively and linearly associated with adverse lipid and inflammatory profiles in offspring, largely because of the association of GWG with offspring adiposity (Fraser et al. 2010). A very recent study of 12,775 children (aged 2–9 years) from the 8 European countries (Dello Russo et al. 2013) also showed that indices of glucose metabolism, namely, blood glucose, serum insulin and HOMA index, and systolic blood pressure significantly increased across tertiles of GWG, but these differences were no longer evident after adjustment for current child BMI. These studies suggest that higher maternal GWG (especially excessive weight gain) is likely to influence offspring metabolic status in early life, mainly throughout its effects on adiposity. A number of recent and ongoing studies have addressed ways to limit gestational weight gain (e.g., the UPBEAT trial, Poston et al. 2013). Future follow-up of these children will be important to determine the effects of maternal GWG on short- and long-term metabolic outcomes.

6.3.2.2 Dietary Intake in Pregnancy

In animal models, dietary manipulation in pregnancy can result in small offspring that display shortened life-span (Aihie-Sayer et al. 2001, Ozanne and Hales 2004), obesity (Breier et al. 2001, Ozanne et al. 2004), hypertension (Vickers et al. 2000, Langley-Evans et al. 2003), diabetes (Vickers et al. 2000), and alteration in the hypothalamic–pituitary–adrenal (HPA) axis (Langley-Evans et al. 1996a, Hawkins et al. 1999). For example, maternal high fat or cholesterol overfeeding during pregnancy and lactation in rodents resulted in an offspring phenotype that closely resembled the human MetS (Langley-Evans 1996, Armitage et al. 2005). In humans, the evidence is less clear, although important findings regarding the role of maternal diet, at specific stages of gestation, on subsequent disease susceptibility have come from follow-up studies of children who were conceived and born during periods of famine. One of the most well known of these is the Dutch Hunger Winter. This was a period of extreme food shortage in the western Netherlands that occurred during the last 5–6 months of World War II (November 1944–May 1945) (Painter et al. 2005, Roseboom et al. 2006). The mean caloric rations during the famine were as low as 400–800 kcal/day. In an analysis of a subset of 783 men and women aged 57–59 years, exposure to famine during gestation was not associated with the risk of the MetS (OR = 1.2; 95% CI: 0.9, 1.7) in adult life (de Rooij et al. 2007), but it was associated with higher triacylglycerol concentration (0.1 g/L; 95% CI: 0.0, 0.2 g/L) and lower HDL-cholesterol concentration (men only: −0.08 mmol/L; 95% CI: −0.14, 0.00 mmol/L). According to the series of the studies on the Dutch famine, exposure during early gestation was associated with a preference for fatty foods, a more atherogenic lipid profile, increased risk for coronary heart disease, disturbed blood coagulation, obesity (women only), increased stress responsiveness, and increased risk of breast cancer (women only) compared to those not exposed to the famine. In comparison, famine exposure in mid gestation was associated with obstructive airways disease and microalbuminuria (Painter et al. 2005, Roseboom et al. 2006).

The analyses from the study of the Chinese famine (1959–1961) have provided further insights on the long-term consequences of famine exposure during early life. In contrast to the Dutch famine, which was a period of acute starvation of a well-nourished population (Painter et al. 2005, Roseboom et al. 2006), the Chinese famine was a period of chronic starvation principally affecting an impoverished rural population. In comparison with unexposed subjects, men and women who had been exposed to the famine during fetal life had a markedly higher risk of developing MetS in adulthood (OR = 3.13; 95% CI: 1.24, 7.89). These associations were even stronger if they had a Western dietary pattern, characterized by high consumption of meat, eggs, dairy, sugary beverages, edible oils, and low intake of vegetables, or were overweight (BMI ≥ 24 kg/m^2) (Li et al. 2011). This finding is consistent with the hypothesis that it is the *mismatch* between the early and later environments that is particularly important in determining the risk of metabolic disease in later life (Gluckman et al. 2005, Godfrey et al. 2007). In another study from the Chinese famine, gender differences in the consequence of famine exposure during fetal life were described. Women who were exposed in fetal life had a significantly higher risk of MetS than control women who were unexposed (OR = 1.87; 95% CI: 1.15, 3.012), but this association was not observed in men (Zheng et al. 2012). These gender differences in the effects of famine and the multiple mechanisms involved are not clearly understood. Apart from differences in sex steroids, these effects may reflect variations in activation of the HPA axis, different responses to oxidative stress, faster postnatal growth rate, mortality selection, and cultural backgrounds (e.g., son preference) (Zheng et al. 2012). Further investigations are needed to elucidate the biological processes that underlie the gender difference in susceptibility to develop MetS.

6.3.2.3 Other Maternal Factors

Although most epidemiological research of early life influences on MetS in the offspring has focused on the adverse programming effects of inadequate nutrition, there is also evidence that maternal overnutrition may result in an offspring phenotype susceptible to the MetS. Gestational diabetes mellitus (GDM) and maternal gestational hyperglycemia may be associated with glucose oversupply to the fetus, which has long-term effects. Children of GDM mothers are more likely to be overweight or obese, and to have greater central adiposity (Boney et al. 2005, Wright et al. 2009, Egeland and Meltzer 2010, West et al. 2011, Yessoufou and Moutairou 2011). Lower insulin sensitivity and/or impaired glucose tolerance, high blood pressure, and dyslipidemia are also more common among children born to women with GDM (Tam et al. 2008, Egeland and Meltzer 2010, West et al. 2011, Yessoufou and Moutairou 2011). For example, Boney et al. demonstrated that large-for-gestational-age (LGA) offspring born to diabetic mothers were at significant risk of developing childhood MetS (Boney et al. 2005). The risk of developing MetS from 6 to 11 years of age was not different between children who were LGA and appropriate-for-gestational age (AGA) offspring of mothers without GDM, but was significantly different between LGA and AGA offspring of the mothers with GDM, with a 3.6-fold greater risk among LGA children by 11 years. In another study examining the combined effects of maternal GDM and child weight status, Chandler-Laney et al. showed that intrauterine exposure to gestational diabetes was associated with greater central adiposity and insulin secretion and lower HDL-cholesterol in the children, irrespective of current weight status (Chandler-Laney et al. 2012). Additionally, they observed an interaction of overweight with intrauterine exposure to GDM, which suggests that excess weight gain among children of GDM mothers may further contribute to metabolic risk.

6.4 BIRTH WEIGHT, SIZE AT BIRTH, AND METABOLIC SYNDROME

Birth weight is commonly used in epidemiological studies as a summary measure of intrauterine growth, and an indirect marker of the fetal nutritional environment. A substantial body of epidemiological literature documents an association of birth weight with later MetS. The first studies from historical cohorts were published in 1993 (Barker et al. 1993). Among 407 men born in Hertfordshire, England, between 1920 and 1930, and 266 men and women born in Preston, between 1935 and 1943, Barker et al. found that the risk of developing syndrome X was more than 10 times greater among men whose birth weight were less than 2.95 kg (6.5 lb) when compared with men whose birth weights were more than 4.31 kg (9.5 lb) (Barker et al. 1993). There have been many subsequent studies, and Silveira and Horta (2008) and Nobili et al. (2008) reviewed those published data. In the review of studies published from 1996 to 2006, Silveira and Horta found that 9 out of 11 reported an inverse relationship between birth weight and MetS (Silveira and Horta 2008). This was evident after adjusting for socioeconomic factors, and unlikely to be explained by differences in adult lifestyle. The pooled odds ratio of low birth weight (>2.5 kg) in comparison with normal birth weight (<3.4 kg) on the development of MetS was 2.53 (95% CI: 1.57, 4.08).

6.5 POSTNATAL NUTRITION AND METABOLIC SYNDROME

6.5.1 POSTNATAL GROWTH

Catch-up growth, following intrauterine restriction, is generally defined as a growth with a velocity above the statistical limits of normality for age during a defined period of time, and most often, is characterized by disproportionately higher rate of fat gain relative to lean tissue gain (Saenger et al. 2007). The effect of faster gain throughout childhood on health outcomes, particularly the risk of obesity, later in life has been reported in different populations and at different ages. The effect has been seen for faster linear growth and for growth from as early as the first month of life (Lanigan and Singhal 2009).

For example, in a Swedish birth cohort, faster weight gain in the first 6 months was shown to be independently associated with a clustered metabolic risk score (comprising fasting TG, HDL-cholesterol, glucose and insulin concentrations, blood pressure, and waist circumference) in adolescents (at the age of 17 years) (Ekelund et al. 2007). More recently, a study from the Netherlands has shown consistent findings: greater gains in weight relative to length SD score in the first 3 months of life were associated with an increased prevalence of MetS (OR=2.51; 95% CI: 1.20, 5.25) and higher prevalence of low HDL-cholesterol (OR=1.49; 95% CI: 1.06, 2.08), increased level of CRP, and lower insulin sensitivity at 21 years. The timing of the period of rapid growth is of key importance, as in this study, there were no associations with weight gain during later periods in the first year of life (Kerkhof et al. 2012). There is also other observational evidence to highlight the effects of rapid weight gain in the first 3 month of life on risk of MetS (Ekelund et al. 2007, Khuc et al. 2012). Overall variation in the pattern of early growth could have major implications for long-term MetS risk and cardiovascular risk factors.

These effects do not appear to be confined to infants who were small at birth, as faster early growth has been shown to be associated with cardiovascular disease risk factors such as insulin resistance in term infants of both normal (Dunger et al. 2007) and low birth weight (Soto et al. 2003). In the latter study, infants with faster weight gain were found to have low insulin sensitivity at 1 year of age, raising the possibility that insulin resistance could be the first component of the MetS to emerge, and may in turn be implicated in the development of other cardiovascular risk factors.

6.5.2 INFANT FEEDING—BREASTFEEDING VERSUS FORMULA MILK

The earlier findings described that rapid growth in postnatal life is linked to the MetS and its components, and highlights the role of early nutrition as a potential determinant of disease risk in later life. It is increasingly recognized that nutrition in early postnatal life may have long-term, as well as short-term, physiological effects in both human and animal studies (Plagemann et al. 2012); in particular, breastfeeding may protect against development of MetS and related diseases.

6.5.2.1 Types of Milk Feeding

To date, there has only been one published study that has investigated the effect of breastfeeding on risk of MetS. In a small study of healthy Chilean adolescents aged 17 years ($n=357$), longer duration of exclusive breastfeeding (≥90 days) was associated with a lower MetS risk score (calculating by the average of five variables of HDL-cholesterol, the mean of the systolic and diastolic blood pressure measurements, waist circumference, fasting serum triglyceride and glucose) ($\beta=-0.16$, 95% CI: −0.29, −0.04) (Khuc et al. 2012). Importantly, this effect was independent of weight gain in the first three months of life, suggesting that the protective effect of breastfeeding on the risk of MetS was mediated by other factors associated with breastfeeding such as differences in the composition of breast milk (Bartok and Ventura 2009, Koletzko et al. 2009). However, to address this, further data are needed.

6.5.2.2 Types of Milk Feeding and Components of Metabolic Syndrome

In contrast to the lack of evidence to link infant nutrition to risk of MetS, a large number of epidemiological studies have been published showing long-term effects of breastfeeding on individual components of the MetS. Several comprehensive meta-analyses have been published (Owen et al. 2002, 2003, 2005a,b, 2006, 2008, Arenz et al. 2004, Harder et al. 2005, Martin et al. 2005, Plagemann and Harder 2005).

A meta-analysis of 9 studies of children, all from developed countries, with over 69,000 participants showed that breast-fed infants had a 22% lower risk of obesity in childhood (5–18 years) compared to formula-fed infants (pooled adjusted OR=0.78; 95% CI: 0.71, 0.85) (Arenz et al. 2004). The protective association of breastfeeding was confirmed in three other meta-analyses of children and adults (Owen et al. 2005a,b, Plagemann and Harder 2005). According to a meta-analysis of 17 studies based in developed countries conducted by Harder and colleagues, they estimated that the risk of overweight was reduced by 4% for each month of breastfeeding (OR=0.96 per month of breastfeeding; 95% CI: 0.94, 0.98) and this effect lasted up to 9 months regardless of the definition of overweight and age at follow-up (Harder et al. 2005). Although the association between early feeding and later body size may be influenced by confounding factors, such as maternal body size, maternal smoking, and socioeconomic factors, causality is strongly supported by the existence of a dose–response relation between the duration of breastfeeding and later over-weight risk.

Whilst obesity is regarded as the central pathogenic component of cardiometabolic disease, other studies have been published on the long-term effects of breastfeeding on single compo-nents of the MetS. Much attention has been paid to the effect of marked differences in early exposure to dietary cholesterol when comparing breast and formula-fed infants, because breast milk has higher cholesterol content. A meta-analysis that examined the lifecourse relationship between infant feeding and blood cholesterol showed that mean total cholesterol concentrations in breast-fed subjects, compared with those in formula-fed subjects, were higher in infancy ($\Delta = 0.64$ mmol/L; 95% CI: 0.49, 0.79), similar in childhood ($\Delta = 0.00$ mmol/L; 95% CI: −0.07, 0.07), but lower in adult life ($\Delta = -0.18$ mmol/L; 95% CI: −0.30, −0.06) (Owen et al. 2002). Patterns for LDL-cholesterol were similar to those for total cholesterol. Additionally, the influence of exclusive breastfeeding, examined in a subsequent meta-analysis, showed a clear difference in total choles-terol level in adulthood ($\Delta = -0.15$ mmol/L; 95% CI: −0.23, −0.06) compared with formula feeding (Owen et al. 2008).

Type and patterns of infant milk feeding have been linked to offspring blood pressure. Owen et al. summarized 24 studies published between 1972 and 2002 examining the association between infant feeding and blood pressure in later life. The pooled mean difference in systolic blood pres-sure (SBP) was 1.1 mmHg (95% CI: 0.4, 1.8) lower in adults who had been breast-fed compared with those formula-fed; effects on diastolic blood pressure were much smaller (Owen et al. 2003). A further meta-analysis showed a similar result (pooled difference in SBP: −1.4 mmHg; 95% CI: −2.2, −0.6) (Martin et al. 2005). The protective effect of breastfeeding on later blood pressure was also supported by the results of a randomized trial. Singhal et al. examined blood pressure in 216 adolescents who were born preterm, and observed that subjects randomized to receive breast milk had a lower mean arterial blood pressure than those who were fed with preterm formula milk (Singhal et al. 2001).

Finally, in terms of associations with the risk of type 2 diabetes in later life, a meta-analysis of 7 studies with 76,744 subjects showed that breastfeeding, compared with formula feeding, in infancy reduced the subsequent risk of type 2 diabetes by nearly 40% (OR = 0.61; 95% CI: 0.44, 0.85) (Owen et al. 2006). There is no strong evidence to suggest effects of early feeding on adult levels of blood glucose and blood insulin, although further data are needed.

The variety of protective effects of breastfeeding may be attributable to differences in the com-position of breast milk, as compared to formula milk. In particular, the amino acid, protein, choles-terol, and PUFA contents, as well as immunoglobulins, nucleotide, or hormones present in breast milk may be important. In addition, early exposure to breast milk may have long-term effects on dietary behavior, such as self-regulation of energy intake, taste preferences, and food choice, in later life (behavioral programming) (Cohen et al. 1994, Dewey 2001, Mennella 2009, Robinson et al. 2013). Robinson et al. demonstrated that early dietary exposures have lifelong influence on food choice, and showed that older men and women (aged 59–73 years) who had been breast-fed in infancy, compared with the other types of milk feeding, tended to have a higher score of healthy dietary pattern, characterized by greater consumption of fruit, vegetables, whole meal cereals and oily fish, and low consumption of refined cereals, sugar, and full-fat dairy products (Robinson et al. 2013). Further investigation of the adult dietary patterns of breast-fed and bottle-fed subjects is needed to confirm the long-term effects of breastfeeding on food preferences and dietary patterns.

6.5.3 Infant Feeding—Weaning and Introduction of Solid Foods

In comparison with types of milk feeding in infancy, there is little knowledge about the influence of variation in weaning practice on long-term health. The age at introduction of solid foods and the type of first solids are often documented, but the assessment of food and nutrient intake during later infancy is less common (Cohen et al. 1994, Marriott et al. 2008, 2009), and the process of weaning is not well described. Some observational studies from Western countries have found that early introduction of solid food was associated with greater weight gain in infancy (Lin et al. 2013), and early introduction of solid food has been positively associated with later obesity in early preschool children (Brophy et al. 2009, Hawkins et al. 2009), especially in formula-fed infants (Huh et al. 2011). However, other observational studies did not find any association (Burdette et al. 2006, Neutzling et al. 2009, Schack-Nielsen et al. 2010). An important observation is that weaning practice, including the timing of introduction of solid food, and type of weaning diet is linked to the pattern of milk feeding in earlier infancy (Cohen et al. 1994). Breast-fed babies are commonly introduced to solid foods later than infants who are formula-fed (Noble and Emmett 2006), and factors that related to the duration of breastfeeding, such as maternal education, also influence the nature of the weaning diet (Robinson et al. 2007). Further investigation of the influence of infant nutrition, with consideration of pattern of milk feeding and solid foods, on later risk of MetS is needed.

6.6 SUMMARY

A substantial body of evidence from experimental and epidemiological studies suggests an important influence of nutrition in early life on later risk of metabolic syndrome. In particular, the strongest evidence is for links with poor maternal nutrition, impaired fetal growth, rapid weight gain in early childhood and not being breast-fed. The effects of early nutrition and growth on later metabolic condition may track from childhood to adulthood and amplify with age. Additionally, recent evidence suggests that the long-term consequences of adverse condition during early development may not be limited to one generation, but may lead to poor health in the generations to follow (Drake and Walker 2004, Roseboom and Watson 2012). Although animal studies provide multiple biologically plausible mechanisms for nutritional programming in early life, many questions remain unresolved. A better understanding of the programming mechanisms is a prerequisite for developing early life interventions to prevent metabolic syndrome and type 2 diabetes in the future.

REFERENCES

Aihie Sayer, A., Dunn, R., Langley-Evans, S., and Cooper, C. 2001. Prenatal exposure to a maternal low protein diet shortens life span in rats. *Gerontology* 47: 9–14.

Arenz, S., Rückerl, R., Koletzko, B., and von Kries, R. 2004. Breast-feeding and childhood obesity—A systematic review. *Int J Obes Relat Metab Disord* 28: 1247–1256.

Armitage, J. A., Taylor, P. D., and Poston, L. 2005. Experimental models of developmental programming: Consequences of exposure to an energy rich diet during development. *J Physiol* 565: 3–8.

Barker, D. J., Eriksson, J. G., Forsén, T., and Osmond, C. 2002. Fetal origins of adult disease: Strength of effects and biological basis. *Int J Epidemiol* 31: 1235–1239.

Barker, D. J., Hales, C. N., Fall, C. H., Osmond, C., Phipps, K., and Clark, P. M. 1993. Type 2 (non-insulin-dependent) diabetes mellitus, hypertension and hyperlipidaemia (syndrome X): Relation to reduced fetal growth. *Diabetologia* 36: 62–67.

Barker, D. J., Winter, P. D., Osmond, C., Margetts, B., and Simmonds, S. J. 1989. Weight in infancy and death from ischaemic heart disease. *Lancet* 2: 577–580.

Bartok, C. J. and Ventura, A. K. 2009. Mechanisms underlying the association between breastfeeding and obesity. *Int J Pediat Obes* 4: 196–204.

Boney, C. M., Verma, A., Tucker, R., and Vohr, B. R. 2005. Metabolic syndrome in childhood: Association with birth weight, maternal obesity, and gestational diabetes mellitus. *Pediatrics* 115: e290–e296.

Breier, B. H., Vickers, M. H., Ikenasio, B. A., Chan, K. Y., and Wong, W. P. 2001. Fetal programming of appetite and obesity. *Mol Cell Endocrinol* 185: 73–79.

Brophy, S., Cooksey, R., Gravenor, M. B. et al. 2009. Risk factors for childhood obesity at age 5: Analysis of the Millennium Cohort Study. *BMC Public Health* 9: 467.

Burdette, H. L., Whitaker, R. C., Hall, W. C., and Daniels, S. R. 2006. Breastfeeding, introduction of complementary foods, and adiposity at 5 y of age. *Am J Clin Nutr* 83: 550–558.

Chandler-Laney, P. C., Bush, N. C., Granger, W. M., Rouse, D. J., Mancuso, M. S., and Gower, B. A. 2012. Overweight status and intrauterine exposure to gestational diabetes are associated with children's metabolic health. *Pediatr Obes* 7: 44–52.

Cohen, R. J., Brown, K. H., Canahuati, J., Rivera, L. L., and Dewey, K. G. 1994. Effects of age of introduction of complementary foods on infant breast milk intake, total energy intake, and growth: A randomised intervention study in Honduras. *Lancet* 344: 288–293.

Crozier, S. R., Inskip, H. M., Godfrey, K. M. et al. 2010. Weight gain in pregnancy and childhood body composition: Findings from the Southampton Women's Survey. *Am J Clin Nutr* 91: 1745–1751.

de Rooij, S. R., Painter, R. C., Holleman, F., Bossuyt, P. M., and Roseboom, T. J. 2007. The metabolic syndrome in adults prenatally exposed to the Dutch famine. *Am J Clin Nutr* 86: 1219–1224.

Dello Russo, M., Ahrens, W., De Vriendt, T. et al. 2013. Gestational weight gain and adiposity, fat distribution, metabolic profile, and blood pressure in offspring: The IDEFICS project. *Int J Obes (Lond)* 37: 914–919.

Dewey, K. G. 2001. Nutrition, growth, and complementary feeding of the breastfed infant. *Pediatr Clin North Am* 48: 87–104.

Drake, A. J. and Walker, B. R. 2004. The intergenerational effects of fetal programming: Non-genomic mechanisms for the inheritance of low birth weight and cardiovascular risk. *J Endocrinol* 180: 1–16.

Dunger, D. B., Salgin, B., and Ong, K. K. 2007. Session 7: Early nutrition and later health early developmental pathways of obesity and diabetes risk. *Proc Nutr Soc* 66: 451–457.

Edwards, L. and McMillen, I. 2002. Periconceptual nutrition programs development of the cardiovascular system in the fetal sheep. *Am J Physiol Regul Integr Comp Physiol* 283: 669–679.

Egeland, G. M. and Meltzer, S. J. 2010. Following in mother's footsteps? Mother–daughter risks for insulin resistance and cardiovascular disease 15 years after gestational diabetes. *Diabet Med* 27: 257–265.

Ekelund, U., Ong, K. K., Linné, Y. et al. 2007. Association of weight gain in infancy and early childhood with metabolic risk in young adults. *J Clin Endocrinol Metab* 92: 98–103.

Ensenauer, R., Chmitorz, A., Riedel, C. et al. 2013. Effects of suboptimal or excessive gestational weight gain on childhood overweight and abdominal adiposity: Results from a retrospective cohort study. *Int J Obes (Lond)* 37: 505–512.

Fernández-Gonzalez, R., Moreira, P., Bilbao, A. et al. 2004. Long-term effect of in vitro culture of mouse embryos with serum on mRNA expression of imprinting genes, development, and behavior. *Proc Natl Acad Sci USA* 101: 5880–5885.

Fraser, A., Tilling, K., Macdonald-Wallis, C. et al. 2010. Association of maternal weight gain in pregnancy with offspring obesity and metabolic and vascular traits in childhood. *Circulation* 121: 2557–2564.

Gardner, D. S., Pearce, S., Dandrea, J. et al. 2004. Peri-implantation undernutrition programs blunted angiotensin II evoked baroreflex responses in young adult sheep. *Hypertension* 43: 1290–1296.

Gluckman, P. D., Hanson, M. A., Spencer, H. G., and Bateson, P. 2005. Environmental influences during development and their later consequences for health and disease: Implications for the interpretation of empirical studies. *Proc Biol Sci* 272: 671–677.

Godfrey, K. M. 2002. The role of the placenta in fetal programming—A review. *Placenta* 23(Suppl A): S20–S27 (Review).

Godfrey, K. M. 2006. The "Developmental Origins" hypothesis: Epidemiology. In *Developmental Origins of Health and Disease–A Biomedical Perspective*. P. D. Gluckman and M. A. Hanson, eds. Cambridge University Press, Cambridge, U.K., pp. 6–32.

Godfrey, K. M., Lillycrop, K. A., Burdge, G. C., Gluckman, P. D., and Hanson, M. A. 2007. Genetic mechanisms and the mismatch concept of the developmental origins of health and disease. *Pediatr Res* 61: 5R–10R.

Hales, C. N. and Barker, D. J. 1992. Type 2 (non-insulin-dependent) diabetes mellitus: The thrifty phenotype hypothesis. *Diabetologia* 35: 595–601.

Hales, C. N., Barker, D. J., Clark, P. M. et al. 1991. Fetal and infant growth and impaired glucose tolerance at age 64. *BMJ* 303(6809): 1019–1022.

Harder, T., Bergmann, R., Kallischnigg, G., and Plagemann, A. 2005. Duration of breastfeeding and risk of overweight: A meta-analysis. *Am J Epidemiol* 162: 397–403.

Hawkins, P., Steyn, C., McGarrigle, H. H. et al. 1999. Effect of maternal nutrient restriction in early gestation on development of the hypothalamic–pituitary–adrenal axis in fetal sheep at 0.8–0.9 of gestation. *J Endocrinol* 163: 553–561.

Hawkins, S. S., Cole, T. J., Law, C., and Millennium Cohort Study Child Health Group. 2009. An ecological systems approach to examining risk factors for early childhood overweight: Findings from the UK Millennium Cohort Study. *J Epidemiol Community Health* 63: 147–155.

Huh, S. Y., Rifas-Shiman, S. L., Taveras, E. M., Oken, E., and Gillman, M. W. 2011. Timing of solid food introduction and risk of obesity in preschool-aged children. *Pediatrics* 127: e544–e551.

Jeffery, A. N., Metcalf, B. S., Hosking, J., Murphy, M. J., Voss, L. D., and Wilkin, T. J. 2006. Little evidence for early programming of weight and insulin resistance for contemporary children: EarlyBird Diabetes Study report 19. *Pediatrics* 118: 1118–1123.

Kerkhof, G. F., Leunissen, R. W., and Hokken-Koelega, A. C. 2012. Early origins of the metabolic syndrome: Role of small size at birth, early postnatal weight gain, and adult IGF-I. *J Clin Endocrinol Metab* 97: 2637–2643.

Khuc, K., Blanco, E., Burrows, R. et al. 2012. Adolescent metabolic syndrome risk is increased with higher infancy weight gain and decreased with longer breast feeding. *Int J Pediatr* 2012: 478610.

Koletzko, B., von Kries, R., Monasterolo, R. C. et al. 2009. Can infant feeding choices modulate later obesity risk? *Am J Clin Nutr* 89: S1502–S1508.

Kwong, W., Wild, A., Roberts, P., Willis, A., and Fleming, T. 2000. Maternal undernutrition during the preimplantation period of rat development causes blastocyst abnormalities and programming of postnatal hypertension. *Development* 127: 4195–4202.

Langley-Evans, S. C. 1996. Intrauterine programming of hypertension in the rat: nutrient interactions. *Comp Biochem Physiol A Physiol* 114: 327–333.

Langley-Evans, S. C., Gardner, D. S., and Jackson, A. A. 1996a. Maternal protein restriction influences the programming of the rat hypothalamic–pituitary–adrenal axis. *J Nutr* 126: 1578–1585.

Langley-Evans, S. C., Langley-Evans, A. J., and Marchand, M. C. 2003. Nutritional programming of blood pressure and renal morphology. *Arch Physiol Biochem* 111: 8–16.

Langley-Evans, S. C., Welham, S. J., Sherman, R. C., and Jackson, A. A. 1996b. Weanling rats exposed to maternal low-protein diets during discrete periods of gestation exhibit differing severity of hypertension. *Clin Sci* 91: 607–615.

Lanigan, J. and Singhal, A. 2009. Early nutrition and long-term health: A practical approach. *Proc Nutr Soc* 68: 422–429.

Li, Y., Jaddoe, V. W., Qi, L. et al. 2011. Exposure to the Chinese famine in early life and the risk of metabolic syndrome in adulthood. *Diabetes Care* 34: 1014–1018.

Lillycrop, K. A. and Burdge, G. C. 2011. Epigenetic changes in early life and future risk of obesity. *Int J Obes (Lond)* 35: 72–83.

Lin, S. L., Leung, G. M., Lam, T. H., and Schooling, C. M. 2013. Timing of solid food introduction and obesity: Hong Kong's "Children of 1997" birth cohort. *Pediatrics* 131: e1459–e1467.

Lucas, A. 1991. Programming by early nutrition in man. *Ciba Found Symp* 156: 38–50.

Mamun, A. A., O'Callaghan, M., Callaway, L., Williams, G., Najman, J., and Lawlor, D. A. 2009. Associations of gestational weight gain with offspring body mass index and blood pressure at 21 years of age: Evidence from a birth cohort study. *Circulation* 119: 1720–1727.

Marriott, L. D., Inskip, H. M., Borland, S. E. et al. 2009. What do babies eat? Evaluation of a food frequency questionnaire to assess the diets of infants aged 12 months. *Public Health Nutr* 12: 967–972.

Marriott, L. D., Robinson, S. M., Poole, J. et al. 2008. What do babies eat? Evaluation of a food frequency questionnaire to assess the diets of infants aged 6 months. *Public Health Nutr* 11: 751–756.

Martin, R. M., Gunnell, D., and Smith, G. D. 2005. Breastfeeding in infancy and blood pressure in later life: Systematic review and meta-analysis. *Am J Epidemiol* 161: 15–26.

McCance, R. A. 1962. Food, growth and time. *Lancet* 2: 621–626.

Mennella, J. A. 2009. Flavour programming during breastfeeding. *Adv Exp Med Biol* 639: 113–120.

Moreira, P., Padez, C., Mourao-Carvalhal, I., and Rosado, V. 2007. Maternal weight gain during pregnancy and overweight in Portuguese children. *Int J Obes* 31: 608–614.

Neutzling, M. B., Hallal, P. R., Araújo, C. L. et al. 2009. Infant feeding and obesity at 11 years: Prospective birth cohort study. *Int J Pediatr Obes* 4: 143–149.

Nobili, V., Alisi, A., Panera, N., and Agostoni, C. 2008. Low birth weight and catch-up-growth associated with metabolic syndrome: A ten year systematic review. *Pediatr Endocrinol Rev* 6: 241–247.

Noble, S. and Emmett, P. 2006. Differences in weaning practice, food and nutrient intake between breast- and formula-fed 4-month-old infants in England. *J Hum Nutr Diet* 19: 303–313.

Oken, E., Rifas-Shiman, S. L., Field, A. E., Frazier, A. L., and Gillman, M. W. 2008. Maternal gestational weight gain and offspring weight in adolescence. *Obstet Gynecol* 112: 999–1006.

Oken, E., Taveras, E. M., Kleinman, K. P., Rich-Edwards, J. W., and Gillman, M. W. 2007. Gestational weight gain and child adiposity at age 3 years. *Am J Obstet Gynecol* 196: 322.

Owen, C. G., Martin, R. M., Whincup, P. H., Davey-Smith, G., Gillman, M. W., and Cook, D. G. 2005a. The effect of breastfeeding on mean body mass index throughout life: A quantitative review of published and unpublished observational evidence. *Am J Clin Nutr* 82: 1298–1307.

Owen, C. G., Martin, R. M., Whincup, P. H., Smith, G. D., and Cook, D. G. 2005b. Effect of infant feeding on the risk of obesity across the life course: A quantitative review of published evidence. *Pediatrics* 115: 1367–1377.

Owen, C. G., Martin, R. M., Whincup, P. H., Smith, G. D., and Cook, D. G. 2006. Does breastfeeding influence risk of type 2 diabetes in later life? A quantitative analysis of published evidence. *Am J Clin Nutr* 84: 1043–1054.

Owen, C. G., Whincup, P. H., Gilg, J. A., and Cook, D. G. 2003. Effect of breast feeding in infancy on blood pressure in later life: Systematic review and meta-analysis. *BMJ* 327: 1189–1195.

Owen, C. G., Whincup, P. H., Kaye, S. J. et al. 2008. Does initial breastfeeding lead to lower blood cholesterol in adult life? A quantitative review of the evidence. *Am J Clin Nutr* 88: 305–314.

Owen, C. G., Whincup, P. H., Odoki, K., Gilg, J. A., and Cook, D. G. 2002. Infant feeding and blood cholesterol: A study in adolescents and a systematic review. *Pediatrics* 110: 597–608.

Ozanne, S. E. and Hales, C. N. 2004. Lifespan: Catch-up growth and obesity in male mice. *Nature* 427: 411–412.

Ozanne, S. E., Lewis, R., Jennings, B. J, and Hales, C. N. 2004. Early programming of weight gain in mice prevents the induction of obesity by a highly palatable diet. *Clin Sci* 106: 141–145.

Painter, R. C., Roseboom, T. J., and Bleker, O. P. 2005. Prenatal exposure to the Dutch famine and disease in later life: An overview. *Reprod Toxicol* 20: 345–352.

Plagemann, A. and Harder T. 2005. Breast feeding and the risk of obesity and related metabolic diseases in the child. *Metab Syndr Relat Disord* 3: 222–232.

Plagemann, A., Harder, T., Rake, A. et al. 1999. Perinatal elevation of hypothalamic insulin, acquired malformation of hypothalamic galaninergic neurons, and syndrome x-like alterations in adulthood of neonatally overfed rats. *Brain Res* 836: 146–155.

Plagemann, A., Harder, T., Schellong, K., Schulz, S., and Stupin, J. H. 2012. Early postnatal life as a critical time window for determination of long-term metabolic health. *Best Pract Res Clin Endocrinol Metab* 26: 641–653.

Plagemann, A., Heidrich, I., Götz, F., Rohde, W., and Dörner, G. 1992. Obesity and enhanced diabetes and cardiovascular risk in adult rats due to early postnatal overfeeding. *Exp Clin Endocrinol* 99: 154–158.

Poston, L., Briley, A. L., Barr, S. et al. 2013. Developing a complex intervention for diet and activity behaviour change in obese pregnant women (the UPBEAT trial); assessment of behavioural change and process evaluation in a pilot randomised controlled trial. *BMC Pregn Childbirth* 13: 148.

Rinaudo, P. and Wang, E. 2012. Fetal programming and metabolic syndrome. *Annu Rev Physiol* 74: 107–130.

Robinson, S., Marriott, L., Poole, J. et al. 2007. Dietary patterns in infancy: The importance of maternal and family influences on feeding practice. *Br J Nutr* 98: 1029–1037.

Robinson, S., Ntani, G., Simmonds, S. et al. 2013. Type of milk feeding in infancy and health behaviours in adult life: Findings from the Hertfordshire Cohort Study. *Br J Nutr* 109: 1114–1122.

Roseboom, T., de Rooij, S., and Painter, R. 2006. The Dutch famine and its long-term consequences for adult health. *Early Hum Dev* 82: 485–491.

Roseboom, T. J. and Watson, E. D. 2012. The next generation of disease risk: Are the effects of prenatal nutrition transmitted across generations? Evidence from animal and human studies. *Placenta* 33(Suppl 2): e40–e44.

Saenger, P., Czernichow, P., Hughes, I., and Reiter, E. O. 2007. Small for gestational age: Short stature and beyond. *Endocr Rev* 28: 219–251.

Schack-Nielsen, L., Sørensen, T. I., Mortensen, E. L., and Michaelsen, K. F. 2010. Late introduction of complementary feeding, rather than duration of breastfeeding, may protect against adult overweight. *Am J Clin Nutr* 91: 619–627.

Silveira, V. M. and Horta, B. L. 2008. Birth weight and metabolic syndrome in adults: Meta-analysis. *Rev Saude Publica* 42: 10–18.

Singhal, A., Cole, T. J., and Lucas, A. 2001. Early nutrition in preterm infants and later blood pressure: Two cohorts after randomised trials. *Lancet* 357: 413–419.

Soto, N., Bazaes, R. A., Peña, V. et al. 2003. Insulin sensitivity and secretion are related to catch-up growth in small-for-gestational-age infants at age 1 year: Results from a prospective cohort. *J Clin Endocrinol Metab* 88: 3645–3650.

Stuebe, A. M., Forman, M. R., and Michels, K. B. 2009. Maternal-recalled gestational weight gain, pre-pregnancy body mass index, and obesity in the daughter. *Int J Obes (Lond)* 33: 743–752.

Tam, W. H., Ma, R. C., Yang, X. et al. 2008. Glucose intolerance and cardiometabolic risk in children exposed to maternal gestational diabetes mellitus in utero. *Pediatrics* 122: 1229–1234.

Tsadok, M. A., Friedlander, Y., Paltiel, O. et al. 2011. Obesity and blood pressure in 17-year-old offspring of mothers with gestational diabetes: Insights from the Jerusalem Perinatal Study. *Exp Diabetes Res* 2011: 906154.

Yessoufou, A. and Moutairou, K. 2011. Maternal diabetes in pregnancy: Early and long-term outcomes on the offspring and the concept of "metabolic memory". *Exp Diabetes Res* 2011: 218598.

You, S., Götz, F., Rohde, W., and Dörner, G. 1990. Early postnatal overfeeding and diabetes susceptibility. *Exp Clin Endocrinol* 96: 301–306.

Vickers, M., Breier, B., Cutfield, W., Hofman, P., and Gluckman, P. 2000. Fetal origins of hyperphagia, obesity, and hypertension and postnatal amplification by hypercaloric nutrition. *Am J Physiol Endocrinol Metabol* 279: E83–E87.

Wrotniak, B. H., Shults, J., Butts, S., and Stettler, N. 2008. Gestational weight gain and risk of overweight in the offspring at age 7 y in a multicenter, multiethnic cohort study. *Am J Clin Nutr* 87: 1818–1824.

West, N. A., Crume, T. L., Maligie, M. A., and Dabelea, D. 2011. Cardiovascular risk factors in children exposed to maternal diabetes in utero. *Diabetologia* 54: 504–507.

Wright, C. S., Rifas-Shiman, S. L., Rich-Edwards, J. W., Taveras, E. M., Gillman, M. W., and Oken, E. 2009. Intrauterine exposure to gestational diabetes, child adiposity, and blood pressure. *Am J Hypertens* 22: 215–220.

Zheng, X., Wang, Y., Ren, W. et al. 2012. Risk of metabolic syndrome in adults exposed to the great Chinese famine during the fetal life and early childhood. *Eur J Clin Nutr* 66: 231–236.

7 Metabolic Syndrome in Children and Adolescents

Jacqueline Isaura Alvarez Leite

CONTENTS

7.1 INTRODUCTION

Overweight and obesity in childhood and adolescents are important health concerns. The increasing prevalence of youth obesity has led to an intensive effort to identify children and adolescents at risk for development of adult cardiovascular disease (CVD) and type 2 diabetes mellitus (T2DM).

The metabolic syndrome (MetS) represents a cluster of potent risk factors for T2DM, dyslipidemia, and atherosclerosis. Fat distribution seems to be the metabolic link among MetS and those disorders.

MetS is now as much a pediatric condition as an adult condition (Weiss et al. 2013). The prevalence of pediatric MetS in 12–19-year olds varies according to age and gender and body mass index (BMI), and has been increasing in most of studies in the last two decades (Kelly et al. 2011). Studies in different countries have shown the prevalence of MetS in both eutrophic or obese children/adolescents (Atabek et al. 2006, Bokor et al. 2008, Braga-Tavares and Fonseca 2010, Caceres et al. 2008, Calcaterra et al. 2008, Chung et al. 2013, Cizmecioglu et al. 2009, Di Bonito et al. 2010, Ekelund et al. 2009, Eyzaguirre et al. 2012, Ford et al. 2008, Fu et al. 2007, Halley et al. 2007, Kiess et al. 2009, Molnar 2004, Papoutsakis et al. 2012, Park et al. 2010, Pirkola et al. 2008, Reinehr et al. 2009, Sangun et al. 2011, Santibhavank 2007, Sartorio et al. 2007, Sen et al. 2008, Seo et al. 2008, Taha et al. 2009, Tailor et al. 2010, Wang et al. 2013). The results of some of them are shown in Table 7.1.

In a systematic analysis including 85 publications (Friend et al. 2013), the median prevalence of MetS in whole populations was 3.3% (range 0%–19.2%), in overweight children was 11.9% (range 2.8%–29.3%), and in obese populations was 29.2% (range 10%–66%). It also confirmed the higher prevalence in obese compared to eutrophic and overweight children as well as in boys compared to girls.

TABLE 7.1

Prevalence of MetS in Children and Adolescents according to the Atherosclerosis Treatment Panel III, The International Diabetes Federation Definitions in Different Populations

Reference	Number of Children and Adolescents	Criteria of MetS	Prevalence
Agirbasli et al. (2006)	1,385 Turkish	ATP III	2.2% all students, 21% (OV/OB)
Atabek et al. (2006)	169 Obese	WHO	27.2%
Barzin et al. (2012)	5,439 Tehran	Cook et al.	Boys: 16.5%; Girls: 6%
Bokor et al. (2008)	1,241 European	de Ferranti et al., WHO, ATP, and IDF	37.4%, 31.4%, 20.3%, and 16.4%
Braga-Tavares and Fonseca (2010)	237 Overweight/obese	Cook et al., de Ferranti et al., IDF	15.6%, 34.9%, and 8.9%
Brufani et al. (2011)	439 Italian obese	ATP III	21% adolescents, 12% children
Bueno et al. (2006)	103 Spanish	Cook and de Ferranti	29.9% and 50%
Caceres et al. (2008)	61 Obese Bolivian	ATP III	36%
Calcaterra et al. (2008)	191 Caucasian obese	ATP III	13.9% all, 12% moderate, 31% severe obesity
Chen et al. (2012)	19,593 Chinese	IDF	0.2% normal, 10% moderate obese, 27.6% severe obesity
Chung et al. (2013)	5,652 Korean	—	1998: 7.5%; 2001: 9.8%; 2005: 10.9%; 2008: 6.7%
Cizmecioglu et al. (2009)	2,491 Schoolchildren	IDF	2.3%
Cook et al. (2003)	2,430 U.S.	ATP III	4.2% (all), 28.7% (overweight)
Di Bonito et al. (2010)	724 Children	Cook et al., Jolliffe et al., and de Ferranti et al.	11%, 12%, and 24%
Duncan et al. (2004)	991 U.S. American	ATP III	6.4% (all), 32.1% (overweight)
Ekelund et al. (2009)	3193 European	IDF	0.2% (10 year old), 1.4% (15 year old)
Eyzaguirre et al. (2012)	1,002 Patients overweight/obese	Boney criteria	6.6%
Ford et al. (2005)	2,014	IDF	4.5%
Fu et al. (2007)	348 Obese	ATP III	10.3%
Halley Castillo et al. (2007)	1,366 Mexicans	ATP III	Age 7–9 years: 31.5; age 10–14 years: 36.3; age 15–19 years: 25.8
Mehairi et al. (2013)	1,018 Emirati	IDF	13% all (21% boys, 6% girls)
Nasreddine et al. (2012)	263 Lebaneses	IDF	21.2% of obese, 3.8% of overweight, and 1.2% of normal weight
Papoutsakis et al. (2012)	1,138 Greek	IDF	0.7%
Pirkola et al. (2008)	5,665 Finnish adolescent	IDF	2.4%
Rizzo et al. (2013)	321 Brazilian	IDF	18%
Sangun et al. (2011)	614 Turkish obese child and adolescent	WHO, Cook and IDF	39%, 34%, and 33%

(*Continued*)

TABLE 7.1 (*Continued*)
Prevalence of MetS in Children and Adolescents according to the Atherosclerosis Treatment Panel III, The International Diabetes Federation Definitions in Different Populations

Reference	Number of Children and Adolescents	Criteria of MetS	Prevalence
Wang et al. (2013)	373 Chinese school children	IDF and ATP III	*IDF*: 14.3% (obese), 3.7% (overweight); *ATP III*: 32.3% (obese), 8.4% (overweight)
Xu et al. (2012)	8,764 Chinese	IDF	0.05% (normal), 0.9% (overweight), 6.6% (obese)
Hosseinpanah et al. (2013)	1,424 Iranian	IDF	13.3%, 14.6% after 10 years follow-up

Sources: de Ferranti, S.D. et al., *Circulation*, 110, 2494, 2004; Wilding, J., *BMJ*, 346, f2777, 2013.

MetS, metabolic syndrome; ATP III, The Atherosclerosis Treatment Panel III; IDF, The International Diabetes Federation; WHO, World Health Organization; OV/OB, prevalence in overweight and obese individuals.

7.2 RISK FACTORS

The predisposing factors for the development of MetS in childhood or adolescence have been studied. Several studies have shown that gestational and birth characteristics are related to trends of MetS (Brufani et al. 2011, Cetin et al. 2013, Efstathiou et al. 2012, Guerrero-Romero et al. 2010, Harville et al. 2012). However, the results were not conclusive. High maternal BMI and low levels of cardiorespiratory fitness and physical activity have been described as independent contributors of the MetS (Ekelund et al. 2009). Some studies analyzing children at high risk for MetS concluded that the coexistence of low birth weight, abdominal adiposity, small head circumference, and parental history of overweight or obesity may be useful for detection of children at risk of developing MetS in adolescence (Brufani et al. 2011, Efstathiou et al. 2012). Babies born large for gestational age also are at high risk of MetS and its components, mainly abnormal lipid profile (low HDL-C and high triglycerides) (Eyzaguirre et al. 2012, Guerrero-Romero et al. 2010). A study analyzing 1262 children and adolescents aged 7–15 years found that both low and high birth weight, in combination with positive familiar history of diabetes in the maternal branch, were determinants of MetS in adolescence (Guerrero-Romero et al. 2010).

In the Prediction of Metabolic Syndrome in Adolescence (PREMA) study, the factors independently associated with MetS in adolescence were birth weight and birth head circumference <10th percentile and parental overweight or obesity (Efstathiou et al. 2012).

Another study based on longitudinal data from "The Muscatine Study" examined the association between childhood/adolescent risk factor measurements and the MetS in adulthood (Burns et al. 2009). The results showed that about 30% of women and 37.0% of men were classified as having MetS. In those with MetS, BMI, systolic blood pressure, and triglycerides were higher at the time they participated in the school survey examinations. The BMI was the strongest childhood predictor of adult MetS, suggesting that early identification of at risk children may reduce the burden of atherosclerotic CVD and T2DM in adults (Burns et al. 2009).

7.3 DEFINITION

Until now, there is no consensus regarding the definition and consequently, the diagnosis of MetS in children and adolescents. The diagnosis of MetS before adulthood is controversial because of the lack of standardized diagnostic criteria and dichotomous definitions.

Certainly, the main core of MetS in adults (high blood pressure, obesity, dyslipidemia, insulin resistance) will be part of this pediatric diagnosis. Efforts have been done to define which cut-offs must be adopted for that. Components used to define childhood MetS are the same used in adult (waist circumference [WC], fasting glucose, blood pressure, high-density lipoprotein cholesterol [HDL-C], and triglycerides) with modifications to be adapted to childhood pattern. The Atherosclerosis Treatment Panel (ATP) III released in 2001 has done the basis for several definitions of MetS in adolescents. According to ATP III, MetS is defined for adults when three or more of the following alterations are present: WC higher than 102 and 88 cm for men and women, respectively; high systolic (>130 mm/Hg) or diastolic (>85 mm/Hg) blood pressure (BP); HDL-C levels lower than 40 for men and 50 mg/dL for women, hypertriglyceridemia (>1.7 mmol/L or 150 mg/dL), and fasting glucose higher than 5.6 mmol/L or 100 mg/dL. The first definition of MetS for the children and adolescents was proposed by Cook et al. (2003) and was based on NCEP/ATP III criteria (Table 7.2). In 2004, Weiss et al. defined MetS using BMI instead WC as obesity assessment, a range of glycemia between 140 and 200 mg/dL and the 95th percentile for TAG and blood pressure and the 5th percentile as cut point for HDL-C.

In 2007, the International Diabetes Federation (IDF) publishes its definition for children and adolescents (Zimmet et al. 2007). According to IDF, the high WC is a sine qua non condition for the diagnosis of MetS and uses different WC cut points based on ethnicity. According to the IDF definition, for a child to be defined as having MetS, she/he must have increased WC plus any two of the following four factors: raised fasting glycemia or previously diagnosed type 2 diabetes, raised blood triglycerides, reduced HDL-C, raised blood pressure, or specific treatment for those abnormalities (Table 7.3).

WC is an independent factor linked to insulin resistance, dyslipidemia, and high blood pressure in children and adolescents, and the presence of abdominal fat is a key point in the establishment of insulin resistance (Biltoft and Muir 2009, Bostanci et al. 2012, Brufani et al. 2011, Caceres et al. 2008, Lee et al. 2008, Marcovecchio and Chiarelli 2013). However, the main differences between IDF and ATP III definitions are that in the former, the presence of higher WC is an obligatory condition for MetS diagnosis, although in ATP III, it has the same importance as that of the other four components. American Heart Association (AHA) MetS definition was published in 2005 and

---

TABLE 7.2

Definitions of the MetS before the International Diabetes Federation Definition

	Components of the MetS[a]				
Definition	Obesity	Blood Pressure	TAG	HDL	Glucose Intolerance
Cook et al. (2003)	WC ≥ 90th p. for age and sex specific	≥ 90th p. for age, sex, and height specific	≥ 110 mg/dL	≤ 40 mg/dL	Fasting glucose ≥ 110 mg/dL
de Ferranti et al. (2004)	WC ≥ 75th p. for age, sex, and ethnicity	≥ 90th p. for age and sex	≥ 110 mg/dL	≤ 50 mg/dL	Fasting glucose ≥ 110 mg/dL
Cruz and Goran (2004)	WC ≥ 90th p. for age, sex, and ethnicity	≥ 90th p. for age and sex	90th p. for age and sex	10th p. for age and sex	Impaired glucose tolerance
Ford et al. (2005)	WC ≥ 90th p. for age, sex, and ethnicity	≥ 90th p. for age and sex	≥ 110 mg/dL	≤ 40 mg/dL	Fasting glucose ≥ 110 mg/dL
Weiss et al. (2004)	BMI z score ≥ 2 for age and sex	95th p. for age and sex	≥ 95th p. for age and sex	≤ 5th p. for age and sex	Glycemia ≥ 140 mg/dL but ≤ 200 mg/dL at 2 h

BMI, Body mass index; WC, waist circumference; TAG, triglycerides; p., percentile; HDL, high-density lipoprotein.

[a] The presence of three or more components defines MetS.

TABLE 7.3

International Diabetes Federation Definition of MetS in Children and Adolescents

	Age 6–10 Years	Age 10–16 Years	>16 Years
Waist circumference	90th percentile	90th percentile or adult cutoff if lower	Europid: >94 cm (♂), >80 cm (♀); South and Southeast Asian, Japanese, South and Central Americans: >90 cm (♂), >80 cm (♀).
Triglycerides		>1.7 mmol/L (150 mg/dL)	>1.7 mmol/L (>150 mg/dL)[a]
HDL		<1.03 mmol/L (40 mg/dL)	<1.03 mmol/L (40 mg/dL) in (♂) and <1.29 mmol/L (50 mg/dL) in (♀)[a]
Blood pressure		Systolic > 130 or diastolic > 85 mmHg	Systolic > 130 or diastolic > 85 mmHg[a]
Blood glucose		>5.6 mmol/L (100 mg/dL) or T2DM	>5.6 mmol/L (100 mg/dL) or T2DM

Source: International Diabetes Federation, The IDF consensus definition of the MetS in children and adolescents, 2007, 24p. HDL, high-density lipoprotein.

[a] Or specific treatment. MetS cannot be diagnosed, but further measurements should be made if there is a family history of MetS, type 2 diabetes mellitus (T2DM), dyslipidemia, CVD, hypertension and/or obesity.

considered diagnostic criteria similar to ATP III. In AHA definition, the presence of abdominal obesity is not mandatory. In 2009, IDF and AHA representatives held discussions to harmonize the definitions of MetS in adults (Alberti et al. 2009). After that, IDF accepted that abdominal obesity should be one of the diagnosis criteria adjusting its MetS definition.

The early detection and immediate treatment of MetS in the childhood is vital to prevent the comorbidities linked to this syndrome in adulthood, particularly CVD and T2DM. In pediatric definition, the adoption of percentiles as cut point of WC is due to the constant changes in body composition of children and adolescents. The percentiles of WC in the specific age groups and the increase of WC are present when values are higher than 90th or 95th (Table 7.4).

The IDF definition of MetS considers three age groups: 6–10 years, 10–16 years, and older than 16 years. Children younger than 6 years were not considered, because the data are insufficient to define the components of MetS. In children between 6 and 10 years with obesity or WC above 90th percentile, weight reduction should be counseled and the child assessed frequently. In children aged 10 years or older, MetS can be diagnosed by high WC associated to, at least, two of the follow clinical features: elevated triglycerides, low HDL-C, high blood pressure, or increased plasma glucose. The specific cut points for triglycerides, HDL-C, and high blood pressure were not defined. In those older than 16 years, the IDF adult criteria can be used. The earlier definition is dated before the 2009 statement, when IDF still considered WC a mandatory component for MetS in adult population.

In children or adolescents, the use of a continuous MetS score rather than the dichotomous definition could be more appropriate for epidemiological research (Eisenmann 2008, Marcovecchio and Chiarelli 2013, Okosun et al. 2010). This score allows each subject to have a continuous value with lower and higher values, indicating a better and poorer MetS profile, respectively.

MetS score can be calculated using standardized residuals (z score) of mean arterial BP (MAP), triglyceride, glucose, WC, and HDL-C (Eisenmann 2003, 2007, 2008). Some authors claim that risk score is a more robust measure of MetS than a categorical measure, because it is more sensitive and has a statistical power higher than categorical measures of MetS (Okosun et al. 2010). However, future research is needed to validate the use of continuous MetS score in children and adolescents (Eisenmann 2008).

TABLE 7.4

Percentiles of Waist Circumference in Children and Adolescents

Age (Years)	Percentile for Boys				Percentile for Girls			
	10th	50th	75th	90th	10th	50th	75th	90th
6	51.2	56.3	60.7	67.1	50.5	56.3	60.4	66.2
7	52.9	58.5	63.4	70.6	52.0	58.4	63.0	69.4
8	54.6	60.7	66.2	74.1	53.5	60.4	65.6	72.6
9	56.3	62.9	68.9	77.6	55.0	62.5	68.2	75.8
10	58.0	65.1	71.6	81.0	56.5	64.6	70.8	78.9
11	59.7	67.2	74.4	84.5	58.1	66.6	73.4	82.1
12	61.4	69.4	77.1	88.0	59.6	68.7	76.0	85.3
13	63.1	71.6	79.8	91.5	61.1	70.8	78.6	88.5
14	64.8	73.8	82.6	95.0	62.6	72.9	81.2	91.7
15	66.5	76.0	85.3	98.4	64.1	74.9	83.8	94.8
16	68.2	78.1	88.0	101.9	65.6	77.0	86.4	98.0

Source: Data from Fernandez, J.R. et al., *J. Pediatr.*, 145, 439, 2004.
Values are presented in cm.

7.4 PREVENTION AND TREATMENT

Since MetS is more frequently seen in the obese population, prevention of obesity is the most important strategy for preventing MetS. Subject in risk of MetS can be initially identified after measure of body weight and WC, and results of blood pressure, lipid profile, and fasting glycemia will confirm the diagnosis of MetS. Risk factors associated to the MetS that are excluded from the definition such and hyperuricemia, insulinemia, and inflammatory markers (adipokines, C reactive protein, etc.) could be also evaluated (DeBoer et al. 2011, Denzer et al. 2003, Ford et al. 2005, 2007, Gilardini et al. 2006, Koulouridis et al. 2010, Kong et al. 2013, Lambert et al. 2004, Tang et al. 2010). Familial history of diabetes, hypertension, and obesity will highlight the genetic and environmental risks in which child/adolescent is engaged; in case of confirmation of MetS, drive the main treatment strategies.

As for adults, the aim of the treatment is to reverse or reduce the cluster components of MetS and the risk of T2DM and infarct (Urakami et al. 2009). Reduction of central adiposity is the main goal of treatment.

Children and adolescents have the advantage of a higher metabolism and constant development, permitting a faster weight control without altering drastically the amount of food intake. However, for this same reason, these individuals need a closer follow-up to avoid nutritional deficiencies or inadequacies that will compromise body development.

Treatment of MetS is primordially composed by diet and exercises. According to IDF (2007), primary management for MetS includes moderate energy restriction (sufficient to acquire a 5%–10% of weight loss in the first year), increase of physical activity, and improvement of food quality (International Diabetes Federation 2007).

With regard to obesity and weight loss, IDF in 2007 (Barlow 2007) established recommendations on the assessment, prevention, and treatment of child and adolescent with overweight and obesity.

Familial history for obesity, type 2 diabetes, hypertension, and other CVDs (especially infarct or stroke) should be assessed mainly in all overweight and obese children/adolescents.

In children/adolescents whose BMI is above 85th percentile, the treatment is based in stages. The first stage aims to maintain the actual body weight. The child should be allowed to self-regulate his or her meals and avoid restrictive behaviors. It is expected that the BMI decreases as the child grows. The main recommendations are to improve food quality, stimulate physical activity, reduce sedentary habits, and reinforce the familial support for those dietary behaviors. Physical activity should be performed at least 1 h a day, and diet should contain five servings of fruits and vegetables and have limited sugar-sweetened beverages. Sedentary behavior should be avoided or limited, which includes hours of television and/or DVD watching, and playing video games. Nowadays, electronic games that need subject physical movement are permitted, mainly in case of children with limited or restricted access to open-air activities.

If the goals of stage 1 were not reached after 6 months, the stage 2 should be initiated. In this stage, the goal is still weight maintenance that results in decreases in BMI. Recommendations are based on the implementation of a structured weight management with improvement of dietary and physical activity behaviors. A dietary plan containing adequate distribution of nutrient divided in daily meals and snacks should be prescribed. The intake of a diet rich in calcium, high in fiber, and calories from fat, carbohydrate, and protein proportions for age according to dietary reference intakes is also recommended. Weight loss, if present, should be restricted to 1 lb (0.45 kg)/month in children aged 2–11 years, or an average of 2 lb (1 kg)/week in older.

Stage 3 is indicated if the goals of body weight were not reached after a period of 6 months. It comprises a comprehensive multidisciplinary protocol. Although physicians or health care professional, at this level of intervention, could conduct the previous stages, the patient should optimally be referred to a multidisciplinary obesity care team with a special involvement of primary care-givers/families for behavioral modification in children under 12 years. This category food and activity monitoring and development of short-term diet are recommended. As in stage 2, the goal is the weight maintenance or gradual weight loss until BMI is less than 85th percentile. Weight loss rate should not exceed 1 lb (0.45 kg)/month in children aged 2–5 years, or 2 lb (1 kg)/week in older ones.

The stage 4 (tertiary care protocol) is recommended for children/adolescents presenting BMI > 99th percentile or 95th percentile with significant comorbidities, which were not successful with stage 3 recommendations. Children/adolescents should be assisted by professionals with expertise in childhood obesity. The therapy includes continued diet and activity counseling and meal replacement and very-low-calorie diets, if necessary. Medication and surgery could be indicated only for older adolescents and in very specific cases individuals. The recommendations based on BMI and age range are presented in Table 7.5.

TABLE 7.5
Goals of Obesity and Overweight Treatments on Stage 4 Based on BMI and Age Range

Percentile BMI	6–11 Years	12–18 Years
85th–94th	Weight maintenance until BMI <85th or slowing of weight gain	Weight maintenance until BMI <85th or slowing of weight gain
95th–98th	Body weight should be maintained until BMI <85th or gradual weight loss (1 lb (0.45 kg)/month)[a]	Weight loss until BMI <85th. Weight loss 2 lb (1 kg)/week[a]
>99th	Weight loss of 2 lb (1 kg)/week[a]	Weight loss of 2 lb (1 kg)/week[a,b]

Source: Barlow, S.E., *Pediatrics*, 120(Suppl 4), S164, 2007.

BMI, body mass index.

[a] Greater weight loss should be avoided and the causes of excessive weight loss investigated.

[b] Primary care physicians and other allied healthcare providers may begin treatment with stages 1, 2, or 3 as indicated based on patient's/family's readiness to change.

The Expert Panel on Integrated Guidelines for Cardiovascular Health and Risk Reduction in Children and Adolescents in 2011 published its recommendations for prevention and treatment of MetS. The presence in children/adolescents of any combination of multiple risk factors for CVD should intensify the lifestyle modification related to overweight/obesity. In turn, in the presence of obesity, evaluation of all other cardiovascular risk factors including family history of premature CVD), hypertension, dyslipidemia, diabetes mellitus (DM), and tobacco exposure should be carried out. If the obesity is associated to any other major cardiovascular risk factor, an intensive program for weight reduction should be started and specific pharmacologic therapy assessed. Special attention should be given to the evaluation for T2DM, liver disorders, and left ventricular and hypoventilation syndrome.

7.4.1 DIETARY STRATEGIES

Diet is the core of treatment of MetS and its components in both adults and children/adolescents (Casazza et al. 2009, de la Iglesia et al. 2014). Diet composition keeps the same macronutrient distribution recommended for health population that contains about 55%, 15%, and 30% of total energy as carbohydrates, proteins, and lipids, respectively. However, one study in adults with MetS showed that a low glycemic load carbohydrates (40% kcal), protein-rich (30% kcal) diet reinforcing, n−3 fatty acids, and natural antioxidant food consumption induced a reduction of BMI and WC that was not seen with isoenergetic standard diet after 4 month of self-monitoring (de la Iglesia et al. 2014). Fiber intake was the dietary component that contributed most to the improvement of anthropometric data.

In fact, fiber intake has been showed as a protective factor of MetS also in children and adolescents (Carlson et al. 2011, Dorgan et al. 2011). Dietary fiber, rather than saturated fat or cholesterol intakes, is associated with MetS in adolescents. These findings suggest that in adolescents, it is more important to emphasize inclusion of fiber-rich, plant-based foods instead of emphasizing on fat- or cholesterol-restricted foods (Carlson et al. 2011).

The increase on fiber consumption should not be accompanied by increases on total carbohydrate intake, since it was positively related to WC, triglyceridemia, and glycemia in a pediatric study (Casazza et al. 2009).

The effect of dietary protein and glycemic index (GI) on MetS in children from eight European centers was investigated (Damsgaard et al. 2013). The results showed that high protein intake reduced WC, lipid profile, blood pressure, and serum insulin, all important components of MetS, suggesting the beneficial effect of high-protein diets. No consistent effect of GI was seen in MetS score. However, another study comparing low glycemic load and low fat diets in a group of 113 obese children (Mirza et al. 2013) showed a similar decreased BMI z score in WC and in systolic blood pressure in both groups.

A recent study compared the Dietary Approaches to Stop Hypertension (DASH) diet and usual dietary advice (UDA) on the MetS in 60 adolescents for 6 weeks (Saneei et al. 2013). DASH diet recommends intake of fruits, vegetables, and low-fat dairy products, limiting saturated fats, total fats, and cholesterol consumption. Intergroup differences in weight, WC, and BMI were not found after 6 weeks of diet introduction. However, compared with the UDA group, adolescents in the DASH group experienced a significant reduction in the prevalence of the MetS and high blood pressure (Saneei et al. 2013).

A large Finnish study evaluated the association of food frequency and physical activity in 2128 individuals aged 3–18 years at the baseline with a follow-up of 27 years (Jaaskelainen et al. 2012). The results showed that the frequency of vegetable consumption in childhood was inversely associated with adult MetS, family history of T2DM, and hypertension. Associations with the other childhood lifestyle factors were not found, suggesting that the higher intake of vegetables in childhood has an important beneficial effect on MetS and its components in adulthood and deserves special concern during infancy.

7.4.2 Physical Activity

Physical activity is defined as body movement produced by contraction of skeletal muscle that increases energy expenditure above a basal level. The influence of diet and physical activity on cardiometabolic outcomes in children has not been clearly established. However, it is also well established that keeping a routine of physical activity increases HDL-C, and reduces body weight, blood pressure, and insulin resistance, all components of MetS. Moreover, it has been shown that physical activity is inversely associated with the risk of MetS in children and adolescents even after age and BMI adjustment (Eisenmann 2007, Ekelund et al. 2009, Jaaskelainen et al. 2012, Kelishadi et al. 2007, Mark and Janssen 2008, Martinez-Gomez et al. 2009).

Activities of a moderate/vigorous intensity are necessary to achieve health benefits. Children and adolescents should maintain moderate-intensity physical activity at least 5 days a week and 20–60 min/day to get most of the health benefits. Nonetheless, some benefits are seen with only 30 min/day. Aerobic exercises should contribute mostly in the exercising period although force activities should be incorporated on at least 2–3 days of the week (Expert Panel on Integrated Guidelines for Cardiovascular Health and Risk Reduction in Children and Adolescents 2011, Janssen and LeBlanc 2010).

Systematic reviews addressed to physical activity and MetS in children and adolescents are less frequent than in adult population. Two systematic reviews and meta-analysis investigating the effect of exercise on visceral adiposity in adult subjects were published in the last years (Ismail et al. 2011, Vissers et al. 2013). In both studies, aerobic exercise of moderate-to-vigorous intensity presented the best effect in reducing central adiposity.

In a recent publication (Gardner et al. 2013), the daily ambulation of 250 children, adolescents, and young adults with and without MetS (10–30 years) was assessed. The results show that children, adolescents, and young adults with MetS ambulate more slowly and take fewer strides throughout the day than those without MetS, and these data are associated with adiposity levels. The clinical significance is that individual with MetS should be encouraged to ambulate faster and for at least 30 additional min/day to reduce body fatness and to improve glucose, triglyceride, and HDL cholesterol profiles (Gardner et al. 2013).

A study analyzing 202 American children aged 7–12 years from different ethnic groups shows that physical activity and sedentary life style were positively associated with HDL-C and glucose concentration, respectively (Casazza et al. 2009).

The role of physical activity improving MetS and its components (WC, triglyceride, HDL-C, and blood pressure) seems to be independent of changes in BMI, as suggested by a study analyzing 4811 Iranian students (Kelishadi et al. 2007).

The association of BMI percentile and leisure-time physical activity with continuous MetS risk score was assessed in 12–17-year-old American children (Okosun et al. 2010). Continuous MetS risk score was calculated using standardized residuals of arterial blood pressure, triglycerides, glucose, WC, and HDL-C.

The authors found that increased BMI percentile and leisure-time physical activity were associated with continuously increased and decreased MetS risk score, respectively. With regard to BMI, there was a gradient of continuously increasing MetS risk score from healthy weight to overweight and obesity categories. A gradient of continuously decreasing MetS risk score from sedentary to moderate and vigorous leisure-time physical activity levels was also observed.

7.4.3 Pharmacotherapy

As mentioned earlier, MetS treatment consists essentially of lifestyle modifications such as diet quality improvement and exercise routine. Drugs and surgery are rarely indicated in children and adolescents. Although there is no pharmacological treatment specific for MetS, MetS components such as hypertension, glucose intolerance or diabetes, and dyslipidemia should be treated with the therapeutic scheme approved for each age group. In those patients in whom hypertension could not be controlled with exercises and DASH diet, drug therapy should be started, according to pediatric guideline for hypertension (Moyer and Force 2013).

Hypertriglyceridemia generally responds well to dietary strategies, weight loss, and lifestyle modifications. Drug therapy is initiated when triglyceridemia reaches 500 mg/dL due to the risk of pancreatitis. Fatty acid ω−3 therapy is able to reduce triglycerides in about 40% and increases HDL-C about 10%–15% (Chan and Cho 2009). In children with severe dyslipidemias, multiple medications should be considered and they should be assisted by a lipid specialist.

Regarding obesity, orlistat is the only antiobesity drug approved for this population. Orlistat is an inhibitor of pancreatic lipase, preventing the absorption of about 30% of dietary fat. Its use is limited by its weak efficacy in reducing weight and by gastrointestinal side effects, mainly steatorrhea. Several groups and government institution have revised the safety of orlistat after reports of severe liver injury. Nonetheless, its use is still approved in United States for adolescents aged 12–18 years old with BMI 2 units higher than the 95th percentile for age and gender (Catoira et al. 2011, Wilding 2013).

Sibutramine is an inhibitor of norepinephrine and serotonin (5-HT) reuptakes that function as a sacietogenic agent. Its main adverse effects are tachycardia, insomnia, elevation of blood pressure, headache, dizziness, dry mouth, and constipation. Sibutramine in the United States was approved to be used in adolescents older than 16 years, but in 2003, it was withdrawn from the American market (Martinez-Gomez et al. 2009). However, the SCOUT trial, a 5-year, randomized, double-blind, placebo-controlled multicenter trial involving 10,744 subjects with obesity, type 2 diabetes, and history of CVD demonstrated a 16% increase in the risk of serious heart events, including nonfatal heart attack, nonfatal stroke, and death, in a group of patients given sibutramine compared with another given placebo. These results were responsible for the prohibition of sibutramine prescription in Europe and other countries. Despite the final results of the SCOUT trial not showing an increased cardiovascular mortality, sibutramine was withdrawn from the U.S. market by FDA in October 2010 and restricted to specific obesity cases in other countries (Di Dalmazi et al. 2013).

Metformin is a safe and well-known oral hypoglycemic drug. Its main effects are reduction of gluconeogenesis, increase of insulin-mediated glucose clearance, and inhibition of fatty acid oxidation. Moreover, it is particularly interesting in MetS, because, besides improving insulin resistance, it has a beneficial effect in reducing BMI and abdominal fat (WC) (Catoira et al. 2011, Iughetti et al. 2011).

7.4.4 BARIATRIC SURGERY

Bariatric surgical procedures comprise procedures such as laparoscopic adjustable gastric banding and Roux-en-Y gastric bypass. The most common surgical techniques are gastric banding, gastric bypass, and sleeve gastrectomy, rather than disabsorptive procedures (Lennerz et al. 2014). The main concern about adolescents is not the efficacy or short-term safety of bariatric surgery but the inability to obtain appropriate consent, the dependence on a caregiver, the risks of elective major surgeries, long-term compliance, and unknown long-term effects. The indications are the same for adults (Lennerz et al. 2014). Adolescents who have reached physical maturity (Tanner stage 4 or 5) and are emotionally and cognitively mature are qualified for bariatric surgery if their BMI ≥50 or ≥40 with comorbidities after confirmation of lack of success of achieving weight loss with all other methods.

7.5 CONCLUSION

MetS is prevalent in childhood and adolescence and is associated with cardiovascular risks as well as in adulthood. The main strategies to prevent or to treat MetS are mainly the combat against overweight and the implementation of good lifestyle. The main strategies to treat metabolic syndrome in children are to introduce healthy dietary habits and to avoid a sedentary life style. Preventing weight gain or maintaining the actual weight is the main goal of most children. Weight loss therapies as well as pharmacological and surgical treatments are reserved for very specific cases.

REFERENCES

Agirbasli, M., Cakir, S., Ozme, S., Ciliv, G. 2006. Metabolic syndrome in Turkish children and adolescents. *Metabolism* 55:1002–1006.

Alberti, K.G., Eckel, R.H., Grundy, S.M. et al. 2009. Harmonizing the metabolic syndrome: A joint interim statement of the International Diabetes Federation Task Force on Epidemiology and Prevention; National Heart, Lung, and Blood Institute; American Heart Association; World Heart Federation; International Atherosclerosis Society; and International Association for the Study of Obesity. *Circulation* 120:1640–1645.

Atabek, M.E., Pirgon, O., Kurtoglu, S. 2006. Prevalence of metabolic syndrome in obese Turkish children and adolescents. *Diabetes Res Clin Pract* 72:315–321.

Barlow, S.E. 2007. Expert committee recommendations regarding the prevention, assessment, and treatment of child and adolescent overweight and obesity: Summary report. *Pediatrics* 120(Suppl 4):S164–S192.

Barzin, M., Hosseinpanah, F., Saber, H., Sarbakhsh, P., Nakhoda, K., Azizi, F. 2012. Gender differences time trends for metabolic syndrome and its components among Tehranian children and adolescents. *Cholesterol* 2012:804643.

Biltoft, C.A., Muir, A. 2009. The metabolic syndrome in children and adolescents: A clinician's guide. *Adolesc Med State Art Rev* 20:109–120, ix.

Bokor, S., Frelut, M.L., Vania, A. et al. 2008. Prevalence of metabolic syndrome in European obese children. *Int J Pediatr Obes* 3(Suppl 2):3–8.

Bostanci, B.K., Civilibal, M., Elevli, M., Duru, N.S. 2012. Ambulatory blood pressure monitoring and cardiac hypertrophy in children with metabolic syndrome. *Pediatr Nephrol* 27(10):1929–1935.

Braga-Tavares, H., Fonseca, H. August 2010. Prevalence of metabolic syndrome in a Portuguese obese adolescent population according to three different definitions. *Eur J Pediatr* 169(8):935–940.

Brufani, C., Fintini, D., Giordano, U., Tozzi, A.E., Barbetti, F., Cappa, M. 2011. Metabolic syndrome in Italian obese children and adolescents: Stronger association with central fat depot than with insulin sensitivity and birth weight. *Int J Hypertens* 2011:257168.

Bueno, G., Bueno, O., Moreno, L.A. et al. 2006. Diversity of metabolic syndrome risk factors in obese children and adolescents. *J Physiol Biochem* 62:125–133.

Burns, T.L., Letuchy, E.M., Paulos, R., Witt, J. 2009. Childhood predictors of the metabolic syndrome in middle-aged adults: The Muscatine study. *J Pediatr* 155(S5):e17–e26.

Caceres, M., Teran, C.G., Rodriguez, S., Medina, M. 2008. Prevalence of insulin resistance and its association with metabolic syndrome criteria among Bolivian children and adolescents with obesity. *BMC Pediatr* 8:31.

Calcaterra, V., Klersy, C., Muratori, T. et al. 2008. Prevalence of metabolic syndrome (MS) in children and adolescents with varying degrees of obesity. *Clin Endocrinol (Oxf)* 68:868–872.

Carlson, J.J., Eisenmann, J.C., Norman, G.J., Ortiz, K.A., Young, P.C. 2011. Dietary fiber and nutrient density are inversely associated with the metabolic syndrome in US adolescents. *J Am Diet Assoc* 111:1688–1695.

Casazza, K., Dulin-Keita, A., Gower, B.A., Fernandez, J.R. 2009. Differential influence of diet and physical activity on components of metabolic syndrome in a multiethnic sample of children. *J Am Diet Assoc* 109:236–244.

Catoira, N., Nagel, M., Di Girolamo, G., Gonzalez, C.D. 2011. Pharmacological treatment of obesity in children and adolescents: Current status and perspectives. *Expert Opin Pharmacother* 11:2973–2983.

Cetin, C., Ucar, A., Bas, F. et al. 2013. Are metabolic syndrome antecedents in prepubertal children associated with being born idiopathic large for gestational age? *Pediatr Diabetes* 14(8):585–592.

Chan, E.J., Cho, L. 2009. What can we expect from omega-3 fatty acids? *Cleve Clin J Med* 76:245–251.

Chen, F., Wang, Y., Shan, X. et al. 2012. Association between childhood obesity and metabolic syndrome: Evidence from a large sample of Chinese children and adolescents. *PLoS One* 7:e47380.

Chung, J.Y., Kang, H.T., Shin, Y.H., Lee, H.R., Park, B.J., Lee, Y.J. 2013. Prevalence of metabolic syndrome in children and adolescents—The recent trends in South Korea. *J Pediatr Endocrinol Metab* 26(1–2):105–110.

Cizmecioglu, F.M., Etiler, N., Hamzaoglu, O., Hatun, S. 2009. Prevalence of metabolic syndrome in schoolchildren and adolescents in Turkey: A population-based study. *J Pediatr Endocrinol Metab* 22(8):703–714.

Cook, S., Weitzman, M., Auinger, P., Nguyen, M., Dietz, W.H. 2003. Prevalence of a metabolic syndrome phenotype in adolescents: Findings from the third National Health and Nutrition Examination Survey, 1988–1994. *Arch Pediatr Adolesc Med* 157:821–827.

Cruz, M.L., Goran, M.I. 2004. The metabolic syndrome in children and adolescents. *Curr Diabetes Rep* 4:53–62.

Damsgaard, C.T., Papadaki, A., Jensen, S.M. et al. 2013. Higher protein diets consumed ad libitum improve cardiovascular risk markers in children of overweight parents from eight European countries. *J Nutr* 143:810–817.

DeBoer, M.D., Gurka, M.J., Sumner, A.E. 2011. Diagnosis of the metabolic syndrome is associated with disproportionately high levels of high-sensitivity C-reactive protein in non-Hispanic black adolescents: An analysis of NHANES 1999–2008. *Diabetes Care* 34(3):734–740.

Denzer, C., Muche, R., Mayer, H., Heinze, E., Debatin, K.M., Wabitsch, M. 2003. Serum uric acid levels in obese children and adolescents: Linkage to testosterone levels and pre-metabolic syndrome. *J Pediatr Endocrinol Metab* 16:1225–1232.

Di Dalmazi, G., Vicennati, V., Pasquali, R., Pagotto, U. 2013. The unrelenting fall of the pharmacological treatment of obesity. *Endocrine* 44(3):598–609.

Dorgan, J.F., Liu, L., Barton, B.A. et al. 2011. Adolescent diet and metabolic syndrome in young women: Results of the Dietary Intervention Study in Children (DISC) follow-up study. *J Clin Endocrinol Metab* 96:E1999–E2008.

Duncan, G.E., Li, S.M., Zhou, X.H. 2004. Prevalence and trends of a metabolic syndrome phenotype among U.S. Adolescents, 1999–2000. *Diabetes Care* 27:2438–2443.

de Ferranti, S.D., Gauvreau, K., Ludwig, D.S., Neufeld, E.J., Newburger, J.W., Rifai, N. 2004. Prevalence of the metabolic syndrome in American adolescents: Findings from the Third National Health and Nutrition Examination Survey. *Circulation* 110:2494–2497.

de la Iglesia, R., Lopez-Legarrea, P., Abete, I. et al. 2014. A new dietary strategy for long-term treatment of the metabolic syndrome is compared with the American Heart Association (AHA) guidelines: The MEtabolic Syndrome REduction in NAvarra (RESMENA) project. *Br J Nutr* 111(4):643–652.

Di Bonito, P., Forziato, C., Sanguigno, E. et al. 2010. Prevalence of the metabolic syndrome using ATP-derived definitions and its relation to insulin-resistance in a cohort of Italian outpatient children. *J Endocrinol Invest* 33(11):806–809.

Efstathiou, S.P., Skeva, I.I., Zorbala, E., Georgiou, E., Mountokalakis, T.D. February 21, 2012. Metabolic syndrome in adolescence: Can it be predicted from natal and parental profile? The Prediction of Metabolic Syndrome in Adolescence (PREMA) study. *Circulation* 125(7):902–910.

Eisenmann, J.C. 2003. Secular trends in variables associated with the metabolic syndrome of North American children and adolescents: A review and synthesis. *Am J Hum Biol* 15:786–794.

Eisenmann, J.C. 2007. Aerobic fitness, fatness and the metabolic syndrome in children and adolescents. *Acta Paediatr* 96:1723–1729.

Eisenmann, J.C. 2008. On the use of a continuous metabolic syndrome score in pediatric research. *Cardiovasc Diabetol* 7:17.

Ekelund, U., Anderssen, S., Andersen, L.B. et al. 2009. Prevalence and correlates of the metabolic syndrome in a population-based sample of European youth. *Am J Clin Nutr* 89(1):90–96.

Expert panel on integrated guidelines for cardiovascular health and risk reduction in children and adolescents: Summary report. 2011. *Pediatrics* 128(Suppl 5):S213–S256.

Eyzaguirre, F., Bancalari, R., Roman, R. et al. 2012. Prevalence of components of the metabolic syndrome according to birthweight among overweight and obese children and adolescents. *J Pediatr Endocrinol Metab* 25:51–56.

Fernandez, J.R., Redden, D.T., Pietrobelli, A., Allison, D.B. 2004. Waist circumference percentiles in nationally representative samples of African-American, European-American, and Mexican-American children and adolescents. *J Pediatr* 145:439–444.

Ford, E.S., Ajani, U.A., Mokdad, A.H. 2005. The metabolic syndrome and concentrations of C-reactive protein among U.S. youth. *Diabetes Care* 28:878–881.

Ford, E.S., Li, C., Cook, S., Choi, H.K. 2007. Serum concentrations of uric acid and the metabolic syndrome among US children and adolescents. *Circulation* 115:2526–2532.

Ford, E.S., Li, C., Zhao, G., Pearson, W.S., Mokdad, A.H. 2008. Prevalence of the metabolic syndrome among U.S. adolescents using the definition from the International Diabetes Federation. *Diabetes Care* 31(3):587–589.

Friend, A., Craig, L., Turner, S. 2013. The prevalence of metabolic syndrome in children: A systematic review of the literature. *Metab Syndr Relat Disord* 11:71–80.

Fu, J.F., Liang, L., Zou, C.C. et al. 2007. Prevalence of the metabolic syndrome in Zhejiang Chinese obese children and adolescents and the effect of metformin combined with lifestyle intervention. *Int J Obes (Lond)* 31:15–22.

Gardner, A.W., Parker, D.E., Krishnan, S., Chalmers, L.J. 2013. Metabolic syndrome and daily ambulation in children, adolescents, and young adults. *Med Sci Sports Exerc* 45:163–169.

Gilardini, L., McTernan, P.G., Girola, A. et al. 2006. Adiponectin is a candidate marker of metabolic syndrome in obese children and adolescents. *Atherosclerosis* 189:401–407.

Guerrero-Romero, F., Aradillas-Garcia, C., Simental-Mendia, L.E., Monreal-Escalante, E., de la Cruz Mendoza, E., Rodriguez-Moran, M. 2010. Birth weight, family history of diabetes, and metabolic syndrome in children and adolescents. *J Pediatr* 156(5):719–723.

Halley Castillo, E., Borges, G., Talavera, J.O. et al. 2007. Body mass index and the prevalence of metabolic syndrome among children and adolescents in two Mexican populations. *J Adolesc Health* 40:521–526.

Harville, E.W., Srinivasan, S., Chen, W., Berenson, G.S. December 2012. Is the metabolic syndrome a "small baby" syndrome? The Bogalusa heart study. *Metab Syndr Relat Disord* 10(6):413–421.

Hosseinpanah, F., Asghari, G., Barzin, M., Ghareh, S., Azizi, F. 2013. Adolescence metabolic syndrome or adiposity and early adult metabolic syndrome. *J Pediatr* 163(6):1663–1669.

International Diabetes Federation. 2007. The IDF consensus definition of the metabolic syndrome in children and adolescents, 24p.

Ismail, I., Keating, S.E., Baker, M.K., Johnson, N.A. 2011. A systematic review and meta-analysis of the effect of aerobic vs. resistance exercise training on visceral fat. *Obes Rev* 13:68–91.

Iughetti, L., China, M., Berri, R., Predieri, B. 2011. Pharmacological treatment of obesity in children and adolescents: Present and future. *J Obes* 2011:928165.

Jaaskelainen, P., Magnussen, C.G., Pahkala, K. et al. 2012. Childhood nutrition in predicting metabolic syndrome in adults: The cardiovascular risk in Young Finns Study. *Diabetes Care* 35:1937–1943.

Janssen, I., LeBlanc, A.G. 2010. Systematic review of the health benefits of physical activity and fitness in school-aged children and youth. *Int J Behav Nutr Phys Activ* 7:40.

Kelishadi, R., Razaghi, E.M., Gouya, M.M. et al. 2007. Association of physical activity and the metabolic syndrome in children and adolescents: CASPIAN Study. *Horm Res* 67:46–52.

Kelly, A.S., Steinberger, J., Jacobs, D.R., Hong, C.P., Moran, A., Sinaiko, A.R. 2011. Predicting cardiovascular risk in young adulthood from the metabolic syndrome, its component risk factors, and a cluster score in childhood. *Int J Pediatr Obes* 6(2–2):e283–e289.

Kiess, W., Bluher, S., Kapellen, T., Korner, A. 2009. Metabolic syndrome in children and adolescents: Prevalence, public health issue, and time for initiative. *J Pediatr Gastroenterol Nutr* 49:268–271.

Kong, A.P., Choi, K.C., Ho, C.S. et al. 2013. Associations of uric acid and gamma-glutamyltransferase (GGT) with obesity and components of metabolic syndrome in children and adolescents. *Pediatr Obes* 8(5):351–357.

Koulouridis, E., Georgalidis, K., Kostimpa, I., Koulouridis, I., Krokida, A., Houliara, D. 2010. Metabolic syndrome risk factors and estimated glomerular filtration rate among children and adolescents. *Pediatr Nephrol* 25:491–498.

Lambert, M., Delvin, E.E., Paradis, G., O'Loughlin, J., Hanley, J.A., Levy, E. 2004. C-reactive protein and features of the metabolic syndrome in a population-based sample of children and adolescents. *Clin Chem* 50:1762–1768.

Lee, S., Bacha, F., Gungor, N., Arslanian, S. 2008. Comparison of different definitions of pediatric metabolic syndrome: Relation to abdominal adiposity, insulin resistance, adiponectin, and inflammatory biomarkers. *J Pediatr* 152:177–184.

Lennerz, B.S., Wabitsch, M., Lippert, H. et al. 2014. Bariatric surgery in adolescents and young adults safety and effectiveness in a cohort of 345 patients. *Int J Obes (Lond)* 38(3):334–340.

Marcovecchio, M.L., Chiarelli, F. 2013. Metabolic syndrome in youth: Chimera or useful concept? *Curr Diabetes Rep* 13(1):56–62.

Mark, A.E., Janssen, I. 2008. Relationship between screen time and metabolic syndrome in adolescents. *J Public Health (Oxf)* 30:153–160.

Martinez-Gomez, D., Eisenmann, J.C., Moya, J.M., Gomez-Martinez, S., Marcos, A., Veiga, O.L. 2009. The role of physical activity and fitness on the metabolic syndrome in adolescents: Effect of different scores. The AFINOS Study. *J Physiol Biochem* 65(3):277–289.

Mehairi, A.E., Khouri, A.A., Naqbi, M.M. et al. 2013. Metabolic syndrome among Emirati adolescents: A school-based study. *PLoS One* 8(2):e56159.

Mirza, N.M., Palmer, M.G., Sinclair, K.B. et al. 2013. Effects of a low glycemic load or a low-fat dietary intervention on body weight in obese Hispanic American children and adolescents: A randomized controlled trial. *Am J Clin Nutr* 97:276–285.

Molnar, D. 2004. The prevalence of the metabolic syndrome and type 2 diabetes mellitus in children and adolescents. *Int J Obes Relat Metab Disord* 28(Suppl 3):S70–S74.

Moyer, V.A., Force, U.S.P.S.T. 2013. Screening for primary hypertension in children and adolescents: U.S. Preventive Services Task Force recommendation statement. *Ann Intern Med* 159:613–619.

Nasreddine, L., Naja, F., Tabet, M. et al. 2012. Obesity is associated with insulin resistance and components of the metabolic syndrome in Lebanese adolescents. *Ann Hum Biol* 39(2):122–128.

Okosun, I.S., Boltri, J.M., Lyn, R., Davis-Smith, M. 2010. Continuous metabolic syndrome risk score, body mass index percentile, and leisure time physical activity in American children. *J Clin Hypertens (Greenwich)* 12:636–644.

Papoutsakis, C., Yannakoulia, M., Ntalla, I., Dedoussis, G.V. 2012. Metabolic syndrome in a Mediterranean pediatric cohort: Prevalence using International Diabetes Federation-derived criteria and associations with adiponectin and leptin. *Metabolism* 61(2):140–145.

Park, J., Hilmers, D.C., Mendoza, J.A., Stuff, J.E., Liu, Y., Nicklas, T.A. 2010. Prevalence of metabolic syndrome and obesity in adolescents aged 12 to 19 years: Comparison between the United States and Korea. *J Korean Med Sci* 25(1):75–82.

Pirkola, J., Tammelin, T., Bloigu, A. et al. 2008. Prevalence of metabolic syndrome at age 16 using the International Diabetes Federation paediatric definition. *Arch Dis Child* 93(11):945–951.

Reinehr, T., Kleber, M., Toschke, A.M. 2009. Lifestyle intervention in obese children is associated with a decrease of the metabolic syndrome prevalence. *Atherosclerosis* 207(1):174–180.

Saneei, P., Hashemipour, M., Kelishadi, R., Rajaei, S., Esmaillzadeh, A. 2013. Effects of recommendations to follow the Dietary Approaches to Stop Hypertension (DASH) diet v. usual dietary advice on childhood metabolic syndrome: A randomised cross-over clinical trial. *Br J Nutr* 111(12):2250–2259.

Sangun, O., Dundar, B., Kosker, M., Pirgon, O., Dundar, N. 2011. Prevalence of metabolic syndrome in obese children and adolescents using three different criteria and evaluation of risk factors. *J Clin Res Pediatr Endocrinol* 3:70–76.

Santibhavank, P. 2007. Prevalence of metabolic syndrome in Nakhon Sawan population. *J Med Assoc Thai* 90(6):1109–1115.

Sartorio, A., Agosti, F., De Col, A., Mornati, D., Francescato, M.P., Lazzer, S. 2007. Prevalence of the metabolic syndrome in Caucasian obese children and adolescents: Comparison between three different definition criteria. *Diabetes Res Clin Pract* 77:341–342.

Sen, Y., Kandemir, N., Alikasifoglu, A., Gonc, N., Ozon, A. 2008. Prevalence and risk factors of metabolic syndrome in obese children and adolescents: The role of the severity of obesity. *Eur J Pediatr* 167:1183–1189.

Seo, S.J., Lee, H.Y., Lee, S.W. 2008. The prevalence of the metabolic syndrome in Korean children and adolescents: Comparisons of the criteria of Cook et al., Cruz and Goran, and ferranti et al. *Yonsei Med J* 49:563–572.

Rizzo, A.C., Goldberg, T.B., Silva, C.C., Kurokawa, C.S., Nunes, H.R., Corrente, J.E. 2013. Metabolic syndrome risk factors in overweight, obese, and extremely obese Brazilian adolescents. *Nutr J* 12:19.

Taha, D., Ahmed, O., bin Sadiq, B. 2009. The prevalence of metabolic syndrome and cardiovascular risk factors in a group of obese Saudi children and adolescents: A hospital-based study. *Ann Saudi Med* 29:357–360.

Tailor, A.M., Peeters, P.H., Norat, T., Vineis, P., Romaguera, D. 2010. An update on the prevalence of the metabolic syndrome in children and adolescents. *Int J Pediatr Obes* 5:202–213.

Tang, L., Kubota, M., Nagai, A., Mamemoto, K., Tokuda, M. 2010. Hyperuricemia in obese children and adolescents: The relationship with metabolic syndrome. *Pediatr Rep* 2:e12.

Urakami, T., Suzuki, J., Yoshida, A. et al. 2009. Prevalence of components of the metabolic syndrome in schoolchildren with newly diagnosed type 2 diabetes mellitus. *Pediatr Diabetes* 10:508–512.

Vissers, D., Hens, W., Taeymans, J., Baeyens, J.P., Poortmans, J., Van Gaal, L. 2013. The effect of exercise on visceral adipose tissue in overweight adults: A systematic review and meta-analysis. *PLoS One* 8:e56415.

Wang, Q., Yin, J., Xu, L. et al. 2013. Prevalence of metabolic syndrome in a cohort of Chinese schoolchildren: Comparison of two definitions and assessment of adipokines as components by factor analysis. *BMC Public Health* 13:249.

Weiss, R., Bremer, A. A., Lustig, R. H. 2013. What is metabolic syndrome, and why are children getting it? *Ann N Y Acad Sci* 1281:123–40.

Weiss, R., Dziura, J., Burgert, T.S. et al. 2004. Obesity and the metabolic syndrome in children and adolescents. *N Engl J Med* 350:2362–2374.

Wilding, J. 2013. Orlistat: Should we worry about liver inflammation? *BMJ* 346:f2777.

Xu, H., Li, Y., Liu, A., Zhang, Q., Hu, X., Fang, H., Li, T., Guo, H., Li, Y., Xu, G., Ma, J., Du, L., Ma, G. 2012. Prevalence of the metabolic syndrome among children from six cities of China. *BMC Public Health* 12:13.

Zimmet, P., Alberti, G., Kaufman, F., Tajima, N., Silink, M., Arslanian, S., Wong, G., Bennett, P., Shaw, J., Caprio, S. 2007. International Diabetes Federation Task Force on Epidemiology and Prevention of Diabetes. The metabolic syndrome in children and adolescents. *Lancet* 369(9579):2059–61.

Section III

Demographic Determinants and Lifestyle Changes in Metabolic Syndrome

8 Social Class and Gender Determinants in Metabolic Syndrome

Guilherme Figueiredo Marquezine

CONTENTS

8.1 INTRODUCTION

It has long been observed that certain metabolic disorders tend to cluster together in individuals. As a matter of fact, independent scientists have reported an association between hypertension, hyperglycemia, and gout as early as the 1920s (Kylin 1923). Almost 30 years later, the role of gender differentiation on visceral obesity made its first appearance on the medical literature (Vague 1947), opening way for our understanding of the role of obesity on triglycerides and hypertension (Albrink et al. 1980) and insulin resistance (Reaven 1988). Reaven (1988) coined the term *Syndrome X* to describe the association between resistance to insulin-mediated glucose uptake, hypertension, type 2 diabetes (T2D), and cardiovascular disease (CVD).

Even though hardly anybody doubts the association between obesity and metabolic syndrome (MetS) components that could increase the risk of developing T2D or coronary disease, it's surprising that definitive criteria and respective cutoffs have not yet been chosen. Several organizations have published their own definitions. The World Health Organization (WHO) first described the MetS in 1988, and it focused on the presence of insulin resistance and microalbuminuria, besides glucose intolerance or the presence of T2D and dyslipidemia (Alberti and Zimmet 1998). In 2001, the National Cholesterol Education Program's Adult Treatment Program III (NCEP:ATPIII) definition was published, and neither insulin resistance nor glucose intolerance was a necessary criterion to characterize the syndrome (Executive Summary of The Third Report of The National Cholesterol Education Program 2001). Five years later, the International Diabetes Federation (IDF) introduced different cutoffs for waist circumference based on ethnicity (Alberti et al. 2005). Interestingly, most definitions take into account redundant characteristics known to be associated to insulin resistance (glucose intolerance, hypertriglyceridemia, low levels of HDL cholesterol and hypertension) and one that is not: obesity or abdominal circumference.

Since the first definition, the MetS has been proposed to predict CVD better than its components could individually. Another popular application is T2D risk stratification. Despite literally thousands of citations per year in the last decade, scientists still argue several limitations and implications regarding this condition. What the best components would be in terms of predictive value or whether different cutoffs for one or more variables would affect its performance have been evaluated over time, but there is still no consensus on which variables to use and how they could lead to better assessment of the patient. There are even a few arguments against its capacity for risk stratification in CVD or T2D compared to other tools (Kahn et al. 2005) or T2D (Stern et al. 2004).

In terms of etiology and pathophysiology, there has been plenty of discussion and research trying to elucidate if MetS is more than just risk factor clustering. The syndrome itself has been closely associated with insulin resistance, and it should, since most of its components individually are a result of lacking insulin action at different metabolic sites, like glucose intolerance, hypertriglyceridemia, low HDL cholesterol, and arterial hypertension. It is not surprising the syndrome itself and most of its components are closely related with insulin resistance and even obesity, the only component that is not directly caused by insulin resistance, is actually one of possible causes of the process. Regardless of our lack of full understanding of the physiopathological mechanisms, one interesting topic that has a clear influence on MetS incidence on a given population is the effect of social factors.

8.2 METABOLIC SYNDROME AND SOCIOECONOMIC STATUS

Socioeconomic status (SES) is a measure of access to material and social resources, as well as prestige-based measures that represent a person's status in a social hierarchy (Yang et al. 2012). Adult SES takes into consideration educational level, income, and occupation, and has been widely associated with obesity prevalence and intensity, MetS, and cardiovascular endpoints in both children and adults.

There's good reason to believe that the recent increase in body weight and obesity worldwide is a likely cause of the increasing prevalence of insulin resistance and the MetS (Reaven 1988, Eckel et al. 2005). Even though not every obese person is metabolically unhealthy, most of them are insulin resistant (Stefan et al. 2008), which is possibly driven by the combination of obesity, sedentarism, and consumption of an atherogenic diet (Grundy et al. 2005).

One of the earliest studies on obesity and socioeconomic variables found a strong inverse association of SES and obesity, especially in women (Moore et al. 1962). Specifically, obesity was six times more prevalent among women of lower SES than among those of upper SES. Another interesting conclusion by the same group in a similar study is the great importance of parental SES, also called SES of origin, on establishing directionality in the relationship between social variables and mental health (Srole et al. 1965). Their study also showed that this variable, SES of origin, is almost as strongly associated with obesity as was the individual's own SES. Those conclusions make SES and SES of origin as well as some other related conditions independent variables associated with obesity.

Two prospective studies followed people from birth into adulthood and provided even stronger evidence that SES directly influenced the risk of obesity. One study (Braddon et al. 1986) showed that social class was strongly associated with body mass at adult age. Interestingly, both men and women who in childhood lived in higher nonmanual work social classes were significantly more likely to be in categories of normal to underweight body mass at an adult age. Other social variables associated with obesity were never being married, parity, and low educational level.

Two different longitudinal studies in England found similar results (Peckham et al. 1983, Power and Moynihan 1988). They showed no significant differences between overweight and obesity by SES in children. By the time they were adults, SES had already become a clear influence on obesity risk. A more recent and broad review on the subject of how socioeconomic variables could influence obesity included 333 studies on the subject (McLaren 2007) and categorized their findings relative to gender. In women, 63% of reviewed studies showed negative associations between body size and Human Development Index (HDI), which is an indicator developed by the United Nations Development Program (www.undp.org) to characterize and rank countries on variables such as life expectancy at birth, adult literacy, school enrolment, and standards of living based on gross domestic product. Education and area-level indicators especially showed negative associations with obesity (72% and 71%, respectively), meaning the lower the HDI, the higher the propensity for obesity. Another particularly interesting issue shown in this review is that as one moved from high-HDI countries to medium and to low HDI status, the percentage of studies with positive associations between HDI and obesity also increased, from 3% in high-HDI countries to 43% in medium-HDI countries and 94% in low-HDI countries. Considering studies from medium- to low-HDI countries, this positive association with obesity was particularly strong for income (71%) and material possessions (86%) as an indicator of SES. Interestingly, the association of socioeconomic variables to body weight and obesity risk was not observed in men in most of the 333 studies.

There are a few studies looking at this question that have taken place in Brazil. One of them studied the association of MetS and several social markers in São Carlos, Southeast Brazil, in a cross-sectional home survey involving 1116 adults aged 30–70 years (Gronner et al. 2011). There were a high proportion of people who met IDF MetS criteria, around 45% for men and women equally. Progressing age, skin color, and high BMI were significantly associated with MetS. People with low education level had the highest risk of developing MetS, a little over 2.5 times compared to people with the higher education levels. Gender was not significantly associated with MetS in this cohort. Table 8.1 lists this study's main results and statistics.

TABLE 8.1

Estimated Crude and Age/Gender/Skin Color–Adjusted Odds Ratio (OR) of Metabolic Syndrome Prevalence according to IDF Criteria in Relation to Different Levels of Demographic-Related Factors in an Urban Population Aged 30–79 Years in the Southeastern Region of Brazil

Characteristics	N (%)	Crude OR (95%CI)	Age/Gender/Skin Color-Adjusted OR (95%CI)
Age groups (years)			
30–39	63 (11.73)	Reference	Reference
40–49	111 (20.67)	2.15 (1.47–3.16)	—
50–59	140 (26.07)	2.68 (1.85–3.89)	—
60–69	117 (21.79)	4.64 (3.06–7.04)	—
70–79	106 (19.74)	4.77 (3.11–7.32)	—
Gender			
Female	342 (63.69)	Reference	Reference
Male	195 (36.31)	1.07 (0.84–1.37)	—
Skin color			
Non-white	145 (27.57)	Reference	Reference
White	381 (72.43)	1.65 (1.28–2.14)	—
Family income (minimal national wages)			
<2	93 (19.14)	Reference	Reference
2–5	286 (58.85)	1.31 (0.82–1.56)	1.18 (0.84–1.66)
5–10	86 (17.70)	0.99 (0.66–1.48)	0.92 (0.61–1.41)
>10	21 (4.32)	0.64 (0.35–1.16)	0.57 (0.30–1.07)
Educational level			
Higher	29 (6.09)	Reference	Reference
Middle	94 (19.75)	1.38 (0.83–2.30)	1.64 (0.96–2.80)
Fundamental	353 (74.16)	2.51 (1.58–4.00)	2.41 (1.47–3.96)
Smoking			
No	421 (79.73)	1.25 (0.94–1.66)	1.10 (0.81–1.48)
Yes	107 (20.27)	Reference	Reference
BMI			
<25	90 (16.76)	Reference	Reference
≥25	447 (83.24)	5.68 (4.30–7.51)	6.33 (4.68–8.54)

IDF, International Diabetes Federation; BMI, body mass index.

TABLE 8.2

Metabolic Syndrome and Metabolic Syndrome Components' Prevalence according to Social Class in an Urban General Population in Southeast Brazil

	Fasting Glucose, ≥110 mg/dL or T2D	Triglycerides, ≥150 mg/dL	HDL-c, <40 mg/dL Men; <50 Women	Waist, <102 cm Men; <88 Women	Hypertension, ≥ 130/85 or Medication	MetS Prevalence
A	28 (8.38)	59 (12.19)	78 (9.20)	26 (10.20)	56 (7.70)	32 (8.06)
B	78 (23.35)	135 (27.89)	225 (26.53)	56 (21.96)	172 (23.66)	89 (22.42)
C	114 (34.13)	150 (30.99)	264 (31.13)	80 (31.37)	229 (31.50)	132 (33.25)
D + E	114 (34.13)	139 (28.72)	281 (33.14)	93 (36.47)	270 (37.14)	144 (36.27)
Linear by linear p value	0.02	0.07	0.03	0.05	<0.001	0.01
Total	334	483	848	255	727	397

MetS, metabolic syndrome; T2D, type 2 diabetes.

Another Brazilian study regarding this subject took place in Vitoria, another Southeastern city in Brazil (Marquezine et al. 2008). This cohort enrolled 1507 adults from the general population. MetS prevalence was somewhat similar to numbers described in developed countries (25% for men and women), although it was more common in younger men and older women. Following many previous reports, the most frequent components of the syndrome were, in decreasing order, arterial hypertension, low HDL-c, high triglycerides, altered fasting glucose or diabetes, and finally, obesity, in men. Of note, women had a different distribution, as follows: low HDL-c, arterial hypertension, high triglycerides, and obesity and, finally, fasting hyperglycemia or diabetes. In this study, higher social class was a protective variable against MetS presence and for each of its components individually. Low social class increased the risk of MetS in a dose-dependent manner (Table 8.2).

8.3   FINAL CONSIDERATIONS

So far, it becomes clear that several socioeconomic factors tend to increase health risks over time, especially T2D and CVD. Low SES may signify low income, fewer years of formal study, poor career prospects, or greater risks of unemployment. Any of these factors will determine and influence one's ability to consume goods and services, such as healthier food and health services, and ability to change and maintain better habits. Income differences, even above the poverty line, may lead to differential access to social participation and social capital. Low SES can also influence health-related variables through higher exposure to occupational hazards, both physical and psychological (Elovainio et al. 2011). Moreover, the relation between SES and health may not be unidirectional, as health problems can certainly affect one's ability to work and maintain his income and impair his career prospects, as well as increase debt and expenses.

The association between SES and health is reciprocal, bound in a reinforcing cycle in which it is difficult to determine the direction of causality. These conclusions have been populating scientific studies for the last decades and should drive further research aiming to better identify those at high risk of CVD. Also, better understanding of these relations could help us define more efficient measures to lessen the burden of those belonging to the lower part of the socioeconomic pyramid and could justify even stronger measures to guarantee access to education and work.

REFERENCES

Alberti, K.G., Zimmet, P.Z. 1998. Definition, diagnosis and classification of diabetes mellitus and its complications. Part 1: Diagnosis and classification of diabetes mellitus provisional report of a WHO consultation. *Diabet Med* 15(7):539–553.

Alberti, K.G., Zimmet, P., Shaw, J. 2005. The metabolic syndrome—A new worldwide definition. *Lancet* 366(9491):1059–1062.

Albrink, M.J., Krauss, R.M., Lindgrem, F.T., von der Groeben, J., Pan, S., Wood, P.D. 1980. Intercorrelations among plasma high density lipoprotein, obesity and triglycerides in a normal population. *Lipids* 15(9):668–676.

Braddon, F.E., Rodgers, B., Wadsworth, M.E., Davies, J.M. 1986. Onset of obesity in a 36 year birth cohort study. *BMJ* 293(6542):299–303.

Eckel, R.H., Grundy, S.M., Zimmet, P.Z. 2005. The metabolic syndrome. *Lancet* 365(9468):1415–1428.

Elovainio, M., Ferrie, J.E., Singh-Manoux, A., Shipley, M., Batty, G.D., Head, J. et al. 2011. Socioeconomic differences in cardiometabolic factors: Social causation or health-related selection? Evidence from the Whitehall II Cohort Study, 1991–2004. *Am J Epidemiol* 174(7):779–789.

Executive Summary of The Third Report of The National Cholesterol Education Program (NCEP). 2001. Expert panel on detection, evaluation, and treatment of high blood cholesterol in adults (adult treatment panel III). *JAMA* 285(19):2486–2497.

Gronner, M.F., Bosi, P.L., Carvalho, A.M., Casale, G., Contrera, D., Pereira, M.A. et al. 2011. Prevalence of metabolic syndrome and its association with educational inequalities among Brazilian adults: A population-based study. *Braz J Med Biol Res* 44:713–719.

Grundy, S.M., Cleeman, J.I., Daniels, S.R., Donato, K.A., Eckel, R.H., Franklin, B.A. et al. 2005. Diagnosis and management of the metabolic syndrome: An American Heart Association/National Heart, Lung, and Blood Institute Scientific Statement. *Circulation* 112(17):2735–2752.

Kahn, R., Buse, J., Ferrannini, E., Stern, M. 2005. The metabolic syndrome: Time for a critical appraisal. Joint statement from the American Diabetes Association and the European Association for the Study of Diabetes. *Diabetes Care* 28(9):2289–2304.

Kylin, E.S. 1923. Hypertonie-hyperglykamie-hyperurikamiesyndrome. *Zentralblatt fur innere Medizin* 44:105–127.

McLaren, L. 2007. Socioeconomic status and obesity. *Epidemiol Rev* 29(1):29–48.

Marquezine, G.F., Oliveira, C.M., Pereira, A.C., Krieger, J.E., Mill, J.G. 2008. Metabolic syndrome determinants in an urban population from Brazil: Social class and gender-specific interaction. *Int J Cardiol* 129(2):259–265.

Moore, M.E., Stunkard, A., Srole, L. 1962. Obesity, social class, and mental illness. *JAMA* 181(11):962–966.

Peckham, C.S., Stark, O., Simonite, V., Wolff, O.H. 1983. Prevalence of obesity in British children born in 1946 and 1958. *BMJ* 286(6373):1237–1242.

Power, C., Moynihan, C. 1988. Social class and changes in weight-for-height between childhood and early adulthood. *Int J Obes* 12(5):445–453.

Reaven, G.M. 1988. Banting lecture 1988. Role of insulin resistance in human disease. *Diabetes* 37(12):1595–1607.

Srole, L., Langner, T.S., Michael, S.T., Opler, M.K., Rennie, TA. 1965. Mental Health in the metropolis. *Int J Psychiatry* 1:64–76.

Stefan, N., Kantartzis, K., Machann, J., Schick, F., Thamer, C., Rittig, K. et al. 2008. Identification and characterization of metabolically benign obesity in humans. *Arch Intern Med* 168(15):1609–1616.

Stern, M.P., Williams, K., González-Villalpando, C., Hunt, K.J., Haffner, S.M. 2004. Does the metabolic syndrome improve identification of individuals at risk of type 2 diabetes and/or cardiovascular disease? *Diabetes Care* 27(11):2676–2681.

Vague, J. 1947. La differenciation sexuelle, facteur determinant des formes de l'obesite. *Presse Med* 30:339–340.

Yang, X., Tao, Q., Sun, F., Zhan, S. 2012. The impact of socioeconomic status on the incidence of metabolic syndrome in a Taiwanese health screening population. *Int J Public Health* 57(3):551–559.

9 Lifestyle Changes and Physical Activity in Metabolic Syndrome

Leandro Arthur Diehl

CONTENTS

9.1 INTRODUCTION

Lifestyle intervention programs encompassing exercise and healthy diets for weight loss are widely used for the treatment of metabolic syndrome (MetS), obesity, and type 2 diabetes (T2DM). The specific role of physical activity as a determinant of health or disease, as well as other lifestyle interventions for improving MetS, will be reviewed in this chapter.

9.2 LIFESTYLE AND SEDENTARISM AS RISK FACTORS FOR METABOLIC SYNDROME

Abdominal obesity is the body fat parameter most closely associated with the MetS [1]. The worldwide obesity epidemic has been the most important driving force in the growing numbers of MetS [2]. Although inherited factors truly can determine increased susceptibility to obesity, insulin resistance, and MetS, it is more likely that the environmental factors linked to lifestyle (diet and physical activity, socioeconomic status) are the main culprits for the overwhelming increase in the prevalence of overweight, obesity, and MetS observed in the last two to three decades [3].

Sedentarism is associated and probably can produce many of the major criteria for the diagnosis of MetS (dysglycemia, high blood pressure, atherogenic lipid profile, abdominal obesity) [4]. In a cross-sectional study with middle-aged men, subjects who used to engage in at least 3 h/week of moderate-intensity leisure-time physical activity were almost 40% less likely to present MetS than those who did less than 1 h/week. The strongest predictor of MetS risk, however, was poor cardio-respiratory fitness (maximal aerobic capacity, $VO_{2max} < 29.1$ mL/kg/min): middle-aged men in this category were seven times more likely to present MetS than the subgroup with a better physical conditioning ($VO_{2max} \geq 35.5$ mL/kg/min) [4].

Among a large Chinese study with men and women from 50 to 70 years old, total physical activity (jogging, tai chi, or dancing) was strongly associated with lower risk of MetS, independent of body weight. In this study, a dose–response effect was found: for each 1 h/week increment in tai chi and dancing, there was a 5% or 9% (respectively) lower risk of MetS [5].

The Copenhagen City Heart Study have shown that the intensity of leisure-time physical activity, walking and jogging, was more important than the volume of physical activity, regarding the prevention of MetS [6].

Reaven, who has found the same results in every one of them, reviewed other studies, with different populations of apparently healthy individuals: poor cardiorespiratory fitness, usually assessed by measuring VO_{2max}, is associated with higher insulin resistance, independent of age and obesity [7]. According to that author, "the convergence of the facts that overweight/obese individuals tend to be less physically active and that decreased activity is associated with insulin resistance supports the notion that the adverse impact of obesity may, at least partly, be due to obesity-related sedentary lifestyle, rather than obesity, per se" [7]. However, this distinction among physical inactivity or body weight excess as the main *villain* may be considered by some as clinically irrelevant, since both obesity and sedentarism are regarded as prejudicial and should be actively fought against, by people who need or want to prevent MetS, T2DM, and cardiovascular disease (CVD).

9.3   LIFESTYLE CHANGES AND PHYSICAL ACTIVITY IN THE TREATMENT OF METABOLIC SYNDROME

Lifestyle changes are cornerstone for the treatment of excess body weight, which is a major trigger for the metabolic disturbances seen in MetS. Thus, the association of regular physical activity and a dietary plan for weight loss and prevention of complications (T2DM, CVD) is considered as the first-choice therapy for MetS, obesity, and insulin resistance [2,8,9]. Effective weight reduction improves all risk factors associated with MetS (dyslipidemia, hypertension, insulin resistance), and it will further reduce the risk for new T2DM [2,10]. Unfortunately, currently available pharmacological options for weight reduction have only mild-to-moderate and little lasting effectiveness for the treatment of obesity. In the other hand, bariatric surgery has been increasingly used to treat severe obesity. Results of bariatric surgery in severely obese patients with MetS are very encouraging, since 95% of patients are rendered free of MetS 1 year after the surgery [11]; however, studies with longer follow-ups are needed to clarify the role of bariatric surgery in the management of MetS in people with and without morbid obesity. Dietary approaches for weight loss and for the management of MetS are reviewed in other chapters of this book.

The importance of increased physical activity for achieving clinically significant weight loss cannot be overstressed, but there is also evidence supporting the idea that regular moderate physical activity, by itself, even if not associated with weight loss, is able to induce improvements in all risk factors of the MetS [12], although it may be difficult, many times, to separate the effects of physical activity from the effects of weight loss [3]. Nevertheless, physical activity is universally proposed as an important approach for global CVD risk modification [3,13], since extensive evidence supports exercise and physical activity as very effective ways to reduce the incidence of coronary heart disease [14] and to promote general health [12]. We will review in the next sections the main categories of benefits generated by physical activity in patients with MetS, according to currently available evidence.

9.3.1 Physical Activity and Metabolic Syndrome

There is substantial evidence supporting the role of physical activity, usually associated with mild-to-moderate weight loss, in reducing the risk of new (incident) cases of MetS, increasing the odds of resolution of MetS in people who were already diagnosed with this condition, and reducing the overall prevalence of MetS, in populations at high risk for T2DM [8].

The Finnish Diabetes Prevention Study (DPS) was a trial designed to demonstrate the effect of a lifestyle intervention for the prevention of new cases of T2DM, in middle-aged patients with impaired glucose tolerance (IGT) [15]. A post hoc analysis of a subgroup of DPS subjects, from whom 73% presented MetS at baseline, has shown that a detailed and individualized dietary and exercise counseling aimed to increase leisure-time moderate-to-vigorous physical activity was sufficient to induce substantial clinical benefits in comparison with the control group, with a 47% lower likelihood of developing new MetS, and a 55% higher likelihood of MetS resolution, after 4 years of follow-up. Interestingly, despite the fact that patients in the intervention group have lost 6 kg in average, and patients in the control group have gained 2 kg, the lower risk of MetS associated with increased physical activity was independent of diet and body mass index (BMI) changes. Of the components of MetS, increased leisure-time physical activity was associated more strongly with improvement of glycemia [16].

In the Diabetes Prevention Program (DPP) trial, which included only patients with IGT and high risk of T2DM, from whom 53% had MetS at baseline, the patients were randomized to intensive lifestyle changes (diet + aerobic exercise–induced weight loss), metformin, or placebo. After 3 years of intervention, among the subjects who already had MetS at baseline, there was resolution of MetS in 38% of subjects in lifestyle group, 23% of metformin, and 18% of placebo group. Among the DPP subjects who did not present MetS at baseline, a 41% reduction in the incidence of MetS was observed in the group who underwent intensive lifestyle changes, compared with 17% in the group treated with metformin. The researchers observed that "the dramatic effect of lifestyle on both the prevention of incident MetS and reduction of its overall prevalence appears to be most strongly related to a reduction in waist circumference and in blood pressure and not […] a correction of the lipid abnormalities" [17]. A lower risk of T2DM, however, was present even after 10 years of follow-up, in the original lifestyle and metformin groups [18]. However, as IGT was an inclusion criteria in this study, we cannot infer whether these results can be generalized to a population with normal glucose tolerance.

Regarding resistance (isometric) exercise, the benefits of decreasing MetS risk are much less clear than those of aerobic (isotonic) exercise. A large prospective study with more than 3000 men of varying age (from 20 to 80), initially free of MetS, has found that the risk of incident MetS was inversely associated with the degree of muscular strength, independent of age, body size, or other risk factors. The researchers concluded by saying that "presumably […] resistance exercise training should be considered in primary prevention of MetS." However, the association between muscular strength and MetS risk was very attenuated when further adjusted for cardiorespiratory fitness, underlining the interrelatedness of those two functional measures [19]. Resistance training can also produce reductions in abdominal fat and therefore indirectly improve metabolic abnormalities [20]. More important than determining whether each isolated exercise modality can improve or prevent MetS, however, is to assess the combined effects of resistance and aerobic exercise as complementary parts of a well-balanced physical activity program. Further prospective studies are needed to answer this relevant question.

9.3.2 Physical Activity and Insulin Resistance

Although there are no definitive criteria for clinically categorizing an individual as insulin resistant or insulin sensitive, most subjects with MetS present some degree of insulin resistance [21], which is considered as an underlying mechanism of the clinical and metabolic abnormalities seen in the syndrome [22].

Physical activity can improve glucose metabolism by stimulating glucose uptake in skeletal muscle, via non-insulin-dependent mechanisms (enhancement of the expression and translocation of muscle glucose transporter, GLUT4), and also by improving tissular insulin action, partly by decreasing intra-abdominal fat, reducing free fatty acids that interfere with insulin action, and improving insulin sensitivity [3,22]. This effect can be seen after a single session of exercise, but in these cases, it lasts 24 h maximum. For this reason, in order to have maximal improvement in insulin-mediated glucose homeostasis, an individual would need to do aerobic exercise regularly (most days of the week) [23]. The effect of exercise is more long-lasting if accompanied by weight loss [24].

A trial that compared equal volumes of either continuous moderate exercise (at 70% of highest measured heart rate, H_{fmax}) or aerobic interval training (at 90% of H_{fmax}), three times a week for 16 weeks, in middle-aged subjects with MetS, has found a more pronounced improvement in insulin signaling, blood glucose, lipogenesis, and endothelial function, with aerobic interval training, with the same reduction in body weight [25].

Resistance training is also effective for improving glucose metabolism. A study assessing the effects of twice-weekly progressive resistance training in older men (mean age: 66) with T2DM has shown a significant (46%) increase in insulin sensitivity, even reducing fasting plasma glucose by 7%. In this study, subjects had a 10% decrease in visceral and subcutaneous abdominal fat, after 16 weeks, with no significant changes in BMI [20].

Yoga exercise was also associated with significant improvements in body fat, insulin sensitivity, and adiponectin levels, in Korean postmenopausal women [26].

9.3.3 PHYSICAL ACTIVITY AND RISK OF TYPE 2 DIABETES

Lifestyle intervention, including dietary modification, physical exercise, and weight loss, is long acknowledged as the first option of approach to reduce the risk of incident T2DM in patients of high risk (*prediabetes*: IGT or impaired fasting glucose) [27].

In the DPP study, a lifestyle intervention, which included an ongoing support program targeting a 7% body weight loss and 150 min/week of moderate aerobic physical activity (walking), has been shown to be more effective than a pharmacological approach (metformin) for the reduction of incidence of T2DM (58% versus 31% risk reduction, respectively) after 3 years [28]. The same degree of protection against the development of T2DM was seen in the Finnish DPS: 58% less diabetes after 3 years in the group of men and women with IGT who underwent lifestyle change. In this trial, the lifestyle group presented a 3.5 kg net weight loss, compared with a 0.8 kg net weight loss in the control group; however, even in the subgroup of patients who did not lose significant body weight (<5% loss), the reduction in diabetes risk was substantial (80%) if the patient did adhere to the proposed physical activity program, which further illustrates the impact of exercise on diabetes risk [29].

The Chinese Da Qing Study was even more interesting, for the evaluation of the role of physical exercise for the prevention of T2DM, since it has randomized high-risk men and women (all with IGT) to four different interventions: diet only, exercise only, diet + exercise, and control. Every three arms of active intervention presented lower incidences of T2DM at 6 years compared with the control group, with a risk reduction of 31% for diet alone, 46% for exercise alone, and 42% for diet + exercise [30]. The changes in body weight observed during the active intervention period did not differ significantly by group.

In a longer time frame, follow-up studies of the three larger clinical trials of lifestyle intervention have shown sustained reduction in the rate of conversion from prediabetes to T2DM: 43% risk reduction at 20 years in the Da Qing study; [31] 43% risk reduction at 7 years in the Finnish DPS; [32] and 34% reduction at 10 years in the U.S. Diabetes Prevention Program Outcomes Study, a follow-up of DPP (18).

9.3.4 PHYSICAL ACTIVITY AND BLOOD PRESSURE

A number of studies suggest that aerobic exercise can have a modest antihypertensive effect. In a trial with men with MetS and mild (Stage I) hypertension, a single session of light-intensity aerobic exercise (cycling, at 40% of VO_2 peak) was associated with a reduction of 8 mmHg in systolic and 5 mmHg in diastolic blood pressures [33].

In a meta-analysis of randomized controlled trials, this effect was confirmed: aerobic exercise reduced about 4 mmHg in systolic and 3 mmHg in diastolic blood pressures [34]. Although this effect can be considered small, it can possibly be potentialized by the concomitant adoption of other lifestyle changes, such as sodium restriction, dietary modification (e.g., DASH diet), or weight loss [3]. From all proposed nonpharmacological interventions, however, weight loss remains the most potent lifestyle modification for blood pressure reduction [35].

9.3.5 PHYSICAL ACTIVITY AND PLASMA LIPIDS

Physical activity is regarded as an important component of the therapeutic lifestyle change recommendations for CVD risk reduction for patients with MetS [36]. Increased physical activity can reduce triglycerides and improve HDL-cholesterol plasma levels, but results regarding LDL-cholesterol are less uniform among different studies [3]. Even so, exercise can have an acute effect of reducing postprandial triglyceride excursions, potentially providing additional protection against atherogenesis [37].

The ApoB/ApoA-I ratio, considered an independent risk factor for coronary artery disease, was improved by 8 weeks of an exercise program individualized at the point where fat oxidation was maximal, in obese children (mean age 13) [38].

9.3.6 PHYSICAL ACTIVITY, ENDOTHELIAL FUNCTION, AND INFLAMMATION

Some plasma biomarkers of chronic inflammation (e.g., high sensitivity C-reactive protein, hs-CRP) and endothelial dysfunction (e.g., tumor necrosis factor-alpha, TNF-α) have been increasingly recognized as additional risk factors for CVD [39]. Also, those markers are commonly higher in people with MetS than in people not affected by the syndrome.

Among a cohort of subjects with a recent coronary event, patients with MetS have 77% higher levels of hs-CRP compared with those with no MetS, and the levels of hs-CRP were related to the number of metabolic derangements present. In the same study, those patients who completed a 3-month program of cardiac rehabilitation and exercise training have had a significant reduction in hs-CRP, almost by half, independent of statin use or weight loss [40].

A trial of a twice-weekly progressive aerobic exercise program in older sedentary patients with T2DM has shown no change in plasma levels of hs-CRP or TNF-α after 6 months, but a marked reduction in plasma P-selectin and ICAM-1 (other biomarkers of endothelial function), as well as a reduction in uric acid by 33%, and an increase in HDL-cholesterol by 12%, with no significant body weight changes, potentially contributing to a reduction of the cardiovascular risk in these patients [41].

The effect of different modalities of physical activity on inflammatory markers does not seem to be the same. In a trial with patients with MetS and T2DM, three different interventions were compared: low-intensity physical activity, high-intensity aerobic exercise, or aerobic + resistance exercise, with the same caloric expenditure, during 12 months. Body fat, insulin sensitivity, plasma lipids, and hs-CRP were improved only in the last two groups, while other inflammation markers (IL-6, TNF-α, and interferon-gamma) improved only in the aerobic + resistance group. Changes in VO_{2max} and the exercise modalities were strong predictors of hs-CRP reduction, independent of body weight changes [42]. Therefore, long-term high-intensity (preferably mixed, aerobic + resistance) training, in addition to daytime physical activity, appears to be the best for a significant anti-inflammatory effect of exercise in type 2 diabetic patients with MetS [42].

9.3.7 PHYSICAL ACTIVITY AND LIVER ENZYMES

Nonalcoholic fatty liver disease is the most common cause of abnormal liver function tests in the Western world. It encompasses a spectrum of liver disease, from a simple fatty infiltration to chronic hepatitis (nonalcoholic steatohepatitis, or NASH), that can chronically evolve to cirrhosis, liver failure, and hepatocellular carcinoma. Insulin resistance, visceral adiposity, and MetS are predisposing factors for fatty liver disease. The management of fatty liver disease includes lifestyle changes (dietary modification, physical activity, weight loss) and, occasionally, insulin-sensitizing drugs [43].

A 12-week lifestyle intervention comprising a hypocaloric diet for weight loss, alone or combined with aerobic exercise training, has shown to significantly reduce plasma liver enzymes (a surrogate marker of liver injury) in obese men and women with MetS (mean BMI 33 kg/m^2). Body weight loss averaged 8% for diet alone and 9% for diet + exercise. Alanine aminotransferase reduction was directly related to the loss of abdominal fat. In this study, the improvement in liver enzymes and abdominal fat was roughly the same in both intervention groups (diet alone and diet + exercise), leading the authors to conclude that "exercise training did not confer significant incremental benefits in this study" [44].

9.3.8 PHYSICAL ACTIVITY AND OVARIAN FUNCTION

Polycystic ovary syndrome (PCOS) is the most common endocrine disorder in women of reproductive age. PCOS is characterized by the presence of polycystic ovaries, menstrual dysfunction, and biochemical or clinical hyperandrogenism, in the absence of other endocrine abnormalities. Many studies show an increased prevalence of obesity, insulin resistance, MetS, T2DM, and cardiovascular risk factors, among women with PCOS. The management of this condition should include lifestyle changes (diet, exercise) for weight loss and amelioration of ovarian function and comorbidities [45].

The specific role of physical exercise, independent of body weight changes, for clinical or metabolic benefits, however, is not very clear, since there are limited studies addressing this question. Yet, the available evidence suggests a beneficial effect of exercise, either alone or in combination with energy restriction, in cardiorespiratory fitness, body composition, insulin sensitivity, menstrual cyclicity, ovulation, self-esteem, quality of life, and depression. The main effect of regular exercise by itself appears to be an additional improvement in body composition, but this effect may have substantial long-term implications for the prevention of disease in women with PCOS [45].

A trial that compared three different lifestyle interventions in obese women with PCOS (diet alone, exercise alone, or diet + exercise) has found significant improvement in BMI, menstrual pattern, and ovulation, with no changes in insulin sensitivity measurements (HOMA index) in all three groups, with no difference among them [46].

9.3.9 PHYSICAL ACTIVITY AND MORTALITY

Higher cardiorespiratory fitness and increased self-reported physical activity have been shown to be inversely related to cardiovascular mortality and to the incidence of T2DM, even with amounts of exercise as low as 1 h/week in one study [47–49].

In a prospective trial with middle-aged men with T2DM, a sedentary lifestyle and poor aerobic capacity (assessed by a maximal exercise test) were associated with a two times higher risk for all-cause mortality, in comparison with physically active fit men, and this association was independent of other factors (such as overweight, smoking status, age, baseline CVD, plasma glucose, dyslipidemia, and parental history of CVD) [49]. In fact, in obese individuals, a low level of physical fitness seems to be a better predictor of all-cause mortality than cholesterol levels, smoking status, or blood pressure, and is similar to having had a previous cardiovascular event [50].

The HUNT 2 was another large prospective study, conducted in Norway, to assess the impact of different levels of physical activity and MetS on all-cause and cardiovascular mortality. In that study, MetS was associated with a 35% higher all-cause mortality, and with a 78% higher cardiovascular mortality in younger (less than 65) subjects, but that association was absent in the older (65 or more) population. Among MetS subjects, however, higher levels of self-reported physical activity at baseline were associated with a reduced risk of all-cause mortality, either in the younger (hazard ratio 0.52) or in the older group (hazard ratio 0.59). Cardiovascular mortality was reduced in the same manner. There was a dose–risk association between reported levels of physical activity and mortality, but more than that, the reduction in mortality was observed even in subjects who reported low levels of physical activity (less than 3 h/week of light-intensity exercise), in comparison with inactive subjects. According to the authors of that study, those "results strongly indicate that physical activity should be recommended to people with MetS to reduce their risk of premature death" [51].

9.3.10   Other Benefits of Physical Activity

Nocturnal GH secretion, which is often reduced in patients with abdominal obesity and MetS, is improved by exercise training in obese adults with MetS, and this may contribute to a better lipid profile and gain of lean (muscle) mass in that population [52]. Also, regular physical activity is widely known to enhance quality of life and psychological well-being [53].

9.4   RECOMMENDATIONS OF PHYSICAL ACTIVITY FOR METABOLIC SYNDROME

Current guidelines recommend practical, regular, and moderate regimens of physical activity for the prevention of MetS, T2DM, CVD, and mortality [13,23]. Usually, MetS patients are stimulated to engage in moderate-intensity exercise a minimum of 150 minutes/week, divided among three to five sessions. A practical and common approach for patient orientation is to recommend brisk walking, 30 min/day or more, on most, and preferably all, days of the week [13,23,35]. Although this volume of exercise (at least 2.5 h/week of moderate activity) is already able to reduce all-cause and cardiovascular mortality, the longer the duration of physical activity performed over the week, the greater the observed benefits [54]. Similar results, however, can also be obtained by performing 1–1.5 h/week (20 min/session, 3–5 days of the week) of vigorous-intensity aerobic exercise training [54].

For practical effects, *moderate*-intensity physical activity is defined as an activity performed at 40%–59% of VO_2 or heart rate reserve. *Vigorous*-intensity physical activity, in the other hand, is performed at 60%–85% of VO_2 or heart rate reserve [54].

Sedentary activities in leisure time should be replaced by more active behavior: jogging, swimming, dancing, biking, etc., and the patients should be encouraged to progressively increase their activity as tolerated, since there is a dose–response relation between physical activity and health [2,13,23]. Lifestyle-common activities such as walking briskly, climbing stairs, and doing more housework and gardening work are other examples of aerobic exercises, which must be encouraged. Exercising with family or friends tends to improve patients' motivation [54].

In addition to aerobic exercise training, it is recommended that every adult should perform activities that maintain or increase muscular strength and endurance a minimum of 2 days each week [23].

However, there are some safety issues that must be taken into account, in the moment of prescribing a given exercise program to any patient with MetS with a higher cardiovascular risk profile (e.g., older subjects with T2DM or previous CVD). A thorough history and physical examination, as well as a resting electrocardiogram, and other more sensitive tests if necessary, should be performed before those patients start exercising [53]. Starting slow (light-intensity aerobic exercising, short-session duration) is recommended in sedentary subjects and those with cardiovascular risk factors [54]. Resistance training can be done with caution (such as lifting small weights, from 2 to 5 kg). Before engaging in a more intense activity (running), an exercise stress test is better advised [53].

Patients with very high levels of blood pressure, or with severe (proliferative) diabetic retinopathy, must avoid exercises with increased intra-abdominal pressure (heavy weight lifting, Valsalva-like maneuvers). Patients with severe diabetic polyneuropathy with a loss of sensation in the feet should avoid running [53].

In patients with known CVD, available data do not allow definition of an aerobic exercise training weekly volume as precise as that indicated for healthy subjects, and exercise prescription must be tailored to the clinical profile of the patient. However, even in the more limited patients, small amounts of properly supervised physical activity are beneficial to maintain independent living [53].

Some guidelines also recommend that the health professionals themselves should personally engage in an active lifestyle, in order to gain familiarity "with the issues involved in maintaining lifelong physical activity and to set a positive example for patients and the public" [13], based on the idea that this might increase the odds for healthcare providers to recommend physical activity to their patients, although evidence supporting this idea is lacking. However, continued physician encouragement and support may definitely help the patients in the long term [53].

9.5 OTHER LIFESTYLE CHANGES IN METABOLIC SYNDROME

9.5.1 PSYCHOTHERAPY AND COGNITIVE THERAPIES

A large number of published recommendations encourage people with body weight excess to engage in a low-calorie diet and increase physical activity in order to lose weight and improve health, but adherence to those recommendations is usually suboptimal, and weight regain is extremely common. Thus, cognitive approaches, such as behavior modification, were proposed as a way to promote behavior change more effectively [55].

Behavior modification consists of a set of behavior change strategies derived from experimental analysis of human behavior and designed to incrementally develop and sustain desirable behaviors or to decrease the frequency of undesirable behaviors. Behavioral modification for weight loss, therefore, is based on the premise that learned behaviors contributing to excessive or inadequate food intake or sedentary habits predominate, but can be modified to produce weight reduction [56].

Three distinct phases of behavior change were proposed: identifying motivation for change, implementing change strategies, and developing relapse-prevention strategies to ensure long-term change [57]. Several studies report good results with these behavioral approaches, regarding short-term and long-term lifestyle modification and weight loss outcomes [55].

Cognitive therapy, or cognitive-behavioral therapy, is another approach to promote lifestyle modification and weight loss, which is founded upon the premise that the manner in which people think about themselves or about a given event impacts how they will emotionally and behaviorally respond to the event. Many publications have highlighted the impact of cognitive thoughts and beliefs on body weight and weight loss, and have recommended increasing the focus on cognitive change to enhance weight loss and weight loss maintenance [55].

A systematic review of the efficacy of behavioral and cognitive interventions has shown significantly greater weight reductions when they are used along with common lifestyle modifications, with an additional weight loss of 2.5–4.9 kg, and supports their adoption in weight loss treatments, in combination with dietary and exercise strategies, in order to improve both short- and long-term outcomes [58].

9.5.2 MIND–BODY THERAPIES

A thorough review of the effects of mind–body therapies on insulin resistance and other metabolic abnormalities compatible with MetS was conducted by Innes et al. [59]. They report an extensive number of studies that should lend support to beneficial effects of mind–body therapies, such as qigong (a Chinese practice, which involves rhythmic breathing coordinated with slow stylized repetition of fluid movement and a calm mindful state) and yoga, on MetS components such as serum lipids, glucose tolerance, blood pressure, body weight, oxidative stress, inflammation, sympathetic activation, and several measures of stress, depression, and quality of life, in both healthy and chronically ill populations. Tai chi chuan (tai chi) is another mind–body therapy originally from ancient Asia, which seems to be an effective intervention for improving stress, depression, and quality of life [59].

However, most studies on those therapies are small and have major methodological limitations, such as the lack of a control arm. Besides, there is no evidence on the effect of those therapies on clinical (*hard*) outcomes, such as cardiovascular events or mortality. Also, as the vast majority of those studies were conducted in Asian countries, with Eastern populations, it may be difficult to generalize their results to ethnically diverse Western populations. However, all those mind–body therapies are relatively low cost, safe, and may have beneficial impacts on psychological or physical well-being, so they can be integrated into a lifestyle program intended to promote good health, along with other interventions (physical activity, healthy diet, weight loss) better known to have beneficial effects on clinical outcomes.

REFERENCES

1. Carr, D. B., Utzschneider, K. M., Hull, R. L. et al. 2004. Intra-abdominal fat is a major determinant of the Treatment Panel III criteria for the metabolic syndrome. *Diabetes* 53:2087–2094.
2. Eckel, R. H., Alberti, K. G. M. M., Grundy, S. M., and Zimmet, P. Z. 2010. The metabolic syndrome. *Lancet* 16(375):181–183.
3. Cornier, M.-A., Dabelea, D., Hernandez, T. L. et al. 2008. The metabolic syndrome. *Endocrine Reviews* 29:777–822.
4. Lakka, T. A., Laaksonen, D. E., Lakka, H. et al. 2003. Sedentary lifestyle, poor cardiorespiratory fitness, and the metabolic syndrome. *Medicine and Science in Sports and Exercise* 35:1279–1286.
5. Chen, M., He, M., Min, X. et al. 2013. Different physical activity subtypes and risk of metabolic syndrome in middle-aged and older Chinese people. *PloS One* 8(1) (January):e53258. http://www.plosone.org/article/info%3Adoi%2F10.1371%2Fjournal.pone.0053258.
6. Laursen, A. H., Kristiansen, O. P., Marott, J. L., Schnohr, P., and Prescott, E. January 2012. Intensity versus duration of physical activity: Implications for the metabolic syndrome. A prospective cohort study. *BMJ Open* 2(5):e001711. Available from: http://bmjopen.bmj.com/content/2/5/e001711.full.
7. Reaven, G. M. 2008. Insulin resistance: The link between obesity and cardiovascular disease. *Endocrinology and Metabolism Clinics of North America* 37:581–601.
8. Grundy, S. M., Cleeman, J. I., Daniels, S. R. et al. 2005. Diagnosis and management of the metabolic syndrome: An American Heart Association/National Heart, Lung, and Blood Institute Scientific Statement. *Circulation* 112:2735–2752.
9. Alberti, K. G. M. M., Zimmet, P., and Shaw, J. 2006. Metabolic syndrome—A new world-wide definition. A Consensus Statement from the International Diabetes Federation. *Diabetic Medicine* 23:469–480.
10. Pasanisi, F., Contaldo, F., De Simone, G., and Mancini, M. 2001. Benefits of sustained moderate weight loss in obesity. *Nutrition, Metabolism, and Cardiovascular Diseases* 11:401–406.
11. Lee, W.-J., Huang, M.-T., Wang, W., Lin, C.-M., Chen, T.-C., and Lai, I.-R. 2004. Effects of obesity surgery on the metabolic syndrome. *Archives of Surgery* 139:1088–1092.
12. Carroll, S. and Dudfield, M. 2004. What is the relationship between exercise and metabolic abnormalities? *Sports Medicine* 34:371–418.
13. Thompson, P.D., Buchner, D., Pina, I. L. et al. 2003. Exercise and physical activity in the prevention and treatment of atherosclerotic cardiovascular disease: a statement from the Council on Clinical Cardiology (Subcommittee on Exercise, Rehabilitation, and Prevention) and the Council on Nutrition, Physical Activity, and Metabolism (Subcommittee on Physical Activity). *Circulation* 107:3109–3116.

14. U. S. Department of Health and Human Services. 1996. Physical activity and health: A report of the surgeon general. Atlanta, GA: U. S. Department of Health and Human Services, Centers for Disease Control and Prevention.

15. Laaksonen, D. E., Lindstro, J., Lakka, T. A. et al. 2005. Physical activity in the prevention of type 2 diabetes—The Finnish Diabetes Prevention Study. *Diabetes* 54:158–165.

16. Ilanne-Parikka, P., Laaksonen, D. E., Eriksson, J. G. et al. 2010. Leisure-time physical activity and the metabolic syndrome in the Finnish Diabetes Prevention Study. *Diabetes Care* 33:1610–1607.

17. Orchard, T. J., Temprosa, M., Goldberg, R. et al. 2005. The effect of metformin and intensive lifestyle intervention on the metabolic syndrome: The Diabetes Prevention Program randomized trial. *Annals of Internal Medicine* 142:611–619.

18. Knowler, W. C., Fowler, S. E., Hamman, R. F. et al. 2009. 10-year follow-up of diabetes incidence and weight loss in the Diabetes Prevention Program Outcomes Study. *Lancet* 374:1677–1686.

19. Jurca, R., Lamonte, M. J., Barlow, C. E., Kampert, J. B., Church, T. S., and Blair, S. N. 2005. Association of muscular strength with incidence of metabolic syndrome in men. *Medicine and Science in Sports and Exercise* 37:1849–1855.

20. Ibañez, J., Izquierdo, M., Argüelles, I. et al. 2005. Twice-weekly progressive resistance training decreases abdominal fat and improves insulin sensitivity in older men with type 2 diabetes. *Diabetes Care* 28:662–667.

21. McLaughlin, T., Abbasi, F., Cheal, K., Chu, J., Lamendola, C., and Reaven, G. 2003. Use of metabolic markers to identify overweight individuals who are insulin resistant. *Annals of Internal Medicine* 139:802–809.

22. Gallagher, E. J., LeRoith, D., and Karnieli, E. 2008. The metabolic syndrome—From insulin resistance to obesity and diabetes. *Endocrinology and Metabolism Clinics of North America* 37:559–579.

23. Haskell, W. L., Lee, I.-M., Pate, R. R. et al. 2007. Physical activity and public health: updated recommendation for adults from the American College of Sports Medicine and the American Heart Association. *Medicine and Science in Sports and Exercise* 39:1423–1434.

24. Dengel, D. R., Pratley, R. E., Hagberg, J. M., Rogus, E. M., and Goldberg, A. P. 1996. Distinct effects of aerobic exercise training and weight loss on glucose homeostasis in obese sedentary men. *Journal of Applied Physiology* 81:318–325.

25. Tjønna, A. E., Lee, S. J., Rognmo, Ø. et al. 2008. Aerobic interval training versus continuous moderate exercise as a treatment for the metabolic syndrome: A pilot study. *Circulation* 118:346–354.

26. Lee, J. A., Kim, J. W., and Kim, D. Y. 2012. Effects of yoga exercise on serum adiponectin and metabolic syndrome factors in obese postmenopausal women. *Menopause* 19:296–301.

27. American Diabetes Association. 2013. Standards of Medical Care in Diabetes—2013. *Diabetes Care* 36(Suppl. 1):S11–S66.

28. Knowler, W. C., Barrett-Connor, E., Fowler, S. E. et al. 2002. Reduction in the incidence of type 2 diabetes with lifestyle intervention or metformin. *New England Journal of Medicine* 346:393–403.

29. Tuomilehto, J., Lindstrom, J., Eriksson, J. G., et al. 2001. Prevention of type 2 diabetes mellitus by changes in lifestyle among subjects with impaired glucose tolerance. *New England Journal of Medicine* 344:1343–1350.

30. Pan, X. R., Li, G. W., Hu, Y. H. et al. 1997. Effects of diet and exercise in preventing NIDDM in people with impaired glucose tolerance. The Da Qing IGT and Diabetes Study. *Diabetes Care* 20:537–544.

31. Li, G., Zhang, P., Wang, J. et al. 2008. The long-term effect of lifestyle interventions to prevent diabetes in the China Da Qing Diabetes Prevention Study: A 20-year follow-up study. *Lancet* 371:1783–1789.

32. Lindström, J., Ilanne-Parikka, P., Peltonen, M. et al. 2006. Sustained reduction in the incidence of type 2 diabetes by lifestyle intervention: Follow-up of the Finnish Diabetes Prevention Study. *Lancet* 368:1673–1679.

33. Pescatello, L. S., Blanchard, B. E., Van Heest, J. L., Maresh, C. M., Gordish-Dressman, H., and Thompson, P. D. June 2008. The metabolic syndrome and the immediate antihypertensive effects of aerobic exercise: A randomized control design. *BMC Cardiovascular Disorders* 8(12):1–10. http://www.biomedcentral.com/1471-2261/8/12.

34. Whelton, S. P., Chin, A., Xin, X., and He, J. 2002. Effect of aerobic exercise on blood pressure: A meta-analysis of randomized, controlled trials. *Annals of Internal Medicine* 136:493–503.

35. Chobanian, A. V., Bakris, G. L., Black, H. R. et al. 2003. Seventh report of the Joint National Committee on prevention, detection, evaluation and treatment of high blood pressure (JNC 7). *JAMA* 289:2560–2572.

36. Stone, N. J., Bilek, S., and Rosenbaum, S. 2005. Recent National Cholesterol Education Program Adult Treatment Panel III update: Adjustments and options. *The American Journal of Cardiology* 96:53E–59E.

37. Katsanos, C. S. 2006. Prescribing aerobic exercise for the regulation of postprandial lipid metabolism: current research and recommendations. *Sports Medicine* 36:547–560.

38. Ben Ounis, O., Elloumi, M., Makni, E. et al. 2010. Exercise improves the ApoB/ApoA-I ratio, a marker of the metabolic syndrome in obese children. *Acta Paediatrica* 99:1679–1685.

39. Lind, L. 2003. Circulating markers of inflammation and atherosclerosis. *Atherosclerosis* 169:203–214.

40. Milani, R. V. and Lavie, C. J. 2003. Prevalence and profile of metabolic syndrome in patients following acute coronary events and effects of therapeutic lifestyle change with cardiac rehabilitation. *The American Journal of Cardiology* 92:50–54.

41. Zoppini, G., Targher, G., Zamboni, C. et al. 2006. Effects of moderate-intensity exercise training on plasma biomarkers of inflammation and endothelial dysfunction in older patients with type 2 diabetes. *Nutrition, Metabolism, and Cardiovascular Diseases* 16:543–549.

42. Balducci, S., Zanuso, S., Nicolucci, A. et al. 2010. Anti-inflammatory effect of exercise training in subjects with type 2 diabetes and the metabolic syndrome is dependent on exercise modalities and independent of weight loss. *Nutrition, Metabolism, and Cardiovascular Diseases* 20:608–617.

43. Kopec, K. L. and Burns, D. 2011. Nonalcoholic fatty liver disease: A review of the spectrum of disease, diagnosis, and therapy. *Nutrition in Clinical Practice* 26:565–576.

44. Straznicky, N., and Lambert, E. 2012. The effects of dietary weight loss with or without exercise training on liver enzymes in obese metabolic syndrome subjects. *Diabetes, Obesity and Metabolism* 14:139–148.

45. Thomson, R. L., Buckley, J. D., and Brinkworth, G. D. 2011. Exercise for the treatment and management of overweight women with polycystic ovary syndrome: A review of the literature. *Obesity Reviews* 12:e202–e210.

46. Nybacka, Å., Carlström, K., Ståhle, A., Nyrén, S., Hellström, P. M., and Hirschberg, A. L. 2011. Randomized comparison of the influence of dietary management and/or physical exercise on ovarian function and metabolic parameters in overweight women with polycystic ovary syndrome. *Fertility and Sterility* 96:1508–1513.

47. Ardern, C. I., Katzmarzyk, P. T., Janssen, I., Church, T. S., and Blair, S. N. 2005. Revised Adult Treatment Panel III guidelines and cardiovascular disease mortality in men attending a preventive medical clinic. *Circulation* 112:1478–1485.

48. Oguma, Y. and Shinoda-Tagawa, T. 2004. Physical activity decreases cardiovascular disease risk in women: Review and meta-analysis. *American Journal of Preventive Medicine* 26:407–418.

49. Wei, M., Gibbons, L. W., Kampert, J. B., Nichaman, M. Z., and Blair, S. N. 2000. Low cardiorespiratory fitness and physical inactivity as predictors of mortality in men with type 2 diabetes. *Annals of Internal Medicine* 132:605–611.

50. Wei, M., Kampert, J. B., Barlow, C. E. et al. 1999. Relationship between low cardiorespiratory fitness and mortality in normal-weight, overweight, and obese men. *JAMA* 282:1547–1553.

51. Stensvold, D., Nauman, J., Nilsen, T. I. L., Wisløff, U., Slørdahl, S. A., and Vatten, L. 2011. Even low level of physical activity is associated with reduced mortality among people with metabolic syndrome, a population based study (the HUNT 2 study, Norway). *BMC Medicine* 9:109. http://www.biomedcentral.com/1741-7015/9/109.

52. Irving, B. A., Weltman, J. Y., Patrie, J. T. et al. 2009. Effects of exercise training intensity on nocturnal growth hormone secretion in obese adults with the metabolic syndrome. *Journal of Clinical Endocrinology and Metabolism* 94:1979–1986.

53. Moser, M. and Sowers, J. 2010. *Clinical Management of Cardiovascular Risk Factors in Diabetes*. 4th ed. West Islip, NY: Professional Communications, Inc.

54. Perk, J., De Backer, G., Gohlke, H. et al. 2012. European Guidelines on cardiovascular disease prevention in clinical practice (version 2012). The Fifth Joint Task Force of the European Society of Cardiology and Other Societies on Cardiovascular Disease Prevention in Clinical Practice. *European Heart Journal* 33:1635–1701.

55. Van Dorsten, B., and Lindley, E. M. 2008. Cognitive and behavioral approaches in the treatment of obesity. *Endocrinology and Metabolism Clinics of North America* 37:905–922.

56. Jeffery, R. W., Drewnowski, A., Epstein, L. H. et al. 2000. Long-term maintenance of weight loss: Current status. *Health Psychology* 19(Suppl 1):5–16.

57. Brownell, K., Marlatt, G., Lichtenstein, E., and Wilson, G. 1986. Understanding and preventing relapse. *American Psychologist* 41:765–782.

58. Shaw, K., O'Rourke, P., Del Mar, C., and Kenardy, J. 2005. Psychological interventions for overweight or obesity. *Cochrane Database of Systematic Reviews* 2:CD003818. http://onlinelibrary.wiley.com/doi/10.1002/14651858.CD003818.pub2/pdf.
59. Innes, K. E., Selfe, T. K., and Taylor, A. G. 2008. Menopause, the metabolic syndrome, and mind-body therapies. *Menopause* 15:1005–1013.

Section IV

Specific Conditions Related to Metabolic Syndrome

10 Metabolic Syndrome in Rheumatoid Arthritis

*Flávia Troncon Rosa, Tatiana Mayumi Veiga Iriyoda,
Elis Carolina de Souza Fatel, Ana Paula Kallaur,
Andréa Name Colado Simão, and Isaias Dichi*

CONTENTS

10.1 INTRODUCTION

Rheumatoid Arthritis (RA) is an autoimmune chronic inflammatory disease of unknown etiology (Aletaha et al. 2010). The prevalence of RA in adult population is approximately 0.5%–1%. It is observed in all ethnic groups (Alarcón 1995), with a female predominance, especially in patients between the fourth and sixth decades of life (Silman et al. 2002). In Brazil, a multicenter study also found prevalence of RA in adults ranging from 0.2% to 1.0% (Marques Neto et al. 1993).

The diagnosis of RA is established considering clinical findings and laboratory tests. Signs and symptoms include complaints of pain, swelling, and limitation of movement; polyarticular impairment (more than four joints), involvement of the wrists, metacarpophalangeal and proximal interphalangeal; symmetric arthritis; and morning stiffness, characterized by stiffness and swelling sensation perceived especially in the morning, lasting more than 1 h (Woolf 2003, Mota et al. 2011). As a systemic disease, fever, malaise, fatigue, myalgia, and weight loss can be present. Also, extra-articular manifestations, such as rheumatoid nodules, Sjogren's syndrome, episcleritis and scleritis, interstitial lung disease, pericardial involvement, systemic vasculitis, and Felty's syndrome can be observed in patients with severe RA, with polyarticular impairment and positive serology for the autoantibodies rheumatoid factor (RF) and anticitrullinated protein antibody (ACPA) (tested as anticyclic citrullinated peptide (anti-CCP)) (Vallbracht et al. 2004, Turesson et al. 2007, Goeldner et al. 2011). RF is an antibody that acts against the Fc portion of the immunoglobulin G (IgG) and affects approximately 70%–80% of AR patients and increased levels determine the aggressiveness of the disease and a poor prognosis (Wolfe et al. 1991, Visser et al. 1996, Vittecoq et al. 2003, Renaudineau et al. 2005). The anti-CCP emerged as a diagnostic tool, as sensitive (70%–75%) and more specific (95%) than RF to a precocious detection of the disease (Raza et al. 2005, van der Helm-van Mil et al. 2005, Klareskog et al. 2008).

TABLE 10.1

The 2010 American College of Rheumatology/European League Against Rheumatism Classification Criteria for Rheumatoid Arthritis

Target population (Who should be tested?):

(1) Patients who have at least 1 joint with definite clinical synovitis (swelling)

(2) Patients who with the synovitis not better explained by another disease

	Score
Classification criteria for RA (score-based algorithm: add score of categories A–D; a score of 6/10 is needed for classification of a patient as having definite RA)	
A. Joint involvement[a]	
1 large joint	0
2–10 large joints	1
1–3 small joints (with or without involvement of large joints)[b]	2
4–10 small joints (with or without involvement of large joints)	3
>10 joints (at least 1 small joint)	5
B. Serology (at least 1 test result is needed for classification)	
Negative RF and negative ACPA	0
Low-positive RF or low-positive ACPA	2
High-positive RF or high-positive ACPA	3
C. Acute-phase reactants (at least 1 test result is needed for classification)	
Normal CRP and normal ESR	0
Abnormal CRP or abnormal ESR	1
D. Duration of symptoms	
<6 weeks	0
≥6 weeks	1

Source: Data from Aletaha, D. et al., *Arthritis Rheum.*, 69(9), 1580, 2010.

RF, rheumatoid factor; ACPA, anti-citrullinated protein antibody; CRP, C-reactive protein; ESR, erythrocyte sedimentation rate.

[a] Joint involvement refers to any swollen or tender joint on examination, which may be confirmed by imaging evidence of synovitis. Distal interphalangeal joints, first carpometacarpal joints, and first metatarsophalangeal joints are excluded from assessment. "Large joints" refers to shoulders, elbows, hips, knees, and ankles.

[b] "Small joints" refers to the metacarpophalangeal joints, proximal interphalangeal joints, second through fifth metatarsophalangeal joints, thumb interphalangeal joints, and wrists.

A new classification of RA was developed by the American College of Rheumatology (ACR) and the European League Against Rheumatism (EULAR). The new classification focus on features at earlier stages of disease since its progression can lead to severe deformity, disability, and premature mortality. Treating patients at a stage where evolution of joint destruction can still be prevented would be ideal (Seven et al. 2008, Aletaha et al. 2010). ACR/EULAR 2010 criteria (Table 10.1) aims to identify factors among patients with undifferentiated and recent inflammatory synovitis that could indicate patients at risk of persistence or structural damage and recommend earlier interventions with antirheumatic drugs (Arnett et al. 1988, Aletaha et al. 2010).

The course of RA varies from mild to severe and the disease activity can be monitored by indices that take into account a simplified count of tender and swollen joints (28 joints), inflammatory markers (ESR and/or CRP), as well as patient visual analog scale regarding pain, and patient and physician visual analog scale regarding disease activity (van der Heijde et al. 1993, van Gestel et al. 1998, Smolen et al. 2003, Aletaha et al. 2005, Siegel et al. 2005). The indices Disease Activity Score 28 (DAS 28), Simplified Disease Activity Index (SDAI), and Clinical Disease Activity Index (CDAI) are shown in Table 10.2.

TABLE 10.2

Calculation and Total Value of the Combined Disease Activity Indices

Elements	SDAI	CDAI	DAS28 (with 4 Variables)
Number of swollen joints	Simple sum (0–28)	Simple sum (0–28)	Square root of the simple sum
Number of tender joints	Simple sum (0–28)	Simple sum (0–28)	Square root of the simple sum
Acute-phase reactants	CRP (0.1–10 mg/dL)	—	ESR (2–100 mm) or CRP (0.1–10 mg/dL) logarithmic transformation
Global health assessment (patient)		—	(0–100 mm)
Disease activity assessment (patient)	(0–10 cm)	(0–10 cm)	—
Disease activity assessment (physician)	(0–10 cm)	(0–10 cm)	—
Total index (index range)	Simple sum (0.1–86)	Simple sum (0–76)	Requires inserting number in the calculator (0.49–9.07)

Source: Data from Mota, L.M.H. et al., *Rev. Bras. Reumatol.*, 51(3), 197, 2011.

SDAI, Simplified disease activity index; CDAI, Clinical disease activity index; DAS28, disease activity score (28 joints); CRP, C-reactive protein; ESR, erythrocyte sedimentation rate.

The precocious diagnosis and treatment reduce articular destruction, preserve function, and improve quality of life and survival rate of patients (ACR Guidelines 2002, Kalpakcioglu and Îenel 2008). There are evidences on the benefits in both the disease course and the impact of treatment on outcomes when starting treatment early. Besides the joint impairment, RA patients have increased risk to develop comorbidities such as systemic arterial hypertension, dyslipidemia and diabetes. Also, 50% of death in RA patients are due to cardiovascular diseases. These explain the recent and increasing interest in studying Metabolic Syndrome in this specific group (Zhang et al. 2013).

10.2   PREVALENCE OF METABOLIC SYNDROME IN RA

RA has been associated to increased prevalence of metabolic syndrome (MetS). However, it is complex to determine the real prevalence because criteria for MetS definition vary from different organizations (Table 10.3). Moreover, different study design and sample size make interpretation and comparison of results difficult.

The first study to show increased prevalence of MetS in RA patients was developed by Chung et al. (2008a). The authors compared RA patients to a control group paired by age, ethnicity, sex, and body mass index (BMI). They applied WHO definition and found that MetS was more frequent in patients with long time duration of RA (42%) compared to patients with recent diagnosis (30%) and healthy controls (11%) (P < 0.001) [OR = 4.29 (95% CI: 1.68–10.96), p = 0.002 for precocious RA and OR = 9.6 (95% CI: 3.5–26.6), p < 0.001 for long lasting RA]. A Brazilian study found significant differences between RA patients and a control group (39.2% versus 19.5%, p < 0.001) (Cunha et al. 2012). Also, recent meta-analysis involving a total of 2283 cases and 4403 controls identified a significant association between RA and risk of MetS, with an overall OR of 1.24 (95% CI, 1.03–1.50) (Zhang et al. 2013).

However, results concerning this issue are conflicting. Karvounaris et al. (2007) did not found significant difference between cases and controls regarding the presence of MetS in RA. The authors studied 200 patients and 400 controls. The MetS prevalence, defined by National Cholesterol Education Program – Adult Treatment Panel (NCEP/ATP III 2001), was 44% in RA patients and 41% in controls. Another study investigated 45 patients versus 48 controls without systemic rheumatic disease. The prevalence of MetS was 55% and 46%, respectively, also without significant difference (La Montagna et al. 2007). Applying the same definition criteria, Giles et al. (2010) designed a case-control study with 131 cases and 121 controls. They also found no differences between case and control groups (36 versus 27%).

TABLE 10.3

Metabolic Syndrome Definition by International Diabetes Federation (IDF), World Health Organization (WHO) and National Cholesterol Education Program's Adult Treatment Panel III (NCEP/ATP III) and European Group for the Study of Insulin Resistance (EGIR)

Parameters	NCEP ATP III 2004	IDF 2005	EGIR 1999	WHO 1999 Modified	AACE 2003
Required		Waist ≥94 cm (m) ≥80 cm (w)[b]	IR or fasting hyperinsulinemia at the top of the 25th percentile	IR: HOMA at the top of the 25th pct, fasting glycemia ≥110 or DM	At high risk for IR[a] or BMI ≥25 or waist ≥ 102 (m)≥ 88 (w)
Number of abnormalities	≥3 of:	≥2 of:	≥2 of:	≥2 of:	≥2 of:
Glucose	≥100 mg/dL or treatment	≥100 mg/dL or DM diagnosis	110–125 mg/dL		≥110 mg/dL; ≥140 (2 h after glucose)
HDL-c	<40 (m); <50 (w) or treatment[c]	<40 (m); <50 (w) or treatment	<40 mg/dL	<35 (m); <40 (w)	<40 (m); <50 (w)
Triglycerides	≥150 mg/dL or treatment[c]	≥150 mg/dL or treatment	Or ≥180 mg/dL or treatment for dyslipidemia	Or ≥150 mg/dL	≥150 mg/dL
Obesity (waist circumference)	≥102 cm (m) ≥88 cm (w)		≥94 cm (m) ≥80 cm (w)	≥94 cm (m) ≥88 cm (w)	
Hypertension	≥130/85 mmHg or treatment	≥130/85 mmHg or treatment	≥140/90 mmHg or treatment	≥140/90 mmHg or treatment	≥130/85 mmHg

Source: Data from Cunha, V.R. et al., *Rev. Bras. Reumatol.*, 51(3), 260, 2011.

m, men; w, women; NCEP, National Cholesterol Education Program; IDF, International Diabetes Federation; EGIR, Group for the Study of Insulin Resistance; WHO, World Health Organization; AACE, American Association of Clinical Endocrinologists; HDL-c, high-density lipoprotein cholesterol; HOMA, homeostasis model assessment; BMI, body mass index; SAH, systemic arterial hypertension; IR, insulin resistance; DM, diabetes mellitus.

[a] At high risk for IR, indicated by the presence of at least one of the following: diagnosis of CVD, hypertension, polycystic ovary syndrome, nonalcoholic fatty liver disease, or acanthosis nigricans; family history of type 2 diabetes, hypertension, or CVD; history of gestational diabetes or glucose intolerance; nonwhite ethnicity; sedentary lifestyle; BMI = 25 kg/m² or waist circumference = 94 cm for men and = 80 cm for women; and age de 40 years.

[b] For South-Asian and Chinese patients, waist ≥90 cm (men) or ≥80 cm (women); for Japanese patients, waist ≥90 (men) or ≥80 cm (women).

[c] Treatment with one or more fibrates or niacin.

Studies without control groups observed diverse results for MetS prevalence in RA. Elkan et al. (2009) used the International Diabetes Federation (IDF) criteria and found a prevalence of 20% for women and 63% for men. Toms et al. (2009) compared five definition criteria (NCEP/ATP III 2001, NCEP/ATP III 2004, IDF 2005, WHO 1999 and EGIR 1999) to evaluate the prevalence of MetS in 400 patients. Highest prevalence was observed by IDF definition reaching 45.3% and the lowest (12.1%) by EGIR definition.

10.3   CAUSES OF METABOLIC SYNDROME IN RA

Although the increased prevalence of MetS evidenced in RA patients, the exact causes are not conclusive. The role of disease activity and duration, inflammation process, oxidative stress, and glucocorticoids treatment has been investigated (Cunha et al. 2011).

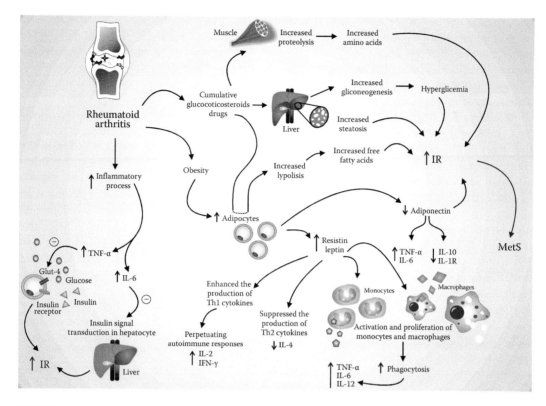

FIGURE 10.1 Interplay between rheumatoid arthritis proinflammatory state and metabolic syndrome.

Several studies suggest that the proinflammatory state in RA contributes to the development of MetS (Borges et al. 2007, Chung et al. 2008b). The abundance of inflammatory cytokines results in insulin resistance (IR), the main metabolic disturbance of MetS (Eckel et al. 2005, La Montagna et al. 2007, Zhang et al. 2013) (Figure 10.1).

Inflammation, as measured by interleukin (IL)-6 and TNF-α, explained a substantially greater proportion of the variance in homeostatic model assessment index (HOMA), regardless of age, race, sex, BMI, and current use of corticosteroids. This reinforces the concept that in patients with RA, specific mediators of inflammation play a key role in the pathogenesis of IR (Chung et al. 2008b). The association between TNF-α and HOMA index in patients with RA is consistent with findings in the general population. TNF-α antagonists have improved insulin sensitivity in some studies (Kiortsis et al. 2005, Huvers et al. 2007), but not in others (Di Rocco et al. 2004). IL-6 can either increase or reduce IR (Carey et al. 2004, Heliovaara et al. 2005), but long-term exposure to IL-6 is more likely to induce it (Mooney 2007).

Dessein et al. (2002) showed increased IR and reduced levels of high-density lipoprotein (HDL) in RA compared to patients diagnosed with osteoarthritis (OA), and both variables correlated to C-reactive protein levels (CRP). However, controlling for CRP, the differences in IR between groups disappeared and in HDL cholesterol attenuated, which indicates that CRP contributed to variance in IR and HDL. Besides that, the same research group investigated the contribution of some factors to impaired insulin sensitivity and beta cell function in RA and found abdominal obesity as the main predictor of IR (Dessein et al. 2006). On the other hand, Chung et al. (2008b) demonstrated that IR was independently associated to markers of inflammation and to disease characteristics.

In this direction, studying the relationship of MetS with disease activity and the functional status in patients with RA, Karakoc et al. (2012) found that the frequency of MetS was higher in patients with impaired functional status. Also, a positive correlation was observed between DAS28 scores and hypertension in patients with RA. However, a limitation is that the relationship between medication and MetS has not been investigated in this study. Cunha et al. (2012) found that DAS28 scores were significantly higher in RA patients with MetS than in those without, but they did not observe differences concerning disease duration, presence of RF, or extra-articular manifestations. The association of changes in insulin sensitivity, pancreatic β cell function, or MetS with disease activity remains controversial (Dessein et al. 2006, Chung et al. 2008b, Shahin et al. 2010).

Regarding RA treatment, chronic users of glucocorticoids (GC) and treatment-naive patients have similar parameters of insulin sensitivity and pancreatic beta cell function. However, cumulative doses of GC have negative impact on the status of glucose tolerance and insulin sensitivity (Buttgereit 2011, Hoes et al. 2011). The use of oral prednisone and frequent intramuscular, intra-articular, and intravenous GC doses were associated to the presence of IR, but not to obesity, dyslipidemia, or hypertension (Cunha et al. 2012). However, it was not evidenced by Toms et al. (2008). The authors studied the prevalence of MetS according to GC exposure [no or limited exposure (<3 months); low-dose long-term exposure (<7.5 mg/day); and medium-dose long-term exposure (≥7.5 mg to 30 mg/day)] and reported presence of MS in 40.1% of 398 patients with RA without associations with long-term GC exposure. Some studies have found weak association (Chung et al. 2007, Chung et al. 2008a) or no association (Dessein et al. 2006, El Magadmi et al. 2006) between GC and presence of MetS or IR in patients with RA (or Systemic Lupus Erythematosus) suggesting that perhaps the best control of inflammation can counteract the deleterious effect of GC on glucose metabolism (Chung et al. 2008b). The use of methotrexate was independently associated with reduced risk to MetS and it was suggested as a good first-line anti-rheumatic drug in RA patients at high risk of developing the syndrome (Toms et al. 2009). Also, findings from Dessein et al. (2008) study indicate that when GC is used sparingly and according to disease activity, they may not adversely affect insulin sensitivity in RA.

The adipose tissue may also play a role in the relationship between MetS and RA. Obesity is highly prevalent in RA patients with a concomitant cachexia condition characterized by increased fat mass and reduced fat-free mass (Roubenoff 2009). Adipose tissue is now considered more than a lipid storage tissue but also an endocrine organ that secrete various hormones and molecules named adipokines that mediate immune response and inflammation (Lago et al. 2007). Recent studies revealed that adipokines such as leptin and adiponectin are involved in inflammation and immune response regulation and may play a role in the pathogenesis of inflammatory joint diseases (Tilg and Moschen 2006, Toussirot et al. 2007). They exert modulatory actions on cells involved in rheumatic disease, including cartilage, synovium, bone, and various immune cells (Gómez et al. 2011).

Leptin is a protein produced mainly by adipose tissue cells and its levels correlate with body mass. This hormone acts in the control of appetite and energy expenditure, but also has proinflammatory activity through the activation and proliferation of monocytes and macrophages, phagocytic function, and increased production of proinflammatory cytokines such as TNF-α, IL-6, and IL-12. Leptin enhances the production of Th1 cytokines that acts perpetuating autoimmune responses such as IL-2 and Interferon-γ and suppresses the production of Th2 cytokines, such as IL-4 (Lord et al. 2002, Palmer and Gabay 2003; La Cava and Matarese 2004, Otero et al. 2005, Bernotiene et al. 2006). Adiponectin is a protein synthesized primarily by adipocytes. It is associated with lipid and glucose metabolism (Berg et al. 2002, Guziket al. 2006, Brochu-Gaudreau et al. 2010). It exerts anti-inflammatory effect by reducing the production and activity of TNF-α and IL-6, and also induces the production of anti-inflammatory mediators such as IL-10 and IL-1 receptor antagonist (IL-1 RA) (Wolf et al. 2004, Toussirotet al. 2007).

The adipokines are associated to obesity, IR, inflammation and coronary artery disease in the general population (Rho et al. 2010). These associations are related to increased levels of leptin and decreased levels of adiponectin (Tilg and Moschen 2006, Martin et al. 2008, Rho et al. 2010). Studies on the role of adipokines in RA are controversial. Data comparing leptin levels from RA patients to normal controls (or patients with osteoarthritis) showed even similar results (Anders et al. 1999,

Popa et al. 2005, Hizmetli et al. 2007, Targojska-Stdpniak et al. 2008), but also low (Tokarczyk-Knapik et al. 2002) or high concentrations (Salazar-Paramo et al. 2001, Bokarewa et al. 2003). Otero et al. (2006) found increased levels of adiponectin and leptin in patients with RA, while Nagashima et al. (2008) found no significant differences compared to healthy controls.

There are few published studies on the association of MetS with adipokine levels in patients with inflammatory arthritis. According to Rho et al. (2010), leptin is associated with IR in RA patients, even after adjustment for BMI, inflammation, and cardiovascular risk factors. However, unexpectedly, adiponectin had no association with IR in RA. The study of Kontunen et al. (2011) did not found differences in leptin or adiponectin levels between RA patients without MetS and control group, while in patients with MetS leptin levels were significantly elevated (even after adjustment for BMI) and adiponectin reduced. These data suggest that these adipokynes are associated with MetS, but not directly with arthritis. In addition, no correlation between leptin and adiponectin, IL-6 and C-reactive protein was found (Kontunen et al. 2011).

Moreover, studies have shown that D vitamin deficiency is associated to cardiovascular risk factors such as MetS and IR (Chiu et al. 2004, Martins et al. 2007, Reis et al. 2007, Ford et al. 2009, Liu et al. 2009, Lu et al. 2009) and suboptimal levels of vitamin D are noted to be common in RA, with a prevalence varying from 40% to 60% (Haque and Bartlett 2010, Rossini et al. 2010, Kerr et al. 2011). Although still scarce, some studies have suggested that hypovitaminosis D is associated with MetS in patients with RA (Baker et al. 2012, Goshayeshi et al. 2012, Haque et al. 2012). Vitamin D is considered an immunomodulator and could reduce the risk of MetS by reducing RA-associated inflammation (Michos and Melamed 2008, Zittermann et al. 2009).

Currently, MetS is a worldwide public health problem. Although obesity and IR comprise the leading causes of MetS, many other pathophysiological mechanisms, like proinflammatory adipocytokines, hyperuricemia, nitric oxide, and oxidative stress, may contribute to the potential cardiovascular risk factors related to the syndrome (Simão 2012). Patients diagnosed with RA present reduced life expectancy and the cardiovascular disease seems to be the main cause of death. These patients have increased risk (up to four times) to have myocardial acute infarction (del Rincon et al. 2001, Dessein et al. 2004, Karvounaris et al. 2007). Chung et al. (2008a) in addition to assessing the prevalence of MetS also evaluated atherosclerosis development by detection of coronary calcification by computed tomography. The RA group with MetS presented increased risk for arterial calcifications (OR = 2.02, IC 95%: 1.03–3.97, p = 0.04). Altogether, these data determine the importance to investigate nutrition interventions to help counteract MetS and risk factors for cardiovascular disease.

10.4 NUTRITIONAL INTERVENTIONS IN METABOLIC SYNDROME AND RA

The influence of nutrition on molecular and cellular metabolism has been widely studied and its interference in pathological inflammatory process has been evidenced. Therefore, treatment of inflammatory diseases such as AR could benefit from nutritional interventions or diets in which anti-inflammatory bioactive compounds or foods were included (González Cernadas et al. 2014). A nonsystematic revision in studies from 2003 to 2013 suggests that polyunsaturated fatty acids (PUFA), olive oil, and Mediterranean diet are promising treatment coadjuvants. The authors found that PUFA produced clinical improvement and inhibitory effects over the AR inflammatory response, olive oil reduced inflammatory markers and inhibited oxidative stress, and Mediterranean diet decreased both pain and disease activity. Finally, limited and contradictory evidence is found regarding the effectiveness of antioxidants (González Cernadas et al. 2014).

10.5 LONG-CHAIN ω-3 PUFA AND FISH OIL

In the last years, epidemiological and clinical studies have demonstrated the efficacy of fish oil supplementation in inflammatory diseases (Dichi et al. 2000, Barbosa et al. 2003, Hagfors et al. 2005) and, particularly, in RA (Berbert et al. 2005, James et al. 2010, Miles and Calder 2012). Fish oil provides two long-chain fatty acids referred to as eicosapentaenoic acid (EPA, 20:5 ω3) and docosahexaenoic acid (DHA, 22:6 ω3). These fatty acids are precursors of inflammatory mediators that are weak platelet aggregator and vasoconstrictor (thromboxane A3), weak inducers of inflammation (leukotriene B5), and strong vasodilators (prostacyclin PGI3), featuring its antiatherogenic activity. EPA promotes the inhibition of arachidonic acid (AA, 20:4 ω6) conversion to its metabolites, particularly leukotriene B4, a potent inducer of inflammation and of leukocyte adherence and chemotaxis. It also inhibits proinflammatory cytokines production, such as IL-1 and TNF-α, involved in the joint pathology of RA (James et al. 2010, Wall et al. 2010).

Due to its effect on RA inflammatory response, dietary long-chain ω-3 PUFA seems also to have a protective role on RA development. Di Giuseppe et al. (2013), studying the Swedish Mammography Cohort (SMC) of among 32,232 women, found that consumption of dietary long-chain ω-3 PUFAs of 0.21 g/day was associated with a 35% decreased risk of developing RA and intake consistently higher than 0.21 g/day [corresponding to at least one serving per week of fatty fish (e.g., salmon) or four servings per week of lean fish (e.g., cod)] was associated with a 52% decreased risk. Also, consistent long-term consumption of 1 or more serving of fish per week compared with less than 1 serving was associated with a 29% decrease in RA risk.

In patients with established disease, the most evident benefits of the use of ω-3 fatty acids from fish oil are reduction of joint pain and swelling, decrease in the duration of morning stiffness, improvement of pain and disease activity, and decreased use of nonsteroidal anti-inflammatory drugs (Berbert et al. 2005, Miles and Calder 2012). On the other hand, few reports were found evaluating the effects of ω-3 fatty acids on criteria for MetS in RA, although increased prevalence of MetS in these patients is nowadays demonstrated.

The use of marine ω-3 fatty acids for the management of hypertriglyceridemia is clinically effective. Different formulations have been studied and showed that dosages of 4 g/day in the form of 2 ethyl ester (ω-3-EE and EPA-EE) achieved clinically significant reductions in TG levels in patients with severe hypertriglyceridemia (Ballantyne et al. 2012). The efficacy and safety of ω-3 in the free fatty acid form was also tested and supplementation with 2, 3, and 4 g/day demonstrated reductions of approximately 25% in TG compared to olive oil, and lowered levels of non-high-density lipoprotein cholesterol (non-HDL-C), total cholesterol-to-HDL-C ratio, very-low-density lipoprotein cholesterol, remnant-like particle cholesterol, apolipoprotein CIII, lipoprotein-associated phospholipase A2, and arachidonic acid (Kastelein et al. 2014). In RA, only one study was found evaluating the effect of fish oil (FO) supplements on HDL-C, Apo-AI, malondialdehyde (MDA), arylesterase (Aryl), and paraoxonase 1 (PON1) activity. Ninety RA patients were randomly allocated into two groups that were treated with one FO pearl (1 g) daily or placebo for 3 months in addition to conventional treatment. The authors evidenced increased serum levels of HDL-C, Aryl, and PON1 activity. Moreover, significant correlations between increased PON1 activity and both HDL-C (p = 0.007, r = 0.419) and Apo-AI (p < 0.001, r = 0.742) concentrations as well as between HDL-C and Apo AI levels (p = 0.01, r = 0.403) were found. Although promising, the increments were actually quite small and need confirmation by future studies and higher doses (Ghorbanihaghjo et al. 2012).

Regarding blood pressure control, Simão et al. (2012) observed a decrease in blood pressure in patients with MetS resulting from the ingestion of 3 g/day of fish oil. Furthermore, a meta-analysis of double-blind randomized trials verified systolic and diastolic blood pressure reductions of 1.7 mmHg (95% CI: 0.3, 3.1) and 1.5 mmHg (95% CI: 0.6, 2.3), respectively (Geleijnse et al. 2002).

In contrast, the improvement of insulin sensitivity and glucose homeostasis by ω-3 PUFA observed in animal models of MetS was not found in humans (Flachs et al. 2014).

Besides its valuable support to the traditional pharmacological treatment of RA (Cleland et al. 2006, James et al. 2010), long-chain ω-3 PUFA can possibly prevent development or help to control some criteria of MetS in this specific group.

10.6 OLIVE OIL AND EXTRA-VIRGIN OLIVE OIL

Olive oil is mainly composed of oleic acid plus additional different chemical components such as sterols, alcohols, antioxidants, and other fatty acids of minor relevance. Oleic acid is a n-9 MUFA that is converted to 8,9,11,-eicosatrienoic acid (20:3n-9; ETA) under restriction of n-6 fatty acids. ETA is converted to LTA3, which is a potent inhibitor of LTB4 synthesis. Therefore, oleic acid and its metabolite ETA may exert inflammatory effects through a mechanism similar to that of fish oil, which contains EPA. Because ETA is substantially less unsaturated than EPA, it may have greater chemical stability, which would be an advantage for use as a dietary constituent or supplement (James et al. 1993).

Virgin olive oil is also a rich source of MUFA, but retains all the lipophilic components of the olive fruit, especially the phenolic compounds with strong antioxidant and anti-inflammatory properties. The administration of olive oil with a high phenolic content has been shown to protect against inflammation. Extra-virgin olive oil (EVOO) is a key component of the Mediterranean diet that has been attributed preventive properties with regard to chronic diseases, particularly those with an inflammatory etiology such as heart disease, cancer, and RA (Wahle et al. 2004). The beneficial effects of the Mediterranean diet can be attributed not only to the high-unsaturated content of olive oil, but also to the antioxidant property of its minor elements (carotenoids and phenolic compounds) with high activity. The phenolic compounds are both lipophilic and hydrophilic. The lipophilics include tocopherols, while the hydrophilics include flavonoids, phenolic alcohols and acids, secoiridoids (oleuropein and ligstroside), and lignans (1-acetoxypinoresinol and pinoresinol) (Tripoli et al. 2005).

Olive oil is a nonoxidative dietary component, and the attenuation of the inflammatory process it elicits could explain their beneficial effects on disease risk since oxidative and inflammatory stresses appear to be the underlying factors in the etiology of inflammatory diseases in man. The antioxidant effects of olive oil are probably due to a combination of its high oleic acid content (low oxidation potential compared with linoleic acid) and its content of a variety of plant antioxidants, particularly oleuropein, hydroxytyrosol, and tyrosol (Wahle et al. 2004).

Berbert et al. (2005) evaluated whether supplementation with olive oil during 6 months could improve clinical and laboratory parameters of disease activity in patients with RA who were using fish oil supplements. Forty tree patients were assigned to one of three groups. The first group (G1) received soy oil (placebo), the second group (G2) received fish oil n-3 fatty acids (3 g/day), and the third group (G3) received fish oil n-3 fatty acids (3 g/day) and 6.8 g/day of oleic acid (9.6 mL of olive oil). There was a statistically significant improvement in G2 and G3 in relation to G1 with respect to joint pain intensity, right and left handgrip strength, duration of morning stiffness, onset of fatigue, Ritchie's articular index for pain joints, ability to bend down to pick up clothing from the floor, and getting in and out of a car. G3, but not G2, in relation to G1 showed additional improvements with respect to duration of morning stiffness, patient global assessment, ability to turn faucets on and off, and RF. In addition, G3 showed a significant improvement in patient global assessment in relation to G2. The RF decrease in G3 has a huge clinical significance because patients who have high titers tend to have a more aggressive, destructive course. The authors concluded that ingestion of fish oil n-3 fatty acids relieved several clinical parameters used in the present study. However, patients showed a more precocious and accentuated improvement when fish oil supplements were used in combination with olive oil.

10.7 CRANBERRY

Cranberries (*Vaccinium macrocarpon* Ait.) are fruits with high antioxidant capacity due to its composition of polyphenols, especially flavonoids and ellagic acid. The main flavonoids present in its composition are the anthocyanins, which confer to the fruit pigmentation that varies from red to blue (Tulio et al. 2014), and the proanthocyanidin, also known as condensed tannins (Gu et al. 2004, de la Iglesia et al. 2010). Intervention studies lasting 2–16 weeks have shown beneficial effects of consuming cranberry (as juice or extract) on oxidative stress (Ruel et al. 2005, Basu et al. 2011), lipemia and markers of atherosclerosis (Ruel et al. 2006, Lee et al. 2008), both in healthy people and patients with MetS and type II diabetes mellitus.

A study conducted by Ruel et al. (2006) showed significant increase in HDL cholesterol levels in obese males supplemented with cranberry juice. Moreover, research conducted by Simão et al. (2013) found that daily consumption of 700 mL of low-calorie cranberry juice by MetS patients significantly decreased homocysteine levels and markers of oxidative stress, and increased serum levels of acid folic and anti-inflammatory cytokine adiponectin.

Despite the beneficial effects of these compounds in dyslipidemia, diabetes mellitus, and also in cardiovascular diseases, few controlled trials evaluating their anti-inflammatory action in humans have been found (Rosa et al. 2012) and none in patients with RA.

10.8   DIET INTERVENTION

The Mediterranean diet consumption based on high intake of olive oil, grains, fruits, legumes, nuts, and fish, low intake of meat, and moderate intake of milk was shown to suppress disease activity in patients who have stable and modestly active RA. Compared with an ordinary omnivorous diet, the authors observed a significant improvement after 3 months in the DAS28 score, in the articular function using the Health Assessment Questionnaire (HAQ), and in two dimensions of the health survey of quality of life (SF-36) (Skoldstam et al. 2003). It is widely known the benefits of this diet on MetS, and it would be also favorable to reduce RA patient's risk. In this sense, Elkan et al. (2009) with the aim of finding associations between diet, body composition, lipids, and atheroprotective natural antibodies against phosphorylcholine (anti-PC) in patients with RA applied a semiquantitative Food Frequency Questionnaire (FFQ) and observed that patients compliant with Mediterranean-like diet did not differ in body composition from the rest of the patients, but had a higher content of PUFA in adipose tissue and significantly higher serum levels of the atheroprotective anti-PC.

Moreover, Elkan et al. (2008) investigated the effect of a 1-year gluten-free vegan diet compared to a well-balanced diet on risk factors for atherosclerosis in RA patients. The authors found that the vegan diet in RA induced decreased LDL and oxidized LDL levels and raised levels of natural antibodies of IgA and IgM subclasses to phosphorylcholine (anti-PC). The authors hypothesize that these changes are atheroprotective since LDL and oxLDL are atherogenic proinflammatory, and anti-PC levels are inversely associated with atherosclerosis. However, the vegan diet was based on vegetables, root vegetables, nuts, fruits, buckwheat, millet, corn, rice, and sunflower seeds, as well as sesame milk, that hamper to identify which components of the diet and the underlying mechanisms contributed to the evidenced effects.

10.9   FINAL CONSIDERATIONS

Besides the joint impairment, studies have shown that RA patients have increased risk to develop MetS due to the proinflammatory state of the disease. The high mortality rate among these patients due to cardiovascular disease emphasizes the importance to find out mechanisms to counteract it.

Despite the beneficial effects of bioactive compounds in dyslipidemia, diabetes mellitus, and also in cardiovascular diseases, few controlled trials evaluating their anti-inflammatory action in humans have been found and even less in patients with rheumatoid arthritis. It is widely recognized the benefits of nutrition in chronic disease prevention, including the MetS, such as dietary interventions with variation in macronutrient composition, inclusion of functional foods, foods rich in polyphenols, dietary fiber, and essential fatty acids. However, in RA, this area of study is only beginning.

The application of ω-3 PUFA as adjuvant treatment of RA is well established due to its effects on disease activity and its signs and symptoms. However, further studies should investigate new dietary interventions for the treatment of RA, since anti-inflammatory food or dietary pattern could not only prevent the onset of MetS, but also possibly minimize the effects and activity of autoimmune diseases.

Finally, independent of the treatment choice, it is important that RA patients with associated comorbidities be monitored by a multidisciplinary team, with the active participation of a rheumatologist, to achieve better results in those of difficult control.

REFERENCES

ACR. 2002. American College of Rheumatology Subcommittee on Rheumatoid Arthritis Guidelines. Guidelines for the management of rheumatoid arthritis. *Arthritis Rheum.* 46:328–346.

Alarcón, G. S. 1995. Epidemiology of rheumatoid arthritis. *Rheum Dis Clin North Am.* 21:589–604.

Aletaha D., Nell, V. P., Stamm, T. et al. 2005. Acute phase reactants add little to composite disease activity indices for rheumatoid arthritis: Validation of a clinical activity score. *Arthritis Res Ther.* 7:R796–R806.

Aletaha, D., Neogi, T., Silman, A. J. et al. 2010. Rheumatoid arthritis classification criteria: An American College of Rheumatology/European League against Rheumatism collaborative initiative. *Arthritis Rheum.* 69(9):1580–1588.

Anders, H., Rihl, M., Heufelder, A., Loch, O., Schattenkirchner, M. 1999. Leptin serum levels are not correlated with disease activity in patients with rheumatoid arthritis. *Metabolism.* 48:745–748.

Arnett, F. C., Edworthy, S. M., Bloch, D. A. et al. 1988. The American Rheumatism Association 1987 revised criteria for the classification of rheumatoid arthritis. *Arthritis Rheum.* 31(3):315–324.

Baker, J. F., Mehta, N. N., Baker, D. G. et al. 2012. Vitamin D, metabolic dyslipidemia, and metabolic syndrome in rheumatoid arthritis. *Am J Med.* 125(10):1036.e-9–1036.e15.

Ballantyne, C. M. I., Bays, H. E., Kastelein, J. J. et al. 2012. Efficacy and safety of eicosapentaenoic acid ethyl ester (AMR101) therapy in statin-treated patients with persistent high triglycerides (from the ANCHOR study). *Am J Cardiol.* 110(7):984–992.

Barbosa, D. S., Cecchini, R., El Kadri, M. Z., Rodríguez, M. A., Burini R. C., Dichi, I. 2003. Decreased oxidative stress in patients with ulcerative colitis supplemented with fish oil omega-3 fatty acids. *Nutrition.* 19(10):837–842.

Basu, A., Betts, N. M., Ortiz, J., Simmons, B., Wu, M., Lyons, T. J. 2011. Low-energy cranberry juice decreases lipid oxidation and increases plasma antioxidant capacity in women with metabolic syndrome. *Nutr Res.* 31:190–196.

Berbert, A. A., Kondo, C. R., Almendra, C. L., Matsuo, T., Dichi, I. 2005. Supplementation of fish oil and olive oil in patients with rheumatoid arthritis. *Nutrition.* 21(2):131–136.

Berg, A. H., Combs, T. P., Scherer, P. E. 2002. ACRP30/adiponectin: An adipokine regulating glucose and lipid metabolism. *Trends Endocrinol. Metab.* 13(2):84–89.

Bernotiene, E., Palmer, G., Gabay, C. 2006. The role of leptin in innate and adaptive immune response. *Arthritis Res Ther.* 8:217–226.

Bokarewa, M., Bokarew, D., Hultgren, O., Tarkowski, A. 2003. Leptin consumption in the inflamed joints of patients with rheumatoid arthritis. *Ann Rheum Dis.* 62:952–956.

Borges, P. K., Gimeno, S. G., Tomita, N. E., Ferreira, S. R. 2007. Prevalence and characteristics associated with metabolic syndrome in Japanese- Brazilians with and without periodontal disease. *Cad Saude Publica.* 23(3):657–668.

Brochu-Gaudreau, K., Rehfeldt, C., Blouin, R., Bordignon, V., Murphy, B. D., Palin, M. F. 2010. Adiponectin action from head to toe. *Endocrine.* 37(1):11–32.

Buttgereit, F. 2011. Do the treatment with glucocorticoids and/or the disease itself drive the impairment in glucose metabolism in patients with rheumatoid arthritis? *Ann Rheum Dis.* 70(11):1881–1883.

Carey, A. L., Febbraio, M. A. 2004. Interleukin-6 and insulin sensitivity: Friend or foe? *Diabetologia.* 47:1135–1142.

Chiu, K. C., Chu, A., Go, V. L., Saad, M. F. 2004. Hypovitaminosis D is associated with insulin resistance and beta cell dysfunction. *Am J Clin Nutr.* 79:820–825.

Chung, C. P., Avalos, I., Oeser, A. et al. 2007. High frequency of the metabolic syndrome in patients with systemic lupus erythematosus: Association with disease characteristics and cardiovascular risk factors. *Ann Rheum Dis.* 66: 208–214.

Chung, C. P., Oeser, A., Solus, J. F. et al. 2008a. Prevalence of the metabolic syndrome is increased in rheumatoid arthritis and is associated with coronary atherosclerosis. *Atherosclerosis.* 196(2):756–763.

Chung, C. P., Oeser, A., Solus, J. F. et al. 2008b. Inflammation-associated insulin resistance: Differential effects in rheumatoid arthritis and systemic lupus erythematosus define potential mechanisms. *Arthritis Rheum.* 58:2105–2112.

Cleland, L. G., Caughey, G. E., James, M. J., Proudman, S. M. 2006. Reduction of cardiovascular risk factors with long-term fish oil treatment in early rheumatoid arthritis. *J Rheumatol.* 33(10):1973–1979.

Cunha, V. R., Brenol, C. V., Brenol, J. C. et al. 2012. Metabolic syndrome prevalence is increased in rheumatoid arthritis patients and is associated with disease activity. *Scand J Rheumatol.* 41(3):186–191.

Cunha, V. R., Brenol, C. V., Brenol, J. C. T., Xavier, R. M. 2011. Rheumatoid arthritis and metabolic syndrome. *Rev Bras Reumatol.* 51(3):260–268.

del Rincon, I. D., Williams, K., Stern, M. P., Freeman, G. L., Escalante, A. 2001. High incidence of cardiovascular events in a rheumatoid arthritis cohort not explained by traditional cardiac risk factors. *Arthritis Rheum.* 44(12):2737–2745.

Dessein, P. H., Joffe, B. I. 2006. Insulin resistance and impaired beta cell function in rheumatoid arthritis. *Arthritis Rheum.* 54:2765–2775.

Dessein, P. H., Joffe, B. I., Stanwix, A. E., Christian, B. F., Veller, M. 2004. Glucocorticoids and insulin sensitivity in rheumatoid arthritis. *J Rheumatol.* 31(5):867–874.

Dessein, P. H., Stanwix, A. E., Joffe, B. I. 2002. Cardiovascular risk in rheumatoid arthritis versus osteoarthritis: Acute phase response related decreased insulin sensitivity and high-density lipoprotein cholesterol as well as clustering of metabolic syndrome features in rheumatoid arthritis. *Arthritis Res.* 4(5):R5.

Di Giuseppe, D., Wallin, A., Bottai, M., Askling, J., Wolk, A. 2014. Long-term intake of dietary long-chain n-3 polyunsaturated fatty acids and risk of rheumatoid arthritis: A prospective cohort study of women. *Ann Rheum Dis.* 73(11):1949–53.

Di Rocco, P., Manco, M., Rosa, G., Greco, A. V., Mingrone, G. 2004. Lowered tumor necrosis factor receptors, but not increased insulin sensitiv- ity, with infliximab. *Obes Res.* 12:734–739.

Dichi, I., Frenhane, P., Dichi, J. B. et al. 2000. Comparison of omega-3 fatty acids and sulfasalazine in ulcerative colitis. *Nutrition.* 16(2):87–90.

Eckel, R. H., Grundy, S. M., Zimmet, P. Z. 2005. The metabolic syndrome. *Lancet.* 365(9468):1415–1428.

Elkan, A. C., Hakansson, N., Frostegard, J., Cederholm, T., Hafstrom, I. 2009. Rheumatoid cachexia is associated with dyslipidemia and low levels of atheroprotective natural antibodies against phosphorylcholine but not with dietary fat in patients with rheumatoid arthritis: A cross- sectional study. *Arthritis Res Ther.* 11(2):R37.

Elkan, A. C., Sjöberg, B., Kolsrud, B., Ringertz, B., Hafström, I., Frostegård, J. 2008. Gluten-free vegan diet induces decreased LDL and oxidized LDL levels and raised atheroprotective natural antibodies against phosphorylcholine in patients with rheumatoid arthritis: A randomized study. *Arthritis Res Ther.* 10(2):R34.

El Magadmi, M., Ahmad, Y., Turkie, W. et al. 2006. Hyperinsulinemia, insulin resistance, and circulating oxidized low density lipoprotein in women with systemic lupus erythematosus. *J Rheumatol.* 33:50–56.

Flachs, P., Rossmeisl, M., Kopecky, J. 2014. The effect of n-3 fatty acids on glucose homeostasis and insulin sensitivity. *Physiol Res.* 63(Suppl. 1):S93–S118.

Ford, E. S., Zhao, G., Li, C., Pearson, W. S. 2009. Serum concentrations of vitamin D and parathyroid hormone and prevalent metabolic syndrome among adults in the United States. *J Diabetes.* 1:296–303.

Geleijnse, J. M., Giltay, E. J., Grobbee, D. E., Donders, A. R., Kok, F. J. 2002. Blood pressure response to fish oil supplementation: Metaregression analysis of randomized trials. *J Hypertens.* 20(8):1493–1499.

Ghorbanihaghjo, A., Kolahi, S., Seifirad, S. et al. 2012. Effect of fish oil supplements on serum paraoxonase activity in female patients with rheumatoid arthritis: A double-blind randomized controlled trial. *Arch Iran Med.* 15(9):549–552.

Giles, J. T., Allison, M., Blumenthal, R. S. et al. 2010. Abdominal adiposity in rheumatoid arthritis: Association with cardiometabolic risk factors and disease characteristics. *Arthritis Rheum.* 62(11):3173–3182.

Goeldner, I., Skare, T. L., de Messias Reason, I. T., Nisihara, R. M., Silva, M. B., da Rosa Utiyama, S. R. 2011. Association of anticyclic citrullinated peptide antibodies with extra-articular manifestations, gender, and tabagism in rheumatoid arthritis patients from southern Brazil. *Clin Rheumatol.* 30(7):975–980.

Gómez, R., Conde, J., Scotece, M., Gómez-Reino, J. J., Lago, F., Gualillo, O. 2011. What's new in our understanding of the role of adipokines in rheumatic diseases? *Nat Rev Rheumatol.* 7(9):528–536.

González Cernadas, L., Rodríguez-Romero, B., Carballo-Costa, L. Importance of nutritional treatment in the inflammatory process of rheumatoid arthritis patients: A review. *Nutr Hosp.* 2014;29(2):237–244.

Goshayeshi, L., Saber, H., Sahebari, M. et al. 2012. Association between metabolic syndrome, BMI, and serum vitamin D concentrations in rheumatoid arthritis. *Clin Rheumatol.* 31(8):1197–203.

Gu, L., Kelm, M. A., Hammerstone, J. F. et al. 2004. Concentrations of proanthocyanidins in common foods and estimations of normal consumption. *J Nutr.* 134: 613–617.

Guzik, T. J., Mangalat, D., Korbut, R. 2006. Adipocytokines—Novel link between inflammation and vascular function? *J Physiol Pharmacol.* 57(4):505–528.

Hagfors, L., Nilsson, I., Sköldstam, L., Johansson, G. 2005. Fat intake and composition of fatty acids in serum phospholipids in a randomized, controlled, Mediterranean dietary intervention study on patients with rheumatoid arthritis. *Nutr Metab* (Lond). 2:26.

Haque, U. J., Bartlett, S. J. 2010. Relationships among vitamin D, disease activity, pain and disability in rheumatoid arthritis. *Clin Exp Rheumatol.* 28:745–747.

Haque, U. J., Bathon, J. M., Giles, J. T. 2012. Association of vitamin D with cardiometabolic risk factors in rheumatoid arthritis. *Arthritis Care Res* (Hoboken). 64(10):1497–1504.

Heliovaara, M. K., Teppo, A. M., Karonen, S. L., Tuominen, J. A., Ebeling, P. 2005. Plasma IL-6 concentration is inversely related to insulin sensitivity, and acute-phase proteins associate with glucose and lipid metabolism in healthy subjects. *Diabetes Obes Metab.* 7:729–736.

Hizmetli, S., Kisa, M., Gokalp, N., Bakici, M. Z. 2007. Are plasma and synovial fluid leptin levels correlated with disease activity in rheumatoid arthritis? *Rheumatol Int.* 27:335–338.

Hoes, J. N., van der Goes, M. C., van Raalte, D. H. et al. 2011. Glucose tolerance, insulin sensitivity and β-cell function in patients with rheumatoid arthritis treated with or without low-to-medium dose glucocorticoids. *Ann Rheum Dis.* 70(11):1887–1894.

Huvers, F. C., Popa, C., Netea, M. G., van den Hoogen, F. H., Tack, C. J. 2007. Improved insulin sensitivity by anti-TNFα antibody treatment in patients with rheumatic diseases. *Ann Rheum Dis.* 66:558–559.

James, M. J., Gibson, R. A., Neumann, M. A., Cleland, L. S. 1993. Effects of dietary supplementation with n-9 eicosatrienoic acid on leukotriene B4 synthesis in rats: A novel approach to inhibition of eicosanoid synthesis. *J Exp Med.* 178:2261–2265.

James, M. J., Proudman, S., Cleland, L. 2010. Fish oil and rheumatoid arthritis: Past, present and future. *Proc Nutr Soc.* 69:316–323.

Kalpakcioglu, B., Înel, K. 2008. The interrelation of glutathione reductase, catalase, glutathione peroxidase, superoxide dismutase, and glucose-6-phosphate in the pathogenesis of rheumatoid arthritis. *Clin Rheumatol.* 27:141–145.

Karakoc, M., Batmaz, I., Sariyildiz, M. A. et al. 2012. The relationship of metabolic syndrome with disease activity and the functional status in patients with rheumatoid arthritis. *J Clin Med Res.* 4(4):279–285.

Karvounaris, S. A., Sidiropoulos, P. I., Papadakis, J. A. et al. 2007. Metabolic syndrome is common among middle-to-older aged Mediterranean patients with rheumatoid arthritis and correlates with disease activity: A retrospective, cross- sectional, controlled, study. *Ann Rheum Dis.* 66(1):28–33.

Kastelein, J. J., Maki, K. C., Susekov, A. et al. 2014. Omega-3 free fatty acids for the treatment of severe hypertriglyceridemia: The EpanoVa fOr Lowering Very high triglyceridEs (EVOLVE) trial. *J Clin Lipidol.* 8(1):94–106.

Kerr, G. S., Sabahi, I., Richards, J. S. et al. 2011. Prevalence of vitamin D insufficiency/deficiency in rheumatoid arthritis and associations with disease severity and activity. *J Rheumatol.* 38:53–59.

Kiortsis, D. N., Mavridis, A. K., Vasakos, S., Nikas, S. N., Drosos, A. A. 2005. Effects of infliximab treatment on insulin resistance in patients with rheumatoid arthritis and ankylosing spondylitis. *Ann Rheum Dis.* 64:765–766.

Klareskog, L., Widhe, M., Hermansson, M., Rönnelid, J. 2008. Antibodies to citrullinated proteins in arthritis: Pathology and promise. *Curr Opin Rheumatol.* 20:300–305.

Kontunen, P., Vuolteenaho, K., Nieminen, R. et al. 2011. Resistin is linked to inflammation, and leptin to metabolic syndrome, in women with inflammatory arthritis. *Scand J Rheumatol.* 40:256–262.

La Cava, A., Matarese, G. 2004. The weight of leptin in immunity. *Nat Rev Immunol.* 4(5):371–379.

La Montagna, G., Cacciapuoti, F., Buono, R. et al. 2007. Insulin resistance is an independent risk factor for atherosclerosis in rheumatoid arthritis. *Diab Vasc Dis Res.* 4(2):130–135.

Lago, F., Dieguez, C., Gómez-Reino, J., Gualillo, O. 2007. Adipokines as emerging mediators of immune response and inflammation. *Nat Clin Pract Rheumatol.* 3(12):716–724.

Lee, I. T., Chan, Y. C., Lin, C. W., Lee, W. J., Sheu, W. H. 2008. Effect of cranberry extracts on lipid profiles in subjects with Type 2 diabetes. *Diabet Med.* 25(12):1473–1477.

Liu, E., Meigs, J. B., Pittas, A. G. et al. 2009. Plasma 25-hydroxyvitamin d is associated with markers of the insulin resistant phenotype in nondiabetic adults. *J Nutr.* 139:329–334.

Lord, G. M., Matarese, G., Howard, J. K., Bloom, S. R., Lechler, R. I. 2002. Leptin inhibits the anti-CD3-driven proliferation of peripheral blood T cells but enhances the production of proinflammatory cytokines. *J Leukoc Biol.* 72(2):330–338.

Lu, L., Yu, Z., Pan, A. et al. 2009. Plasma 25-hydroxyvitamin D concentration and metabolic syndrome among middle-aged and elderly Chinese individuals. *Diabetes Care.* 32:1278–1283.

Marques Neto, J. F., Gonçalves, E. T., Langen, L. F. O. B. et al. 1993. Estudo multicêntrico da prevalência da artrite reumatóide do adulto em amostras da populaçao brasileira/Multicentric study of the prevalence of adult rheumatoid arthritis in Brazilian population samples. *Rev Bras Reumatol.* 33(5):169–173.

Martin, S. S., Qasim, A., Reilly, M. P. 2008. Leptin resistance: A possible interface of inflammation and metabolism in obesity-related cardiovascular disease. *J Am Coll Cardiol.* 52:1201–1210.

Martins, D., Wolf, M., Pan, D. et al. 2007. Prevalence of cardiovascular risk factors and the serum levels of 25-hydroxyvitamin D in the United States: Data from the Third National Health and Nutrition Examination Survey. *Arch Intern Med.* 167:1159–1165.

Michos, E. D., Melamed, M. L. 2008. Vitamin D and cardiovascular disease risk. *Curr Opin Clin Nutr Metab Care.* 11:7–12.

Miles, E. A., Calder, P. C. 2012. Influence of marine n-3 polyunsaturated fatty acids on immune function and a systematic review of their effects on clinical outcomes in rheumatoid arthritis. *Br J Nutr.* 107(Suppl 2):S171–S184.

Mooney, R. A. 2007. Counterpoint: Interleukin-6 does not have a beneficial role in insulin sensitivity and glucose homeostasis. *J Appl Physiol.* 102:816–818.

Mota, L. M. H., Cruz, B. A., Brenol, C. V. et al. 2011. Consenso da Sociedade Brasileira de Reumatologia 2011 para o diagnóstico e avaliação inicial da artrite reumatoide. *Rev Bras Reumatol.* 51(3):197–198.

Nagashima, T., Okubo-Fornbacher, H., Aoki, Y. et al. 2008. Increase in plasma levels of adiponectin after administration of anti-tumor necrosis factor agents in patients with rheumatoid arthritis. *J Rheumatol.* 35:936–938.

Otero, M., Lago, R., Gómez, R. et al. 2006. Changes in plasma levels of fat-derived hormones adiponectin, leptin, resistin and visfatin in patients with rheumatoid arthritis. *Ann Rheum Dis.* 65:1198–1201.

Otero, M., Lago, R., Lago, F. et al. 2005. Leptin, from fat to inflammation: Old questions and new insights. *FEBS Lett.* 579:295–301.

Palmer, G., Gabay, C. 2003. A role for leptin in rheumatic diseases? *Ann Rheum Dis.* 62:913–915.

Popa, C., Netea, M. G., Radstake, T. R. D. S., van Riel, P. L., Barrera, P., van der Meer, J. W. M. 2005. Markers of inflammation are negatively correlated with serum leptin in rheumatoid arthritis. *Ann Rheum Dis.* 64:1195–1198.

Raza, K., Breese, M., Nightingale, P. et al. 2005. Predictive value of antibodies to cyclic citrullinated peptides in patients with very early inflammatory arthritis. *J Rheumatol.* 32:231–238.

Reis, J. P., von Mühlen, M. D., Kritz-Silverstein, D., Wingard, D. L., Barrett-Connor, E. 2007. Vitamin D, parathyroid hormone levels, and the prevalence of metabolic syndrome in community-dwelling older adults. *Diabetes Care.* 30:1549–1555.

Renaudineau, Y., Jamin, C., Saraux, A., Youinou, P. 2005. Rheumatoid factor on a daily basis. *Autoimmunity.* 38:11–16.

Rho, Y. H., Chung, C. P., Solus, J. F. et al. 2010. Adipocytokines, Insulin resistance, and coronary atherosclerosis in rheumatoid arthritis. *Arthritis Rheum.* 62(5):1259–1264.

Rosa, F. T., Zulet, M. Á., Marchini, J. S., Martínez, J. A. 2012. Bioactive compounds with effects on inflammation markers in humans. *Int J Food Sci Nutr.* 63(6):749–765.

Rossini, M., Maddali Bongi, S., La Montagna, G. et al. 2010. Vitamin D deficiency in rheumatoid arthritis: Prevalence, determinants and associations with disease activity and disability. *Arthritis Res Ther.* 12:R216.

Roubenoff, R. 2009. Rheumatoid cachexia: A complication of rheumatoid arthritis moves into the 21st century. *Arthritis Res Ther.* 11(2):108.

Ruel, G., Pomerleau, S., Couture, P., Lamarche, B., Couillard, C. 2005. Changes in plasma antioxidant capacity and oxidized low-density lipoprotein levels in men after short-term cranberry juice consumption. *Metabolism.* 54(7):856–861.

Ruel, G., Pomerleau, S., Couture, P., Lemieux, S., Lamarche, B., Couillard, C. 2006. Favourable impact of low-calorie cranberry juice consumption on plasma HDL-cholesterol concentrations in men. *Br J Nutr.* 96(2):357–364.

Salazar-Paramo, M., Gonzalez-Ortiz, M., Gonzalez-Lopez, L. et al. 2001. Serum leptin levels in patients with rheumatoid arthritis. *J Clin Rheumatol.* 7:57–59.

Seven, A., Güzel, S., Aslan, M., Hamuryudan, V. 2008. Lipid, protein, DNA oxidation and antioxidant status in rheumatoid arthritis. *Clin Biochem.* 41:538–543.

Shahin, D., Eltoraby, E., Mesbah, A. et al. 2010. Insulin resistance in early untreated rheumatoid arthritis patients. *Clin Biochem.* 43:661–665.

Siegel, J. N., Zhen, B. G. 2005. Use of the American College of Rheumatology N (ACR-N) index of improvement in rheumatoid arthritis: Argument in favor. *Arthritis Rheum.* 52:1637–1641.

Silman, A. J., Pearson, J. E. 2002. Epidemiology and genetics of rheumatoid arthritis. *Arthritis Res.* 4:S265–S272.

Simão, A. N. C. 2012. Metabolic syndrome: New targets for an old problem. *Expert Opin Ther Targets.* 16(2):147–150.

Simão, A. N., Lozovoy, M. A., Bahls, L. D. et al. 2012. Blood pressure decrease with ingestion of a soya product (kinako) or fish oil in women with the metabolic syndrome: Role of adiponectin and nitric oxide. *Br J Nutr.* 108(8):1435–1442.

Simão, T. N. l., Lozovoy, M. A., Simão, A. N. et al. 2013. Reduced-energy cranberry juice increases folic acid and adiponectin and reduces homocysteine and oxidative stress in patients with the metabolic syndrome. *Br J Nutr.* 110(10):1885–1894.

Skoldstam, L., Hagfors, L., Johansson, G. 2003. An experimental study of a Mediterranean diet intervention for patients with rheumatoid arthritis. *Ann Rheum Dis.* 62(3):208–214.

Smolen, J. S., Breedveld, F. C., Schiff, M. H. et al. 2003. A simplified disease activity index for rheumatoid arthritis for use in clinical practice. *Rheumatology.* 42:244–257.

Targojska-Stdpniak, B., Majdan, M., Dryglewska, M. 2008. Leptin serum levels in rheumatoid arthritis patients: Relation to disease duration and activity. *Rheumatol Int.* 28:585–591.

Tilg, H., Moschen, A. R. 2006. Adipocytokines: Mediators linking adipose tissue, inflammation and immunity. *Nat Rev Immunol.* 6(10):772–783.

Tokarczyk-Knapik, A., Nowicki, M., Wyromlak, J. 2002. The relation between plasma leptin concentration and body fat mass in patients with rheumatoid arthritis. *Pol Arch Med Wewn.* 108:761–767.

Toms, L. E., Panoulas, V. F., Douglas, K. M. J., Griffiths, H. R., Kitas, G. D. 2008. Lack of association between glucocorticoid use and presence of the metabolic syndrome in patients with rheumatoid arthritis: A cross-sectional study. *Arthritis Res Ther.* 10:R145.

Toms, T. E., Panoulas, V. F., John, H., Douglas, K. M., Kitas, G. D. 2009. Methotrexate therapy associates with reduced prevalence of the metabolic syndrome in rheumatoid arthritis patients over the age of 60- more than just an anti-inflammatory effect? A cross sectional study. *Arthritis Res Ther.* 11(4):R110.

Toussirot, É., Streit, G., Wendling, D. 2007. The contribution of adipose tissue and adipokines to inflammation in joint diseases. *Curr Med Chem.* 14:1095–1100.

Tripoli, E., Giammanco, M., Tabacchi, G., Di Majo, D., Giammanco, S., La Guardia, M. 2005. The phenolic compounds of olive oil: Structure, biological activity and beneficial effects on human health. *Nutr Res Rev.* 18:98–112.

Tulio, A. Z. Jr, Jablonski, J. E., Jackson, L. S., Changm, C., Edirisinghe, I., Burton-Freeman, B. 2014. Phenolic composition, antioxidant properties, and endothelial cell function of red and white cranberry fruits. *Food Chem.* 157:540–552.

Turesson, C., Eberhardt, K., Jacobsson, L. T., Lindqvist, E. 2007. Incidence and predictors of severe extra-articular disease manifestations in an early rheumatoid arthritis inception cohort. *Ann Rheum Dis.* 66(11):1543–1544.

Vallbracht, I., Rieber, J., Oppermann, M., Förger, F., Siebert, U., Helmke, K. 2004. Diagnostic and clinical value of anti-cyclic citrullinated peptide antibodies compared with rheumatoid factor isotypes in rheumatoid arthritis. *Ann Rheum Dis.* 63:1079–1084.

van der Heijde, D. M., van t Hof, M., van Riel, P. L., van de Putte, L. B. 1993. Development of a disease activity score based on judgment in clinical practice by rheumatologists. *J Rheumatol.* 20:579–581.

van der Helm-van Mil, A. H. M, Verpoort, K. N., Breedveld, F. C., Toes, R. E. M., Huizinga, T. W. J. 2005. Antibodies to citrullinated proteins and differences in clinical progression of rheumatoid arthritis. *Arthritis Res Ther.* 7:R949–R958.

van Gestel, A. M., Haagsma, C. J., van Riel, P. L. 1998. Validation of rheumatoid arthritis improvement criteria that include simplified joint counts. *Arthritis Rheum.* 41:1845–1850.

Visser, H., Gelinck, L. B., Kampfraath, A. H., Breedveld, F. C., Hazes, J. M. 1996. Diagnostic and prognostic characteristics of the enzyme linked immunosorbent rheumatoid factor assays in rheumatoid arthritis. *Ann Rheum Dis.* 55:157–161.

Vittecoq, O., Pouplin, S., Krzanowska, K. et al. 2003. Rheumatoid factor is the strongest predictor of radiological progression of rheumatoid arthritis in a three-year prospective study in community-recruited patients. *Rheumatology.* 42(8):939–946.

Wahle, K. W. J., Caruso, D., Ochoa, J. J., Quiles, J. L. 2004, Olive oil and modulation of cell signaling in disease prevention. *Lipids.* 39(12):1223–1231.

Wall, R., Ross, R. P., Fitzgerald, G. F. et al. 2010. Fatty acids from fish: The anti-inflammatory potential of long-chain omega-3 fatty acids. *Nutr Rev.* 68:280–289.

Wolf, A. M., Wolf, D., Rumpold, H., Enrich, B., Tilg, H. 2004. Adiponectin induces the anti-inflammatory cytokines IL-10 and IL-1RA in human leukocytes. *Biochem Biophys Res Commun.* 323(2):630–635.

Wolfe, F., Cathey, M. A., Roberts, F. K. 1991. The latex test revised rheumatoid factor testing in 8,287 rheumatic disease patients. *Arthritis Rheum.* 34:951–960.

Woolf, A. D. 2003. How to assess musculoskeletal conditions. History and physical examination. *Best Pract Res Clin Rheumatol.* 17(3):381–402.

Zhang, J., Fu, L., Shi, J. et al. 2013. The risk of metabolic syndrome in patients with rheumatoid arthritis: A meta-analysis of observational studies. *PLoS One.* 8(10):e78151. doi:10.1371/journal.pone.0078151.

Zittermann, A., Frisch, S., Berthold, H. K. et al. 2009. Vitamin D supplementation enhances the beneficial effects of weight loss on cardiovascular disease risk markers. *Am J Clin Nutr.* 89:1321–1327.

11 Metabolic Syndrome in Systemic Lupus Erythematosus

Tatiana Mayumi Veiga Iriyoda,
Marcell Alysson Batisti Lozovoy, Ana Paula Kallaur,
Andréa Name Colado Simão, and Isaias Dichi

CONTENTS

11.1 INTRODUCTION

Metabolic syndrome (MetS) is a cluster of cardiovascular (CV) risk factors that includes central obesity, dyslipidemia, hypertension, and disturbed glucose metabolism, is highly prevalent (Ford et al. 2002) and an independent predictor of CV morbidity and mortality (Kipp et al. 2004).

MetS has several current definitions (Cornier et al. 2008) and recent criteria set was agreed in an effort to further harmonize the definition (Alberti et al. 2009). MetS is present if three or more of the following five criteria are present: (1) elevated triglycerides ≥1.7 mmol/L (≥150 mg/dL) or drug therapy for hypertriglyceridemia; (2) reduced HDL-cholesterol <1.3 mmol/L (<50 mg/dL) in females or <1.0 mmol/L (<40 mg/dL) in males or drug therapy for reduced HDL-C; (3) elevated blood pressure ≥130/85 mmHg or drug therapy for hypertension; and (4) elevated fasting glucose ≥5.6 mmol/L (≥100 mg/dL) or drug therapy for hyperglycemia; and (5) elevated waist circumference (WC), established according to population-/country-specific thresholds. It is recommended by the International Diabetes Federation (IDF) (Alberti et al. 2005) that the following WCs cut points be used for non-Europeans: ≥94 cm for men and ≥80 cm for women, whereas both IDF and American Heart Association/National Heart, Lung, and Blood Institute (AHA/NHLBI) (Grundy et al. 2005) recommends cut points ≥102 cm for men and ≥88 cm for women for people of European origin.

11.2 PREVALENCE OF METS IN SLE

In the general population, men with MetS are 1.9–3 times more likely to die of any cause, and 2.9–4.2 times more likely to die from coronary heart disease (CHD) (Lakka et al. 2002), whereas women with MetS also have a twofold increased risk of major adverse CV events and death (Kip et al. 2004).

MetS is more prevalent in systemic lupus erythematosus (SLE) patients than in general population and is associated with endothelial injury and coronary atherosclerosis (Mok et al. 2010). More recent observational studies have reported a 16%–38% prevalence of MetS in patients with SLE. Sabio et al. (2008) reported a prevalence of 20%, compared to 13% in controls, whereas Parker et al. (2011) found a prevalence of 30% in a UK SLE cohort, compared to 20% in controls. More recently, Parker et al. (2013) reported that MetS was present in 239/1494 (16%) in a young SLE cohort, predominantly female, and early in the course of their disease. On the other hand, the frequency of MetS was higher in other studies. For example, Negron et al. (2008) studied MetS in 204 lupus patients in Puerto Rico, mean age at study visit 43.6 years, and diagnosed the syndrome in 78 (38.2%) patients. In the study by Telles et al. (2010), 52/162 (32.1%) lupus patients presented with MetS, whereas Lozovoy et al. (2011) reported that 24 of 58 (41.4%) patients met the criteria for MetS compared with 11 of 105 (10.5%) controls. Social class is associated with the prevalence of all the five risk factors that define the syndrome and it has already been observed that the prevalence of MetS is higher among the poorest. In female lupus patients, MetS has been associated with lower income and government health insurance (Marquezine et al. 2008, Negrón et al. 2008, Zonana-Nacach et al. 2008). Moreover, susceptibility factors to the syndrome include genetic and racial factors, aging, endocrine disorders, lifestyle, and diet habits (Grundy 2008). Altogether, these factors could contribute to the differences found in MetS frequency among all mentioned studies.

Chung et al. (2007) compared the prevalence of MetS in 102 patients with SLE and 101 controls using the National Cholesterol Education Program Adult Treatment Panel III (NCEP ATP III) and the World Health Organization (WHO) definitions. MetS was present in 32.4% patients and in 10.9% controls subjects (p < 0.001) using the WHO definition that requires direct determination of insulin resistance (IR), and in 29.4% patients with SLE and in 19.8% controls (p=0.14) using the NCEP definition. The definition of the MetS that requires the direct ascertainment of the presence of IR (the WHO MetS) was more strongly associated with SLE than the NCEP syndrome.

11.3   SYSTEMIC LUPUS ERYTHEMATOSUS AND ATHEROSCLEROSIS

The prevalence of atherosclerosis is increased in patients with SLE, but the causes are not clear (Asanuma et al. 2003, Roman et al. 2003). Accelerated atherosclerosis and premature CV events have been recognized as important causes of morbidity and mortality in lupus patients. Women with SLE have more than fivefold increased risk of clinical CHD events, rising to 50-fold increase in younger patients. Classic Framingham risk factors for CHD, although more prevalent in SLE, do not fully explain this disparity in CHD risk (Manzi et al. 1997, Esdaile et al. 2001, Bruce et al. 2003, Bruce 2005). SLE should therefore be considered an independent risk factor for CHD.

MetS was significantly associated with coronary atherosclerosis in SLE patients after adjustment for age and other vascular risk factors not included in the syndrome. Risk factors identified include older age, male sex, smoking, hypertension, longer disease duration, dyslipidemia, hyperhomocysteinemia, oxidized LDL, and antiphospholipid antibodies (Manzi et al. 1997, Esdaile et al. 2001, Asanuma et al. 2003, Manger et al. 2003, Roman et al. 2003, Bruce 2005, Mok et al. 2006).

11.4   SLE FEATURES AND METS

Lupus features implicated in MetS include inflammatory disease activity, disease damage, and therapeutic exposures, particularly to corticosteroids, although studies to date have been inconsistent (Parker and Bruce 2010). Neither formal measures of disease activity nor damage were associated with the syndrome by some authors (Chung et al. 2007, Parker et al. 2011). In the study of Lozovoy et al. (2011), SLEDAI score presented positive correlation with body mass index (BMI) ($r=0.2636$, $p=0.05$) and WC ($r=0.3190$, $p=0.03$), and the authors showed that C3 and C4 have a strong positive correlation with fasting glucose ($r=0.6140$, $p \leq 0.0001$, and $r=0.6319$, $p \leq 0.0001$, respectively) and

C3 had also a significant direct correlation with C-reactive protein (CRP) (r=0.3085, p=0.02) in patients with SLE. Reduced serum C3 and C4 levels have been considered to be important parameters to define SLE activity; however, components of the complement system can have hepatic synthesis enhanced by inflammatory stimulus and adipose tissue is a direct source of complement factors. Therefore, it can be assumed that C3 and C4 levels in SLE patients, especially those who simultaneously present SLE and MetS, may better reflect a positive acute-phase protein response than SLE disease activity (Lozovoy et al. 2011). A high C3 level has been closely associated with development of MetS, fasting triacylglycerol, CRP, and IR (Onat et al. 2005, Tso et al. 2009). However, Parker et al. (2011) found that low C3 were independently associated with the presence of MetS in SLE.

The Systemic Lupus International Collaborating Clinics Registry for Atherosclerosis inception cohort enrolled 1686 patients with recently diagnosed (<15 months) SLE to examine the association of demographic factors, lupus phenotype, and therapy exposure with the presence of MetS and found that higher daily average prednisolone dose (mg) (OR 1.02, 95% CI 1.00–1.03), older age (years) (OR 1.04, 95% CI 1.03–1.06), Korean (OR 6.33, 95% CI 3.68–10.86) and Hispanic (OR 6.2, 95% CI 3.78–10.12) ethnicity, current renal disease (OR 1.79, 95% CI 1.14–2.80), and immunosuppressant use (OR 1.81, 95% CI 1.18–2.78) were associated with MetS. The relatively high prevalence of MetS at enrolment suggests that the metabolic derangements that contribute to long-term CHD risk characterized by MetS appear early in the course of the disease (Parker et al. 2013).

Long-term and high-dose corticosteroid use is associated with the pro-atherogenic metabolic disturbances characterized by MetS (Ross 1999, Tso et al. 2006). Parker et al. (2013) suggested that in early disease higher doses of corticosteroids play a pivotal role in the development of MetS. Current corticosteroid use was not significantly associated with MetS although past intravenous corticosteroid use was (OR 2.45, 95%CI 1.01–5.97), suggesting that increasing corticosteroid doses have a greater impact on MetS susceptibility than simple exposure status. Some authors did not find an association between prednisone use and MetS (Chung et al. 2007, Zonana-Nacach et al. 2008). The use of immunosuppressive therapies remained a significant predictor of MetS even after adjusting for all clinically correlating factors, such as SLEDAI, renal disease, and corticosteroid use/dose (fully adjusted OR 2.15, 95%CI 1.15–4.00).

11.5 METS AND INFLAMMATION

The role of inflammation in the development of atherosclerosis has been increasingly recognized (Petri et al. 1992), and SLE is associated with higher circulating levels of high sensitivity CRP, interleukin (IL)-18, and tumor necrosis factor alpha (TNF-α), which are associated with IR and endothelial dysfunction and have been implicated in the development of CHD in the general population (Posadas-Romero et al. 2004, Mok 2006). MetS is associated with inflammation that is characterized by increased circulation adipocytokines such as TNF-α, IL-6, leptin, resistin, plasminogen activator inhibitor-1 (PAI-1), and acute-phase reactants such as CRP (Miranda et al. 2005, Grundy 2006, Negrón et al. 2008). Roman et al. (2003) have demonstrated an association between atherosclerosis and less immunosuppressive therapy arguing strongly on the importance of chronic inflammation in SLE patients. Cytokines levels are elevated both in active and inactive periods of SLE, indicating that there is a low-grade chronic inflammation, which can be increased during exacerbation in SLE (Capper et al. 2004). Systemic chronic inflammation has been proposed to have a prominent role in the pathogenesis of IR (Hotamisligil 2000, Capper et al. 2004). The proinflammatory state induces IR, leading to clinical and biochemical manifestations of the MetS. The resistance to insulin action promotes further inflammation through an increase in free fatty acids concentration and interferes with the anti-inflammatory effects of insulin (Escárcega et al. 2006). Inflammatory cytokine TNF-α can induce IR and suppression of Glut4 expression. IL-6 also inhibits insulin signal transduction in hepatocytes (Sidiropoulos et al. 2008) (Figure 11.1).

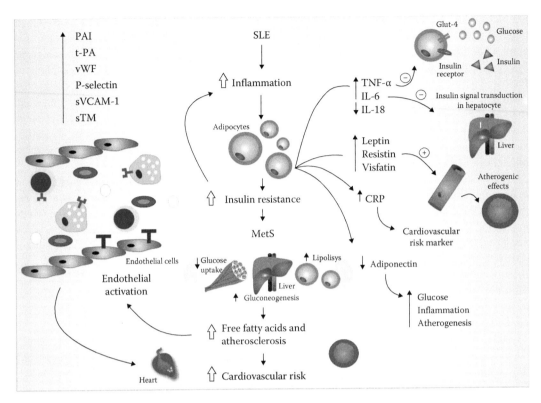

FIGURE 11.1 Systemic lupus erythematosus patients present a proinflammatory state that might induce insulin resistance, leading to a clinical and biochemical manifestations of the metabolic syndrome. The association between inflammation and insulin resistance (IR) is considered to be fundamental to the increased cardiovascular risk attributed to the MetS. This patients have higher circulating levels of TNF-α, interleukin 6 (IL-6), interleukin-18 (IL-18), sensitivity C-reactive protein (sCRP); leptin, resistin, visfatin; and decreased adiponectin. TNF-α can induce insulin resistance and suppression of Glut4 expression. IL-6 also inhibits insulin signal transduction in hepatocytes. Leptin, resistin, and visfatin have pro-inflammatory and atherogenic effects and are associated with insulin resistance, while adiponectin has antidiabetic, anti-inflammatory, and antiatherogenic effects. Adipocytokines may provide a mechanistic link among impaired insulin sensitivity, obesity, chronic inflammation, and atherosclerosis. Endothelial activation is the earliest stage of atherosclerosis, with increased circulating levels of thrombomodulin (sTM), soluble vascular cell adhesion molecule-1 (sVCAM)-1 and P-selectin, von Willebrand factor (vWF), tissue plasminogen activator (t-PA), or plasminogen activator inhibitor type 1 (PAI-1). SLE, systemic lupus erythematosus; MetS, metabolic syndrome; TNF-α, tumor necrosis factor; IL-6, interleukin 6; IL-18, interleukin-18; sCRP, sensitivity C-reactive protein; sTM, thrombomodulin; sVCAM-1, soluble vascular cell adhesion molecule-1; vWF, von Willebrand factor (vWF); t-PA, tissue plasminogen activator (t-PA); PAI-1, plasminogen activator inhibitor type 1.

The association between inflammation and IR is of interest because IR is considered by many to be fundamental to the increased CV risk attributed to the MetS (Lakka et al. 2002, Reilly et al. 2004). In keeping with this notion, data from the general population show that measures of IR provide additional value to the association between the MetS and coronary atherosclerosis (Reilly et al. 2004, Chung et al. 2007). SLE patients are significantly insulin resistant when the later is measured by HOMA estimates (El-Magadmi et al. 2006, Chung et al. 2008, Tso and Huang 2009). El-Magadmi et al. (2006), Posadas-Romero et al. (2004) and Chung et al. (2007) found that insulin levels were higher in patients with SLE but not related to disease activity, use of corticosteroids, or use of antimalarial drugs. The higher prevalence of MetS in SLE despite similar measures of central obesity demonstrated by some authors (El-Magadmi et al. 2004, Sabio et al. 2008,

Bellomio et al. 2009) suggests an alternative clinical phenotype of MetS in SLE (Parker et al. 2011). IR was associated with markers of inflammation such as CRP (r = 0.31, p = 0.001) and erythrocyte sedimentation rate (r = 0.26, p = 0.009). These findings thus link inflammatory markers with reduced insulin sensitivity and suggest a potential mechanism for increased CV risk in SLE (Chung et al. 2007).

Adipose tissue has endocrine functions and is the main source of several mediators, termed adipocytokines, which include leptin, resistin, visfatin, and adiponectin. Adipocytokines may provide a mechanistic link among impaired insulin sensitivity, obesity, chronic inflammation, and atherosclerosis. Leptin, resistin, and visfatin have pro-inflammatory and atherogenic effects and are associated with IR (Guzik et al. 2006, Lago et al. 2007). In contrast, adiponectin has antidiabetic, anti-inflammatory, and antiatherogenic effects (Maahs et al. 2005, Guzik et al. 2006). Chung et al. (2009) found that lower concentrations of adiponectin and higher concentrations of leptin were associated with IR, BMI, and CRP in patients with SLE. Adipocytokines were associated with inflammatory markers, but not with disease activity (measured with the SLEDAI score) and coronary calcification. Vadacca et al. (2009) found that leptin was increased in SLE patients, while resistin, visfatin, and adiponectin did not differ between SLE patients and controls. In SLE patients, leptin correlated with insulin and HOMA-IR levels and with the MetS. This author found a positive correlation between leptin and SLE-specific disease activity indexes.

Endothelial activation is the earliest stage of atherosclerosis. Circulating levels of markers of endothelial activation and injury such as thrombomodulin (sTM), soluble adhesion molecules such as soluble vascular cell adhesion molecule-1 (sVCAM)-1 and P-selectin, von Willebrand factor (vWF), tissue plasminogen activator (t-PA), or plasminogen activator inhibitor type 1 (PAI-1) have been found to be significantly elevated in SLE patients compared with controls (Constans et al. 2003, Ho et al. 2003, Tam et al. 2003, Somers et al. 2005, Svenungsson et al. 2008). Mok et al. (2010) demonstrated significantly higher levels of hsCRP, homocysteine, and sTM in SLE patients with MetS. It indicates that endothelial dysfunction and injury are more serious and CV risk is higher in these patients (Figure 11.1).

11.6   METS AND OXIDATIVE STRESS

Oxidative stress has been implicated in the pathophysiology of CV disease, MetS, and SLE (Nuttall et al. 2003, Simão et al. 2008, Oates 2010, Lozovoy et al. 2011). SLE has a strong inflammatory component and consequently chronic overproduction of reactive oxygen species (ROS) and reactive nitrogen species occurs (RNS). Oxidative stress may contribute to immune cell dysfunction, autoantigen production, and autoantibody reactivity in SLE (Oates 2010). In autoimmune disease, oxidatively modified proteins can generate neo-epitopes from self-proteins, causing aggressive autoimmune attack (Sheikh et al. 2007).

Systemic chronic inflammation and oxidative stress has been proposed to have a prominent role in the pathogenesis of IR (Hotamisligil 2000, Capper et al. 2004, Simão et al. 2008). In 2011, Lozovoy et al. considering patients with SLE and MetS found significantly raised serum uric acid (UA), CRP, lipid hydroperoxides, and protein oxidation when compared with patients with SLE without MetS. Lipid hydroperoxides were correlated with CRP, whereas protein oxidation was associated with WC and UA. SLE disease activity index (SLEDAI) scores were positively correlated with BMI and WC. The authors concluded that inflammatory processes, being overweight/obese, and UA may favor oxidative stress increases in patients with SLE and MetS (Lozovoy et al. 2011). More recently, Lozovoy et al. (2013) showed that SLE patients with IR showed higher advanced oxidation protein products (AOPP) (p = 0,030), and gamma-glutamyltransferase levels (p = 0,001), and lower sulfhydryl groups of proteins (p = 0.0002) and total radical-trapping antioxidant parameter (TRAP) corrected by UA levels (p = 0.04) when compared to SLE patients without IR. However, SLE patients with IR presented lower serum 8-isoprostanes (p = 0.05) and carbonyl protein levels (p = 0.04) when compared to SLE patients without IR.

11.7 DIET AND NUTRITIONAL ASPECTS IN METS RELATED TO SYSTEMIC LUPUS ERYTHEMATOSUS

The nutritional status is extremely important to the immune system balance (Selmi and Tsuneyama 2010), thus dietary guidance is important to improve the prognosis of immune diseases in addition to prevent the progression of CV diseases, considering that CV risk is increased in patients with SLE due to the increased frequency of conditions associated with atherosclerosis, such as obesity, dyslipidemia, diabetes mellitus, and MetS (Bruce 2005).

Although specific reports on nutritional intervention in MetS patients with SLE are still scarce, we may assume that many nutrients recommended to benefit some components of MetS may favor SLE patients, especially those with concomitant MetS.

The Mediterranean diet is one of the most studied dietary patterns in the context of the MetS and other diseases. The traditional Mediterranean diet relies on unrefined cereals, legumes, nuts, fruit, vegetables, olive oil, moderate/high consumption of fish and yoghurt, low/moderate intakes of poultry, low intakes of red/processed meats, and moderate consumption of wine, generally with meals (Keys et al. 1986).

The Mediterranean diet has been shown to have a beneficial effect on all components of the MetS, as described in a recent meta-analysis (Kastorini et al. 2011). There is substantial and consistent evidence from epidemiological studies of an independent protective effect of the Mediterranean diet on inflammatory and endothelial dysfunction markers such as circulating IL-6, CRP, TNF-α, adiponectin, soluble intercellular cell adhesion molecule 1 (sICAM-1), soluble vascular cell adhesion molecule 1 (sVCAM-1), and E-selectin (Esposito et al. 2003, 2004, Chrysohoou et al. 2004, Fung et al. 2005, Estruch et al. 2006, Dai et al. 2008, Fragopoulou et al. 2010).

Weight loss programs targeting energy restriction can be effective approaches to ameliorating numerous MetS parameters (Andersen and Fernandez 2013), while it has also been associated with improved immunity and prolonged lifespan (Dixit 2008). The patient with SLE should be instructed to follow a calorie-restricted diet to prevent and/or treat excessive weight, in addition to a diet with moderate protein content (Klack et al. 2012).

Beneficial effects on MetS parameters have also been observed from intake of specific protein sources. Sardine protein was more effective than casein in diminishing high-fat diet-induced IR, inflammation, and adipose tissue oxidative stress in a fructose-induced rat model of MetS (Madani et al. 2012). In a placebo-controlled crossover trial, consumption of L-arginine-enriched biscuits in combination with a hypocaloric diet reduced body weight, fat mass, plasma glucose, and the proinsulin/insulin ratio in MetS when compared to placebo (Monti et al. 2013).

Among proteins, isoflavones have been indicated for protein supplementation, but L-canavanine, which aggravates SLE symptoms, has been contraindicated. Hong et al. (2008) have shown that the supplementation with isoflavones increased the survival of SLE murine models, inhibiting the production of autoantibodies (anti-dsDNA and anticardiolipin), and reducing the secretion of IFN-γ. L-canavanine is a nonprotein amino acid that can be found in grains (soybean), onion, seeds, alphalpha (major source), and other plants. It can be associated with the appearance of SLE and reactivates the clinical symptoms of the disease and its serological aspects (Petri 2001, Akaogi et al. 2006, Hong et al. 2009).

The dyslipoproteinemia of SLE, similarly to MetS, is characterized by higher levels of triglycerides (TG) and very-low-density lipoprotein cholesterol (VLDL-C) associated with lower levels of high-density lipoprotein cholesterol (HDL-C) (Borba and Bonfá 1997). The inflammatory activity of the disease and several drugs used to treat SLE determine deleterious changes in the lipid profile, the effect of corticosteroids being of particular importance (Petri et al. 1994, Bruce 2005).

A variety of monounsaturated fatty acids (MUFA) and MUFA-rich foods have been found to be protective against MetS and various CVD risk factors (Gillingham et al. 2011), whereas n-3 polyunsaturated fatty acids (PUFA), including α-linoleic acid (ALA), eicosapentanoic acid (EPA), and docohexanoic acid (DHA), have similarly been found to exert beneficial effects on MetS parameters—particularly in regard to inflammation (Robinson and Mazurak 2013). MUFA- and n-3 PUFA-rich diets promote insulin sensitivity (Jans et al. 2012) and postprandial plasma TG and TG-rich lipoprotein clearance when compared to saturated fatty acid–rich diet. ALA has similarly been shown to improve abdominal obesity, IR, dyslipidemia, and vascular function in a high-carbohydrate, high-fat diet–fed rat model of MetS, in addition to improving cardiac and liver inflammation and tissue integrity. Similar beneficial effects were observed in DHA and EPA-fed rats in all parameters other than glucose tolerance (Poudyal et al. 2013).

Dietary lipids can change the balance between Th1 and Th2 cells, favoring the development of autoimmune phenomena (Maki and Newberne 1992, Leiba et al. 2001). DHA significantly reduces the serum levels of anti-dsDNA, regulates IgG renal deposits in NZB/NZW mice, and reduces IL-18 (Halade et al. 2010, Fasset et al. 2010). Mohan and Das (1997) and Pestka et al. (2010) have reported a significant increase in the levels of the antioxidant enzymes with the EPA/DHA supplementation, inducing SLE remission and being beneficial in the treatment of lupus nephritis with cyclophosphamide (Mohan and Das 1997, Duffy et al. 2004, Pestka 2010).

Fish oil, known as one of the major sources of ω-3 PUFA, has anti-inflammatory and antiautoimmune effects due to inhibition of T and B lymphocytes, it suppresses the activity of macrophages and the production of cyclooxygenase metabolites, being significantly beneficial to the clinical, immune, and biochemical status in animal and human models of SLE (Chandrasekar et al. 1995, Patavino and Brady 2001, Duffy et al. 2004, MacLean et al. 2004, Chou 2010, Selmi and Tsuneyama 2010). Supplementation with fish oil as the exclusive source of lipids reduces proteinuria and protects the kidneys against the deleterious effects of free radicals in murine models of lupus nephritis (Chou 2010, Petska 2010).

Flaxseed oil, with 70% of ω-3 PUFA, is a good dietary complement because it reduces proteinuria levels, preserves glomerular filtration and promote a reduction of 11% in total cholesterol levels and of 12% in LDL-C levels. In addition, it reduces anti-dsDNA and anticardiolipin antibodies in mice and suppresses the anti-β2-glycoprotein I in the experimental model of the antiphospholipid syndrome (Leiba et al. 2001, Patavino and Brady 2001, Petri 2001).

One area of recent study has been the investigation of the association between vitamin D status and the MetS. Vitamin D is produced in the skin and obtained from food (cod liver oil, canned salmon, sardines and tuna, fortified milk). Low serum 25-hydroxyvitamin D concentrations are associated with increased body fat (Rosenstreich et al. 1971, Bell et al. 1985, Snijder et al. 2005) and reduced insulin turnover. Several investigations have found that people with impaired glucose tolerance (Boucher 1998, Morris and Zemel 2005) or diabetes (Mathieu et al. 2005) have lower concentrations of serum 25-hydroxyvitamin D than do subjects with normal glucose tolerance. Adequate vitamin D status facilitates the biosynthetic capacity of the β-cell and accelerates the conversion of pro-insulin to insulin. (Bourlon et al. 1999, Ayesha et al. 2001). A recent study found an inverse association between fasting plasma glucose and serum 25-hydroxyvitamin D while controlling for age and BMI (Need et al. 2005). Chiu et al. (2004) found a positive correlation between 25-hydroxyvitamin D and insulin sensitivity index. Future prospective studies investigating biomarkers of vitamin D insufficiency and the risk of incident hypertension are needed, considering the potential limitations of the studies, such as sun exposure and other factors in addition to dietary vitamin D intake as determinants of vitamin D status (Martini and Wood 2006). Hypovitaminosis D has been associated with increased total serum cholesterol concentration; however, there is little mechanistic evidence suggesting a likely mechanism by which vitamin D status could affect the development of dyslipidemia. (Grimes et al. 1996, Chiu et al. 2004, Martini and Wood 2006).

There is compelling evidence that vitamin D status, and specifically 1,25-dihydroxyvitamin D, can affect cytokine production and immunity. The hormonal form of vitamin D can inhibit the production of proinflammatory cytokines, including IL-1, IL-2, IL-6, TNF-α, and others, likely via vitamin D receptor expressed in monocytes and activated T lymphocytes (Muller et al. 1993).

There are controversies about its role in the development of SLE and autoimmune diseases. High consumption of vitamin D ($\geq$37 ng/mL) has been associated with the reduction in the risks for development and severity of some autoimmune diseases, including SLE (Kamen et al. 2006, Wu et al. 2009). Of note, low levels of 25(OH)D are related to the highest scores of inflammatory activity in SLE (SLEDAI) (Wu et al. 2009). Nevertheless, a recent prospective study carried out with 18,000 women during 22 years has found no association between vitamin D intake and risk for SLE, disagreeing with the hypothesis that high vitamin D intake would be associated with protection against SLE (Costenbader et al. 2008).

Patients with SLE have shown several factors that reduce vitamin D levels ($\leq$20 ng/mL): the intense photoprotection of those patients (Patavino and Brady 2001, Costenbader et al. 2008, Cutolo and Otsa 2008, Wu et al. 2009, Knott and Martínez 2010); the relative hypoparathyroidism caused by the high IL-6 levels (mainly in disease activity); the chronic use of steroids, which changes its metabolism leading to the formation of biologically inactive metabolites and decreasing calcium absorption (Cutolo and Otsa 2008, Wright et al. 2009, Tolosa et al. 2010); and the use of hydroxychloroquine that seems to reduce the conversion of vitamin D2 into D3, its biologically more active form. At last, antibodies anti–vitamin D have also been described (Cutolo and Otsa 2008, Wu et al. 2009). Some studies have also suggested that excessive weight is an important risk factor for vitamin D deficiency in SLE (Cutolo and Otsa 2008, Wright et al. 2009, Tolosa et al. 2010).

Antioxidant- and phytonutrient-rich foods and supplements have been associated with lower incidence of MetS and MetS parameters (Puchau et al. 2010, Beydoun et al. 2011, Li et al. 2013). While supplementation of vitamins A, C, and E protected against sodium-induced MetS in albino rats by improving plasma lipids (dyslipidemia), insulin sensitivity, and antioxidant defenses (Bilbis et al. 2012), antioxidant supplementation (vitamins C and E, β-carotene, selenium, and zinc) for 7.5 years did not appear to influence the risk of developing MetS in French SU.VI.MAX study participants (Czernichow et al. 2009). However, serum β-carotene and vitamin C were negatively associated with risk of developing MetS, whereas serum zinc was positively associated with MetS risk, suggesting that diets containing antioxidant-rich foods are still protective against MetS development (Czernichow et al. 2009). Although results remain inconclusive, numerous flavonoids and polyphenols have been shown to improve parameters of MetS, including markers of dyslipidemia, endothelial dysfunction, hypertension, obesity and energy expenditure, and IR (Schini-Kerth et al. 2010, Galleano et al. 2012).

Kinoshita et al. (2010) have shown that patients treated with metabolites of vitamin A improved their proteinuria, their high levels of anti-dsDNA, and low titers of complements, with no side effects, suggesting that retinoids can be promising for the treatment of lupus nephritis.

Studies with mice have suggested that vitamin C reduces IgG and anti-dsDNA levels and that its insufficient consumption can maintain oxidative stress and induce inflammation in the active phase of disease (Minami et al. 2003). Tam et al. (2005) have shown that daily supplementation of vitamin C with vitamin E was associated with a small reduction in lipid peroxidation, without affecting other markers of oxidative stress or endothelial function in patients with SLE.

Some studies with MRL/lpr mice have shown that treatment with vitamin E supplementation modulates the levels of inflammatory cytokines, delays the appearance of autoimmunity, and increases survival (Costenbader et al. 2010), but the treatment in patients with SLE is still controversial (Brown 2000).

A diet rich in selenium, a natural antioxidant, increases anti-inflammatory properties, with a reduction in anti-dsDNA antibodies, improving the activity of natural killer cells and survival in murine models of SLE (Brown 2000, Patavino and Brady 2001, Chou 2010). It can have a significant effect on the maturation of T cells and on the response of T cell–dependent autoantibodies (Hong et al. 2009).

MetS parameters have been shown to be ameliorated by intake of both soluble and insoluble fibers (Papathanasopoulos and Camilleri 2010, Cloetens et al. 2012). Adequate intake of dietary fibers is recommended, because it lowers postprandial glycemia and lipids and protects against

CV diseases (Pereira et al. 2004, Dietary Guidelines for Americans 2005). Minami et al. (2011) have also reported that fiber intake was inversely proportional to the SLE severity risk and that fiber intake is inversely associated with the plasma levels of homocysteine and of the inflammatory markers IL-6 and CRP.

Several studies have assessed the effects of dairy consumption on MetS, as dairy products are rich sources of protein and micronutrients (van Meijl et al. 2008). Rideout et al. (2013) compared the effects of low- (no more than two servings per day) vs. high-dairy (four servings per day) consumption for 6 months in a randomized, crossover intervention in MetS. At the end of the intervention, both low- and high-dairy diets were equally effective in lowering plasma glucose and lipids and in reducing blood pressure; however, high-dairy intake resulted in lower plasma insulin and IR when compared to low-dairy intake (Siri-Tarino et al. 2010).

An adequate consumption of calcium is extremely important in SLE, particularly in patients with a reduction in bone mineral density either associated or not with corticotherapy and regardless of disease duration (Shah et al. 2004, Schmajuk et al. 2010). The American College of Rheumatology (ACR) has suggested that patients receiving more than 5 mg of prednisone daily, for 3 months, should begin to receive calcium and vitamin D prophylactically, and undergo assessment of bone density and of the use of other medications. Supplementation of calcium (>1500 mg) and vitamin D (20 μg or 800 UI) is indicated in cases of difficulty in obtaining those nutrients from the diet (Brown 2000, Aghdassi et al. 2010).

11.8 CONCLUSION

In conclusion, patients with SLE have a high prevalence of MetS and this syndrome may constitute a common link between the increased CV risk and higher levels of inflammation (Chung et al. 2007). The syndrome is associated not only with traditional CV risk factors, confirming the clustering of risk factors for CHD, but also with lupus characteristics (Telles et al. 2010). This aspect is relevant in clinical practice since MetS can be modified with appropriate pharmacological interventions and certain changes in lifestyle, which could prevent or delay the development of accelerated atherosclerosis in these patients (Sabio et al. 2009). It must be assumed that the adequate diet for the treatment of SLE is mainly aimed at reducing the risk for CV and atherosclerotic diseases, in addition to reducing the inflammatory factors and improving the immune function (Klack et al. 2012).

REFERENCES

Aghdassi, E., Morrison, S., Landolt-Marticorena, C. et al. 2010. The use of micronutrient supplements is not associated with better quality of life and disease activity in Canadian patients with systemic lupus erythematosus. *J Rheumatol.* 37(1):87–90.

Akaogi, J., Barker, T., Kuroda, Y. et al. 2006. Role of non-protein amino acid L-canavanine in autoimmunity. *Autoimmun Rev.* 5(6):429–435.

Alberti, K.G., Eckel, R.H., Grundy, S.M. et al. 2009. Harmonizing the metabolic syndrome: A joint interim statement of the International Diabetes Federation Task Force on Epidemiology and Prevention; National Heart, Lung, and Blood Institute; American Heart Association; World Heart Federation; International Atherosclerosis Society; and international association for the Study of Obesity. *Circulation* 120:1640–1645.

Alberti, K.G., Zimmet, P., Shaw, J. 2005. IDF Epidemiology Task Force Consensus Group. The MetS: A new worldwide definition. *Lancet* 366:1059–1062.

Andersen, C.J., Fernandez, M.L. September 2013. Dietary strategies to reduce metabolic syndrome. *Rev Endocr Metab Disord.* 14(3):241–254.

Asanuma, Y., Oeser, A., Shintani, A.K. et al. 2003. Premature coronary-artery atherosclerosis in systemic lupus erythematosus. *N Engl J Med.* 349:2407–2415.

Ayesha, I., Bala, T.S., Reddy, C.V., Raghuramulu, N. 2001. Vitamin D deficiency reduces insulin secretion and turnover in rats. *Diabetes Nutr Metab.* 14:78–84.

Bell, N.H., Epstein, S., Greene, A., Shary, J., Oexmann, M.J., Shaw, S. 1985. Evidence for alteration of the vitamin D-endocrine system in obese subjects. *J Clin Invest.* 76:370–373.

Bellomio, V., Spindler, A., Lucero, E. et al. 2009. Metabolic syndrome in Argentinean patients with systemic lupus erythematosus. *Lupus.* 18:1019–1025.

Beydoun, M.A., Shroff, M.R., Chen, X., Beydoun, H.A., Wang, Y., Zonderman, A.B. 2011. Serum antioxidant status is associated with metabolic syndrome among U.S. adults in recent national surveys. *J Nutr.* 141:903–913.

Bilbis, L.S., Muhammad, S.A., Saidu, Y., Adamu, Y. 2012. Effect of vitamins A, C, and E supplementation in the treatment of metabolic syndrome in albino rats. *Biochem Res Int.* 2012:678582.

Borba, E.F., Bonfá, E. 1997. Dyslipoproteinemias in systemic lupus erythematosus: Influence of disease, activity, and anticardiolipin antibodies. *Lupus.* 6(6):533–539.

Boucher, B.J. 1998. Inadequate vitamin D status: Does it contribute to the disorders comprising syndrome 'X'? *Br J Nutr.* 79:315–327.

Bourlon, P.M., Billaudel, B., Faure-Dussert, A. 1999. Influence of vitamin D3 deficiency and 1,25 dihydroxyvitamin D3 on de novo insulin biosynthesis in the islets of the rat endocrine pancreas. *J Endocrinol.* 160:87–95.

Brown, A.C. 2000. Lupus erythematosus and nutrition: A review of the literature. *J Ren Nutr.* 10(4):170–183.

Bruce, I.N. 2005. "Not only...but also": Factors that contribute to accelerated atherosclerosis and premature coronary heart disease in systemic lupus erythematosus. *Rheumatology.* 44:1492–1502.

Bruce, I.N., Urowitz, M.B., Gladman, D.D., Ibanez, D., Steiner, G. 2003. Risk factors for coronary heart disease in women with systemic lupus erythematosus: The Toronto Risk Factor Study. *Arthritis Rheum.* 48:3159–3167.

Capper, E.R., Maskill, J.K., Gordon, C., Blakemore, A.L. 2004. Interleukin (IL)-10, IL-1ra and Il-12 profiles in active and quiescent systemic lupus erythematosus: Could longitudinal studies reveal patients subgroups of differing pathology. *Clin Exp Immunol.* 138:348–356.

Chandrasekar, B., Troyer, D.A., Venkatraman, J.T., Fernandes, G. 1995. Dietary omega-3 lipids delay the onset and progression of autoimmune lupus nephritis by inhibiting transforming growth factor beta mRNA and protein expression. *J Autoimmun.* 8(3):381–393.

Chiu, K.C., Chu, A., Go, V.L., Saad, M.F. 2004. Hypovitaminosis D is associated with insulin resistance and beta cell dysfunction. *Am J Clin Nutr.* 79:820–825.

Chou, C.T. 2010. Alternative therapies: What role do they have in the management of lupus? *Lupus.* 19(12):1425–1429.

Chrysohoou, C., Panagiotakos, D.B., Pitsavos, C., Das, U.N., Stefanadis, C. 2004. Adherence to the Mediterranean diet attenuates inflammation and coagulation process in healthy adults: The ATTICA Study. *J Am Coll Cardiol.* 44:152–158.

Chung, C.P., Avalos, I., Oeser, A. et al. 2007. High prevalence of the metabolic syndrome in patients with systemic lupus erythematosus: Association with disease characteristics and cardiovascular risk factors. *Ann Rheum Dis.* 66:208–214.

Chung, C.P., Long, A.G., Solus, J.F. et al. 2009. Adipocytokines in systemic lupus erythematosus: Relationship to inflammation, insulin resistance and coronary atherosclerosis. *Lupus.* 18:799–806.

Chung, C.P., Oeser, A., Solus, J.F. et al. 2008. Inflammation-associated insulin resistance: Differential effects in rheumatoid arthritis and systemic lupus erythematosus define potential mechanisms. *Arthritis Rheum.* 58:2105–2112.

Cloetens, L., Ulmius, M., Johansson-Persson, A., Akesson, B., Onning, G. 2012. Role of dietary beta-glucans in the prevention of the metabolic syndrome. *Nutr Rev.* 70:444–458.

Constans, J., Dupuy, R., Blann, A.D. et al. 2003. Anti-endothelial cell autoantibodies and soluble markers of endothelial cell dysfunction in systemic lupus erythematosus. *J Rheumatol.* 30:1963–1966.

Cornier, M.A., Dabelea, D., Hernandez, T.L. et al. 2008. The metabolic syndrome. *Endocr Rev.* 29:777–822.

Costenbader, K.H., Feskanich, D., Holmes, M., Karlson, E.W., Benito-Garcia, E. 2008. Vitamin D intake and risks of systemic lupus erythematosus and rheumatoid arthritis in women. *Ann Rheum Dis* 67(4):530–535.

Costenbader, K.H., Kang, J.H., Karlson, E.W. 2010. Antioxidant intake and risks of rheumatoid arthritis and systemic lupus erythematosus in women. *Am J Epidemiol.* 172(2):205–216.

Cutolo, M., Otsa, K. 2008. Vitamin D, immunity and lupus. *Lupus.* 17(1):6–10.

Czernichow, S., Vergnaud, A.C., Galan, P. et al. 2009. Effects of long-term antioxidant supplementation and association of serum antioxidant concentrations with risk of metabolic syndrome in adults. *Am J Clin Nutr.* 90:329–335.

Dai, J., Miller, A.H., Bremner, J.D. et al. 2008. Adherence to the Mediterranean diet is inversely associated with circulating interleukin-6 among middle-aged men: A twin study. *Circulation.* 117:169–175.

Dixit, V.D. 2008. Adipose-immune interactions during obesity and caloric restriction: Reciprocal mechanisms regulating immunity and health span. *J Leukoc Biol.* 84:882–892.

Duffy, E.M., Meenagh, G.K., McMillan, S.A., Strain, J.J., Hannigan, B.M., Bell, A.L. 2004. The clinical effect of dietary supplementation with omega-3 fish oil and/or copper in systemic lupus erythematosus. *J Rheumatol.* 31(8):1551–1556.

El-Magadmi, M., Ahmad, Y., Turkie, W. et al. 2006. Hyperinsulinemia, insulin resistance, and circulating oxidized low density lipoprotein in women with systemic lupus erythematosus. *J Rheumatol.* 33:50–56.

Escárcega, R.O., García-Carrasco, M., Fuentes-Alexandro, S. et al. 2006. Insulin resistance, chronic inflammatory state and the link with systemic lupus eryhtematosus-related coronary disease. *Autoimmunity Rev.* 6:48–53.

Esdaile, J.M., Abrahamowicz, M., Grodzicky, T., Li, Y., Panaritis, C., Berger, R.D. 2001. Traditional Framingham risk factors fail to fully account for accelerated atherosclerosis in systemic lupus erythematosus. *Arthritis Rheum.* 44:2331–2337.

Esposito, K., Marfella, R., Ciotola, M. et al. 2004. Effect of a Mediterranean-style diet on endothelial dysfunction and markers of vascular inflammation in the metabolic syndrome: A randomized trial. *JAMA.* 292:1440–1446.

Esposito, K., Pontillo, A., Di, P.C. et al. 2003. Effect of weight loss and lifestyle changes on vascular inflammatory markers in obese women: A randomized trial. *JAMA.* 289:1799–1804.

Estruch, R., Martinez-Gonzalez, M.A., Corella, D. et al. 2006. Effects of a Mediterranean-style diet on cardiovascular risk factors: A randomized trial. *Ann Intern Med.*145:1–11.

Fassett, R.G., Gobe, G.C., Peake, J.M., Coombes, J.S. 2010. Omega-3 polyunsaturated fatty acids in the treatment of kidney disease. *Am J Kidney Dis.* 56(4):728–742.

Ford, E.S., Giles, W.H., Dietz, W.H. 2002. Prevalence of the metabolic syndrome among US adults: Findings from the third National Health and Nutrition Examination Survey. *JAMA.* 287:356–359.

Fragopoulou, E., Panagiotakos, D.B., Pitsavos, C. et al. 2010. The association between adherence to the Mediterranean diet and adiponectin levels among healthy adults: The ATTICA study. *J Nutr Biochem.* 21:285–289.

Fung, T.T., McCullough, M.L., Newby, P.K. et al. 2005. Diet-quality scores and plasma concentrations of markers of inflammation and endothelial dysfunction. *Am J Clin Nutr.* 82:163–173.

Galleano, M., Calabro, V., Prince, P.D. et al. 2012. Flavonoids and metabolic syndrome. *Ann N Y Acad Sci.* 1259:87–94.

Gillingham, L.G., Harris-Janz, S., Jones, P.J. 2011. Dietary monounsaturated fatty acids are protective against metabolic syndrome and cardiovascular disease risk factors. *Lipids.* 46:209–228.

Grimes, D.S., Hindle, E., Dyer, T. 1996. Sunlight, cholesterol and coronary heart disease. *QJM.* 89:579–589.

Grundy, S.M. 2006. Metabolic syndrome: Connecting and reconciling cardiovascular and diabetes worlds. *J Am Coll Cardiol.* 47:1093–1100.

Grundy, S.M. 2008. Metabolic syndrome pandemic. *Artherioscler Thromb Vasc Biol.* 28:629–636.

Grundy, S.M., Cleeman, J.I., Daniels, S.R. et al. 2005. American Heart Association; National Heart, Lung, and Blood Institute. Diagnosis and management of the metabolic syndrome: An American Heart Association/ National Heart, Lung, and Blood Institute Scientific Statement. *Circulation.* 112:2735–2752.

Guzik, T.J., Mangalat, D., Korbut, R. 2006. Adipocytokines—Novel link between inflammation and vascular function. *J Physiol Pharmacol.* 57:505–528.

Halade, G.V., Rahman, M.M., Bhattacharya, A., Barnes, J.L., Chandrasekar, B., Fernandes, G. 2010. Docosahexaenoic acid-enriched fish oil attenuates kidney disease and prolongs median and maximal life span of autoimmune lupus-prone mice. *J Immunol.* 184(9):5280–5286.

Ho, C.Y., Wong, C.K., Li, E.K., Tam, L.S., Lam, C.W. 2003. Elevated plasma concentrations of nitric oxide, soluble thrombomodulin and soluble vascular cell adhesion molecule-1 in patients with systemic lupus erythematosus. *Rheumatology* (Oxford). 42:117–122.

Hong, Y., Wang, T., Huang, C., Cheng, W., Lin, B. 2008. Soy isoflavones supplementation alleviates disease severity in autoimmune-prone MRL-lpr/lpr mice. *Lupus.* 17(9):814–821.

Hong, Y.H., Huang, C.J., Wang, S.C., Lin, B.F. 2009. The ethyl acetate extract of alphalpha sprout ameliorates disease severity of autoimmune-prone MRL-lpr/lpr mice. *Lupus.* 18(3):206–215.

Hotamisligil, G.S. 2000. Molecular mechanisms of insulin resistance and the role of the adipocyte. *Int J Obes Relat Metab Disord.* 24:23–27.

Jans, A., van Hees, A.M., Gjelstad, I.M. et al. 2012. Impact of dietary fat quantity and quality on skeletal muscle fatty acid metabolism in subjects with the metabolic syndrome. *Metabolism.* 61:1554–1565.

Kamen, D.L., Cooper, G.S., Bouali, H., Shaftman, S.R., Hollis, B.W., Gilkeson, G.S. 2006. Vitamin D deficiency in systemic lupus erythematosus. *Autoimmun Rev.* 5(2):114–117.

Kastorini, C.M., Milionis, H.J., Esposito, K., Giugliano, D., Goudevenos, J.A., Panagiotakos, D.B. 2011. The effect of Mediterranean diet on metabolic syndrome and its components: A meta-analysis of 50 studies and 534,906 individuals. *J Am Coll Cardiol.* 57:1299–1313.

Keys, A., Menotti, A., Karvonen, M.J. et al. 1986. The diet and 15-year death rate in the seven countries study. *Am J Epidemiol.* 124:903–915.

Kinoshita, K., Kishimoto, K., Shimazu, H. et al. 2010. Successful treatment with retinoids in patients with lupus nephritis. *Am J Kidney Dis.* 55(2):344–347.

Kip, K.E., Marroquin, O.C., Kelley, D.E. et al. 2004. Clinical importance of obesity versus the metabolic syndrome in cardiovascular risk in women: A report from the Women's Ischemia Syndrome Evaluation (WISE) study. *Circulation.* 109:706–713.

Klack, K., Bonfa, E., Neto, E.F.B. 2012. Diet and nutritional aspects in systemic lupus erythematosus. *Rev Bras Reumatol.* 52(3):384–408.

Knott, H.M., Martínez, J.D. 2010. Innovative management of lupus erythematosus. *Dermatol Clin.* 28(3):489–499.

Lago, F., Dieguez, C., Gomez-Reino, J., Gualillo, O. 2007. The emerging role of adipokines as mediators of inflammation and immune responses. *Cytokine Growth Factor Rev.* 18:313–325.

Lakka, H.M., Laaksonen, D.E., Lakka, T.A. et al. 2002. The metabolic syndrome and total and cardiovascular disease mortality in middle-aged men. *JAMA.* 288:2709–2716.

Leiba, A., Amital, H., Gershwin, M.E., Shoenfeld, Y. 2001. Diet and lupus. *Lupus.* 10(3):246–248.

Li, Y., Guo, H., Wu, M., Liu, M. 2013. Serum and dietary antioxidant status is associated with lower prevalence of the metabolic syndrome in a study in Shanghai, China. *Asia Pac J Clin Nutr.* 22:60–68.

Li, Y.C. 2005. Vitamin D and the renin-angiotensin system. In: Feldman, D., Pike, J.W., Glorieux, F.H., eds. *Vitamin D.*, Vol 1. Amsterdam, the Netherlands: Elsevier Academic Press, pp. 871–882.

Lozovoy, M.A.B., Simão, A.N.C., Hohmann, M.S.N. et al. 2011. Inflammatory biomarkers and oxidative stress measurements in patients with systemic lupus erythematosus with or without metabolic syndrome. *Lupus.* 20:1356–1364.

Maahs, D.M., Ogden, L.G., Kinney, G.L. et al. 2005. Low plasma adiponectin levels predict progression of coronary artery calcification. *Circulation.* 111:747–753.

MacLean, C.H., Mojica, W.A., Morton, S.C. et al. 2004. Effects of omega-3 fatty acids on lipids and glycemic control in type II diabetes and the metabolic syndrome and on inflammatory bowel disease, rheumatoid arthritis, renal disease, systemic lupus erythematosus, and osteoporosis. *Evid Rep Technol Assess.* (Summ) (89):1–4.

Madani, Z., Louchami, K., Sener, A., Malaisse, W.J., Ait Yahia, D. 2012. Dietary sardine protein lowers insulin resistance, leptin and TNF-alpha and beneficially affects adipose tissue oxidative stress in rats with fructose-induced metabolic syndrome. *Int J Mol Med.* 29:311–318.

Maki, P.A., Newberne, P.M. 1992. Dietary lipids and immune function. *J Nutr.* 122(3 Suppl):610–614.

Manger, K., Kusus, M., Forster, C. et al. 2003. Factors associated with coronary artery calcification in young female patients with SLE. *Ann Rheum Dis.* 62:846–850.

Manzi, S., Meilahn, E.N., Rairie, J.E. et al. 1997. Age-specific incidence rates of myocardial infarction and angina in women with systemic lupus erythematosus: Comparison with the Framingham study. *Am J Epidemiol.* 145:408–415.

Marquezine, G.F., Oliveira, C.M., Pereira, A.C., Krieger, J.E., Mill, J.G. 2008. Metabolic syndrome determinants in an urban population from Brazil: Social class and gender-specific interaction. *Int J Cardiol.* 129:259–265.

Martini, L.A., Wood, R.J. 2006. Vitamin D status and the metabolic syndrome. *Nutr Rev.* 64(11):479–486.

Mathieu, C., Gysemans, C., Giulietti, A., Bouillon, R. 2005. Vitamin D and diabetes. *Diabetologia.* 48:1247–1257.

Minami, Y., Hirabayashi, Y., Nagata, C., Ishii, T., Harigae, H., Sasaki, T. 2011. Intakes of vitamin B6 and dietary fiber and clinical course of systemic lupus erythematosus: A prospective study of Japanese female patients. *J Epidemiol.* 21(4):246–254.

Minami, Y., Sasaki, T., Arai, Y., Kurisu, Y., Hisamichi, S. 2003. Diet and systemic lupus erythematosus: A 4 year prospective study of Japanese patients. *J Rheumatol.* 30(4):747–754.

Miranda, P.J., De-Fronzo, R.A., Califf, R.M., Guyton, J.R. 2005. Metabolic syndrome: Definition, pathophysiology, and mechanisms. *Am Heart J.* 149:33–45.

Mohan, I.K., Das, U.N. 1997. Oxidant stress, anti-oxidants and essential fatty acids in systemic lupus erythematosus. *Prostaglandins Leukot Essent Fatty Acids.* 56(3):193–198.

Mok, C.C. 2006. Accelerated atherosclerosis, arterial thromboembolism and preventive strategies in systemic lupus erythematosus. *Scand J Rheumatol.* 35:85–95.

Mok, C.C., Poon, W. L., Lai, J.P.S. et al. 2010. Metabolic syndrome, endothelial injury, and subclinical atherosclerosis in patients with systemic lupus erythematosus. *Scand J Rheumatol.* 39:42–49.

Monti, L.D., Casiraghi, M.C., Setola, E. et al. 2013. L-arginine enriched biscuits improve endothelial function and glucose metabolism: A pilot study in healthy subjects and a cross-over study in subjects with impaired glucose tolerance and metabolic syndrome. *Metabolism.* 62:255–264.

Morris, K.L., Zemel, M.B. 2005. 1,25-dihydroxyvitamin D3 modulation of adipocyte glucocorticoid function. *Obes Res.* 13:670–677.

Muller, K., Odum, N., Bendtzen, K. 1993. 1,25-dihydroxyvita- min D3 selectively reduces interleukin-2 levels and proliferation of human T cell lines in vitro. *Immunol Lett.* 35:177–182.

Need, A.G., O'Loughlin, P.D., Horowitz, M., Nordin, B.E. 2005. Relationship between fasting serum glucose, age, body mass index and serum 25 hydroxyvitamin D in postmenopausal women. *Clin Endocrinol* (Oxford). 62:738 –741.

Negrón, A.M., Molina, M.J., Mayor, A.M., Rodriguez, V.E., Vilá, L.M. 2008. Factors associated with metabolic syndrome in patients with systemic lupus erythematosus from Puerto Rico. *Lupus.* 17:348–354.

Nuttall, S.L., Heaton, S., Piper, M.K., Martin, U., Gordon, C. 2003. Cardiovascular risk in systemic lupus erythematosus—Evidence of increased oxidative stress and dyslipidemia. *Rheumatology.* 42:758–762.

Oates, J.C. 2010. The biology of reactive intermediates in systemic lupus erythematosus. *Autoimmunity.* 43:56–63.

Onat, A., Uzunlar, B., Hergenc, G. et al. 2005. Cross-sectional study of complement C3 as a coronary risk factor among men and women. *Clin Sci.* 108:129–135.

Papathanasopoulos, A., Camilleri, M. 2010. Dietary fiber supplements: Effects in obesity and metabolic syndrome and relationship to gastrointestinal functions. *Gastroenterology.* 138(65–72):e61–e62.

Parker, B., Ahmad, Y., Shelmerdine, J. et al. 2011. An analysis of the metabolic syndrome phenotype in systemic lupus erythematosus. *Lupus.* 20:1459–1465.

Parker, B., Bruce, I.N. 2010. The metabolic syndrome in systemic lupus erythematosus. *Rheum Dis Clin North Am.* 36:81–97.

Parker, B., Urowitz, M.B., Gladman, D.D. et al. August 2013. Clinical associations of the metabolic syndrome in systemic lupus erythematosus: Data from an international inception cohort. *Ann Rheum Dis.* 72(8):1308–1314.

Patavino, T., Brady, D.M. 2001. Natural medicine and nutritional therapy as an alternative treatment in systemic lupus erythematosus. *Altern Med Rev.* 6(5):460–471.

Pereira, M.A., O'Reilly, E., Augustsson, K. et al. 2004. Dietary fiber and risk of coronary heart disease: A pooled analysis of cohort studies. *Arch Intern Med.* 164(4):370–376.

Petri, M. 2001. Diet and systemic lupus erythematosus: From mouse and monkey to woman? *Lupus.* 10(11):775–777.

Petri, M., Lakata, C., Magder, L., Goldman, D. 1994. Effect of prednisone and hydroxychloroquine on coronary artery disease risk factors in systemic lupus erythematosus: A longitudinal data analysis. *Am J Med.* 96(3):254–259.

Petri, M., Spence, D., Bone, L.R. et al. 1992. Coronary artery disease risk factors in the Johns Hopkins Lupus Cohort: Prevalence, recognition by patients, and preventive practices. *Medicine.* 71:291–302.

Pestka, J.J. 2010. N-3 polyunsaturated fatty acids and autoimmune-mediated glomerulonephritis. *Prostaglandins Leukot Essent Fatty Acids.* 82(4–6):251–258.

Posadas-Romero, C., Torres-Tamayo, M., Zamora-Gonzalez, J. et al. 2004. High insulin levels and increased low-density lipoprotein oxidizability in pediatric patients with systemic lupus erythematosus. *Arthritis Rheum.* 50:160–165.

Poudyal, H., Panchal, S.K., Ward, L.C., Brown, L. 2013. Effects of ALA, EPA and DHA in high-carbohydrate, high-fat diet-induced metabolic syndrome in rats. *J Nutr Biochem.* 24:1041–1052.

Puchau, B., Zulet, M.A., de Echavarri, A.G., Hermsdorff, H.H., Martinez, J.A. 2010. Dietary total antioxidant capacity is negatively associated with some metabolic syndrome features in healthy young adults. *Nutrition.* 26:534–541.

Reilly, M.P., Wolfe, M.L., Rhodes, T., Girman, C., Mehta, N., Rader, D.J. 2004. Measures of insulin resistance add incremental value to the clinical diagnosis of metabolic syndrome in association with coronary atherosclerosis. *Circulation.* 110:803–809.

Rideout, T.C., Marinangeli, C.P., Martin, H., Browne, R.W., Rempel, C.B. 2013. Consumption of low-fat dairy foods for 6 months improves insulin resistance without adversely affecting lipids or bodyweight in healthy adults: A randomized free-living cross-over study. *Nutr J.* 12:56.

Robinson, L.E., Mazurak, V.C. 2013. N-3 polyunsaturated fatty acids: Relationship to inflammation in healthy adults and adults exhibiting features of metabolic syndrome. *Lipids.* 48:319–332.

Roman, M.J., Shanker, B.A., Davis, A. et al. 2003. Prevalence and correlates of accelerated atherosclerosis in systemic lupus erythematosus. *N Engl J Med.* 349:2399–2406.

Rosenstreich, S.J., Rich, C., Volwiler, W. 1971. Deposition in and release of vitamin D3 from body fat: Evidence for a storage site in the rat. *J Clin Invest.* 50:679–687.

Ross, R. 1999. Atherosclerosis is an inflammatory disease. *Am Heart J.* 138:S419–S420.

Sabio, J.M., Vargas-Hitos, J., Zamora-Pasadas, M. et al. 2009. Metabolic syndrome is associated with increased arterial stiffness and biomarkers of subclinical atherosclerosis in patients with Systemic Lupus Erythematosus. *J Rheumatol.* 36:2204–2211.

Sabio, J.M., Zamora-Pasadas, M., Jimenez-Jaimez, J. et al. 2008. Metabolic syndrome in patients with systemic lupus erythematosus from Southern Spain. *Lupus.* 7:849–859.

Schini-Kerth, V.B., Auger, C., Kim, J.H., Etienne-Selloum, N., Chataigneau, T. 2010. Nutritional improvement of the endothelial control of vascular tone by polyphenols: Role of NO and EDHF. *Pflugers Arch.* 459:853–862.

Schmajuk, G., Yelin, E., Chakravarty, E., Nelson, L.M., Panapolis, P., Yazdany, J. 2010. Osteoporosis screening, prevention, and treatment in systemic lupus erythematosus: Application of the systemic lupus erythematosus quality indicators. *Arthritis Care Res* (Hoboken). 62(7):993–1001.

Selmi, C., Tsuneyama, K. 2010. Nutrition, geoepidemiology, and autoimmunity. *Autoimmun Rev.* 9(5):A267–A270.

Shah, M., Adams-Huet, B., Kavanaugh, A., Coyle, Y., Lipsky, P. 2004. Nutrient intake and diet quality in patients with systemic lupus erythematosus on a culturally sensitive cholesterol lowering dietary program. *J Rheumatol.* 31(1):71–75.

Sheikh, Z., Ahmad, R., Sheikh, N., Ali, R. 2007. Enhanced recognition of reactive oxygen species damage human serum albumin by circulating systemic lupus erythematosus autoantibodies. *Autoimmunity.* 40:512–520.

Sidiropoulos, P.I., Karvounaris, S.A., Boumpas, D.T. 2008. Metabolic syndrome in rheumatic diseases: Epidemiology, pathophysiology, and clinical implications. *Arth Res Ther.* 10:207–215.

Simão, A.N.C., Dichi, J.B., Barbosa, D.S., Cecchini, R., Dichi, I. 2008. Influence of uric acid and g-glutamyltransferase on total antioxidant capacity an oxidative stress in patients with metabolic syndrome. *Nutrition.* 24:675–681.

Siri-Tarino, P.W., Sun, Q., Hu, F.B., Krauss, R.M. 2010. Meta-analysis of prospective cohort studies evaluating the association of saturated fat with cardiovascular disease. *Am J Clin Nutr.* 91:535–546.

Snijder, M.B., van Dam, R.M., Visser, M. et al. 2005. Adiposity in relation to vitamin D status and parathyroid hormone levels: A population-based study in older men and women. *J Clin Endocrinol Metab.* 90:4119–4123.

Somers, E.C., Marder, W., Kaplan, M.J., Brook, R.D., McCune, W.J. 2005. Plasminogen activator inhibitor-1 is associated with impaired endothelial function in women with systemic lupus erythema-tosus. *Ann N Y Acad Sci.* 1051:271–280.

Svenungsson, E., Cederholm, A., Jensen-Urstad, K., Fei, G.Z., deFaire, U., Frostegard, J. 2008. Endothelial function and markersof endothelial activation in relation to cardiovascular disease in systemic lupus erythematosus. *Scand J Rheumatol.* 37:352–359.

Tam, L.S., Fan, B., Li, E.K. et al. 2003. Patients with systemic lupus erythematosus show increased platelet activation and endothelial dysfunction induced by acute hyper-homocysteinemia. *J Rheumatol.* 30:1479–1484.

Tam, L.S., Li, E.K., Leung, V.Y. et al. 2005. Effects of vitamins C and E on oxidative stress markers and endothelial function in patients with systemic lupus erythematosus: A double blind placebo controlled pilot study. *J Rheumatol.* 32(2):275–282.

Telles, R.W., Lanna, C.C.D., Ferreira, G.A., Ribeiro, A.L. 2010. Metabolic syndrome in patients with systemic lupus erythematosus. *Lupus.* 19:803–809.

Toloza, S.M., Cole, D.E., Gladman, D.D., Ibañez, D., Urowitz, M.B. 2010. Vitamin D insufficiency in a large female SLE cohort. *Lupus.* 19(1):13–19.

Tso, T.K., Huang, W.N. 2009. Elevation of fasting insulin and its association with cardiovascular disease risk in women with systemic lupus erythematosus. *Rheumatol Int.* 29:735–742.

Tso, T.K., Huang, W.N., Huang, H.Y. et al. 2006. Elevation of plasma interleukin-18 concentration is associated with insulin levels in patients with systemic lupus erythematosus. *Lupus.* 15:207–212.

US Department of Health and Human Services, US Department of Agriculture. Dietary Guidelines for Americans. 2005. Available from: http://www.health.gov/DietaryGuidelines/dga2005/document.

Vadacca, M., Margiotta, D., Rigon, A. et al. 2009. Adipokines and systemic Lupus Erythematosus: Relationship with metabolic syndrome and cardiovascular disease risk factors. *J Rheumatol.* 36:295–297.

van Meijl, L.E., Vrolix, R., Mensink, R.P. 2008. Dairy product consumption and the metabolic syndrome. *Nutr Res Rev.* 21:148–157.

Wright, T.B., Shults, J., Leonard, M.B., Zemel, B.S., Burnham, J.M. 2009. Hypovitaminosis D is associated with greater body mass index and disease activity in pediatric systemic lupus erythematosus. *J Pediatr.* 155(2):260–265.

Wu, P.W., Rhew, E.Y., Dyer, A.R. et al. 2009. 25-hydroxyvitamin D and cardiovascular risk factors in women with systemic lupus erythematosus. *Arthritis Rheum.* 61(10):1387–1395.

Zonana-Nacach, A., Santana-Sahagún, E., Jiménez-Balderas, F.J., Camargo-Coronel, A. 2008. Prevalence and factors associated with metabolic syndrome in patients with rheumatoid arthritis and systemic lupus erythematosus. *J Clin Rheumatol.* 14:74–77.

12 Metabolic Syndrome Post Liver Transplantation

Lucilene Rezende Anastácio, Suzana Mantovani, and Maria Isabel Toulson Davison Correia

CONTENTS

12.1 INTRODUCTION

Liver transplantation is a life-saving as well as a life-changing procedure for patients with advanced chronic liver disease, hepatocellular carcinoma, and acute liver failure (Kallwitz 2012).

Survival rates after liver transplantation have reached 85% at 5 years post transplant and as high as 56% at 20 years post transplant, in the two last decades. However, the improved survival of patients following liver transplantation (LTx) has been accompanied by an increased prevalence and incidence of chronic diseases over that of the general population (Adam and Hoti 2009, Duffy et al. 2010). Metabolic disorders are significantly higher in this subgroup of individuals, affecting more than half of the patients (Bianchi et al. 2008, Hanoueh et al. 2008, Kallwitz 2012, Laryea et al. 2007).

Hypertension, which is described in up to 77% of these patients, is the most common metabolic disorder (Stegal et al. 1995). Excessive weight is described, by the third year after the operation, in up to 70% of them (Richards et al. 2005). In the first year after orthotopic liver transplantation (OLTx), obesity rates can reach up to 41% (Richards et al. 2005). In addition, glucose intolerance can affect up to 60% (Bianchi et al. 2008, Duffy et al. 2010), and 13%–38% become diabetic (Anastácio et al. 2013). Hypertriglyceridemia and low high-density lipoprotein levels are also highly prevalent after OLTx and can, respectively, affect up to 69% and 50% of post–liver transplant patients (Anastácio et al. 2010).

All these disorders were recognized recently as being interrelated, and together, they result in the metabolic syndrome (MetS), prevalent in these population, affecting 44%–58% of the patients (Bianchi et al. 2007, Hanoueh et al. 2008, Anastácio et al. 2011a,b). MetS is a strong risk factor for cardiovascular disease and also for liver damage in both the general (Kip et al. 2004, Marchesini et al. 2003) and the liver transplant population (Lunati et al. 2013, Sprintzl et al. 2013).

Considering these numbers, the prevention of excessive weight gain and the critical aspects associated with MetS in post–liver transplant patients should be treated as importantly as graft rejection or hepatic failure prevention, which place these patients at higher risk of mortality. Moreover, it should be mandatorily a teamwork approach of these patients since some of the MetS components can be reversed by adequate lifestyle modification attitudes, such as diet and exercise counseling.

12.2 LIVER TRANSPLANTATION

LTx is a life-saving procedure for patients with chronic end-stage liver disease and selected patients with acute liver failure, as well as few cancer cases. Surgical techniques have undergone major changes, in the last years, and there has been an improvement in the understanding of pre- and post-transplantation physiology. Furthermore, the introduction of newer and more effective immunosuppressive drugs and strategies for preventing post-transplantation infections has contributed to reach higher survival rates (Varma et al. 2011).

In 1997, the American Society of Transplant Physicians and the American Association for the Study of the Liver Disease put forward the minimal listing criteria for patients with end-stage liver disease. To qualify for the listing, the patient's expected survival should be ≤90% within 1 year without transplantation. Overall, LTx should lead to prolonged survival and improved quality of life (Varma et al. 2011).

12.3 METABOLIC SYNDROME

There are many definitions for MetS in the literature. The criteria used by the National Cholesterol Program Education, Adult Treatment Panel III adapted by the National Heart, Lung and Blood Institute/American Heart Association (NHLBI/AHA) (Grundy et al. 2004) and International Diabetes Federation (IDF) (Alberti et al. 2006) are detailed in Table 12.1.

The prevalence of MetS in the general population is approximately 30% (Ford et al. 2002), while it is significantly higher in the transplant population regardless of the transplanted organ. In patients undergoing kidney transplantation, the prevalence of the syndrome varies from 16.7% to 63%

TABLE 12.1

International Diabetes Federation (IDF) and American Heart Association (AHA) Criteria for the Definition of Metabolic Syndrome

MetS Criteria—MetS Components	IDF(2006)—Abdominal Obesity + Two or More Components	NHLBI/AHA(2005)—At least Three Components
Waist circumference	≥90 cm (man)	≥102 cm (man)
	≥80 cm (woman)[a]	≥88 cm (woman)
Blood fast glucose	≥100 mg/dL and/or diabetes treatment	≥100 mg/dL and/or diabetes treatment
Blood pressure	≥130 mmHg (SBP) and/or ≥85 mmHg (DBP) and/or hypertension treatment	≥140 mmHg (SBP) and/or ≥90 mmHg (DBP) and/or hypertension treatment
Triglycerides	≥150 mg/dL and/or hypertriglyceridemia treatment	≥150 mg/dL and/or hypertriglyceridemia treatment
HDL	<40 mg/dL (man)	<40 mg/dL (man)
	<50 mg/dL (woman)	<50 mg/dL (woman)

DBP, diastolic blood pressure; SBD, systolic blood pressure.

[a] Abdominal obesity cut points for South Americans.

(de Vries et al. 2004), and in patients undergoing heart transplantation, it is 42.3% (Cordero et al. 2006). In patients who have undergone kidney transplantation, the risk factors and implications of the problem have been well described, such as older age (de Vries et al. 2004), male sex (Courivaud et al. 2007), shorter time since the operation (Bellinghieri et al. 2009), and higher body mass index (BMI) prior to transplantation (Bellinghieri et al. 2009). The presence of MetS in these patients affects the function of the graft (Courivaud et al. 2007) and increases the rate of coronary artery calcification (Adeseun et al. 2008), which increases the chance of atherosclerotic events when compared to those patients without the syndrome.

In liver transplant recipients, Laryea et al. (2007) documented MetS rates of 58%, Bianchi et al. (2008) showed rates of 44%, and Hanouneh et al. (2008) of 50%. In Brazil, our group has diagnosed, among 148 patients who underwent LTx, a prevalence of 50% (IDF criteria) and 38.5% (NHLBI/ AHA criteria) (Anastácio et al. 2011a,b).

As in the overall population and in renal transplant patients, the syndrome is also a risk factor for higher morbidity and mortality among liver transplant patients. Laryea et al. (2007) demonstrated that liver transplant recipients were more likely to have major vascular events (including stroke, transient ischemic attack, myocardial infarction, acute coronary syndrome, and sudden cardiac death) if they had MetS. The rates of these events were significantly higher in patients with MetS relative to those without it at 30% vs. 8% (p < 0.01). MetS has been considered an independent risk factor for fibrosis in patients with recurrent hepatitis C virus (de Vries et al. 2004), and it also promoted elevation of hepatic transaminases in patients undergoing LTx due to cryptogenic cirrhosis (Angelico et al. 2003).

The risk factors for the syndrome *per se* remain unclear. Older age was directly related to the syndrome in the study by Laryea et al. (2007), but not in the study of Bianchi et al. (2008). Alcohol-related liver disease, cryptogenic cirrhosis, and hepatitis C infection have also been associated with MetS (Laryea et al. 2007) but not in all cases (Bianchi et al. 2008). Due to the aggressive immunosuppressive regime in the early postoperative period, patients usually present with high blood glucose, triglycerides, and blood pressure, even if they are still malnourished. In our study (Anastácio et al. 2011a,b), for both the IDF and the NHLBI/AHA classifications, the independent factors associated with MetS were older age, shorter time since transplantation, and history of excessive weight prior to OLTx. Other predictors for MetS by IDF criteria were alcohol abuse as the indication for OLTx, physical activity reduction as the cause of weight gain after transplantation, and calcium intake below recommended levels. The presence of MetS (NHLBI/AHA) was also associated with decreased intake of potassium, fiber, and folic acid.

In summary, the classical risk factors, which are included in the definition of MetS or which directly affect it, include higher pre-transplant BMI and higher post-transplant weight; higher blood fasting glucose and presence of pre-LTx diabetes; and higher blood pressure, higher triglycerides, and lower HDL levels. Post-transplant changes in BMI have also been directly associated with the syndrome, although weight gain alone is not considered a predictive risk factor for it. Logically, weight gain is critical for the recovery of the patients' overall nutritional status, and it will not cause metabolic disorders if it does not lead to overweight or obesity. All factors associated with MetS and its components are detailed in Table 12.2.

Known as a post-transplant complication, MetS may already be present in the pre-transplant setting as it is important to recognize that complications of advanced stage of liver disease can confound the diagnosis in this phase. For instance, the presence of ascites alters waist circumference. Vasodilation and decreased effective circulating volume found with portal hypertension result in lowered systemic blood pressure. Metabolic dysfunction observed with end stages of liver disease immediately prior to transplant can result in lowered serum glucose and lipid values. A study evaluating the MetS prior to LTx found a rate of 5.4% (Laish et al. 2011). Pre-transplant rates for hypertension were 9%–19%, diabetes 10%–22%, dyslipidemia 3%–43%, and obesity 11%–38% (Kallwitz 2012).

TABLE 12.2

Factors Associated with Metabolic Syndrome and Its Components in Liver Transplant Recipients

	Obesity	Diabetes	Hypertension	Dyslipidemia	Metabolic Syndrome
Immunosuppressive medication — Yes	Steroids Cyclosporine	Tacrolimus	Cyclosporine Steroids	Cyclosporine Sirolimus + cyclosporine Tacrolimus	Cyclosporine, tacrolimus, steroids 14,16
Immunosuppressive medication — No	Steroids Cyclosporine	Tacrolimus without steroids	Cyclosporine with low steroids doses	Sirolimus	
Other associated factors	Older age Chronic liver disease Previous history of excessive weight Physical inactivity Greater donor BMI Being married	Older age Obesity Hepatitis viral C infection Alcohol-related disease indication for transplantation Familiar history of diabetes Hispanic and black ethnicity Male gender	Older age Male gender Familiar history of hypertension Renal disease	Weight gain Hepatocellular liver disease Renal dysfunction	Older age 16 Alcohol-related liver disease 16 Cryptogenic cirrhosis 16 Hepatitis C infection 16 Higher pre-transplant BMI 16 Presence of pre–liver transplantation diabetes 14 Post-transplant changes in BMI 14

Source: Data from Anastácio et al., *Clin. Nutr.*, 29, 175, 2010.

12.4 INDIVIDUAL RISK FACTORS FOR METABOLIC SYNDROME AFTER LIVER TRANSPLANTATION

12.4.1 OBESITY

Weight gain after LTx is critical for the recovery of the nutritional status of patients. However, these patients typically gain more than they should. Richards et al. (2005) in a study with 597 patients observed that the median weight gain of LTx patients increased from 1.8 kg at 6 months to 9.5 kg at 3 years after LTx, and the median weight gain at 1 year was 5.1 kg, leading to a prevalence of nearly 70% of patients with excessive body weight (BMI > 25 kg/m^2).

The incidence of obesity within 1 year of LTx varies from 15.5% to 40.7% (Anastácio et al. 2011a,b, Richards et al. 2005) depending on the definition used, and it continues to grow over the years post transplantation (Anastácio et al. 2013). However, in most patients, the greatest relative weight gain occurs in the first year after transplantation. In our own experience (Anastácio et al. 2011a,b), 69.9% of patients were overweight and 37.8% were obese. Some degree of abdominal obesity was seen in 88% of patients.

Several factors have been implicated as risk factors for weight gain after liver transplantation. In our study (Anastácio et al. 2011a,b), independent risk factors for overweight, obesity, and abdominal obesity after LTx included greater BMI before liver disease, weight gain since LTx, family history of overweight, smoking, working, being married, having less time since transplantation, lower calcium intake, and less sleeping hours.

Some authors have raised the possibility that resting energy expenditure (REE) may be altered in these patients causing the changes in weight. Plank et al. (2001) followed 14 patients throughout the first year after surgery and reported that the REE changed significantly, peaking at around day 10 after surgery, when it averaged 42% above predicted. This hypermetabolism resolved slowly. After 30 days since surgery, the REE began to fall significantly and reached its lowest value a year after transplantation. Nevertheless, only in this period, the measured REE was similar to the predicted REE values. They also observed that total body fat returned to preoperative levels within 3 months. However, the restoration of protein stores occurred slowly and incompletely. Only 54% of the protein lost in the early postoperative phase was regained after 12 months.

Richardson et al. (2001) followed 23 patients up to 9 months after LTx. They found a significant drop in measured REE in comparison to pre-LTx and to controls. The measured REE after LTx was above the predicted REE, in contrast to the study of Plank et al. (2001). These authors also found hypometabolism as a strong predictor of greater fat mass gain after LTx, although this association was not always observed.

A recent study from our group has shown that REE was elevated at 30 days and reduced at the end of the study (1 year of patient follow-up, after LTx). Increases in body weight and fat mass were observed, and these were most likely related to positive energy balance at all times after LTx, as well as an increase in fat intake. After multivariate analyses, the REE before transplantation and triceps skinfold thickness were positively associated, and the cumulative dose of prednisone was negatively associated with REE after LTx. Percentage of fat intake and fat mass before LTx were also associated with hypometabolism post transplantation (Ferreira et al. 2013).

Another important risk factor widely believed to be associated with weight gain is the immunosuppressive medication. However, this association remains controversial in the literature. In some studies, higher steroid intake was associated with obesity (Everhart et al. 1998) and greater post-transplant weight gain (Canaznello et al. 1997), while in others, it was not (Ferreira et al. 2013, Richardson et al. 2001). In some studies, cyclosporine was associated with this disorder (Canzanello et al. 1997), but this was not observed in other studies (Rabkin et al. 2002). The fact that cyclosporine is related to greater weight gain and obesity could be due to higher steroid intake associated with it, when compared to the use of tacrolimus (Ferreira et al. 2013). Thus, the benefit of steroid intake as a treatment for weight gain after LTx comes into question.

Although the contribution of the earlier risk factors remains a point of question among liver recipients, various studies have shown that obesity is a multifactor disease as in the general population. Thus, weight gain is associated with older age, previous history of excessive weight, or higher BMI levels prior to transplantation (Ferreira et al. 2013, Anastácio et al. 2011a,b, 2013). Greater weight gain has also been observed in patients displaying physical inactivity, those with a greater donor BMI, and patients who were married (Anastácio et al. 2011a,b, 2013).

Although Everhart et al. (1998) found a weak correlation between donor BMI and pre-transplant receptor BMI, this might be due to the need for compatibility of body sizes. Thus, it is possible that a graft of a heavier donor just matches a heavier receptor. Another explanation for the influence of the donor BMI on greater weight gain after LTx is that changes in body composition after LTx may be a result of failure to monitor energy intake through the brain–liver axis, since the donor's liver is removed from the vagal afferent nerve and then *related* to another vagal nerve. Marital status is also associated with body changes in the general and transplant population (Sobal et al. 2003), and it is suggested that marriage may lead to increased body weight as a consequence of greater food intake, because the couple eats together, and this influences the diet of each other. Furthermore, it can also be hypothesized that after LTx, married patients receive excessive spouse care.

Even though some predictors for post–liver transplant obesity appear to be unmodified, as in the general population, physical inactivity and excessive food intake play an important role in the incidence of overweight and obesity. Patients often stop exercising or retire while severely ill on the transplant waiting list. After the transplant, most do not return to work (Anastácio et al. 2011a,b, 2013). It is well established that the majority of post-transplant patients (76%) are sedentary or perform minimal physical daily activity (Painter et al. 2001). Food intake in liver transplant recipients has not been fully assessed, but three studies have not shown association between diet intake and weight changes (Koutsovasilis et al. 2009, Kransnoff et al. 2006, Richardson et al. 2001). This was possibly due to the used methods, since these usually assess current and not chronic diet eating patterns. Our own data support that there is in fact inadequate food intake with bad eating patterns in most of the patients (Anastácio et al. 2011a,b).

The role of steroids on weight gain suggests that they could enhance appetite and stimulate the intake of sweet and high-fat foods. Thus, patients are likely to consume excessive calories. In addition, patients are free from their pre-transplant dietary restrictions and have decreased anorexia, related to an increased sense of well-being, as well as eagerness to regain the lost weight (Anastácio et al. 2010). Additionally, patients are likely to return to old dietary habits, as it has been described by some authors who have stated that a previous history of obesity contributes to weight gain after LTx (Everhart et al. 1998, Anastácio et al. 2011a,b, 2012, 2013, Richardson et al. 2001).

There are several implications of obesity in LTx. Studies have shown that donor and receptor obesity influence the outcome of surgery. Pre-transplant obese patients may be more likely, after surgery, to have primary graft nonfunction and delayed graft function, and they also present with higher risk of death (Malik et al. 2009, Pelletier et al. 2007). However, this has not been a universal finding (Leonard et al. 2008). Obesity is considered a predictor of hepatic steatosis in deceased (Escartin et al. 2005) and living donors (Rinella et al. 2001), and weight loss has been advocated as a way to reduce the amount of liver fat of the last ones (Hwang et al. 2004, Nakamuta et al. 2005, Perkins 2006). The donor's fatty liver is strongly linked to decreased allograft function and patient survival, and its presence is the main cause for liver discarding (Escartin et al. 2005).

In the late post-surgery period, obesity can also affect the graft. Seo et al. (2007) observed that 83% of patients who developed nonalcoholic fatty liver disease (NAFLD) gained weight greater than 10% of pre-transplantation BMI, compared to 25% of patients with no significant post-LTx NAFLD. Lim et al. (2007) also noticed that liver transplant recipients who developed nonalcoholic steatohepatitis had significantly higher BMI (32.5 ± 4.3 kg/m^2) than others (22.9 ± 0.7 kg/m^2).

12.4.2 Impaired Fasting Glucose and Diabetes

Impaired fasting glucose levels and diabetes have been described in two-thirds of liver transplant recipients (Bianchi et al. 2008, Laryea et al. 2007). When compared to the general population, a higher prevalence of post-transplant diabetes mellitus has been observed in liver transplant recipients (Kallwitz 2012). Much of this altered glucose metabolism can be related to immunosuppression with both calcineurin inhibitors and steroids playing a major role.

Glucose intolerance is a well-established side effect of corticosteroid therapy by inducing insulin resistance and enhancing hepatic gluconeogenesis. Tacrolimus has been reported as more diabetogenic than cyclosporine (Bianchi et al. 2008), but the incidence of diabetes after LTx in tacrolimus-treated patients appears to be lower in steroid-free regimens (van Hooff et al. 2007). The diabetogenic effects of cyclosporine and tacrolimus include reduced insulin secretion, increased insulin resistance, and toxic effects in the β-pancreatic cells. However, this appears to be reversible, since the prevalence of diabetes decreases with time, coincident with tapering and discontinuation of the immunosuppressive drugs over the early postoperative period. Therefore, persistent diabetes appears to be related to many other factors such as obesity, hepatitis C infection, alcohol-related disease indications for transplantation, family history of diabetes, older age, ethnicity (Hispanic and black), and the male sex (Anastácio et al. 2010).

12.4.3 Arterial Hypertension

It has been shown that up to 77% of post–liver transplant patients can be hypertensive (Anastácio et al. 2010); this is primarily due to immunosuppressive treatments and renal disease, especially in the early months after LTx. Other factors such as older age, sex, and a family history of hypertension have been associated with elevated blood pressure (Bianchi et al. 2008).

Both cyclosporine and tacrolimus lead to renal vasoconstriction and nephrotoxicity, but cyclosporine appears to be more hypertensive (Bianchi et al. 2008). However, it has been suggested that cyclosporine is more hypertensive than tacrolimus only in cases of higher doses of steroids, as it occurs in the first months of transplantation. Steroids are related to hypertension in post–liver transplant patients because they can induce vasoconstriction (Mells and Neuberger 2009).

12.4.4 Dyslipidemia

Dyslipidemia is herein described as the modifications in triglycerides and HDL levels, as they are components of the MetS. The onset of hypertriglyceridemia occurs early after LTx, and by 1 month to 1 year, nearly 70% of patients have developed high triglyceride levels (Anastácio et al. 2010). Predictive factors for hypertriglyceridemia are pre-LTx hepatocellular liver disease and post-LTx renal dysfunction. Greater weight gain has also been associated with hypertriglyceridemia (Canzanello et al. 1998). It has been observed that hypertriglyceridemia is higher in patients taking cyclosporine than in the ones taking tacrolimus. However, Dehghani et al. (2007) have shown that it is higher in those taking tacrolimus in comparison to the ones taking cyclosporine.

Abnormal HDL levels are described in the literature in nearly half of liver transplant recipients. The risk factors associated with the high number of patients with low levels of HDL have not yet been well established. All that is known, in the liver transplant population, is that low levels of HDL are unrelated to the type of calcineurin inhibitor used (Bianchi et al. 2008).

Mammalian Target of Rapamycin inhibitor (M-TOR) immunosuppressive therapy (i.e., sirolimus/everolimus) is strongly associated with hypercholesterolemia in renal transplanted patients (Kahan 2000), but sirolimus use did not affect triglycerides and HDL levels in liver transplant patients in comparison to other immunosuppressive treatments (Kniepeiss et al. 2004). In the study of Trotter et al. (2001), patients using sirolimus presented only with hypertriglyceridemia when this treatment was associated with cyclosporine.

12.5 CONCLUSION

Metabolic disorders and MetS are highly prevalent in liver transplant patients. Some of the risk factors are inherent to the overall treatment. However, others such as inadequate dietary intake and physical activity are highly reported and, most importantly, may be modifiable. Therefore, prevention rests upon the knowledge of these factors, which should carefully be addressed by an interdisciplinary team approach. The main goals should be to engage liver transplant patients in advising lifestyle modifications and to create new therapeutic strategies. On the other hand, those factors such as the use of immunosuppression after transplantation are unavoidable. Therefore, it is important to be aware of this in order to early identify patients at higher risk to developed MetS.

REFERENCES

Adam, R., Hoti, E. 2009. Liver transplantation: The current situation. *Semin Liver Dis* 29:3–18.

Adeseun, G.A, Rivera, M.E., Thota, S., Joffe, M., Rosas, S.E. 2008. Metabolic syndrome and coronary artery calcification in renal transplant recipients. *Transplantation* 86:728–732.

Alberti, K.G., Zimmet, P., Shaw, J. 2006. Metabolic syndrome—A new world-wide definition. A consensus statement from the international diabetes federation. *Diabet Med* 23:469–480.

Anastácio, L.R., Ribeiro, H.S., Ferreira, L.G. et al. 2013. Incidence and risk factors for diabetes, hypertension and obesity after liver transplantation. *Nutr Hosp* 28:643–648.

Anastácio, L.R., Ferreira, L.G., Liboredo, J.C. et al. 2012. Overweight, obesity and weight gain up to three years after liver transplantation. *Nutr Hosp* 27:1351–1356.

Anastácio, L.R., Ferreira, L.G., Ribeiro, H.S., Liboredo, C.J., Lima, A.S., Correia, M.I. 2011a. Metabolic syndrome after liver transplantation: Prevalence and predictive factors. *Nutrition* 27:1–7.

Anastácio, L.R., Ferreira, L.G., Ribeiro, H.S., Lima, A.S., Vilela, E.G., Correia, M.I. 2011b. Body composition and overweight of liver transplant recipients. *Transplantation* 92:947–951.

Anastácio, L.R., Lima, A.S., Correia, M.I. 2010. Metabolic syndrome and its components after liver transplantation: Incidence, prevalence, risk factors, and implications. *Clin Nutr* 29:175–179.

Angelico, F., Del Ben, M., Francioso, S. et al. 2003. Recurrence of insulin resistant metabolic syndrome following liver transplantation. *Eur J Gastroenterol Hepatol* 15:99–102.

Bellinghieri, G., Bernardi, A., Piva, M. et al. 2009. Metabolic syndrome after kidney transplantation. *J Ren Nutr* 19:105–110.

Bianchi, G., Marchesini, G., Marzocchi, R. et al. 2008. Metabolic syndrome in liver transplantation: Relation to etiology and immunosuppression. *Liver Transplant* 14:1648–1654.

Canzanello, V.J., Textor, S.C., Taler, S.J., et al. 1998. Late hypertension after liver transplantation: A comparison of cyclosporine and tacrolimus (FK506). *Liver Transplantation a Surgery* 4:328–334.

Canzanello, V.J., Schwartz, L., Taler, S.J. et al. 1997. Evolution of cardiovascular risk after liver transplantation: A comparison of cyclosporine A and tacrolimus (FK506). *Liver Transplant Surg* 3:1–9.

Cordero, F.A., Gavira, J.J., Alegria-Barrero, E. et al. 2006. Prevalence of metabolic syndrome in heart transplant patients: Role of previous cardiopathy and years since the procedure—The TRACA study. *J Heart Lung Transplant* 25:1192–1198.

Courivaud, C., Kazory, A., Simula-Faivre, D., Chalopin, J.M., Ducloux, D. 2007. Metabolic syndrome and atherosclerotic events in renal transplant recipients. *Transplantation* 83:1577–1581.

de Vries, A.P., Bakker, S.J., van Son, W.J. et al. 2004. Metabolic syndrome is associated with impaired long-term renal allograft function; not all component criteria contribute equally. *Am J Transplant* 4:1675–1683.

Dehghani, S.M., Taghavi, S.A., Eshraghian, A. et al. 2007. Hyperlipidemia in Iranian liver transplant recipients: Prevalence and risk factors. *J Gastroenterol* 42:769–774.

Duffy, J.P., Kao, K., Ko, C.Y. et al. 2010. Long-term patient outcome and quality of life after liver transplantation: Analysis of 20-year survivors. *Ann Surg* 252:652–661.

Escartin, A., Castro, E., Dopazo, C., Bueno, J., Bilbao, I., Margarit, C. 2005. Analysis of discarded livers for transplantation. *Transplant Proc* 37:3859–3860.

Everhart, J.E., Lombardero, M., Lake, J.R., Wiesner, R.H., Zetterman, R.K., Hoofnagle, J.H. 1998. Weight change and obesity after liver transplantation: Incidence and risk factors. *Liver Transplant Surg* 4:285–296.

Ford, E.D., Giles, W.H., Dietz, W.H. 2002. Prevalence of the metabolic syndrome among US adults: Findings from the third National Health and nutrition Examination Survey. *Journal of the Medical Association* 287: 356–359.

Ferreira, L.G., Santos, L.F., Anastácio, L.R., Lima, A.S., Correia, M.I. 2013. Resting energy expenditure, body composition, and dietary intake: A longitudinal study before and after liver transplantation. *Transplantation* 96(6):579–585.

Grundy, S.M., Brewer Jr., H.B., Cleeman, J.I., Smith Jr., S.C., Lenfant, C. 2004. Definition of metabolic syndrome. Report of the National Heart, Lung, and Blood Institute/American Heart Association conference on scientific issues related to definition. *Circulation* 109:433–438.

Hanouneh, I.A., Feldstein, A.E., McCullough, A.J. et al. 2008. The significance of metabolic syndrome in the setting of recurrent hepatitis C after liver transplantation. *Liver Transplant* 14:1287–1293.

Hwang, S., Lee, S.G., Jang, S.J. et al. 2004. The effect of donor weight reduction on hepatic steatosis for living donor liver transplantation. *Liver Transplant* 10:721–725.

Kahan, B.D. 2000. Efficacy of sirolimus compared with azathioprine for reduction of acute renal allograft rejection: A randomized multicentre study. The Rapamune US Study Group. *Lancet* 356:194–202.

Kallwitz, E.R. 2012. Metabolic syndrome after liver transplantation: Preventable illness or common consequence? *World J Gastroenterol* 18:3627–3634.

Kip, K.E., Marroquin, O.C., Kelley, D.E. et al. 2004. Clinical importance of obesity versus the metabolic syndrome in cardiovascular risk in women: A report from the Women's Ischemia Syndrome Evaluation (WISE) study. *Circulation* 109:706–713.

Kniepeiss, D., Iberer, F., Schaffellner, S., Jakoby, E., Duller, D., Tscheliessnigg, K. 2004. Dyslipidemia during sirolimus therapy in patients after liver transplantation. *Clin Transplant* 18:642–646.

Koutsovasilis, A., Protopsaltis, J., Triposkiadis, F. et al. 2009. Comparative performance of three metabolic syndrome definitions in the prediction of acute coronary syndrome. *Intern Med* 48:179–187.

Krasnoff, J.B., Vintro, A.Q., Ascher, N.L. et al. 2006. A randomized trial of exercise and dietary counseling after liver transplantation. *Am J Transplant* 6:1896–1905.

Laish, I., Braun, M., Mor, E., Sulkes, J., Harif, Y., Ben Ari, Z. 2011. Metabolic syndrome in liver transplant recipients: Prevalence, risk factors, and association with cardiovascular events. *Liver Transplant* 17:15–22.

Laryea, M., Watt, K.D., Molinari, M. et al. 2007. Metabolic syndrome in liver transplant recipients: Prevalence and association with major vascular events. *Liver Transplant* 13:1109–1114.

Leonard, J., Heimbach, J.K., Malinchoc, M., Watt, K., Charlton, M. 2008. The impact of obesity on long-term outcomes in liver transplant recipients-results of the NIDDK liver transplant database. *Am J Transplant* 8:667–672.

Lim, L.G., Cheng, C.L., Wee, A. et al. 2007. Prevalence and clinical associations of posttransplant fatty liver disease. *Liver Int* 27:76–80.

Lunati, M.E., Grancini, V., Agnelli, F. et al. 2013. Metabolic syndrome after liver transplantation: Short-term prevalence and pre- and post-operative risk factors. *Dig Liver Dis* 45(10):833–839. doi:pii: S1590–8658(13)00109-6. 10.1016/j.dld.2013.03.009.

Malik, S.M., deVera, M.E., Fontes, P., Shaikh, O., Ahmad, J. 2009. Outcome after liver transplantation for NASH cirrhosis. *Am J Transplant* 9:782–793.

Marchesini, G., Bugianesi, E., Forlani, G. et al. 2003. Nonalcoholic fatty liver, steatohepatitis, and the metabolic syndrome. *Hepatology* 37:917–923.

Mells, G., Neuberger, J. 2009. Long-term care of the liver allograft recipient. *Semin Liver Dis* 29:102–120.

Nakamuta, M., Morizono, S., Soejima, Y. et al. 2005. Short-term intensive treatment for donors with hepatic steatosis in living donor liver transplantation. *Transplantation* 80:608–612.

Painter, P., Krasnoff, J., Paul, S.M., Ascher, N.L. 2001. Physical activity and health-related quality of life in liver transplant recipients. *Liver Transplant* 7:213–219.

Pelletier, S.J., Schaubel, D.E., Wei, G. et al. 2007. Effect of body mass index on the survival benefit of liver transplantation. *Liver Transplant* 13:1678–1683.

Perkins, J.D. 2006. Saying "Yes" to obese living liver donors. Short-term intensive treatment for donors with hepatic steatosis in living-donor liver transplantation. *Liver Transplant* 12:1012–1013.

Plank, L.D., Metzger, D.J., McCall, J.L. et al. 2001. Sequential changes in the metabolic response to orthotopic liver transplantation during the first year after surgery. *Ann Surg* 234:245–255.

Rabkin, J.M., Corless, C.L., Rosen, H.R., Olyaei, A.J. 2002. Immunosuppression impact on long-term cardiovascular complications after liver transplantation. *Am J Surg* 183:595–599.

Richards, J., Gunson, B., Johnson, J., Neuberger, J. 2005. Weight gain and obesity after liver transplantation. *Transplant Int* 18:461–466.

Richardson, R.A., Garden, O.J., Davidson, H.I. 2001. Reduction in energy expenditure after liver transplantation. *Nutrition* 17:585–589.

Rinella, M.E., Alonso, E., Rao, S. et al. 2001. Body mass index as a predictor of hepatic steatosis in living liver donors. *Liver Transplant* 7:409–414

Sobal, J., Rauschenbach, B., Frongillo, E.A. 2003. Marital status changes and body weight changes: A US longitudinal analysis. *Soc Sci Med* 56:1543–1555.

Seo, S., Maganti, K., Khehra, M. et al. 2007. De novo nonalcoholic fatty liver disease after liver transplantation. *Liver Transplant* 13:844–847.

Stegall, M.D., Everson, G., Schroter, G. et al. 1995. Metabolic complications after liver transplantation: Diabetes, hypercholesterolemia, hypertension, and obesity. *Transplantation* 60: 1057–1060.

Sprinzl, M.F., Weinmann, A., Lohse, N. et al. 2013. Metabolic syndrome and its association with fatty liver disease after orthotopic liver transplantation. *Transplant Int* 26:67–74.

Trotter, J.F., Wachs, M.E., Trouillot, T.E. et al. 2001. Dyslipidemia during sirolimus therapy in liver transplant recipients occurs with concomitant cyclosporine but not tacrolimus. *Liver Transplant* 7:401–408.

van Hooff, J.P., Christiaans, M.H., van Duijnhoven, E.M. 2007. Glucose metabolic disorder after transplantation. *Am J Transplant* 7:1435–1436.

Varma, V., Mehta, N., Kumaran, V., Nundy, S. 2011. Indications and contraindications for liver transplantation. *Int J Hepat* 2011:Article ID 121862, doi:10.4061/2011/121862.

Section V

Effects of Dietary Components in Metabolic Syndrome

13 Olive Oil in Metabolic Syndrome

Javier Sanchez Perona

CONTENTS

13.1 INTRODUCTION

After decades of epidemiological, clinical, and experimental research, consumption of specific dietary patterns has a profound influence on health outcomes. The Mediterranean diet is considered one of the most health-promoting dietary patterns and it has been associated with numerous health benefits. The consequence of the consumption of the Mediterranean diet for centuries is the observed increased longevity and the lower incidence of chronic diseases, including cardiovascular disease, cancer, and neurodegenerative conditions in the countries surrounding the Mediterranean sea (Huang and Sumpio 2008, Lairon 2007, Pérez-Jiminez et al. 2007). The ingredients of the dietary pattern vary somewhat between different cultures of the Mediterranean countries, but they all have olive oil as a common factor, with approximately 90% of world production of olive oil originating in this geographical area (Huang and Sumpio 2008). Since the Seven Countries Study (Keys et al. 1986), the numerous investigations of the contribution of olive oil to the effects on health of the Mediterranean diet have demonstrated that it has a beneficial influence on a wide range of processes and risk factors (Huang and Sumpio 2008, Lairon 2007, Serra-Majem et al. 2004), and thus it is recognized as a key element in this respect. Today, there is a firm and reliable experimental base supporting the beneficial effects of olive oil. In fact, a recent study has demonstrated that long-term consumption of a Mediterranean diet rich in olive oil or nuts can protect against the incidence of major cardiovascular events, like myocardial infarction, stroke, or death from cardiovascular causes, in a population with a high cardiovascular risk (Estruch et al. 2013).

Olive oil, which contains mostly monounsaturated fatty acids (MUFA) in the form of oleic acid (18:1, n-9), provides about 85% of the fat content of the Mediterranean diet (Huang and Sumpio 2008, Pérez-Jimnez et al. 2007). Despite olive oil being firstly considered as neutral in the prevention of cardiovascular disease, due to its high MUFA content, today it is well known that replacing saturated fatty acids (SFA) in the diet by MUFA reduces the risk of coronary heart disease (CHD). Additionally, many other health benefits of MUFA consumption have recently been discovered (Covas 2007, Covas et al. 2009). Apart from olive oil, there are a number of other oleic acid-rich dietary oils obtained from seeds, some of which have been developed by modern biotechnology (Pérez-Jimenez et al. 2007), which can provide an alternative source of dietary MUFA with some of the benefits of olive oil consumption. However, an increasing number of studies point out that the content of oleic acid alone cannot fully explain the impact of olive oil on health. This conclusion has been drawn from studies comparing the effects of diets enriched with olive oil and other MUFA-rich oils, such as high-oleic sunflower oil (HOSO) (Mangas-Cruz et al. 2001, Perona et al. 2004a, 2008, Perona and Ruiz-Gutierrez 2005). Unlike olive oil, HOSO failed to reduce blood pressure in hypertensive patients (Ruiz-Gutierrez et al. 1996) or to protect low-density lipoproteins (LDL) from oxidation (Nicolaiew et al. 1998) in intervention studies in humans comparing these oils. These data supported the idea that the protective effects of olive oil against CHD should not be attributed exclusively to oleic acid, but to some other components of oil. In fact, virgin olive oil can be considered a fruit juice, as it is obtained only by mechanical means, that is, by pressing the fruit. This procedure helps to retain a wide range of potentially beneficial micronutrients, including vitamins, carotenoids, sterols, and phenolic compounds, which are lost during the compulsory refining of seed oils. These minor components, together with the high content of MUFA, make olive oil the quintessential functional food.

The effect of the Mediterranean diet on different components of the metabolic syndrome (MetS) has been studied in detail. Improvements in endothelial function and a reduction in markers of systemic vascular inflammation and coagulation have been reported for a number of years (Chrysohoou et al. 2004, Esposito et al. 2004). Quite surprisingly, olive oil, as a single component, has been studied in less detail. Its role in being a major constituent of the Mediterranean diet has led many authors to conclude that the beneficial effects observed are attributable to this MUFA-rich source. To ascertain the effects of a MUFA-rich fat meal or diet on glycemic control, lipoprotein metabolism, or endothelial dysfunction, olive oil has been used to increase the MUFA content and its percentage contribution to energy. However, the role of the minor components of the oil should not be discarded. The biological activity of olive oil minor components include antiatherogenic, hypotensive, antioxidant, antithrombotic, and even anti-inflammatory activities, which in different concentrations confer its protective effect against cardiovascular disease and the components of MetS.

13.2   OLIVE OIL AND THE MEDITERRANEAN DIET

The Mediterranean area is a broad geographical region, bordering the Mediterranean Sea that has been the settlement of some of the oldest civilizations and cultures of the world: Greeks, Romans, Arabians, etc. These civilizations combined the available foods of the region to create a dietary pattern that has lasted for centuries. However, the Mediterranean culinary culture, regarded as the Mediterranean diet, is not really a diet as it is understood in Western countries, but it is rather a dietary pattern. In addition to social, political, and economic differences among the Mediterranean countries, the concept of the Mediterranean diet is based on dietary habits and a lifestyle, more similar to those of the 1960s in that region than to the ones present today. It typically emphasizes the consumption of fresh fruits and vegetables, cooked vegetables and legumes, grains, and, in moderation, wine, nuts, fish, and dairy products, with large amounts of olive oil and small amounts of meat (Figure 13.1). Trichopoulou and Lagiou (1997) describe the commonality of the various diets of the Mediterranean region, the fact being that olive oil occupies a central position in all of them. Olive oil is used liberally in food preparation, cooking, and serving and therefore is used in significant quantities in the gastronomy of the Mediterranean countries. It is noteworthy that in the Italian and Spanish traditional diets, the daily dietary intake of olive

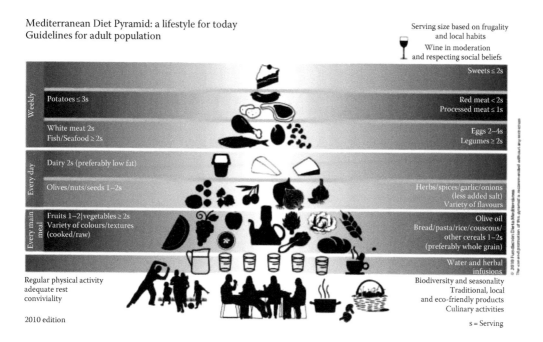

FIGURE 13.1 Representation of the Mediterranean diet pyramid proposed by the Dieta Mediterranea Foundation.

oil is approximately 15–20 g, but in the diet of the inhabitants of the isle of Crete, it can be much higher, reaching 70 g (Zampelas et al. 2004).

In the 1950s, the World Health Organization sponsored the Seven Countries Study to study the possible relationships between the dietary habits of people from different parts of the world and cardiovascular disease. The study lasted for 30 years and involved approximately 13,000 subjects. It was reported that populations throughout the Mediterranean region had a lower risk of suffering from CHD (Keys et al. 1966, 1986), but the main outcome was that people from the cohort of Crete had lower death rates from stroke and heart attack, despite their moderate to high intake of fat (Keys et al. 1966). This impressive finding was attributed to their diet and lifestyle and the term "Mediterranean diet" was born.

Despite the bioactive substances present in virgin olive oil, benefits cannot be expected from just adding quantities of olive oil to an unhealthy diet. A high intake of fresh fruit and vegetables, and particularly tomatoes, are also important components of the Mediterranean diet and have been shown to protect against both heart disease and cancer, which has been attributed to the antioxidant content of these foods. Other relevant components of the Mediterranean pattern are fish and nuts. Oily fish are a source of very long chain n-3 polyunsaturated fatty acids (PUFA), which appear to be beneficial against cardiovascular disease because of the anti-inflammatory and vasodilatory properties of their metabolites, as well as their capacity to reduce plasma triglyceride concentrations. Nuts are rich in MUFA and PUFA and have been reported to reduce cardiovascular risk, ameliorate lipid profile and triglyceride levels, and decrease inflammatory adhesion molecules in patients with hypercholesterolemia (Hu and Willett 2002, Kris-Etherton 1999). Walnuts are particularly rich in 18:3, n-3 (α-linolenic acid), which is a precursor of very long chain PUFA.

Although the Mediterranean diet is still the model for southern Mediterranean populations, many individuals are switching to more "westernized" diets and there is a great concern that the Mediterranean diet is being lost in countries where it was originated. In contrast, countries with no olive tree plantations and no olive oil production are now increasing their olive oil consumption and in some cases are even acquiring Mediterranean-style diets and lifestyles. The published evidence indicates that there are heterogeneous degrees of adherence to the diet. The combination of healthy weight, varied natural and fresh products, physical activities, a relaxed, well-ordered life, and a small dose of sunlight may reduce cardiovascular events, MetS, insulin resistance, diabetes, cancer, and other chronic diseases.

13.3 OLIVE OIL COMPONENTS

13.3.1 MAJOR COMPONENTS

According to the European Union Regulation No 1019/2002, virgin olive oils are those obtained from the fruit of the olive tree by mechanical processes or other physical processes, in conditions, especially thermal ones, that do not cause alterations in the oil, which must not receive any treatment other than washing, decantation, centrifugation, and filtering. This category does not include oils that have been obtained using solvents or by a re-esterification process or any other mixture with oils of different characteristics. The oil obtained in this way will be a natural, fresh, and aromatic juice with different flavors depending on the climatological circumstances of each year, the ground of origin, the variety, and the treatments and technical cares applied. Virgin olive oils are commonly classified according to their organoleptic properties.

Therefore, virgin olive oil is produced by direct pressing or centrifugation of the olive and is considered "extra" when the free acidity, expressed as oleic acid, is lower than 1 g/100 g and organoleptic characteristics (flavor and color) are excellent as assessed by a certified tasting panel. Oils below that standard are named "lampante" and need to be submitted to refination and blended with virgin olive oil before being commercialized. The refination process does not affect greatly the fatty acid composition of the oils but causes important losses of bioactive minor components.

Olive oil components can be divided into two fractions according to their ability to form soaps when it is treated with a strong base. The saponifiable fraction constitutes 98%–99% of the oil and is composed mainly of triglycerides, whereas the unsaponifiable fraction accounts for most of the minor components with important biological activities, except for polyphenols.

Oleic acid is the main component of olive oil, accounting for 55%–83% of total fatty acids, but this concentration depends on the maturation stage, the variety of olive tree, and the growing conditions (Boskou 2000). The content of palmitic (16:0) and linoleic (18.2, n-6) acid ranges from 7.5% to 20% and from 3.5% to 21%, respectively. These fatty acids are present in the oil, esterified in groups of three to a glycerol molecule to form triglycerides. According to the theoretical combination of all fatty acids present in olive oil, it would be possible to find more than 70 molecular species of triglycerides, but in fact only a few are found. The most abundant one is triolein (trioleoyl-glycerol), accounting for about 40%–60% of total triglycerides, followed by dioleoyl-palmitoyl-glycerol (12%–20%) and palmitoyl-oleoyl-linoleoyl-glycerol (5.5%–7.0%). Usually, unsaturated fatty acids, like oleic and linoleic acids, are preferentially found at the central position (sn-2) of the triglyceride molecule. These features are extremely important for all the processes related to the digestion, absorption, transport, and accumulation of olive oil triglycerides, since lipases, the enzymes in charge of hydrolyzing triglycerides, have a preference for the fatty acids in the outer positions (sn-1 and sn-3) of the molecule.

13.3.2 MINOR COMPONENTS

Considering that, as stated before, the beneficial effects of olive oil on cardiovascular disease have traditionally been attributed to its high levels of MUFA, the Federal Drug Administration of the United States permitted a claim on olive oil labels concerning its benefits on health on the basis of its oleic acid content (US FDA Press Release). However, olive oil is not merely a MUFA fat, but it contains other minor components with important biological properties (Covas et al. 2006a,b). The components of the unsaponifiable fraction of virgin olive oil classified in growing order of polarity are hydrocarbons, tocopherols, fatty alcohols, triterpenic alcohols, 4-methylesterols, sterols, triterpenic dialcohols, and polar-colored pigments (chlorophylls and pheophytins). Apart from these hydrophobic substances, probably the most investigated minor components of olive oil are hydrophilic phenolics, among which tyrosol and hydroxytyrosol are the ones that have shown the greatest biological activity. The structure of the most relevant of these minor compounds is depicted in Figure 13.2.

The bioactive compounds contained in the unsaponifiable fraction of virgin olive oil are present usually in the range of mg/kg (ppm) and one of the most abundant is squalene (Guinda et al. 1996), a polyunsaturated triterpene constituted by the condensation of six isoprene units. Its concentration varies from 1200 to 7500 mg/kg of oil, and once it is absorbed it can participate as a precursor

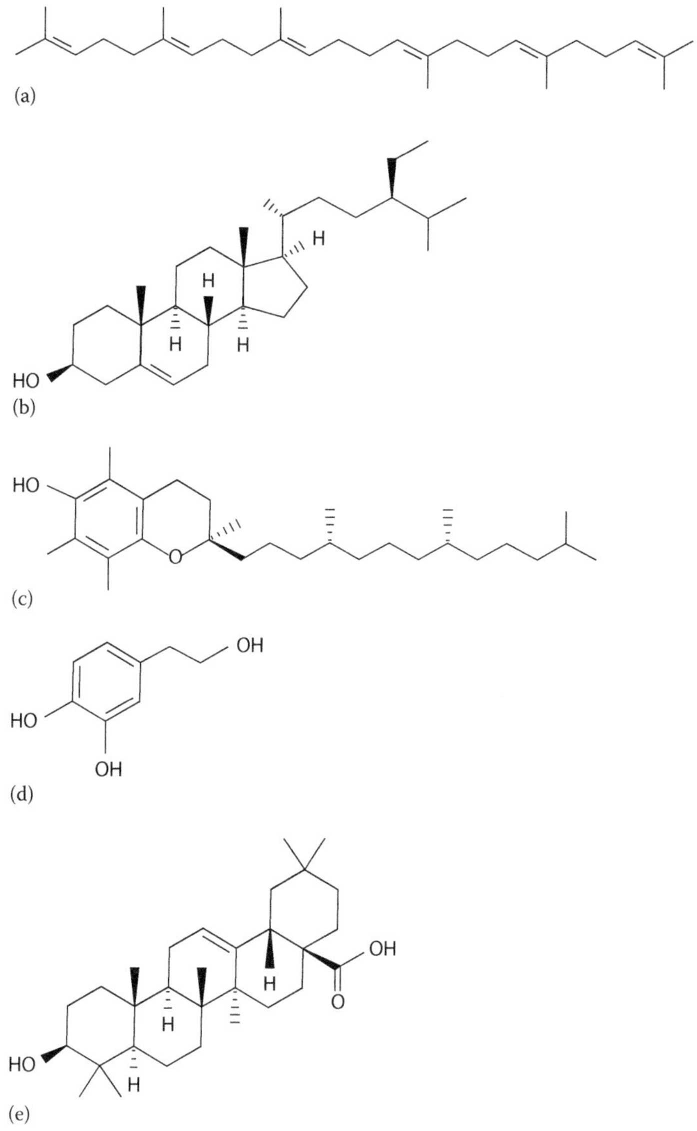

FIGURE 13.2 Chemical structures of some of the most relevant minor components present in olive oil according to their concentration or biological activity. A, squalene; B, beta-sitosterol; C, α-tocopherol; D, hydroxytyrosol; E, oleanolic acid.

in the biosynthesis pathway of cholesterol and steroid hormones. Although it has been suggested that as precursor of cholesterol, dietary squalene could increase plasma cholesterol concentrations, this has not been confirmed (Guillén et al. 2008). Actually, squalene does not consistently behave as a good marker of cholesterol synthesis, probably because the flow of squalene to the cholesterol route is only partial (Tsuchiya et al. 2010). Other olive oil components in this fraction include carotenes such as β-carotene and lycopene, which are found at amounts lower than 1 mg/kg (Su et al. 2002). β-Carotene plays an important role as precursor of vitamin A and lycopene is a potent antioxidant. Both compounds contribute to the yellowish color of the oil, although lycopene is found only in traces. α-Tocopherol, with vitamin E activity, is the most abundant tocopherol in olive oil, although it is found in lower concentrations compared to other seed oils (Herrera and Barbas 2001). Chlorophylls a and b and their oxidation products, pheophytins a and b, are naturally present in olive oil and are responsible for the greenish color. In virgin olive oil from mature olives, chlorophyll levels vary from about 1 to 10 mg/kg, while those of pheophytins are in the range of 0.2–24 mg/kg (Psomiadou and Tsimidou 2001). Phytosterols comprise a major proportion among the unsaponifiable components in all vegetable oils, including virgin olive oil. Therefore, the analysis of the sterol fraction is of importance, not only because it helps the characterization of the varieties from which the oil has been extracted, but also because it aids the identification of adulterations, particularly with other MUFA-rich oils, such as hazelnut oil (Zamora et al. 1994). The phytosterol content varies from one olive oil to another, but it is always below 2600 mg/kg. The main sterol found in virgin olive oil is β-sitosterol (about 95%), but there are other species present, like Δ5-avenasterol, campesterol, Δ7-stigmastenol, stigmasterol, and campestanol. The β-sitosterol content in virgin olive oil ranges from 683 to 2600 mg/kg (Benítez-Sánchez et al. 2003). The terpenic alcohol erythrodiol, which in some cases is accompanied by another triterpenic-tetracyclic, uvaol, is found in the skin of the olive fruit in amounts fluctuating between 100 and 120 mg/kg, but in virgin olive oils the concentration is usually as low as 6–10 mg/kg. Maslinic and oleanolic acids are also pentacyclic triterpenes present in the skin of olive fruits with higher concentrations in pomace olive oil than in virgin olive oil, in which they can be found only in traces. In olive fruits, these terpenic acids are present at concentrations around 681 and 420 mg/kg, respectively (Pérez-Camino and Cert 1999).

Phenolic compounds are soluble in water and constitute the "polar fraction" in virgin olive oil, which explains their absence from both unsaponifiable and glyceridic fractions. In addition to prevent oxidation and to confer virgin olive oil with exceptional thermal stability (Gutfinger 1981, Tsimidou et al. 1992), these substances contribute to the characteristic flavor and taste of the oil. The most abundant phenolic compounds in virgin olive oil are oleuropein- and ligstroside-aglycones and their derivatives, which are formed during the ripening of olive fruits by the enzymatic removal of glucose from their respective oleuropein and ligstroside glycosides. Further degradation of the aglycones generates the simple phenolic compounds hydroxytyrosol and tyrosol, respectively (Owen et al. 2000). Tyrosol, hydroxytyrosol, and their secoiridoid derivatives make up around 90% of the total phenolic content of a virgin olive oil.

13.4 DIETARY FAT, INSULIN RESISTANCE, AND DIABETES

The quality of dietary fat seems to be determinant in the effect of diet on insulin sensitivity. Diets high in SFA consistently impair both insulin sensitivity and blood lipids, while substituting carbohydrates or MUFA for SFA revert these abnormalities in both healthy (Salas et al. 1999, Vessby et al. 2001) and diabetic cohorts (Parillo et al., 1992). Postprandial lipemia and glucose homeostasis are also improved after meals containing MUFA from olive oil compared to meals rich in SFA (Paniagua et al. 2007).

Back in 1988, a study in patients with type 2 diabetes mellitus demonstrated that a high-fat, MUFA-enriched diet (33% of total energy) resulted in lower insulin requirements and lower plasma glucose concentrations compared to a low-fat (25% total energy), high-carbohydrate diet (60% total energy) (Garg et al. 1988). Olive oil, as source of MUFA, has also been compared to PUFA-rich oils, like sunflower oil. In a cross-sectional study performed in the south of Spain, levels of insulin resistance were found to be lower in people who used olive oil than in those who used sunflower oil (Soriguer et al. 2004). The sectional Pizarra study showed that dietary MUFA from olive oil and PUFA contributed to the variability of β-cell function (Rojo-Martinez et al. 2006). Ryan et al. (2000) examined the relationship between changes in membrane fatty acid composition and glucose transport and found a reduction in insulin resistance when a linoleic acid–rich diet was changed to oleic acid–rich diet. This was attributed to a reduction in its fluidity when the membrane was enriched in oleic acid.

After a comprehensive review, Ros (2003) concluded that natural foods and olive oil as the main source of MUFA provided a similar degree of glycemic control than low-fat diets. Nevertheless, high-MUFA diets generally had more favorable effects on proatherogenic alterations associated with the diabetic status, such as dyslipidemia, postprandial lipemia, small LDL concentrations, lipoprotein oxidation, inflammation, thrombosis, and endothelial dysfunction. Of particular interest was the ability of an olive oil–rich Mediterranean diet to improve mild systemic inflammation in subjects with MetS in the study of Esposito et al. (2004) and in the Prevention with Mediterranean Diet (PREDIMED) study (Estruch et al. 2006).

13.5   OLIVE OIL AND THE COMPONENTS OF THE METABOLIC SYNDROME

Epidemiological studies suggest that Western-style dietary patterns promote MetS, while healthy diets rich in fruits, vegetables, grains, fish, and low-fat dairy products, the paradigm of the Mediterranean diet, have a protective role (Esmaillzadeh et al. 2007, Lutsey et al. 2008). Apart from a cross-sectional study by Alvarez-Leon et al. (2003), which did not find a relationship between the adherence to the Mediterranean dietary pattern and the prevalence of MetS, studies that have analyzed that this relationship supports a beneficial effect (Williams et al. 2000). In a cross-sectional substudy of the PREDIMED intervention trial, an inverse relationship between the score of adherence to the Mediterranean diet and the prevalence of MetS was observed in a cohort of 808 individuals with a high cardiovascular risk (Babio et al. 2009). In this study, logistic regression analysis confirmed that the Mediterranean diet supplemented with nuts or virgin olive oil was associated with MetS reversion among individuals who had the syndrome at baseline. Esposito et al. (2004) showed that at the end of a 2-year follow-up, only 44% patients on a Mediterranean diet had features of MetS compared to 87% patients in the control group. It was noteworthy that energy intake was reduced, especially in the Mediterranean diet intervention group, and substantial weight loss was achieved. However, a high-fat Mediterranean diet, as traditionally followed in Mediterranean countries, has only been tested within the PREDIMED study, which compared the effects of two high-fat Mediterranean diets, supplemented with virgin olive oil or mixed nuts, to a low-fat diet in volunteers at high risk for cardiovascular disease. After 1 year, the prevalence of MetS was reduced by 6.7%, 13.7%, and 2.0% in the groups receiving the Mediterranean diet supplemented with virgin olive oil, with nuts, and low-fat diet, respectively. However, incident MetS rates were not significantly different among groups (22.9%, 17.9%, and 23.4%, respectively) (Salas-Salvado et al. 2008). In a cohort of patients with MetS, subjects following a Mediterranean-style diet containing olive oil (n = 90) as compared to a control diet (n = 90) were found to have lower serum concentrations of C-reactive protein (CRP), interleukin-6 (IL-6), and other inflammatory cytokines after 2 years (Esposito et al. 2004). Three shorter-term studies (less than 3 months) involving patients with a high cardiovascular risk or hypercholesterolemic men also showed decreased blood levels of intracellular adhesion molecule-1 (ICAM-1), vascular cell adhesion molecule-1 (VCAM-1), P-selectin, IL-6, and CRP in subjects consuming a Mediterranean-style diet supplemented with virgin olive oil in comparison to a low-fat diet (Estruch et al. 2006, Fuentes et al. 2001, Mena et al. 2009). Therefore, there is sufficient evidence showing that the Mediterranean diet and olive oil, in particular, can have a beneficial effect against proatherogenic factors, but also against the components of MetS (Table 13.1).

TABLE 13.1

Beneficial Effects Related to the Metabolic Syndrome of Dietary Olive Oil Intake and Its Bioactive Components

Effect	Active Components	Reference
Lower cardiovascular mortality	MUFA phenolic compounds	Covas et al. (2009)
		Lairon (2007)
Improved blood lipid profile	MUFA phenolic compounds	Covas et al. (2009)
		Huang and Sumpio (2008)
		Cabello-Moruno et al. (2007)
		Kris-Etherton et al. (1999)
		Covas et al. (2006)
	β-sitosterol	Gylling et al. (2010)
Reduced blood pressure	MUFA phenolic compounds	Covas (2007)
		Bondia-Pons et al. (2007)
Improved insulin sensitivity	MUFA	Salas et al. (1999)
		Vessby et al. (2001)
		Parillo et al. (1992)
Glucose homeostasis	MUFA phenolic-compounds	Paniagua et al. (2007)
		Hamden et al. (2009)
		Jemai et al. (2009)
	α-tocopherol	Shen et al. (2009)

MUFA, monounsaturated fatty acids; α-tocopherol, alpha-tocopherol; β-sitosterol, beta-sitosterol.

13.5.1 OLIVE OIL AND OBESITY

Body mass index (BMI) and waist circumference, which are both used as indicators of the presence of overweight and obesity, correlate positively with insulin resistance and MetS (Clausen et al. 1996, Parker et al. 1993). Actually, waist circumference has been singled out as the most important risk factor in the new International Diabetes Federation definition of MetS. The prevalence of obesity is one of the greatest public health problems in the world, even in developing countries, and it has increased alarmingly in most European countries, especially those around the Mediterranean Sea (Papandreou et al. 2008). These countries have undergone important changes in lifestyle, eating habits, and physical activity in the last years, with increasing dietary consumption of energy, animal proteins, and fatty, affordable food. Obesity increases the risk of diabetes, hypertension, coronary disease, and nonalcoholic hepatic steatosis, either independently or within the context of MetS (Friedman 2004, Kopelman 2000), central adiposity, specifically visceral obesity, being one of the key factors in the pathophysiology of insulin resistance and all the other components of MetS.

Traditionally, nutritional advice for treating obesity has emphasized reducing energy intake by diminishing all kinds of dietary fat, which are replaced with carbohydrates. However, recent studies are pointing out that in Mediterranean countries, restricted energy diets that were relatively high in fat from olive oil may be more effective than the traditional low-fat diet for weight loss in obese persons (Schroder et al. 2004). The Mediterranean patterns show better palatability and compliance, which helps to maintain the weight loss (Shai et al. 2008). Olive oil consumption was associated with nonsignificant lower likelihood of weight gain in a large Mediterranean cohort of 7368 individuals, who were followed for a median period of 28.5 months (Bes-Rastrollo et al. 2006), which is in striking contrast to the consistent association between unhealthy dietary patterns and a higher risk of weight gain and obesity (Bes-Rastrollo et al. 2006, Pereira et al. 2005). Results from the Spanish cohort of the European Prospective Investigation into Cancer and Nutrition (EPIC) study, in 2782 normal-weight individuals, suggested that the adherence to the Mediterranean diet is not associated with the incidence of overweight. Therefore, the investigators suggested that promoting eating habits consistent with the traditional Mediterranean patterns may be useful to combat obesity (Mendez et al. 2006). Similarly, the pilot study of the PREDIMED trial reported a weight loss in a group of 772 subjects with a high cardiovascular risk that received recommendations for a Mediterranean-style diet rich in olive oil, after a 3-month intervention (Estruch et al. 2006). The observed effect was attributed to a satiating effect of olive oil intake. In this regard, recent experimental evidence suggests that mobilization of intestinally derived oleoylethanolamide, a lipid messenger of satiety, is enabled by the uptake of dietary oleic acid (Schwartz et al. 2008).

13.5.2 Olive Oil and Plasma Triglycerides

The last scientific statement from the American Heart Association on triglycerides and cardiovascular disease emphasizes the pivotal role of triglycerides in lipid metabolism and reaffirms that triglyceride is not directly atherogenic but represents an important biomarker of cardiovascular risk because of its association with atherogenic remnant particles and apolipoprotein CIII (Miller et al. 2011). The statement also indicates that knowledge of the metabolic pathways of triglyceride-rich particles and the consequences of hypertriglyceridemia are crucial in understanding the characteristic lipid alterations in diabetes mellitus.

Hypertriglyceridemia that results from either increased production or decreased catabolism of triglyceride-rich lipoproteins (TRL) directly influences LDL and high-density lipoprotein (HDL) composition and metabolism, which gives triglycerides a central role in the pathogenesis of atherosclerosis. A number of studies have demonstrated that TRL can be proatherogenic in different experimental models, like macrophages and endothelial cells, but their remnant particles, a by-product of their partial hydrolysis by lipoprotein lipase (LPL), are ascribed as the most atherogenic of all TRL. These remnants can be isolated from the postprandial plasma of hypertriglyceridemic subjects and they are of intestinal (chylomicron remnants) or liver (very-low-density lipoproteins [VLDL] remnants) origin. Although in the postprandial period, both chylomicrons and VLDL compete for a common lipolytic pathway (Björkegren et al. 1996), this competence is unbalanced, since LPL shows a preference for large chylomicrons, an accumulation of VLDL particles occurs (Björkegren et al. 1996, Cohn et al. 1988, Schneeman et al. 1993).

The size and fatty acid composition of the TRL particles are determinant in the preference of LPL for VLDL or chylomicrons and in the hydrolysis rate of the triglycerides. Chylomicrons enriched in n-6 PUFA are processed by LPL at a faster rate than chylomicrons enriched in SFA, MUFA, or n-3 PUFA, which may contribute to their increased rate of removal from circulation in the postprandial state (Botham et al. 1997). However, Sato et al. (1999) prepared TRL enriched in palmitic, oleic, linoleic, or α-linolenic acids (18:3, n-3), obtained from rats fed palm, olive, safflower, and linseed oils, respectively. They found that the LPL specificity for TRL enriched in oleic acid was higher than that for linoleic acid and was correlated to a reduction in lipoprotein fluidity, suggesting that this effect might enhance the affinity of the particles for the enzyme.

The triglyceride composition of the dietary oils may be a strong determinant of the VLDL lipid composition and therefore may play a role in regulating lipoprotein metabolism (Perona et al. 2004b). In the PREDIMED study, serum triglyceride concentrations were significantly lowered after 3 months of consuming a Mediterranean diet rich in virgin olive oil or nuts but only virgin olive oil was able to reduce the cholesterol and triglyceride content in VLDL. The Mediterranean diet rich in olive oil also modified the triglyceride/apolipoprotein B ratio in VLDL, which was used to estimate particle size (Perona et al. 2010). The intake of olive oil meals leads to the formation of higher-size TRL particles, with a higher triglyceride concentration per particle, compared with fat sources rich in SFA and n-6 PUFA (Jackson et al. 2002, Pérez-Martinez et al. 2011). In vitro studies carried out using artificial chylomicron-like particles (CRLPs) derived from different dietary oils indicate that differences in the fatty acid and triglyceride composition of lipoproteins have differential effects on VLDL secretion by the liver. Secretion of triglycerides into the fraction containing VLDL was unaffected after incubation of hepatocytes with CRLPs obtained from olive oil, but was significantly increased in the cells exposed to palm or corn oil–derived CRLPs. In contrast, olive and corn CRLPs, compared to palm-derived CRLPs (López-Soldado et al. 2009), decreased apolipoprotein B messenger RNA levels.

Minor components of virgin olive oil can also modulate the triglyceride content of VLDL. Administration of olive oils with different phenolic content did not modify the concentrations of serum LDL-cholesterol and triglycerides, but they exerted changes in the cholesterol, and triglyceride composition of VLDL from healthy subjects. Consumption of the olive oil with the highest phenolic content led to increased concentrations of oleic and palmitic acids, as well as decreased content of linoleic acid, in these lipoproteins. In addition, a dose-dependent linear trend was found between the phenolic content in the olive oils and the palmitic and linoleic acid concentrations and their corresponding triglyceride molecular species in VLDL (Perona et al. 2011). Olive oil minor components can also have a role on the fate of plasma triglycerides. Rat hepatocytes incubated with human TRL originated after the intake of virgin olive oil with an increased concentration of bioactive minor components were found to increase the expression of the LDL-receptor gene, although no differences were found in the TRL uptake and VLDL secretion by the cells (Perona et al. 2006, 2008).

13.5.3 Olive Oil and Blood Pressure

Despite our considerable knowledge on diet and blood pressure, some unanswered questions remain. Most studies evaluating the association between diet and risk of hypertension have been conducted in the United States and northern Europe, regions with specific dietary patterns. For that reason, the role of foods less represented in these populations in the prevention of hypertension, such as olive oil, has not been adequately addressed. Only a few controlled experiments in small groups of individuals and a clinical trial have been conducted and suggest that consumption of olive oil could reduce the need for antihypertensive medications on hypertensives (Alonso et al. 2006, Ferrara et al. 2000).

Moreover, few cross-sectional studies carried out to date have related olive consumption and blood pressure. In the Greek cohort of the EPIC study, consumption of olive oil was associated with lower levels of both systolic and diastolic blood pressure (Psaltopoulou et al. 2004), and in the Seguimiento Universidad de Navarra (SUN) study a higher consumption of olive oil was associated with a lower risk of hypertension among men but not among women (Alonso et al. 2004). In this latter study, men in the highest category of olive oil intake presented a 50% lower risk of developing hypertension, as compared to those with the lowest intake. In addition, a significant inverse trend in the association between olive oil consumption and risk of hypertension in men was observed, which was independent of the consumption of fruits and vegetables. The lack of association in women was explained due to the lower number of hypertension cases included in the study (Figure 13.3).

Intervention studies have also reported blood pressure reductions in hypertensive subjects after consumption of virgin olive, regardless the presence of hypercholesterolemia (Perona et al. 2004c, Ruiz-Gutierrez et al. 1996). More recently, supplementation with olive oil rich in phenolic compounds was effective in reducing blood pressure levels in a group of individuals from non-Mediterranean countries (Bondia-Pons et al. 2007). In the PREDIMED trial, after a 3-month follow-up, mean systolic and diastolic blood pressure were significantly reduced in the group allocated to the Mediterranean-type diet supplemented with virgin olive oil (Estruch et al. 2006).

Although the mechanisms of the hypotensive effect of virgin olive oil are still uncertain, changes have been found in the fatty acid composition of the erythrocyte membrane of women with untreated essential hypertension after the intake of diets rich in virgin olive oil (Ruiz-Gutierrez et al. 1996). Virgin olive oil consumption induces significant changes of specific fatty acid moiety

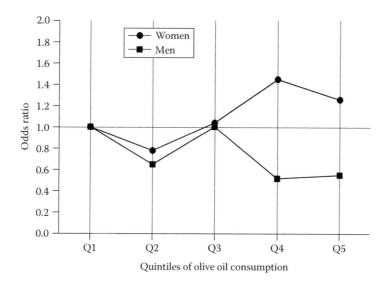

FIGURE 13.3 Odds ratio of hypertension according to olive oil consumption, distributed in quintiles in men and women. Results of the Seguimiento Universidad de Navarra (SUN) study from 1999–2004. Analysis adjusted for age, body mass index, energy intake, alcohol consumption, calcium intake, and physical activity during leisure time. Quintile 1 is comprised of individuals with the lowest olive oil intake, whereas quintile five represents the highest olive oil intake. (Adapted from Alonso, A. et al., *Br. J. Nutr.*, 92, 311, 2004.)

concentrations in plasma membrane phospholipids and cholesterol esters of hypertensive subjects, mainly due to a rise in the proportion of oleic acid. Membrane lipid composition is crucial in regulating membrane structure, influencing the localization and activity of several membrane-associated proteins and processes, such as the activities of the Na^+–Li^+ countertransport, the Na^+–K^+ cotransport, and the Na^+–K^+ ATPase (Muriana et al. 1996). Likewise, G-protein expression, involved in cell signal transduction and the regulation of blood pressure, is also modulated by changes in membrane lipids (Escriba et al. 2003). The reduction in membrane fluidity (high cholesterol/phospholipid ratio) has been associated with the development of hypertension (Tsuda et al. 2000) and with an age-related impaired β-adrenergic-mediated vasorelaxation and G-protein coupling (Martínez et al. 2005, Noble et al. 1999). Therefore, the effects of virgin olive oil, helping to normalize blood pressure in hypertensive patients, could be originated by the modulation of the interaction of G-proteins and other signal-related proteins, in addition or alternatively to membrane fluidity (Perona et al. 2007).

These normotensive effects have been attributed to minor components present in virgin olive oil, such as α-tocopherol, oleuropein, hydroxytyrosol, and tyrosol, all of them with antioxidant and free radical scavenging activities (Tuck and Hayball 2002). These substances could help to revert the imbalance between increased oxidative stress and impaired antioxidant defense that affects endothelial function (Visioli and Galli 1998) and modulate eicosanoid metabolism in endothelial cells (Jialal et al. 2001, Wu et al. 2001). The reduction of blood pressure by virgin olive oil has also been linked to improvements in the endothelial function. This is what was observed in a randomized trial with 180 participants diagnosed with MetS, after 2 years on a Mediterranean-style diet including virgin olive oil (Esposito et al. 2004). In these subjects, blood pressure and platelet aggregation response to L-arginine, the natural precursor of nitric oxide, were improved. The mechanism might also be triggered by other minor components like triterpenic acids and alcohols, which are present in low concentrations in virgin olive oil but in relevant content in pomace olive oil. In isolated thoracic rat aorta, oleanolic acid evoked an endothelium-dependent vasorelaxation, which was mainly mediated by the endothelial production of NO (Rodriguez-Rodriguez et al. 2004).

13.5.4 Olive Oil and HDL-Cholesterol

Apart for the classic function of HDL as shuttle for reverse cholesterol transport, this lipoprotein has an important role in inflammation and oxidative stress (Navab et al. 2009). HDL from healthy rabbits and humans can prevent LDL oxidation and LDL-induced monocyte chemotactic protein-1 (MCP-1) production in cultures of human artery wall cells (Van Lenten et al. 1995). However, in subjects with diabetes or insulin resistance, these features of HDL may be impaired and these lipoproteins can even have a pro-inflammatory role (Navab et al. 2009). Perségol et al. (2007) found that HDL taken from subjects with abdominal obesity and from those with type 1 and type 2 diabetes was defective in reversing the effects of oxidized LDL compared with HDL from normal subjects (Perségol et al. 2006, 2007). According to Roberts et al. (2006), HDL inflammatory properties were increased concomitantly to a fall in HDL-cholesterol levels in men with MetS who were treated with a 3-week residential program of diet and daily aerobic exercise.

Nevertheless, the role of HDL on reverse cholesterol transport is likely the most important mechanism by which HDL reduces cardiovascular risk. The primary structural protein of HDL, apolipoprotein A1, is synthesized and secreted predominantly by the liver and it is rapidly lipidated with phospholipids transported via ATP-binding cassette (ABC) transporter A1 (ABCA1). The nascent pre-β-HDL particle enters into circulation and is an efficient acceptor of cellular cholesterol from peripheral cells such as macrophages, initiating the reverse cholesterol transport pathway. Stimulation of macrophage cholesterol efflux in the form of HDL is one of the mechanisms proposed for the effect of olive oil intake on HDL-cholesterol. In mice, Rosenblat et al. (2008) showed a greater cholesterol efflux from peritoneal macrophages after olive oil consumption. The antiatherogenic affect can be accompanied by reduced macrophage uptake of oxidized LDL via scavenger receptors, which has also been observed in mice consuming virgin olive oil (Miles et al. 2001).

The Mediterranean diet can be helpful in maintaining the concentrations of cholesterol associated to HDL. In the PREDIMED study, participants with the highest adherence to the Mediterranean diet had 47% and 54% lower odds of having low HDL-cholesterol and hypertriglyceridemia, respectively, than those in the lowest quartile (Babio et al. 2009). It is well known that consumption of diets relatively high in MUFA have the advantage of lowering plasma LDL-cholesterol concentrations compared to PUFA without lowering HDL-cholesterol (Mattson and Grundy, 1985). The substitution of a high-SFA diet with a high-MUFA diet can help to lower total and LDL-cholesterol concentrations, while HDL-cholesterol concentrations are higher and triglycerides are lower on a high-MUFA as compared with a low-fat, high-carbohydrate diet (Kris-Etherton et al. 1999).

Therefore, the benefits of MUFA-rich dietary oil, like olive oil, are reflected in the reduction of total/HDL-cholesterol and LDL/HDL-cholesterol ratios, which are indicators of lipid atherogenesis, reflecting the balance of cholesterol transport in and out of the arterial intima (Kannel and Wilson 1992). In fact, in a recent report from the Framingham Offspring Study, total/HDL-cholesterol and LDL/HDL-cholesterol ratios were reported to be the most efficient lipid parameters for predicting CHD (Byung-Ho et al. 2006). The increasing effect of olive oil intake as part of the Mediterranean diet on HDL-cholesterol levels was also observed in the pilot study of the PREDIMED trial. In these subjects, HDL-cholesterol was increased by 2.4 mg/dL in only 3 months (Estruch et al. 2006). In a similar period of time, 4 months, a moderately hypoenergetic Mediterranean diet combined with an exercise program ameliorated body weight and the cardiovascular parameters of MetS in a group of obese women, including HDL-cholesterol concentrations (Andreoli et al. 2008). However, not all intervention studies have found increases in HDL-cholesterol concentrations. In a primary prevention study involving 59 healthy subjects, followed for 4 weeks, the Mediterranean diet decreased both LDL-cholesterol and HDL-cholesterol concentrations in plasma (Pérez-Jiménez et al. 2001). Mezzano et al. (2003) compared the effect of a Mediterranean-type diet and a high-fat diet in two groups of 21 healthy young males over 90 days, failing to find changes in total plasma cholesterol, HDL, and LDL in either study group at any time point. Nevertheless, in these latter studies, the number of participants was lower and the duration of the intervention was shorter.

The effect of olive oil on plasma HDL-cholesterol concentrations has been observed for MUFA-rich dietary oils, regardless of their minor components. Long-term consumption of virgin olive oil and HOSO, both with a high content in oleic acid, modified in a similar way the plasma lipid profile of healthy women, as well as that of normo or hypercholesterolemic hypertensive women (Ruiz-Gutierrez et al., 1996). Interestingly, both oils are capable of significantly increasing the plasma concentration of the cholesterol associated to HDL. However, virgin olive oil phenolic compounds may also increase HDL-cholesterol concentrations. Olive oil with a high phenolic content (366 mg/kg) increased HDL-cholesterol in addition to reducing triglyceride concentrations as compared with olive oil low in polyphenols (Covas et al. 2006a,b).

Virgin olive oil consumption can increase the capacity of serum and HDL to produce cholesterol esters from macrophages after incubation with HDL (whole HDL as wells as HDL2/HDL3 subclasses) isolated from the plasma of healthy volunteers. Three HDL-mediated CE pathways identified (ABCA1, ABCG1, and scavenger receptor class B type I [SR-BI]) were modulated by virgin olive oil consumption. The consequence was an increased release of excess cholesterol from human monocyte-derived macrophages by 44% (Helal et al. 2012).

It has been suggested that there is a connection between the glycemic index and HDL-cholesterol. The intake of carbohydrates with a low glycemic index has been associated with a smaller HDL-cholesterol reduction than the intake of carbohydrates with a higher index. Additionally, the intake of carbohydrates with a high glycemic index was inversely associated with HDL-cholesterol concentrations and positively associated with fasting triglycerides (Katan 1998).

13.5.5   Olive Oil and Glucose

Changes in lifestyle focused to weight loss are also beneficial for diabetes prevention in subjects with impaired glucose tolerance (Schulze et al. 2008, Saaristo et al. 2010). Diets with a low glycemic index, that is, those with a low glucose-raising effect, are associated with improvements of glycemic control and insulin sensitivity (Thomas and Elliott 2009). This is even more relevant in obese subjects, who must increase their insulin secretion in order to reestablish glucose homeostasis following a high-glycemic index meal (Sunehag et al. 2002, Solomon et al. 2009). However, diet can be helpful to restore insulin sensitivity. Animal and human studies have demonstrated that MUFA-rich diets can improve peripheral insulin sensitivity in both healthy (Salas et al. 1999, Vessby et al. 2001) and diabetic (Parillo et al. 1992) individuals.

High-MUFA diets generally have more favorable effects on glucose homeostasis and insulin secretion in nondiabetic subjects (Ros 2003). Administration of MUFA can increase plasma glucagon-like peptide-1 concentrations, which might contribute to increase insulin secretion (Beysen et al. 2002). In addition, β-cell function can be progressively improved in the postprandial state, as the proportion of MUFA with respect to SFA in fatty meals is increased (Lopez et al. 2008). Experimental animal and cell culture studies have shown that SFA are less readily oxidized and accumulate as lipotoxic products that synergize with elevated glucose, thereby impairing β-cell function and eventually causing β-cell death, while MUFA and PUFA appear to prevent these events by directing fat into oxidation or triglycerides rather than to deleterious lipid metabolites such as diglycerides and ceramide (Gaster et al. 2005, Lee et al. 2006).

In the pilot study of the PREDIMED trial, both Mediterranean-style diets, supplemented in virgin olive oil or nuts, reduced plasma glucose levels in all patients as well as improved insulin levels and the homeostasis model assessment (HOMA) index in nondiabetic patients, supporting the beneficial role of the Mediterranean diet on insulin resistance and particularly that of olive oil and nuts (Estruch et al. 2006). Pérez-Jimenez et al. (2001) investigated the effects of a Mediterranean-style diet, a SFA-rich diet, and a low-fat, high-carbohydrate diet in 59 young subjects for 28 days.

Compared to the SFA-rich diet, plasma glucose was significantly decreased and basal and insulin-stimulated 2-deoxiglucose uptake in peripheral monocytes were increased after the Mediterranean and high-carbohydrate diets, indicating an improvement in insulin sensitivity. Additionally, in a cross-sectional study of the general population in Spain, after an oral glucose tolerance test, a favorable association between MUFA intake and insulin secretion was observed, estimated from the HOMA index (Rojo-Martinez et al. 2006).

These results clearly show that diets rich in MUFA tend to improve insulin sensitivity, although not all studies showed a positive effect. The LIPGENE (Diet, genomics and the metabolic syndrome: an integrated nutrition, agro-food, social and economic analysis.) study showed no effect on insulin sensitivity, LDL-cholesterol, or inflammatory markers, after the administration of high-SFA, high-MUFA, and high-carbohydrate diets with or without n-3 PUFA supplementation in patients with MetS (Tierney et al. 2010). In the KANWU study, insulin sensitivity did not improve in healthy subjects when the MUFA content of the diet exceeded 37% of energy (Vessby et al. 2001), indicating potential interaction between fat quality and quantity. This is remarkable as another intervention study in patients with type 2 diabetes mellitus showed that a MUFA-enriched diet, with a 33% of total energy in the form of fat, resulted in lower insulin requirements and lower plasma glucose concentration compared to a low-fat (25% total energy) diet (Garg et al. 1998).

Due to these discrepancies and given that subsequent studies failed to report positive effects of dietary MUFA enrichment and carbohydrate modifications on fasting insulin in diabetics (Bonanome et al. 1991, Garg et al. 1998) or on insulin sensitivity in healthy subjects (Pérez-Jiménez et al. 2001), the American Diabetes Association recommended dividing 60%–70% of energy between carbohydrate and MUFA, depending on individual assessments and establishing desirable goals (American Diabetes Association 2007). These discrepancies may be due to differences and/or insufficient cohort size, diverse clinical characteristics of the cohorts (healthy, impaired fasting glycaemia, MetS, diabetes), the nature of the dietary fat modification (MUFA vs. PUFA; MUFA vs. SFA; MUFA vs. carbohydrate), study duration, measures of insulin sensitivity, and inappropriate study design (Tierney and Roche 2007).

The effect of olive oil minor components on glucose homeostasis and insulin sensitivity has not been extensively addressed. The sterol metabolism is impaired in insulin resistance. Sitosterol and other plant sterols have been found in lower concentrations in plasma of subjects with impaired fasting glucose compared with normoglycemic subjects (Gylling et al. 2010, Sutherland et al. 1992). However, when rats were supplemented with oral β-sitosterol, they showed increased fasting insulin level, decreased fasting glucose level, improved oral glucose tolerance, and increased insulin release from isolated rat pancreatic islet cells (Ivorra et al. 1990). In vitro, β-sitosterol induced glucose uptake and stimulated both adipogenesis and lipolysis in adipocytes. These observations were related to down regulation of GLUT4, Akt, and PI3K genes (Chai et al. 2011). Squalene has been found to correlate with visceral obesity but not with insulin sensitivity in the normoglycemic offspring of patients with type 2 diabetes (Peltola et al. 2006). However, in vitro studies have reported that squalene can enhance glucose-stimulated insulin secretion in β-cells (Tsuchiya et al. 2010). In agreement with these results, Xia et al. (2008) reported that in mouse β-cells, NB-598, an inhibitor of squalene epoxidase, was effective in decreasing insulin secretion by altering the lipid rafts in plasma membrane. Dietary supplementation with α-tocopherol decreased insulin and glucose levels in diet-induced obesity Sprague-Dawley rats (Shen et al. 2009). In dexamethasone-induced glucose intolerant rats, the area under the curve (AUC) of glucose, but not insulin, in an intraperitoneal glucose tolerance test was lowered after a diet supplemented in both vitamin E and C (Williams et al. 2012). In a group of Swedish volunteers, lower serum α-tocopherol concentrations were independently associated with impaired insulin sensitivity and α-tocopherol independently predicted type 2 diabetes during 7 years of follow-up. Maslinic and oleanolic acids, potent triterpenic compounds present in relevant concentrations in pomace olive oil, have been related with glucose homeostasis and insulin sensitivity. Both compounds have shown hypoglycemic effects by reducing insulin resistance in animal models of type 2 diabetes (de Melo et al. 2010, Liu et al. 2007, Somova et al. 2003). In addition, oleanolic acid may promote insulin signal transduction and inhibit oxidative stress-induced hepatic insulin resistance and gluconeogenesis (Wang et al. 2011). There is also some evidence indicating that virgin olive oil phenolics might have also some hypoglycemic effect. Hydroxytyrosol was efficient to prevent hyperglycemia in alloxan-induced diabetic rats. In these animals, glucose concentration in plasma was decreased by 55% compared to untreated diabetic rats. The reduction was concomitant to an enhancement in the oxidant status and the activity of enzymatic defenses (Hamden et al. 2009). Similar results were obtained in the same experimental model by administration of an oleuropein-rich extract (Jemai et al. 2009).

13.6 CONCLUSIONS

Mediterranean diet is being now considered among the scientific community as the most healthy dietary pattern because of the increasing evidence that it can be effective in preventing the onset and development of a number of diseases and pathophysiological processes, including cardiovascular disease, cancer, neurodegenerative disorders, diabetes, and MetS. For many years, scientists have accumulated data on the beneficial effects of the key ingredient of the Mediterranean diet, olive oil, on factors and parameters implicated in atherosclerosis and CHD. Nowadays, it is well known that olive oil consumption can prevent atherogenesis by reducing total and LDL-cholesterol levels, while maintaining HDL-cholesterol, protecting LDL from oxidation, reducing plasma triglycerides, and inducing a good inflammatory and thrombotic status. Some of these factors are also implicated in MetS and recent reports are pointing out to a role of olive oil also in glucose homeostasis, insulin sensitivity, and the other components of MetS. Despite being rich in fat, the Mediterranean diet has not been related with an increase in body weight in epidemiological and intervention studies.

However, the mechanisms and actual components of this dietary oil that are responsible for the observed effects are still uncertain. There is a roughly uniform consensus that the high presence of oleic acid in the oil has an important role, but comparative studies with other dietary oils are showing that there must be other factors influencing the effects of olive oil on health. Several studies are starting to associate minor components of olive oil with some of the observed effects. These components, despite being present in low concentrations in the oil, have potent biological activities as anti-inflammatory, antithrombotic, and antioxidant agents. Nevertheless, the actual cellular and molecular mechanisms by which these components, at the concentrations present in the oil, exert their protective activities are only envisaged. Therefore, there is need of studies at the cellular and molecular level to ascertain the processes involved in these mechanisms in different experimental models.

Additionally, a higher level of evidence is needed in order to confirm the results obtained so far and give recommendations of olive oil intake to the population. Very few randomized controlled trials focused on the role of olive oil and MetS have been carried out to date. The most comprehensive one is probably the PREDIMED study, which has recently published the results of the effects of consuming a Mediterranean diet rich in virgin olive oil or nuts on major cardiovascular events, among which a high number of them present features of MetS. The main outcomes of the PREDIMED study show that in 7447 individuals with a high cardiovascular risk followed for almost 5 years, the Mediterranean diet is helpful to prevent myocardial infarction, stroke, and death from cardiovascular causes. Still, more large-scale clinical trials are needed, as well as meta-analysis of those studies.

Despite all the data supporting the beneficial role of olive oil against cardiovascular disease and MetS, recommendations should be given in the direction of a whole healthy diet including this oil, as there is no sufficient evidence of a protective role of the oil isolated from a healthy dietary pattern, such as the Mediterranean diet.

REFERENCES

Alonso, A., de la Fuente, C., Martín-Arnau, A.M., de Irala, J., Martínez, J.A., Martínez-González, M.A. 2004. Fruit and vegetable consumption is inversely associated with blood pressure in a Mediterranean population with a high vegetable-fat intake: The Seguimiento Universidad de Navarra (SUN) Study. *Br J Nutr* 92:311–319.

Alonso, A., Ruiz-Gutiérrez, V., Martínez-González, M.A. 2006. Monounsaturated fatty acids, olive oil and blood pressure: Epidemiological, clinical and experimental studies. *Public Health Nutr* 9:251–257.

Alvarez-Leon, E.E., Ribas-Barba, L., Serra-Majem, L. 2003. Prevalence of the metabolic syndrome in the population of Canary Islands, Spain. *Med Clin (Barc)* 120:172–174.

Andreoli, A., Lauro, S., Di Daniele, N., Sorge, R., Celi, M., Volpe, S.L. 2008. Effect of a moderately hypoenergetic Mediterranean diet and exercise program on body cell mass and cardiovascular risk factors in obese women. *Eur J Clin Nutr* 62(7):892–897.

Babio, N., Bullo, M., Basora, J. et al. on behalf of the Nureta-PREDIMED investigators. 2009. Adherence to the Mediterranean diet and risk of metabolic syndrome and its components. *Nutr Metab Cardiovasc Dis* 19(8):563–570.

Bénitez-Sánchez, P.L., Camacho, L.M., Aparicio, R. 2003. A comprehensive study of hazelnut oil composition with comparisons to other vegetable oils, particularly olive oil. *Eur Food Res Technol* 218:13–19.

Bes-Rastrollo, M., Sanchez-Villegas, A., de la Fuente, C., de Irala, J., Martinez, J.A., Martinez-Gonzalez, M.A. 2006. Olive oil consumption and weight change: The SUN prospective cohort study. *Lipids* 41:249–256.

Beysen, C., Karpe, F., Fielding, B.A., Clark, A., Levy, J.C., Frayn, K.N. 2002. Interaction between specific fatty acids, GLP-1 and insulin secretion in humans. *Diabetologia* 45:1533–1541.

Bjorkegren, J., Packard, C.J., Hamsten, A. et al. 1996. Accumulation of large very low density lipoprotein in plasma during intravenous infusion of a chylomicron-like triglyceride emulsion reflects competition for a common lipolytic pathway. *J Lipid Res* 37(1):76–86.

Bonanome, A., Visona, A., Lusiani, L. et al. 1991. Carbohydrate and lipid metabolism in patients with non-insulin-dependent diabetes mellitus: Effects of a low-fat, high-carbohydrate diet vs a diet high in monounsaturated fatty acids. *Am J Clin Nutr* 54:586–590.

Bondia-Pons, I., Schröder, H., Covas, M.I. et al. 2007. Moderate consumption of olive oil by healthy European men reduces systolic blood pressure in non-Mediterranean participants. *J Nutr* 137(1):84–87.

Boskou, D. 2000. Olive oil. *World Rev Nutr Diet* 87:56–77.

Botham, K.M., Avella, M., Cantafora, A., Bravo, E. 1997. The lipolysis of chylomicrons derived from different dietary fats by lipoprotein lipase in vitro. *Biochim Biophys Acta* 1349(3):257–263.

Byung-Ho, N., Kannel, W., D'Agostino, R.B. 2006. Search for an optimal atherogenic lipid risk profile: From the Framingham study. *Am J Cardiol* 97:372–375.

Chai, J.W., Lim, S.L., Kanthimathi, M.S., Kuppusamy, U.R. 2011. Gene regulation in β-sitosterol-mediated stimulation of adipogenesis, glucose uptake, and lipid mobilization in rat primary adipocytes. *Genes Nutr* 6(2):181–188.

Chrysohoou, C., Panagiotakos, D.B., Pitsavos, C., Das, U.N., Stefanadis, C. 2004. Adherence to the Mediterranean diet attenuates inflammation and coagulation process in healthy adults: The ATTICA Study. *J Am Coll Cardiol* 44:152–158.

Clausen, J.O., Borch-Johnsen, K., Ibsen, H. et al. 1996. Insulin sensitivity index, acute insulin response, and glucose effectiveness in a population-based sample of 380 young healthy Caucasians. Analysis of the impact of gender, body fat, physical fitness, and life-style factors. *J Clin Invest* 98:1195–1209.

Cohn, J.S., McNamara, J.R., Schaefer, E.J. 1988. Lipoprotein cholesterol concentrations in the plasma of human subjects as measured in the fed and fasted states. *Clin Chem* 34(12):2456–2459.

Covas, M.I. 2007. Olive oil and the cardiovascular system. *Pharmacol Rev* 55:175–186.

Covas, M.I., Konstantinidou, V., Fitó, M. 2009. Olive oil and cardiovscular health. *J Cardiovasc Pharmacol* 54:477–482.

Covas, M.I., Nyyssonen, K., Poulsen, H.E. et al. 2006a. The effect of polyphenols in olive oil on heart disease risk factors: A randomized trial. *Ann Intern Med* 145:333–341.

Covas, M.I., Ruiz-Gutiérrez, V., de la Torre, R. et al. 2006b. Minor components of olive Oil: Evidence to date of health benefits in humans. *Nutr Rev* 64:20–30.

de Melo, C.L., Queiroz, M.G., Fonseca, S.G. et al. 2010. Oleanolic acid, a natural triterpenoid improves blood glucose tolerance in normal mice and ameliorates visceral obesity in mice fed a high-fat diet. *Chem Biol Interact* 185:59–65.

Escribá, P.V., Sánchez-Dominguez, J.M., Alemany, R., Perona, J.S., Ruiz-Gutiérrez, V. 2003. Alteration of lipids, G proteins, and PKC in cell membranes of elderly hypertensives. *Hypertension* 41(1):176–182.

Esmaillzadeh, A., Kimiagar, M., Mehrabi, Y., Azadbakht, L., Hu, F.B., Willett, W.C. 2007. Dietary patterns, insulin resistance, and prevalence of the metabolic syndrome in women. *Am J Clin Nutr* 85:910–918.

Esposito, K., Marfella, R., Ciotola, M. et al. 2004. Effect of a mediterranean-style diet on endothelial dysfunction and markers of vascular inflammation in the metabolic syndrome: A randomized trial. *JAMA* 292:1440–1446.

Estruch, R., Martínez-González, M.A., Corella, D. et al. 2006. Effects of a Mediterranean-style diet on cardiovascular risk factors: A randomized trial. *Ann Intern Med* 145:1–11.

Estruch, R., Ros, E., Salas-Salvadó, J. et al. PREDIMED Study Investigators. 2013. Primary prevention of cardiovascular disease with a Mediterranean diet. *N Engl J Med* 368(14):1279–1290.

European Union. Commission Regulation (EC) No 1019/2002 of 13 June 2002 on marketing standards for olive oil (OJ L 155, 14.6.2002, p. 27).

Ferrara, L.A., Raimondi, A.S., d'Episcopo, L., Guida, L., Dello Russo, A., Marotta, T. 2000. Olive oil and reduced need for antihypertensive medications. *Arch Intern Med* 160:837–842.

Friedman, J.M. 2004. Modern science versus the stigma of obesity. *Nat Med* 10:563–569.

Fuentes, F., López-Miranda, J., Sánchez, E. 2001. Mediterranean and low-fat diets improve endothelial function in hypercholesterolemic men. *Ann Intern Med* 134:1115–1119.

Garg, A., Bonanome, A., Grundy, S.M., Zhang, Z.J., Unger, R.H. 1988. Comparison of a high-carbohydrate diet with a high-monounsaturated-fat diet in patients with non-insulin-dependent diabetes mellitus. *N Engl J Med* 319:829–834.

Gaster, M., Rustan, A.C., Beck-Nielsen, H. 2005. Differential utilization of saturated palmitate and unsaturated oleate: Evidence from cultured myotubes. *Diabetes* 54:648–656.

Guillén, N., Acín, S., Navarro, M.A. et al. 2008. Squalene in a sex-dependent manner modulates atherosclerotic lesion which correlates with hepatic fat content in apoE-knockout male mice. *Atherosclerosis* 197(1):72–83.

Guinda, A., Lanzon, A., Albi, T. 1996. Differences in hydrocarbons of virgin olive oils obtained from several olive varieties. *J Agric Food Chem* 44:1723–1726.

Gutfinger, T. 1981. Plyphenols in olive oils. *J Am Oil Chem Soc* 58:966–968.

Gylling, H., Hallikainen, M., Pihlajamäki, J. et al. 2010. Insulin sensitivity regulates cholesterol metabolism to a greater extent than obesity: Lessons from the METSIM Study. *J Lipid Res* 51(8):2422–2427.

Hamden, K., Allouche, N., Damak, M., Elfeki, A. 2009. Hypoglycemic and antioxidant effects of phenolic extracts and purified hydroxytyrosol from olive mill waste in vitro and in rats. *Chem Biol Interact* 180(3):421–432.

Helal, O., Berrougui, H., Loued, S., Khalil, A. 2012. Extra-virgin olive oil consumption improves the capacity of HDL to mediate cholesterol efflux and increases ABCA1 and ABCG1 expression in human macrophages. *Br J Nutr* 10:1–12.

Herrera, E., Barbas, C. 2001. Vitamin E: Action, metabolism and perspectives. *J Physiol Biochem* 57:43–56.

Hu, F.B., Willett, W.C. 2002. Optimal diets for prevention of coronary heart disease. *JAMA* 288:2569–2578.

Huang, C.L., Sumpio, B.E. 2008. Olive oil, the Mediterranean diet, and cardiovascular health. *J Am Coll Surg* 207:407–416.

Ivorra, M.D., Paya, M., Villar, A. 1990. Effect of beta-sitosterol-3-beta-D-glucoside on insulin secretion in vivo in diabetic rats and in vitro in isolated rat islets of Langerhans. *Pharmazie* 45:271–273.

Jackson, K.G., Robertson, M.D., Fielding, B.A., Frayn, K.N., Williams, C.M. 2002. Measurement of apolipoprotein B-48 in the Svedberg flotation rate (S(f))>400, S(f) 60-400 and S(f) 20-60 lipoprotein fractions reveals novel findings with respect to the effects of dietary fatty acids on triacylglycerol-rich lipoproteins in postmenopausal women. *Clin Sci (Lond)* 103(3):227–237.

Jemai, H., El Feki, A., Sayadi, S. 2009. Antidiabetic and antioxidant effects of hydroxytyrosol and oleuropein from olive leaves in alloxan-diabetic rats. *J Agric Food Chem* 57(19):8798–8804.

Jialal, I., Devaraj, S., Kaul, N. 2001. The effect of alpha-tocopherol on monocyte proatherogenic activity. *J Nutr* 131(2):389S–394S.

Kannel, W.B., Wilson, P.W.F. 1992. Efficacy of lipid profiles in prediction of coronary disease. *Am Heart J* 124:768–774.

Katan, M.B. 1998. Effect of low-fat diets on plasma high-density lipoprotein concentrations. *Am J Clin Nutr* 67(3 Suppl):573S–576S.

Keys, A., Aravanis, C., Blackburn, H.W. et al. 1966. Epidemiological studies related to coronary heart disease: Characteristics of men aged 40–59 in seven countries. *Acta Med Scand Suppl* 460:1–392.

Keys, A., Menotti, A., Karvonen, M.J. et al. 1986. The diet and 15-year death rate in the seven countries study. *Am J Epidemiol* 124:903–915.

Kopelman, P.G. 2000. Obesity as a medical problem. *Nature* 404:635–643.

Kris-Etherton, P. 1999. Monounsaturated fatty acids and risk of cardiovascular disease. *Circulation* 100:1253–1258.

Lairon, D. 2007. Intervention studies on Mediterranean diet and cardiovacular risk. *Mol Nutr Food Res* 51:1209–1214.

Lee, J.S., Pinnamaneni, S.K., Eo, S.J. et al. 2006. Saturated, but not n-6 polyunsaturated, fatty acids induce insulin resistance: Role of intramuscular accumulation of lipid metabolites. *J Appl Physiol* 100:1467–1474.

Liu, J., Sun, H., Duan, W. et al. 2007. Maslinic acid reduces blood glucose in KK-Ay mice. *Biol Pharm Bull* 30:2075–2078.

Lopez, S., Bermudez, B., Pacheco, Y.M., Villar, J., Abia, R., Muriana, F.J. 2008. Distinctive postprandial modulation of beta cell function and insulin sensitivity by dietary fats: Mono-unsaturated compared with saturated fatty acids. *Am J Clin Nutr* 88:638–644.

López-Soldado, I., Avella, M., Botham, K.M. 2009. Differential influence of different dietary fatty acids on very low-density lipoprotein secretion when delivered to hepatocytes in chylomicron remnants. *Metabolism* 58(2):186–195.

Lutsey, P.L., Steffen, L.M., Stevens, J. 2008. Dietary intake and the development of the metabolic syndrome: The Atherosclerosis Risk in Communities study. *Circulation* 117:754–761.

Mangas-Cruz, M.A., Fernández-Moyano, A., Albi, T. et al. 2001. Effects of minor constituents (non-glyceride compounds) of virgin olive oil on plasma lipid concentrations in male Wistar rats. *Clin Nutr* 20(3):211–215.

Martínez, J., Vögler, O., Casas, J. et al. 2005. Membrane structure modulation, protein kinase C alpha activation, and anticancer activity of minerval. *Mol Pharmacol* 67:531–540.

Mattson, F.H., Grundy, S.M. 1985. Comparison of the effects of saturated, monounsaturated and polyunsaturated fatty acids on plasma lipids and lipoproteins in man. *J Lipid Res* 26:684–689.

Mena, M.P., Sacanella, E., Vazquez-Agell, M. et al. 2009. Inhibition of circulating immune cell activation: A molecular antiinflammatory effect of the Mediterranean diet. *Am J Clin Nutr* 89:248–256.

Mendez, M.A., Popkin, B.M., Jakszyn, P. et al. 2006. Adherence to a Mediterranean diet is associated with reduced 3-year incidence of obesity. *J Nutr* 136:2934–2938.

Mezzano, D., Leighton, F., Strobel, P. et al. 2003. Mediterranean diet, but not red wine, is associated with beneficial changes in primary haemostasis. *Eur J Clin Nutr* 57(3):439–446.

Miles, E.A., Wallace, F.A., Calder, P.C. 2001. An olive oil-rich diet reduces scavenger receptor mRNA in murine macrophages. *Br J Nutr* 85(2):185–191.

Miller, M., Stone, N.J., Ballantyne, C. et al. 2011. American Heart Association Clinical Lipidology, Thrombosis, and Prevention Committee of the Council on Nutrition, Physical Activity, and Metabolism; Council on Arteriosclerosis, Thrombosis and Vascular Biology; Council on Cardiovascular Nursing; Council on the Kidney in Cardiovascular Disease. Triglycerides and cardiovascular disease: A scientific statement from the American Heart Association. *Circulation* 123(20):2292–2333.

Muriana, F.J., Villar, J., Ruíz-Gutiérrez, V. 1996. Erythrocyte membrane cholesterol distribution in patients with untreated essential hypertension: Correlation with sodium-lithium countertransport. *J Hypertens* 14(4):443–446.

Navab, M., Anantharamaiah, G.M., Reddy, S.T., Van Lenten, B.J., Fogelman, A.M. 2009. HDL as a biomarker, potential therapeutic target, and therapy. *Diabetes* 58(12):2711–2717.

Nicolaiew, N., Lemort, N., Adorni, L. et al. 1998. Comparison between extra virgin olive oil and oleic acid rich sunflower oil: Effects on postprandial lipemia and LDL susceptibility to oxidation. *Ann Nutr Metab* 42(5):251–260.

Noble, J.M., Thoma, T.H., Ford, G.A. 1999. Effect of age on plasma embrane asymmetry and membrane fluidity in human leukocytes and platelets. *J Gerontol A Biol Sci Med Sci* 54:M601–M606.

Nutrition Recommendations and Interventions for Diabetes. 2007. A position statement of the American Diabetes Association. *Diabetes Care* 30:S48–S65.

Owen, R.W., Mier, W., Giacosa, A., Hull, W.E., Spiegelhalder, B., Bartsch, H. 2000. Phenolic compounds and squalene in olive oils: The concentration and antioxidant potential of total phenols, simple phenols, secoroids, lignans and squalene. *Food Chem Toxicol* 38:647–659.

Paniagua, J.A., de la Sacristana, A.G., Sanchez, E. et al. 2007. A MUFA-rich diet improves posprandial glucose, lipid and GLP-1 responses in insulin-resistant subjects. *J Am Coll Nutr* 26:434–444.

Papandreou, C., Mourad, T.A., Jildeh, C., Abdeen, Z., Philalithis, A., Tzanakis, N. 2008. Obesity in Mediterranean region (1997–2007): A systematic review. *Obes Rev* 9(5):389–399.

Parillo, M., Rivellese, A.A., Ciardullo, A.V. et al. 1992. High-monounsaturated-fat/low-carbohydrate diet improves peripheral insulin sensitivity in non-insulin- dependent diabetic patients. *Metabolism* 41:1373–1378.

Parker, D.R., Weiss, S.T., Troisi, R., Cassano, P.A., Vokonas, P.S., Landsberg, L. 1993. Relationship of dietary saturated fatty acids and body habitus to serum insulin concentrations: The Normative Aging Study. *Am J Clin Nutr* 58:129–136.

Peltola, P., Pihlajamäki, J., Koutnikova, H. et al. 2006. Visceral obesity is associated with high levels of serum squalene. *Obesity* (Silver Spring) 14(7):1155–1163.

Pereira, M.A., Kartashov, A., Ebbeling, C.B. et al. 2005. Fast- food habits, weight gain, and insulin resistance (the CARDIA Study): 15-year prospective analysis. *Lancet* 365:36–42.

Pérez-Camino, M.C., Cert, A. 1999. Quantitative determination of hydroxyl pentacyclic triterpene acids in vegetable oils. *J Agric Food Chem* 47:1558–1562.

Pérez-Jiménez, F., López-Miranda, J., Pinillos, M.D. et al. 2001. A Mediterranean and a high-carbohydrate diet improve glucose metabolism in healthy young persons. *Diabetologia* 44(11):2038–2043.

Pérez-Jimenez, F., Ruano, J., Perez-Martinez, P., Lopez-Segura, F., Lopez-Miranda, J. 2007. The influence of olive oil on human health: Not a question of fat alone. *Mol Nutr Food Res* 51:1199–1208.

Pérez-Martinez, P., Ordovas, J.M., Garcia-Rios, A. et al. 2011. Consumption of diets with different type of fat influences triacylglycerols-rich lipoproteins particle number and size during the postprandial state. *Nutr Metab Cardiovasc Dis* 21(1):39–45.

Perona, J.S., Avella, M., Botham, K.M., Ruiz-Gutierrez, V. 2006. Uptake of triacylglycerol-rich lipoproteins of differing triacylglycerol molecular species and unsaponifiable content by liver cells. *Br J Nutr* 95(5):889–897.

Perona, J.S., Avella, M., Botham, K.M., Ruiz-Gutierrez, V. 2008. Differential modulation of hepatic very low-density lipoprotein secretion by triacylglycerol-rich lipoproteins derived from different oleic-acid rich dietary oils. *Br J Nutr* 99(1):29–36.

Perona, J.S., Cañizares, J., Montero, E., Sánchez-Domínguez, J.M., Catalá, A., Ruiz-Gutiérrez, V. 2004c. Virgin olive oil reduces blood pressure in hypertensive elderly subjects. *Clin Nutr* 23(5):1113–1121.

Perona, J.S., Cañizares, J., Montero, E., Sánchez-Domínguez, J.M., Pacheco, Y.M., Ruiz-Gutierrez, V. 2004b. Dietary virgin olive oil triacylglycerols as an independent determinant of very low-density lipoprotein composition. *Nutrition* 20(6):509–514.

Perona, J.S., Covas, M.I., Fitó, M. et al. 2010. Reduction in systemic and VLDL triacylglycerol concentration after a 3-month Mediterranean-style diet in high-cardiovascular-risk subjects. *J Nutr Biochem* 21(9):892–898.

Perona, J.S., Fitó, M., Covas, M.I., Garcia, M., Ruiz-Gutierrez, V. 2011. Olive oil phenols modulate the triacylglycerol molecular species of human very low-density lipoprotein. A randomized, crossover, controlled trial. *Metabolism* 60(6):893–899.

Perona, J.S., Martínez-González, J., Sanchez-Domínguez, J.M., Badimon, L., Ruiz-Gutierrez, V. 2004a. The unsaponifiable fraction of virgin olive oil in chylomicrons from men improves the balance between vasoprotective and prothrombotic factors released by endothelial cells. *J Nutr* 134(12):3284–3289.

Perona, J.S., Ruiz-Gutierrez, V. 2005. Triacylglycerol molecular species are depleted to different extents in the myocardium of spontaneously hypertensive rats fed two oleic acid-rich oils. *Am J Hypertens* 18(1):72–80.

Perona, J.S., Vögler, O., Sánchez-Domínguez, J.M., Montero, E., Escribá, P.V., Ruiz-Gutierrez, V. 2007. Consumption of virgin olive oil influences membrane lipid composition and regulates intracellular signaling in elderly adults with type 2 diabetes mellitus. *J Gerontol A Biol Sci Med Sci* 62(3):256–263.

Perségol, L., Vergès, B., Foissac, M., Gambert, P., Duvillard, L. 2006. Inability of HDL from type 2 diabetic patients to counteract the inhibitory effect of oxidized LDL on endothelium-dependent vasorelaxation. *Diabetologia* 49:1380–1386.

Perségol, L., Vergès, B., Gambert, P., Duvillard, L. 2007. Inability of HDL from abdominally obese subjects to counteract the inhibitory effect of oxidized LDL on vasorelaxation. *J Lipid Res* 48:1396–1401.

Psaltopoulou, T., Naska, A., Orfanos, P., Trichopoulos, D., Mountokalakis, T., Trichopoulou, A. 2004. Olive oil, the Mediterranean diet, and arterial blood pressure: The Greek European Prospective Investigation into Cancer and Nutrition (EPIC) study. *Am J Clin Nutr* 80:1012–1018.

Psomiadou, E., Tsimidou, M. 2001. Pigments in Greek virgin olive oils: Occurrence and levels. *J Sci Food Agric* 81:640–647.

Roberts, C.K., Ng, C., Hama, S., Eliseo, A.J., Barnard, R.J. 2006. Effect of a short-term diet and exercise intervention on inflammatory/anti-inflammatory properties of HDL in overweight/obese men with cardiovascular risk factors. *J Appl Physiol* 101:1727–1732.

Rodríguez-Rodríguez, R., Herrera, M.D., Perona, J.S., Ruiz-Gutiérrez, V. 2004. Potential vasorelaxant effects of oleanolic acid and erythrodiol, two triterpenoids contained in 'orujo' olive oil, on rat aorta. *Br J Nutr* 92(4):635–642.

Rojo-Martinez, G., Esteva, I., Ruiz de Adana, M.S. et al. 2006. Dietary fatty acids and insulin secretion: A population-based study. *Eur J Clin Nutr* 60:1195–1200.

Ros, E. 2003. Dietary cis-monounsaturated fatty acids and metabolic control in type 2 diabetes. *Am J Clin Nutr* 78:617S–625S.

Rosenblat, M., Volkova, N., Coleman, R., Almagor, Y., Aviram, M. 2008. Antiatherogenicity of extra virgin olive oil and its enrichment with green tea polyphenols in the atherosclerotic apolipoprotein-E-deficient mice: Enhanced macrophage cholesterol efflux. *J Nutr Biochem* 19(8):514–523.

Ruiz-Gutierrez, V., Muriana, F.J., Guerrero, A., Cert, A.M., Villar, J. 1996. Plasma lipids, erythrocyte membrane lipids and blood pressure of hypertensive women after ingestion of dietary oleic acid from two different sources. *J Hypertens* 14(12):1483–1490.

Ryan, M., McInerney, D., Owens, D., Collins, P., Johnson, A., Tomkin, G.H. 2000. Diabetes and the Mediterranean diet: A beneficial effect of oleic acid on insulin sensitivity, adipocyte glucose transport and endothelium-dependent vasoreactivity. *QJM* 93:85–91.

Saaristo, T., Moilanen, L., Korpi-Hyovalti, E. et al. 2010. Lifestyle intervention for prevention of type 2 diabetes in primary health care: One-year follow-up of the Finnish National Diabetes Prevention Program (FIN-D2D). *Diabetes Care* 33(10):2146–2151.

Salas, J., Lopez Miranda, J., Jansen, S. et al. 1999. The diet rich in monounsaturated fat modifies in a beneficial way carbohydrate metabolism and arterial pressure. *Med Clin (Barc)* 113:765–769.

Salas-Salvado, J., Fernandez-Ballart, J., Ros, E. et al. 2008. PREDIMED Study Investigators. Effect of a Mediterranean Diet supplemented with nuts on metabolic syndrome status: One-year results of the PREDIMED randomized trial. *Arch Intern Med* 168:2449–2458.

Sato, K., Takahashi, T., Takahashi, Y., Shiono, H., Katoh, N., Akiba, Y. 1999. Preparation of chylomicrons and VLDL with monoacid-rich triacylglycerol and characterization of kinetic parameters in lipoprotein lipase-mediated hydrolysis in chickens. *J Nutr* 129(1):126–131.

Schneeman, B.O., Kotite, L., Todd, K.M., Havel, R.J. 1993. Relationships between the responses of triglyceride-rich lipoproteins in blood plasma containing apolipoproteins B-48 and B-100 to a fat-containing meal in normolipidemic humans. *Proc Natl Acad Sci USA* 90(5):2069–2073.

Schroder, H., Marrugat, J., Vila, J., Covas, M.I., Elosua, R. 2004. Adherence to the traditional Mediterranean Diet is inversely associated with body mass index and obesity in a Spanish population. *J Nutr* 134:3355–3361.

Schulze, M.B., Schulz, M., Heidemann, C., Schienkiewitz, A., Hoffmann, K., Boeing, H. 2008. Carbohydrate intake and incidence of type 2 diabetes in the European prospective investigation into cancer and nutrition (EPIC)-Potsdam study. *Br J Nutr* 99:1107–1116.

Schwartz, G.J., Fu, J., Astarita, G. et al. 2008. The lipid messenger OEA links dietary fat intake to satiety. *Cell Metab* 8:281–288.

Serra-Majem, L., de la Cruz, J.N., Ribas, L., Salleras, L. 2004. Mediterranean diet and health: Is all the secret in olive oil? *Pathophysiol Haemost Thromb* 33:461–465.

Shai, I., Schwarzfuchs, D., Henkin, Y. et al. 2008. Weight loss with a low-carbohydrate, Mediterranean, or low-fat diet. *N Engl J Med* 359:229–241.

Shen, X., Tang, Q., Wu, J., Feng, Y., Huang, J., Cai, W. 2009. Effect of vitamin E supplementation on oxidative stress in a rat model of diet-induced obesity. *Int J Vitam Nutr Res* 79(4):255–263.

Solomon, T.P., Haus, J.M., Kelly, K.R. et al. 2009. Randomized trial on the effects of a 7-d low-glycemic diet and exercise intervention on insulin resistance in older obese humans. *Am J Clin Nutr* 90:1222–1229.

Somova, L.O., Nadar, A., Rammanan, P., Shode, F.O. 2003. Cardiovascular, antihyperlipidemic and antioxidant effects of oleanolic and ursolic acids in experimental hypertension. *Phytomedicine* 10:115–121.

Soriguer, F., Esteva, I., Rojo-Martinez, G. et al. 2004. Oleic acid from cooking oils is associated with lower insulin resistance in the general population (Pizarra study). *Eur J Endocrinol* 150:33–39.

Su, Q., Rowley, K.G., Itsiopoulus, C., O'Dea, K. 2002. Identification and quantitation of major carotenoids in selected components of the Mediterranean diet: Green leafy vegetables and olive oil. *Eur J Clin Nutr* 56:1149–1154.

Sunehag, A.L., Toffolo, G., Treuth, M.S. et al. 2002. Effects of dietary macronutrient content on glucose metabolism in children. *J Clin Endocrinol Metab* 87:5168–5178.

Sutherland, W.H., Scott, R.S., Lintott, C.J., Robertson, M.C., Stapely, S.A., Cox, C. 1992. Plasma non-cholesterol sterols in patients with non-insulin dependent diabetes mellitus. *Horm Metab Res* 24:172–175.

Thomas, D., Elliott, E.J. 2009. Low glycaemic index, or low glycaemic load, diets for diabetes mellitus. *Cochrane Database Syst Rev* (1):CD006296.

Tierney, A.C., McMonagle, J., Shaw, D.I. et al. 2010. Effects of dietary fat modification on insulin sensitivity and on other risk factors of the metabolic syndrome-LIPGENE: A European randomized dietary intervention study. *Int J Obes (Lond)* 35(6):800–809.

Tierney, A.C., Roche, H.M. 2007. The potential role of olive oil-derived MUFA in insulin sensitivity. *Mol Nutr Food Res* 51:1235–1248.

Trichopoulou, A., Lagiou, P. 1997. Healthy traditional Mediterranean diet: An expression of culture, history, and lifestyle. *Nutr Rev* 55:383–389.

Tsimidou, M., Papadopoulos, G., Boskou, D. 1992. Phenolic-compounds and stability of virgin olive oil. *Food Chem* 45:141–144.

Tsuchiya, M., Hosaka, M., Moriguchi, T. et al. 2010. Cholesterol biosynthesis pathway intermediates and inhibitors regulate glucose-stimulated insulin secretion and secretory granule formation in pancreatic beta-cells. *Endocrinology* 151(10):4705–4716.

Tsuda, K., Kinoshita, Y., Nishio, I., Masuyama, Y. 2000. Role of insulin in the regulation of membrane fluidity of erythrocytes in essential hypertension: An electron paramagnetic resonance investigation. *Am J Hypertens* 13(4 Pt 1):376–382.

Tuck, K.L., Hayball, P.J. 2002. Major phenolic compounds in olive oil: Metabolism and health effects. *J Nutr Biochem* 13(11):636–644.

Van Lenten, B.J., Hama, S.Y., de Beer, F.C. et al. 1995. Anti-inflammatory HDL becomes pro-inflammatory during the acute phase response: Loss of protective effect of HDL against LDL oxidation in aortic wall cell cocultures. *J Clin Invest* 96:2758–2767.

Vessby, B., Unsitupa, M., Hermansen, K. et al. 2001. Substituting dietary saturated for monounsaturated fat impairs insulin sensitivity in healthy men and women: The KANWU Study. *Diabetologia* 44:312–319.

Visioli, F., Galli, C. 1998. The effect of minor constituents of olive oil on cardiovascular disease: New findings. *Nutr Rev* 56(5 Pt 1):142–147.

Wang, X., Li, Y.L., Wu, H. et al. 2011. Antidiabetic effect of oleanolic acid: A promising use of a traditional pharmacological agent. *Phytother Res* 25(7):1031–1040.

Williams, D.B., Wan, Z., Frier, B.C., Bell, R.C., Field, C.J., Wright, D.C. 2012. Dietary supplementation with vitamin E and C attenuates dexamethasone-induced glucose intolerance in rats. *Am J Physiol Regul Integr Comp Physiol* 302(1):R49–R58.

Williams, D.E., Prevost, A.T., Whichelow, M.J., Cox, B.D., Day, N.E., Wareham, N.J. 2000. A cross-sectional study of dietary patterns with glucose intolerance and other features of the metabolic syndrome. *Br J Nutr* 83:257–266.

Wu, D., Hayek, M.G., Meydani, S.N. 2001. Vitamin E and macrophage cyclooxygenase regulation in the aged. *J Nutr* 131:382S–388S.

Xia, F., Xie, L., Mihic, A. et al. 2008. Inhibition of cholesterol biosynthesis impairs insulin secretion and voltage-gated calcium channel function in pancreatic β-cells. *Endocrinology* 149:5136–5145.

Zamora, R., Navarro, J.L., Hidalgo, F.J. 1994. Identification and classification of olive oils by high-resolution c-13 nuclear-magnetic-resonance. *J Am Oil Chem Soc* 7(4):361–364.

Zampelas, A., Kafatos, A.G., Levin, B.E. 2004. Olive oil intake in relation to cardiovascular diseases. *Grasas y Aceites* 55:24–32.

14 Soy and Soy-Based Products

*Marcell Alysson Batisti Lozovoy, Andréa Name Colado Simão,
Ana Paula Kallaur, and Isaias Dichi*

CONTENTS

14.1 INTRODUCTION

Obesity is a metabolic disease of worldwide occurrence and a serious public health problem, being a common form of malnutrition that contributes to the onset of various diseases (Repetto et al. 2003). The excessive accumulation of adipose tissue in obesity may be caused by endocrine, metabolic, or genetic changes, or by changes in energy expenditure factors due to reduced physical activity and increased food intake (Ali et al. 2004). Adipocytes in greater number and volume in obesity have functional aspects in metabolism and energy homeostasis (Rayalam et al. 2008). The central adiposity induces chronic systemic inflammation by increasing the concentration of inflammatory markers, which may be a risk for the onset of metabolic syndrome (MetS) (Duarte et al. 2003, Lee and Pratley 2005). Several adipokines are involved in systemic inflammation such as resistin, adipsin, tumor necrosis factor alpha (TNF-α) and interleukin-1 and -6 (IL1 and IL6), plasminogen factor 1 (PAI-1), and angiotensinogen.

Cardiovascular disease (CVD) is widespread in the modern world and represents one of the main causes of mortality (Hu et al. 2010). Increased blood cholesterol content and oxidative modifications of low-density lipoproteins (Nwose et al. 2013) represent risk factors for the development of CVD. Adequate nutrition is considered effective in the prevention and treatment of CVD (Rudkowska and Jones 2007). The results of epidemiological, clinical, and experimental studies show that soy foods decrease blood cholesterol in individuals with hyperlipidemia as well as mortality rates from CVD in both Asians and Caucasians (Anderson et al. 1995, Messina and Messina 2003, Borodin et al. 2009). Soybeans exert antioxidant effects when people consume soy foods (Bertipaglia et al. 2008, Simão et al. 2010). This effect may also be beneficial for CVD or MetS patients (Bahls et al. 2011).

MetS comprises pathological conditions that include insulin resistance, arterial hypertension, visceral adiposity, and dyslipidemia, which favor the development of CVDs and type 2 diabetes (Reaven 1988). MetS is an independent predictor of cardiovascular morbidity and mortality (Ford et al. 2002, Reilly and Rader 2003, Kip et al. 2004). Abdominal obesity and insulin resistance are the core features of MetS (Reaven 1988).

MetS prevalence motivated the National Cholesterol Education Program on its third panel: *Treatment of High Blood Cholesterol in Adults*—ATP III (Jacobs 2001) to propose clinical criteria to define MetS by the presence of three or more of these altered factors: high blood pressure (BP), dyslipidemia (hypertriglyceridemia, low HDL-c), high plasmatic glucose, and abdominal obesity.

Nutrition has a major role in MetS (Feldeisen and Tucker 2007, Lutsey et al. 2008, Djousse et al. 2010). Several dietary patterns and dietary components have been studied to evaluate their influence on MetS parameters. Therefore, it has been shown that there are nutritional alternatives, which can improve many factors related to MetS. Dietary soy has been recommended for its potential role in CVD, although the recommendation has changed from soy protein or isoflavones to soy products because of their high content of polyunsaturated fats, fiber, vitamins and minerals, and low content of saturated fat (Sacks et al. 2006).

Most studies, which evaluated the effect of soy intake, have been performed on healthy people, hypercholesterolemic, or diabetic patients (Hall et al. 2006, McVeigh et al. 2006, Sacks et al. 2006, Hanachi and Golkho 2008, Sakai and Kogiso 2008). The results of these studies are contradictory (Moutsatsou 2007).

Several studies suggest that soy protein and its phytoestrogens (isoflavones) may have beneficial effects in obesity and correlated dysfunctions. Soy phytoestrogens have numerous physiological activities, particularly in lipid metabolism, playing an important role in hypercholesterolemic and hyperlipidemic patients (Bhathena et al. 2000, Bhathena and Velasquez 2002, Zhan and Ho 2005). In addition, reduction in fat mass can occur through lipolysis and loss of mature fat cells via apoptosis (Rayalam et al. 2008).

This chapter will report the main biological effects of soy, soy-based products, and soy components, and their effects on MetS indicators.

14.2 MAIN BIOLOGICAL EFFECTS OF SOYBEANS AND SOY COMPONENTS

Soybeans (*Glycine max* [L.] Merr) contain an impressive array of biologically active components (Carter et al. 2004). People have been eating soybeans for almost 5000 years. Researchers are interested in both the nutritional value and the potential health benefits of soybeans. This research includes a wide range of areas, such as cancer, coronary heart disease (cardiovascular disease), osteoporosis, cognitive function (memory related), menopausal symptoms, renal function, and many others. Remarkably, seeds of soy contain very high levels of protein, carbohydrate conjugates, fatty acids (soybean oil), amino acids, and inorganic materials (minerals). Among these soybean components, protein and fatty acid content account for about 40% and 20%, respectively. Some molecules with biological effects are the isoflavones, phytic acid, soy lipids, soy phytoalexins, soy saponins, lectins, hemagglutinin, soy toxins, and vitamins (Table 14.1).

Food and Drug Administration recognized soy protein functionality in 1999 (Department of Health and Human Services 1999). It was stated that "diets with low content in saturated fat and cholesterol and that include 25 g soy protein can reduce cardiovascular risk." Similar claims have been approved in several other countries including the United Kingdom (Harland and Haffner 2008).

The American Heart Association recommends the ingestion of soybeans and soy-based products to patients with high cholesterol levels. In Federal Programs of School Feeding, it was reported that soybeans could substitute animal protein until 30% without any prejudice (Messina et al. 2003).

Brazil is one of the main soybean producers of the world (The American Soybean Association 2014). The National Agency for Sanitarian Surveillance (ANVISA—Brazil), an organization that regulates production and commercialization of food and drugs, claimed that a minimum ingestion of 25 g/day soy protein can reduce cholesterol levels; a minimum ingestion of 0.8 g/day phytosterols was also recommended (Agência Nacional de Vigilância Sanitária 2008).

TABLE 14.1
Biological Major Classes of Biochemical Compounds Found in Raw Soybean Grain and Their Effects

Chemical Class	Components	Subcomponents	[1]/g Soy	Biological Effects
Polyphenols	Isoflavones/flavonoids	Genistein (50%)	1.11 mg	Isoflavones have been reported to show estrogenic, antifungal, antitumor, and antimutagenic properties (Miyazawa et al. 1999, Dorge and Sheehan 2002, Rishi 2002).
		Daidzein (40%)	0.37 mg	
		Glycitein (10%)	0.10 mg	
Lipids	Fatty acids	Linoleic and linolenic acids	0.2 g	Generates low inflammatory effect after degradation (Deckelbaum and Torrejon 2012).
	Sterols	β-sitosterol, β-sitostarol, campesterol, campestanol, brassicasterol, stigmasterol, and Δ5-avenasterol, and cholesterol	ND	The lowering of serum cholesterol by plant sterols is believed to be the result of an inhibition of cholesterol absorption in small intestine (Normén et al. 2000).
	Lipid-soluble vitamins	Vitamins A, D, E, and K	ND	Several effects.
	Glycerolipids–glycerophospholipids	Phosphatidyl choline, phosphatidyl ethanolamine, phosphatidyl inositol, and phosphatidylserine	NA	Lecithin has been a popular supplement because of its high choline (N,N,N-trimethylethanol) content. Choline is an essential nutrient that has benefit for heart health and brain development, as choline deficiency plays a role in liver disease, atherosclerosis, and possibly neurological disorders (Kunmen and Van Eck 2012).
	Sphingoglycolipid	Cerebroside and sphingomyelin	NA	Soya-cerebroside was reported to exhibit moderate tyrosinase inhibitory activity and applied for making skin-care cosmetics for the removal of (black) freckles. In humans, sphingomyelin represents ~85% of all sphingolipids in the membranous myelin sheath that surrounds some nerve cell axons (Fuller 2010).
Glycoprotein	Soy phytoalexins	6a-Hydroxyphaseollin	NA	Phytoalexins are known to inhibit bacterial or fungus cell wall biosynthesis, or delay maturation, or disrupt metabolism. Contribute to the prevention and treatment of breast cancer (Tilghman et al. 2013).
		Glycecollins	NA	Besides their antifungal or antibacterial activities, glyceollins have recently been demonstrated to be a novel antiestrogen that bind to the estrogen receptor (ER) and inhibit estrogen-induced tumor progression (Zimmermann et al. 2010).

(Continued)

TABLE 14.1 (*Continued*)
Biological Major Classes of Biochemical Compounds Found in Raw Soybean Grain and Their Effects

Chemical Class	Components	Subcomponents	[1/g Soy]	Biological Effects
Phytoestrogens	Coumestrol	ND	ND	Coumestrol has less estrogen activities than estrogen and therefore may reduce the risk of developing breast or prostate cancer in humans by preventing estradiol binding to estrogen receptor (ER). Coumestrol was reported to inhibit the enzymes involved in the biosynthesis of steroid hormone (aromatase and hydroxysteroid dehydrogenase), and inhibition of these enzymes results in the modulation of hormone production. Coumestrol, a novel ATP competitive and cell permeable CK2 inhibitor with submicromolar IC (50), had inhibition effects on the growth of three cancer cell lines and may represent a promising class of CK2 inhibitors (Liu et al. 2013).
Amphipathic glycosides	Soy saponins	ND	0.02–0.05 g	The blood cholesterol–lowering properties of dietary saponins are of particular interest in human nutrition. Saponins bind cholesterol and bile acids in the gut. Cancer cells have more cholesterol-type compounds in their membranes than normal cells. Soy saponins can bind cholesterol in vitro and thus interfere with cell growth and division (Mac Donald et al. 2005).
Protein	Total	ND	0.365 g	
	Lectins and hemagglutinins	ND	ND	Lectins are plant-derived proteins that are capable of binding to carbohydrate moieties of complex glycoconjugates but do not possess immunoglobulin nature. They typically agglutinate certain animal cells and/or precipitate glycoconjugates. Many members of the lectinic protein family agglutinate red blood cells.
Water-soluble vitamins	Thiamine, riboflavin, niacin, pantothenic acid, biotin, folic acid, inositol, choline, and vitamin C	ND	ND	Several effects.

Source: Adapted from Parh, 2001 and Carter, T.E. Jr. et al., Genetic diversity in soybean, in: Boerma, H.R. and Specht, J.E., eds., *Soybeans: Improvement, Production and Uses*, American Society of Agronomy, Madison, WI, 2004.

NA, not applied; ND, not demonstrated.

14.3 EFFECTS OF SOY, SOY-BASED PRODUCTS, AND SOY COMPONENTS ON METABOLIC SYNDROME PARAMETERS

14.3.1 EFFECTS ON OBESITY

Soy and soy-based products have several effects on obesity. However, the mechanisms whereby soy protein may exert its beneficial effects on obesity are not completely clear. Several lines of evidence suggest that soy protein may favorably affect lipid absorption, insulin resistance, fatty acid metabolism, and other hormonal, cellular, or molecular changes associated with adiposity.

Our group has performed a study in which the role of inflammatory markers was investigated in obese patients with MetS after ingestion of 29 g of kinako (toasted ground soybean) for 90 days (Simão et al. 2012). One of the main findings of that study was an increase in IL-6 levels with kinako ingestion. The current understanding of the role of IL-6 in the context of obesity is ambivalent. IL-6 can be viewed as a proinflammatory cytokine, which induces C-reactive protein secretion, but may also be regarded as an anti-inflammatory cytokine as it induces the synthesis of IL-1 receptor antagonist and the release of soluble TNF receptor, leading to reduced activity of proinflammatory cytokines (Ait-Oufella et al. 2011). There is also growing evidence that IL-6 has a role in inducing lipolysis and decreasing appetite and weight gain, thus controlling obesity-associated pathologies (Berg and Scherer 2005). In addition to IL-6 increase, a significant decrease in waist circumference after kinako ingestion was also found, which favors the latter hypothesis. Soy-based products, due to their high contents of protein and fiber, may have beneficial effects on satiety (Allison et al. 2003). They may even produce weight loss with a decrease in fat mass but not muscle mass in overweight and obese subjects (Deibert et al. 2004).

14.3.2 EFFECTS ON LIPID METABOLISM

Traditional soy foods are high in polyunsaturated fat, and so when substituted for foods high in saturated fat, they can reduce blood cholesterol levels and the risk of coronary heart disease (CHD) (Jakobsen et al. 2009, Mozaffarian et al. 2010). The consumption of soybean or its bioactive compounds has been reported to contribute significantly to reducing cholesterol and triglyceride levels in laboratory animals and humans (Reynolds et al. 2006, Sirtori et al. 2007, Sirtori et al. 2009, Esteves et al. 2011). The beneficial effect on lipemia has been explained by the action of various constituents present in soybean, which act via different mechanisms (Figure 14.1):

- *Amino acid profile*: The high content of arginine and low methionine content can promote higher levels of nitric oxide (NO; Gornik and Creager 2004) and lower levels of homocysteine (Torres et al. 2005), favoring vessel relaxation and reduction of the risk of CVD. There are suggestions that soy protein exerts hypolipidemic and antiatherogenic effects because the relationship between amino acids lysine and arginine alters the insulin/glucagon relationship, which, when elevated, increases the risk of CVD (Demonty et al. 2002, Torres et al. 2005).
- *Action of nondigestible peptide*: The presence of peptides from undigested soybean in the gastrointestinal tract has also explained their hypocholesterolemic effect. Peptides increase the fecal excretion of steroids, elevating the hepatic synthesis of bile acids and receptors of LDL-c, as well as the uptake and oxidation of cholesterol in the liver (Belleville 2002). Hypocholesterolemic effect has been found in peptide Leu-Pro-Tyr-Pro-Arg, a protein fragment derived from soybean glycinin, which reduced serum cholesterol in mice (−25.4% in total cholesterol and −30.6% in LDL-c) (Yoshikawa et al. 2000); this peptide has structural homology to enterostatin (Val-Pro-Asp-Pro-Arg). Although both have hypocholesterolemic activities, enterostatin did not increase fecal excretion of bile acids, suggesting that they may act by different mechanisms (Takenaka et al. 2004).

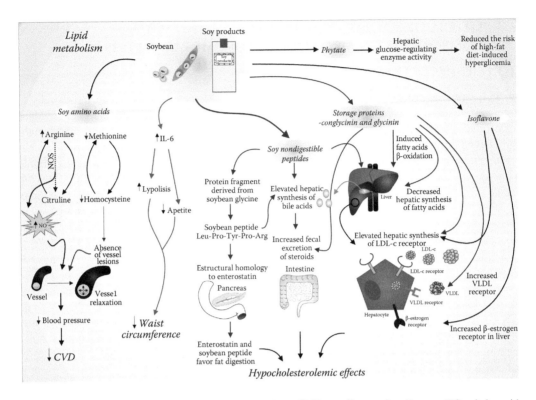

FIGURE 14.1 Soybean compounds in lipid metabolism. CVD, cardiovascular disease; NO, nitric oxide; IL-6, interleukin 6; Leu, leucine; Pro, proline; Tyr, tyrosine; Arg, arginine; LDL-c, low-density lipoprotein cholesterol; VLDL, very low-density lipoprotein.

- *Bioactivity of isoflavones*: Isoflavones, acting on β-estrogen receptors (β-ERs) present in the liver, lead to increased number of hepatic receptors of LDL-c and favors the catabolism of cholesterol and β-oxidation of fatty acids (Dewell et al. 2002, Douglas et al. 2006, Torrezan et al. 2008). The antioxidant effect of isoflavones can act protecting the oxidation of copper-dependent LDL-c and favors a serum lipid profile associated with protection against atherosclerosis (Teixeira Damasceno et al. 2007).
- *Hypolipidemic action of storage proteins*: β-conglycinin and glycinin showed hypolipidemic effect through increased fecal excretion of fatty acids, induction of β-oxidation in the liver, and decreased hepatic synthesis of fatty acids by downregulation of fatty acid synthesis and upregulation of liver VLDL receptors (Duranti et al. 2004, Fukui et al. 2004, Moriyama et al. 2004).
- *Hypolipidemic action of phytate*: Phytate intake improves serum lipid profile and reduces the hepatic lipid depot in the animal model of atherosclerosis (Lee et al. 2007). It is known that phytate exerts an effect on hepatic glucose-regulating enzyme activities and reduces the risk of high-fat diet-induced hyperglycemia (Kim et al. 2011).
- *Hypolipidemic action of β-conglycinin*: It has been shown that soy contents of 7S globulin protein (fraction β-conglycinin) possibly upregulate LDL receptors and thereby reduce serum LDL concentrations (Ferreira et al. 2011).
- The evidences commented earlier show that the beneficial effects of soybean on lipid profile improvement is mediated by various constituents present in the grain, and thus, the intake of whole soybean has potential to exert greater effect in comparison with the supplementation of their components. Some evidence supports this idea. The hypocholesterolemic effect of soy consumption may be attributed not only to the presence of bioactive

compounds (intrinsic effect) but also to replacing animal foods rich in saturated fat and cholesterol (extrinsic effect). A recent study estimated the intrinsic and extrinsic effects of soybean to reduce cholesterol and verified that the combined effects are important to reduce cholesterol in approximately 4% (Jenkins et al. 2010). In fact, the synergistic action of amino acids and isoflavones in improving lipid metabolism has been demonstrated (Bertipaglia et al. 2008).

On the other side, a study performed with a group of postmenopausal women found no significant hypocholesterolemic effect of ingesting soymilk for 4 weeks, despite good adherence of the participants (Beavers et al. 2010). The authors discussed that the baseline cholesterol status, supplement type, dosage, and duration, as well as dietary control, are all potential confounding factors, and they have been identified as determinants of the conflicting results. In contrast, a study performed with MetS women using 35 g/day of textured soy protein (obtained by manufacturing; in this process, 95% of its fat is extracted, with a reduction in many of its nutrients) or soy nut for 12 weeks showed an improvement in lipid profile, mainly in the group of patients that ingested soy nut (Bakhtiary et al. 2012).

The aforementioned data allow suggesting that ingestion of soy or soy products seems to offer more benefits to MetS patients when compared to soy-isolated component.

In the literature, improvement in lipid profile is usually reached with soy ingestion above 50 g/day. However, a previous study has reported that 25 g/day of soy is sufficient to reduce LDL cholesterol and triacylglycerol levels in MetS patients (Bahls et al. 2011). In addition, our group (Simão et al. 2014) has also shown that kinako (29.14 g/day) moderates the effects of high doses (3 g/day) of fish oil n-3 fatty acids on LDL cholesterol and total cholesterol. Other reports have verified an increase in LDL, total cholesterol levels, and glucose levels when fish oil is used in doses above 3 g/day (Jacobson 2008).

Soy seems to favor cholesterol decrease due to the presence of molecular symmetries with the enzyme 3-hydroxy-3-methylglutaryl CoA reductase (HMG-CoA reductase). Therefore, soy is a robust candidate to reproduce, in a weaker way, the characteristic of statins (Pak et al. 2006).

14.3.3 EFFECT ON GLYCEMIC CONTROL

Soybean has shown a potential to exert physiological effects through mechanisms that stimulate insulin production and decrease the glycemic index of diet, suggesting the possibility of preventing and controlling diabetes, obesity, and their metabolic complications. Nevertheless, the effects of soy consumption on glucose metabolism are more controversial than the beneficial effects on lipids and remain uncertain since there are many contradictory publications (Figure 14.2).

Although the beneficial effects of soy and soy-based products are undisputed, some components, such as isoflavones, deserve special attention. The effect of isoflavones in reducing blood glucose may be explained by the stimulus by genistein to pancreatic β cells, which increases insulin production and consequently the glucose uptake by cells (Esteves et al. 2011). These effects has been demonstrated in studies with animals that received genistein (Jonas et al. 1995) and also in an in vitro study, which used adipocytes and insulinoma cells, showing that bioactive compounds formed from isoflavonoids and soy peptides during the fermentation process to produce Meju-activated signaling cascades that stimulated insulin release (Kwon et al. 2011). Meju is one of the soybean fermented products well known to exert many health-promoting activities like anticancer, lowering of BP and serum cholesterol, enhancement of immune function, and promotion of calcium absorption (Messina 1995).

The dietary fiber contained in soybeans is effective in controlling blood glucose (Penha et al. 2007). It can reduce the rate of emptying of the digestive tract, increase the rate of peristalsis of the bowel, and slow down the rate of glucose uptake (Takahashi et al. 2003). In a clinical study, the intake of soybean fiber resulted in decreased blood glucose levels after ingestion of a glucose

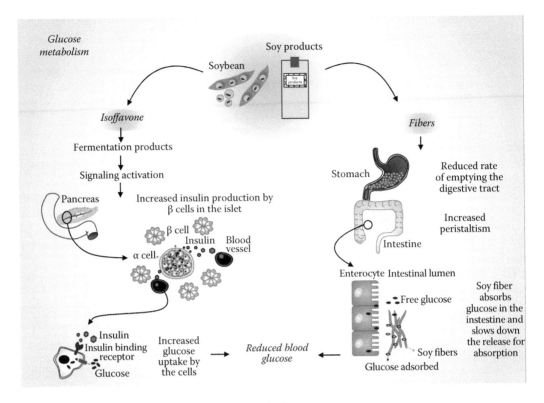

FIGURE 14.2 Soybean compounds in glucose metabolism.

solution; thus, soy fibers may adsorb glucose in the intestine and slows down their release for absorption (Messina et al. 1992). A cake made with whole soybean flour showed low glucose and insulin indexes in a study with a group of 20 individuals (Oku et al. 2009).

Phytate also shows potential in controlling diabetes, as demonstrated by its hypoglycemic effect in diabetic mice (Lee et al. 2007, Kim et al. 2010). Lee (2006) observed that consumption of diets containing phytate reduced high blood glucose levels and glycated hemoglobin in diabetic mice.

In summary, various bioactive soy compounds may act on mechanisms that improve the metabolism of carbohydrates, working in reducing the risk of metabolic complications of obesity and diabetes. However, in diabetic individuals, studies are needed to show whether pancreatic β cells of these individuals are responsive to stimulation of soy isoflavones to increase insulin release.

Azadbakht et al. (2007) reported the effects of two different kinds of soy on the components of the MetS. They randomly assigned to 42 postmenopausal women with MetS a control diet (Dietary Approaches to Stop Hypertension [DASH]), a soy protein diet, or a soy nut diet, each for 8 weeks. Consumption of soy nut reduced fasting plasma glucose more significantly than the soy protein or control diet. Soy nut consumption significantly reduced serum C-peptide concentrations compared with control diet, but consumption of soy protein did not. The soy nut regimen also decreased LDL cholesterol more than did the soy protein period and the control diet. Our group also showed that soy ingestion (25 g/day) reduced serum glucose levels and insulin resistance in patients with MetS and that 29.14 g/day moderates the undesirable effects of high doses of fish oil n-3 fatty acids (3 g/day) on glucose metabolism (Bahls et al. 2011, Simão et al. 2014).

On the other hand, Liu et al. (2010) recently published an interesting placebo-controlled trial, where they investigated the effects of soy protein and isoflavones on glycemic control and insulin sensitivity, in a 6-month control-case trial, with postmenopausal Chinese women with prediabetes or untreated early diabetes. They concluded that the results did not support the hypothesis that soy protein had favorable effects on glycemic control and insulin sensitivity.

14.3.4 Effect on Blood Pressure

Elevated BP results from environmental factors, genetic factors, and interactions among these factors. Among the environmental factors that affect BP, dietary factors have a prominent and likely predominant role (Appel et al. 2006). Several clinical trials and meta-analysis have identified nutritional strategies using soy-based products (Jenkins et al. 2002, He et al. 2005, Yang et al. 2005) as noninvasive approaches to managing and reducing the risk of elevated BP (Figure 14.3).

Simão et al. (2012) studied the effects of soybean (29 g/day) and fish oil on BP in patients with MetS. The group that received fish oil and kinako concomitantly showed a statistically significant decrease in systolic BP, whereas there was a significant decrease in diastolic BP in kinako group and fish oil group after 90 days in relation to the baseline values. These findings were attributed to increasing levels verified in serum adiponectin and NO in the kinako group and in the fish oil group after 90 day.

Fish oil action on NO may result from increased expression of endothelial nitric oxide synthase (eNOS) expression (Nyby et al. 2004), whereas it can be hypothesized that the relative higher amount of NO precursor, arginine, in the amino acid profile of soy protein (Erdman 2001) could explain, at least in part, its effects on NO concentration, as the L-arginine/NO pathway plays a critical role in maintaining normal endothelial function by causing vasodilatation (Bai et al. 2009).

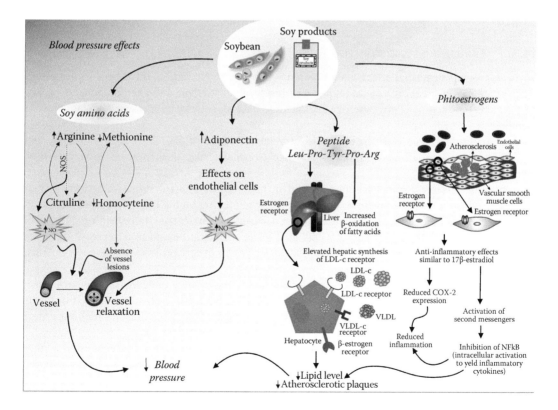

FIGURE 14.3 Soybean compounds in blood pressure. NO, nitric oxide; LDL-c, low-density lipoprotein-cholesterol; VLDL, very-low-density lipoprotein cholesterol; COX-2, cyclooxygenase; NFkB, nuclear factor kappa B; Leu, leucine; Pro, proline; Tyr, tyrosine; Arg: arginine.

In experimental studies, adiponectin has been shown to enhance NO production in cultured aortic endothelial cells (ECs; Tan et al. 2004), to significantly increase eNOS expression (83%) and reduce inducible NO synthase (70%) in hyperlipidemic rats (Li et al. 2007) and to improve obesity-related hypertension in mice (Ohashi et al. 2006). Adiponectin has anti-inflammatory effects and augments blood flow by enhancing NO production and activating eNOS, and it may act as a modulator of vascular remodeling by suppressing smooth muscle cell migration, which possibly plays a role in the regulation of atherosclerosis (Ziemke and Mantzoros 2010). Human studies have also shown that hypoadiponectinemia is closely linked to endothelial dysfunction in healthy (Shimabukuro et al. 2003) and hypertensive subjects (Ouchi et al. 2003).

Other events that could explain the beneficial action of soybeans on cardiovascular system are related to the capacity of phytoestrogens in protecting vascular bed against mechanisms, which lead to high BP; because their similarity with estrogens, phytoestrogens act specially in cells with estrogen receptors (ERs). ERs are present in several tissues and have also been identified in ECs and vascular smooth muscle cells (VSMCs) (Chambliss et al. 2002, Orshal and Khalil 2004, Miller and Duckles 2008, Smiley and Khalil 2009), which could explain the action of phytoestrogens on BP control. Phytoestrogens may also exert vascular anti-inflammatory effects similar to 17β-estradiol (E2) (Dharmappa et al. 2010). Phytoestrogens and other similar E2 molecules can link to β-ER and lead to reduced cyclooxygenase-2 (COX-2) expression through 3 beta-diol (3β-diol) metabolic pathway by enzymes 3α-hydroxysteroid dehydrogenase (HSD), 3β-HSD, and/or 17β-HSD in VSMC, which generates an anti-inflammatory effect (Zuloaga et al. 2012). Another hypothesis is that ER activates the second messenger inositol trisphosphate kinase (IP3K), which could inhibit NFkB, one of the main factors responsible for intracellular activation to yield inflammatory cytokines (Vegeto et al. 2008). This favorable condition expressed by an anti-inflammatory milieu would make the development of atherogenesis and arterial hypertension difficult.

14.3.5 Conclusions and Perspectives

Soybean presents beneficial effects on all parameters of MetS. Nowadays, these benefits are essentially related to ingestion of soy and soy-based products. Nevertheless, some components of soy, such as fibers, protein, and phytosterols, also seem to have an activity on lipid metabolism, glucose metabolism, and BP.

The main importance of fibers seems to be related to lipid profile, since they can delay and reduce fat absorption. However, proteins and isoflavones can also positively interfere with lipid metabolism.

Hypocholesterolemic effect has been found in peptide Leu-Pro-Tyr-Pro-Arg, a protein fragment derived from soybean glycinin, whereas isoflavones acting on the β-ERs present in the liver lead to increased number of hepatic receptors of LDL-c and favors the catabolism of cholesterol and β-oxidation of fatty acids. These events lead to fat mobilization and to a decrease in serum lipid levels. Thus, it is conceivable to suggest that they can at last provoke a reduction in waist circumference.

Soybean action on glucose metabolism is associated to its capacity to decrease glucose absorption and increase insulin production by pancreatic β cells, being these effects produced by fibers and isoflavones, respectively. The aforementioned actions also aid to avoid diabetes mellitus type 2 development.

L-arginine/NO pathway, eNOS induced by adiponectin, and phytoestrogens are all physiopathological mechanisms, which can justify the decrease in BP verified with soybeans and soy-based products.

Although the beneficial effects of soybean, soy-based products, and their components are relatively well known, the exact mechanism or more likely the precise mechanisms, which are responsible for these actions, deserve future studies. In this sense, the complex network, which regulates interaction between adiponectin, NO, and oxidative stress, needs special attention.

REFERENCES

Ali, A. A. Velasquez, M. T., Hansen, C. T., Mohamed, A. I., Bhathena, S. J. 2004. Effects of soybean isoflavones, probiotics, and their interactions on lipid metabolism and endocrine system in an animal model of obesity and diabetes. *J Nutr Biochem* 15(10):583–590.

Allison, D. B., Gadbury, G., Schwartz, L. G. et al. 2003. A novel soy-based meal replacement formula for weight loss among obese individuals: A randomized controlled clinical trial. *Eur J Clin Nutr* 57(4):514–522.

Anderson, J. W., Johnstone, B. M., Cook-Newell, M. E. 1995. Meta-analysis of the effects of soy protein intake on serum lipids. *N Engl J Med* 333(5):276–282.

Agência Nacional de Vigilância Sanitária. 2008. Alimentos com alegações de propriedades funcionais e ou de saúde, novos alimentos/ingredientes, substâncias bioativas e probióticos. http://www.anvisa.gov.br/alimentos/comissoes/tecno_lista_alega.htm (accessed January 2014).

Ait-Oufella, H., Taleb, S., Mallat, Z. et al. 2011. Recent advances on the role of cytokines in atherosclerosis. *Arterioscler Thromb Vasc Biol* 31:969–979.

Appel, L. J., Brands, M. W., Daniels, S. R. et al. 2006. Dietary approaches to prevent and treat hypertension a scientific statement from the American Heart Association. *Hypertension* 47:296–308.

Azadbakht, L., Kimiagar, M., Mehrabi, Y., Esmaillzadeh, A., Hu, F. B., Willett, W. C. 2007. Soy consumption, markers of inflammation, and endothelial function: A cross-over study in postmenopausal women with the metabolic syndrome. *Diabetes Care* 30(4):967–973.

Azadbakht, L., Kimiagar, M., Mehrabi, Y. et al. 2007. Soy inclusion in the diet improves features of the metabolic syndrome: A randomized crossover study in postmenopausal women. *Am J Clin Nutr* 85:735–741.

Bahls, L. D., Venturini, D., Scripes, N. D. E. A. et al. 2011. Evaluation of the intake of a low daily amount of soybeans in oxidative stress, lipid and inflammatory profile, and insulin resistance in patients with metabolic syndrome. *Arq Bras Endocrinol Metab* 55(6):399–405.

Bai, Y., Lun, S., Yang, T., Sun, K., Chen, J., Hui, R. 2009. Increase in fasting vascular endothelial function after short-term oral L-arginine is effective when baseline flow-mediated dilatation is low: A meta-analysis of randomized trials. *Am J Clin Nutr* 89:77–84.

Bakhtiary, A., Yassin, Z., Hanachi, P., Rahmat, A., Ahmad, Z., Jalali, F. 2012. Effects of soy on metabolic biomarkers of cardiovascular disease in elderly women with metabolic syndrome. *Arch Iran Med* 15(8):462–468.

Beavers, K. M., Serra, M. C., Beavers, D. P., Cooke, M. B., Willoughby, D. S. 2010. Soy and the exercise-induced inflammatory response in postmenopausal women. *Appl Physiol Nutr Metab* 35:261–269.

Belleville, J. 2002. Hypocholesterolemic effect of soy protein. *Nutrition* 18(7–8):684–686.

Berg, A. H., Scherer, P. E. 2005. Adipose tissue, inflammation and cardiovascular disease. *Circ Res* 96:939–949.

Bertipaglia, D. S. M., Mandarino, M. G., Cardoso, J. R. et al. 2008. Association between soy and green tea (*Camellia sinensis*) diminishes hypercholesterolemia and increases total plasma antioxidant potential in dyslipidemic subjects. *Nutrition* 24(6):562–568.

Bhathena, S. J. 2000. Dietary fatty acids and fatty acid metabolism in diabetes. In: Chow, C. K., ed. *Fatty Acids in Food and Their Health Implications*, 2nd edn. New York: Marcel Dekker.

Bhathena, J., Velasquez, T. 2002. Beneficial role of dietary phytoestrogens in obesity and diabetes. *Am J Clin Nutr* 76(6):1191–1201.

Borodin, E. A., Menshikova, I. G., Dorovskikh, V. A. et al. 2009. Effects of two-month consumption of 30 g a day of soy protein isolate or skimmed curd protein on blood lipid concentration in Russian adults with hyperlipidemia. *J Nutr Sci Vitaminol* 55(6):492–497.

Carter, T. E. Jr., Nelson, R., Sneller, C. H., Cui, Z. 2004. Genetic diversity in soybean. In: Boerma, H. R., Specht, J. E., eds. *Soybeans: Improvement, Production and Uses*. Madison, WI: American Society of Agronomy.

Chambliss, K. L., Yuhanna, I. S., Anderson, R. G., Mendelsohn, M. E., Shaul, P. W. 2002. ERbeta has nongenomic action in caveolae. *Mol Endocrinol* 16(5):938–946.

Deckelbaum, R. J., Torrejon, C. 2012. The omega-3 fatty acid nutritional landscape: Health benefits and sources. *J Nutr* 142:587S–591S.

Deibert, P., König, D., Schmidt-Trucksaess, A. et al. 2004. Weight loss without losing muscle mass in pre-obese and obese subjects induced by a high-soy-protein diet. *Int J Obes Relat Metab Disord* 28:1349–1352.

Demonty, I., Lamarche, B., Deshaies, Y., Jacques, H. 2002. Role of soy isoflavones in the hypotriglyceridemic effect of soy protein in the rat. *J Nutr Biochem* 13(11):671–677.

Department of Health and Human Services. 1999. Food labeling: Health claims; soy protein and coronary heart disease. Food and Drug Administration, HHS. Final rule. *Fed. Regist* 64:57700–57733.

Dewell, A., Hollenbeck, C. B., Bruce, B. 2002. The effects of soy-derived phytoestrogens on serum lipids and lipoproteins in moderately hypercholesterolemic postmenopausal women. *J Clin Endocrinol Metab* 87(1):118–121.

Dharmappa, K. K., Mohamed, R., Shivaprasad, H. V., Vishwanath, B. S. 2010. Genistein, a potent inhibitor of secretory phospholipase A2: A new insight in down regulation of inflammation. *Inflammopharmacology* 18(1):25–31.

Djousse, L., Padilla, H., Nelson, T. L. 2010. Diet and metabolic syndrome. *Endocr Metab Immune Disord Drug Targets* 10:124–137.

Doerge, D. R., Sheehan, D. M. 2002. Goitrogenic and estrogenic activity of soy isoflavones. *Environ Health Perspect* 110(Suppl 3):349–353.

Douglas, G., Armitage, J. A., Taylor, P. D., Lawson, J. R., Mann, G. E., Poston, L. 2006. Cardiovascular consequences of life-long exposure to dietary isoflavones in the rat. *J Physiol* 571(2):477–487.

Duarte, A. C., Faillace, G., Wadi, M. T., Pinheiro, R. 2003. *Síndrome Metabólica: Semiologia, Bioquímica e Prescrição Nutricional*, 1 edn. Rio de Janeiro, Brazil: Axcel Books do Brasil.

Duranti, M., Lovati, M. R., Dani, V. et al. 2004. The alpha' subunit from soybean 7S globulin lowers plasma lipids and upregulates liver beta-VLDL receptors in rats fed a hypercholesterolemic diet. *J Nutr* 134(6):1334–1339.

Erdman, J. W. Jr. 2001. AHA Science Advisory: Soy protein and cardiovascular disease: A statement for healthcare professionals from the Nutrition Committee on the AHA. *Circulation* 102:2555–2559.

Esteves, E. A., Bressan, J., Costa, N. M. B., Martino, H. S. D., Donkin, S. S., Story, J. A. 2011. Modified soybean affects cholesterol metabolism in rats similarly to a commercial cultivar. *J Med Food* 14(11):1363–1369.

Feldeisen, S. E., Tucker, K. L. 2007. Nutritional strategies in the prevention and treatment of metabolic syndrome. *Appl Physiol Nutr Metab* 32:46–60.

Ferreira, E. D. E. S., Silva, M. A., Demonte, A., Neves, V. A. 2011. Soy beta-conglycinin (7S globulin) reduces plasma and liver cholesterol in rats fed hypercholesterolemic diet. *J Med Food* 14:94–100.

Ford, E. S., Giles, W. H., Dietz, W. H. 2002. Prevalence of the metabolic syndrome among US adults: Findings from the third national Health and Nutrition Examination Survey. *JAMA* 287:356–359.

Fukui, K., Kojima, M., Tachibana, N. et al. 2004. Effects of soybean beta-conglycinin on hepatic lipid metabolism and fecal lipid excretion in normal adult rats. *Biosci Biotechnol Biochem* 68(5):1153–1155.

Fuller, M. 2010. Sphingolipids: The nexus between Gaucher disease and insulin resistance. *Lipids Health Dis* 11(9):113.

Gornik, H. L., Creager, M. A. 2004. Arginine and endothelial and vascular health. *J Nutr* 134(10):2880–2887.

Hall, W. L., Vafeiadou, K., Kallund, J. 2006. Soy-isoflavone-enriched foods and markers of lipid and glucose metabolism in postmenopausal women: Interactions with genotype and equol production. *Am J Clin Nutr* 83:592–600.

Hanachi, P., Golkho, S. 2008. Assessment of soy phytoestrogens and exercise on lipid profiles and menopause symptoms menopausal women. *J Biol Sci* 8:789–793.

Harland, J. I., Haffner, T. A. 2008. Systematic review, meta-analysis and regression of randomised controlled trials reporting an association between an intake of circa 25 g soya protein per day and blood cholesterol. *Atherosclerosis* 200(1):13–27.

He, J., Gu, D., Wu, X. et al. 2005. Effect of soybean protein on blood pressure: A randomized controlled trial. *Arch Intern Med* 143:1–9.

Hu, S. S., Kong, L. Z., Gao, R. L. et al. 2010. Outline of the report on cardiovascular disease in China. *Biomed Environ Sci* 25(3):251–256.

Jacobs Jr., D. R. 2001. Executive summary of the third report of the National Cholesterol Education Program (NCEP) expert panel on detection, evaluation, and high blood cholesterol in adults (Adults Treatment Panel III). *JAMA* 285:2486–2497.

Jacobson, T. A. 2008. Role of n-3 fatty acids in the treatment of hypertriglyceridemia and cardiovascular disease. *Am J Clin Nutr* 87:1981S–1990S.

Jakobsen, M. U., O'reilly, E. J., Heitmann, B. L. et al. 2009. Major types of dietary fat and risk of coronary heart disease: A pooled analysis of 11 cohort studies. *Am J Clin Nutr* 89:1425–1432.

Jenkins, D. J. A., Kendall, C. W. C., Jackson, C. J. C. et al. 2002. Effects of high and low-isoflavone soy foods on blood lipids, oxidized LDL, homocysteine, and blood pressure in hyperlipidemic men and women. *Am J Clin Nutr* 76:365–372.

Jenkins, D. J. A., Mirrahimi, A., Srichaikul, K. et al. 2010. Soy protein reduces serum cholesterol by both intrinsic and food displacement mechanisms. *J Nutr* 140(12):2302–2311.

Jonas, J. C., Plant, T. D., Gilon, P., Detimary, P., Nenquin, M., Henquin, J. C. 1995. Multiple effects and stimulation of insulin secretion by the tyrosine kinase inhibitor genistein in normal mouse islets. *Br J Pharmacol* 114(4):872–880.

Kim, K., Lim, K. M., Kim, C. W. et al. 2011. Black soybean extract can attenuate thrombosis through inhibition of collagen-induced platelet activation. *J Nutr Biochem* 22(10):964–970.

Kim, S. M., Rico, C. W., Lee, S. C., Kang, M. Y. 2010. Modulatory effect of rice bran and phytic acid on glucose metabolism in high fat-fed C57BL/6N mice. *J Clin Biochem Nutr* 47(1):12–17.

Kip, K. E., Marroquin, O. C., Kelley, D. E. et al. 2004. Clinical importance of obesity versus the metabolic syndrome in cardiovascular risk in women: A report from the Women's Ischemia Syndrome Evaluation (WISE) study. *Circulation* 109:706–713.

Kunnen, S., Van Eck, M. 2012. Lecithin: Cholesterol acyltransferase: Old friend or foe in atherosclerosis? *J Lipid Res* 53(9):1783–1799.

Kwon, D. Y., Hong, S. M., Ahn, I. S., Kim, M. J., Yang, H. J., Park, S. 2011. Isoflavonoids and peptides from meju, long-term fermented soybeans, increase insulin sensitivity and exert insulinotropic effects in vitro. *Nutrition* (Burbank, Los Angeles County, Calif.) 27(2):244–252.

Lee, J. S. 2006. Effects of soy protein and genistein on blood glucose, antioxidant enzyme activities, and lipid profile in streptozotocin-induced diabetic rats. *Life Sci* 79(16):1578–1584.

Lee, S. H., Parka, H. J., Chuna, H. K., 2007. Dietary phytic acid improves serum and hepatic lipid levels in aged ICR mice fed a high-cholesterol diet. *Nutr Res* 27(8):505–510.

Lee, Y. H., Pratley, R. E. 2005. The evolving role of inflammation in obesity and the metabolic syndrome. *Curr Diabetes Rep* 5(1)70–75.

Li, R., Wang, W. Q., Zhang, H. et al. 2007. Adiponectin improves endothelial function in hyperlipidemic rats by reducing oxidative/ nitrative stress and differential regulation of eNOS/ iNOS activity. *Am J Physiol Endocrinol Metab* 293(6):E1703–E1708.

Liu, S., Hsieh, D., Yang, Y. L. et al. 2013. Coumestrol from the national cancer Institute's natural product library is a novel inhibitor of protein kinase CK2. *BCM Pharmacol Toxicol* 11(14):36. http://www.ncbi. nlm.nih.gov/pubmed?term=Xu%20Z%5BAuthor%5D&cauthor=true&cauthor_uid=23845105.

Liu, Z. M., Chen, Y. M., Ho, S. C., Ho, Y. P., Woo, J. 2010. Effects of soy protein and isoflavones on glycemic control and insulin sensitivity: A 6-mo double-blind, randomized, placebo-controlled trial in postmenopausal Chinese women with prediabetes or untreated early diabetes. *Am J Clin Nutr* 91:1394–1401.

Lutsey, P. L., Steffen, L. M., Stevens, J. 2008. Dietary intake and the development of the metabolic syndrome: The Atherosclerosis Risk in Communities study. *Circulation* 117:754–761.

Mac Donald, R. S., Guo, J., Copeland, J. et al. 2005. Environmental influences on isoflavones and saponins in soybeans and their role in colon cancer. *J Nutr* 135(5):1239–1242.

McVeigh, B. L., Dillingham, B. L., Lampe, J. W. 2006. Effect of soy protein varying in isoflavone content on serum lipids in healthy young men. *Am J Clin Nutr* 83:244–251.

Messina, M. 1995. Modern applications for an ancient bean: Soybeans and the prevention and treatment of chronic disease. *J Nutr* 125:567S–569S.

Messina, M., Messina, V. 2003. Provisional recommended soy protein and isoflavone intakes for healthy adults: Rationale. *Nutr Today* 38(3):100–109.

Messina, M. J., Persky, V., Setchell, K. D., Barnes, S. 1992. Soy intake and cancer risk: A review of the in vitro and in vivo data. *Nutr Cancer* 21(2):113–131.

Messina, V., Melina, V., Mangels, A. R. 2003. A new food guide for North American vegetarians. *J Am Diet Assoc.* 103(6):771–5.

Miller, V. M., Duckles, S. P. 2008. Vascular actions of estrogens: Functional implications. *Pharmacol Rev* 60(2):210–241.

Miyazawa, M., Sakano, K., Nakamura, S., Kosaka, H. 1999. Antimutagenic activity of isoflavones from soybean seeds (Glycine max merrill). *J Agric Food Chem* 47(4):1346–1349.

Moriyama, T., Kishimoto, K., Nagai, K., et al. 2004. Soybean beta-conglycinin diet suppresses serum triglyceride levels in normal and genetically obese mice by induction of beta-oxidation, downregulation of fatty acid synthase, and inhibition of triglyceride absorption. *Biosci Biotechnol Biochem.* 68(2):352–9.

Moutsatsou, P. 2007. The spectrum of phytoestrogens in nature: Our knowledge is expanding. *Hormones* 6:173–193.

Mozaffarian, D., Micha, R., Wallace, S. 2010. Effects on coronary heart disease of increasing polyunsaturated fat in place of saturated fat: A systematic review and meta-analysis of randomized controlled trials. *PLoS Med* 7(3):e1000252.

Normén, L., Dutta, P. Lia, A., Andersson, H. 2000. Soy sterol esters and beta-sitostanol ester as inhibitors of cholesterol absorption in human small bowel. *Am J Clin Nutr* 71(4):908–913.

Nwose, E. U., Richards, R. S., Digban, K. et al. 2013. Cardiovascular risk assessment in prediabetes and undiagnosed diabetes mellitus study: International collaboration research overview. *N Am J Med Sci* 5(11):625–630.

Nyby, M. D., Abedi, K., Eslami, P. et al. 2004. Dietary fish oil prevents hypertension, oxidative stress and suppression of endothelial nitric oxide synthase expression in fructose-fed rats. *Am J Hypertens* 17:216A.

Ohashi, K., Kihara, S., Ouchi, N. et al. 2006. Adiponectin replenishment ameliorates obesity-related hypertension. *Hypertension* 47:1108–1116.

Oku, T., Nakamura, M., Takasugi, A., Hashiguchi-Ishiguro, M., Tanabe, K., Nakamura, S. 2009. Effects of cake made from whole soy powder on postprandial blood glucose and insulin levels in human subjects. *Int J Food Sci Nutr* 60(s4):224–231.

Orshal, J. M., Khalil, R. A. 2004. Gender, sex hormones, and vascular tone. *Am J Physiol Reg Integr Comp Physiol* 286(2):R233–R249.

Ouchi, N., Ohishi, M., Kihara, S. et al. 2003. Association of hypoadiponectinemia with impaired vasoreactivity. *Hypertension* 42:231–234.

Pak, V. V., Kim, S. H., Koo, M., Lee, N., Shakhidoyatov, K. M., Kwon, D. Y. 2006. Peptide design of a competitive inhibitor for HMG-CoA reductase based on statin structure. *Biopolymers* (Peptide Science) 84:586–594.

Penha, L. A. O., Fonseca, I. C. B., Mandarino, J. M., Benassi, V. T. 2007. Soy as food: Nutritional value, health benefits and organic cultivation. *Bol Cent Pesqui Process Aliment* (Curitiba, PR) 25:91–102 (in Portuguese).

Rayalam, S., Della-Fera, A., Baile, A. A. 2008. Phytochemicals and regulation of adipocyte life cycle. *J Nutr Biochem* 19:717–726.

Reaven, G. M. 1988. Banting Lecture 1988: Role of insulin resistance in human disease. *Diabetes* 37:1595–1607.

Reilly, M. P., Rader, D. J. 2003. The metabolic syndrome: More than the sum of its parts? *Circulation* 108:1546–1551.

Repetto, G., Rizzolli, J., Bonatto, C. 2003. Prevalência, Riscos e Soluções na Obesidade e Sobrepeso: Here, There, and Everywhere. *Arq Bras Endocrinol Metab* 47(6):633–635.

Reynolds, K., Chin, A., Lees, K. A., Nguyen, A., Bujnowski, D., He, J. 2006. A meta-analysis of the effect of soy protein supplementation on serum lipids. *Am J Cardiol* 98(5):633–640.

Rishi, R. K. 2002. Phytoestrogens in health and illness. *Indian J Pharmacol* 34(5):311–320.

Rudkowska, I., Jones, P. J. 2007. Functional foods for the prevention and treatment of cardiovascular diseases: Cholesterol and beyond. *Expert Rev Cardiovasc Ther* 5(3):477–490.

Sacks, F. M., Lichtenstein, A., Van Rorn, L. 2006. Soy protein, isoflavones, and cardiovascular health: An American Heart Association science advisory for professionals from the Nutrition Committee. *Circulation* 113:1034–1044.

Sakai, T., Kogiso, M. 2008. Soy isoflavone and immunity. *J Med Invest* 55:167–173.

Shimabukuro, M., Higa, N., Asahi, T. et al. 2003. Hypoadiponectinemia is closely linked to endothelial dysfunction in men. *J Clin Endocrinol Metab* 88:3236–3240.

Simão, A. N. C., Lozovoy, M. A. B., Bahls, L. D. et al. 2012. Blood pressure decrease with ingestion of a soya product (kinako) or fish oil in women with the metabolic syndrome: Role of adiponectin and nitric oxide. *Br J Nutr* 108:1435–1442.

Simão, A. N. C., Lozovoy, M. A. B., Dichi, I. 2014. Effect of soy product kinako and fish oil on serum lipids and glucose metabolism in women with metabolic syndrome. *Nutrition* 30:112–115.

Simão, A. N., Lozovoy, M. A., Simão, T. N., Dichi, J. B., Matsuo, T., Dichi, I. 2010. Nitric oxide enhancement and blood pressure decrease in patients with metabolic syndrome using soy protein or fish oil. *J Clin Endocrinol Metab* 54(6):540–545.

Sirtori, C. R., Eberini, I., Arnoldi, A. 2007. Hypocholesterolaemic effects of soya proteins: Results of recent studies are predictable from the Anderson meta-analysis data. *Br J Nutr* 97(5):816–822.

Sirtori, C. R., Galli, C., Anderson, J. W., Arnoldi, A. 2009. Nutritional and nutraceutical approaches to dyslipidemia and atherosclerosis prevention: Focus on dietary proteins. *Atherosclerosis* 203(1):8–17.

Smiley, D. A., Khalil, R. A. 2009. Estrogenic compounds, estrogen receptors and vascular cell signaling in the aging blood vessels. *Curr Med Chem* 16(15):1863–1887.

Takahashi, T., Nakamura, A., Kato, M. et al. 2003. Soluble soybean fiber: A 3-month dietary toxicity study in rats. *Food Chem Toxicol* 41(8):1111–1121.

Takenaka, Y., Doyama, N., Maruyama, N., Utsumi, S., Yoshikawa, M. 2004. Introduction of DPR, an enterostatin fragment peptide, into soybean beta-conglycinin alpha' subunit by site-directed mutagenesis. *Biosci Biotechnol Biochem* 68(1):253–256.

Tan, K. C. B., Xu, A., Chow, W. S. et al. 2004. Hypoadiponectinemia is associated with impaired endothelium-dependent vasodilatation. *J Clin Endocrinol Metab* 89:765–769.

Teixeira Damasceno, N. R., Apolinário, E., Dias Flauzino, F., Fernandes, I., Abdalla, D. S. 2007. Soy isoflavones reduce electronegative low-density lipoprotein (LDL−) and anti-LDL−autoantibodies in experimental atherosclerosis. *Eur J Nutr* 46(3):125–132.

The American Soybean Association, 2014. http://soystats.com/international-world-soybean-production/ (Accessed March 21, 2014.)

Tilghman, S. L., Rhodes, L. V., Bratton, M. R. et al. 2013. Phytoalexins, miRNAs and breast cancer: A review of phytochemical-mediated miRNA regulation in breast cancer. *J Health Care Poor Underserved* 24(1 Suppl):36–46.

Torrezan, R., Gomes, R. M., Ferrarese, M. L. et al. 2008. Treatment with isoflavones replaces estradiol effect on the tissue fat accumulation from ovariectomized rats. *Arq Bras Endocrinol Metab* 52(9):1489–1496.

Vegeto, E., Benedusi, V., Maggi, A. 2008. Estrogen anti-inflammatory activity in brain: A therapeutic opportunity for menopause and neurodegenerative diseases. *Front Neuroendocrinol* 29(4):507–519.

Yang, G., Shu, X.-O., Jin, F. et al. 2005. Longitudinal study of soy intake and blood pressure among middle-aged and elderly Chinese women. *Am J Clin Nutr* 81:1012–1017.

Yoshikawa, M., Fujita, H., Matoba, N. et al. 2000. Bioactive peptides derived from food proteins preventing lifestyle-related diseases. *BioFactors* 12(1–4):143–146.

Zhan, S., Ho, S. C. 2005. Meta-analysis of the effects of soy protein containing isoflavones on the lipid profile. *Am J Clin Nutr* 81:397–408.

Ziemke, F., Mantzoros, C. S. 2010. Adiponectin in insulin resistance: Lessons from translational research. *Am J Clin Nutr* 91(1):258S–261S.

Zimmermann, M. C., Tilghman, S. L., Boue, S. M. et al. 2010. Glyceollin I, a novel antiestrogenic phytoalexin isolated from activated soy. *J Pharmacol Exp Ther* 332(1):35–45.

Zuloaga, K. L., O'Connor, D. T., Handa, R. J., Gonzales, R. J. 2012. Estrogen receptor beta dependent attenuation of cytokine-induced cyclooxygenase-2 by androgens in human brain vascular smooth muscle cells and rat mesenteric arteries. *Steroids* 77(8–9):835–844.

15 Omega-3 Polyunsaturated Fatty Acids and Metabolic Syndrome

Philip C. Calder

CONTENTS

15.1 INTRODUCTION

Metabolic syndrome (MetS) has been increasingly recognized over the last two decades, beginning with the description of insulin resistance syndrome, also known as syndrome X (Reaven, 1988). MetS is the combination of abdominal obesity with two out of three of dyslipidemia, hypertension, and hyperglycemia. The cutoff values used in defining MetS have been modified over the years (Table 15.1; National Cholesterol Education Program (NCEP) Expert Panel on Detection, 2001; Alberti et al., 2005, 2009). The number of people with MetS has increased over the last two decades, an increase that is directly associated with the increased prevalence of obesity (Zimmet et al., 2001). It is estimated that MetS affects 10%–25% of adults globally, although in some countries the percentage can be as high as 50% or 60% (Eckel et al., 2005). MetS increases the risk of type 2 diabetes and cardiovascular disease by five- and twofold, respectively (Ford, 2005; Galassi et al., 2006; Gami et al., 2007; Ford et al., 2008; Li et al., 2008; Mottillo et al., 2010; Wild and Byrne, 2011) (Figure 15.1). Hence, strategies to delay or slow the development of MetS or to treat its components are very valuable since they will reduce the risk of future severe disease and the associated personal, social, healthcare, and economic costs. Various pharmaceutical interventions are used to control, with significant success, dyslipidemia, hypertension, and hyperglycemia, so lowering future disease burden (Hanefield et al., 2011). However, diet plays a significant role in predisposition to obesity and also contributes to the development of dyslipidemia, hypertension, and hyperglycemia. Hence, dietary

TABLE 15.1
Cutoff Values for the Different Components of Metabolic Syndrome

	National Cholesterol Education Program (NCEP) Expert Panel on Detection (2001)	Alberti et al. (2005)	Alberti et al. (2009)
Central obesity (Waist circumference [cm])	>102 (men), >88 (women)	≥94 (European men), ≥90 (South Asian or Chinese men), ≥80 (women)	≥102 (North American men), ≥94 (European men), ≥90 (South Asian or Chinese men), ≥88 (North American women), ≥80 (women other than North American)
Blood pressure (mmHg)	≥130/85 or treatment	≥130/85 or treatment	≥130/85 or treatment
Fasting triglycerides (mmol/L)	≥1.7	≥1.7 or treatment	≥1.7 or treatment
Fasting HDL cholesterol (mmol/L)	<1.03 (men), <1.29 (women)	<1.03 (men), <1.29 (women) or treatment	<1.03 (men), <1.29 (women) or treatment
Fasting glucose (mmol/L)	≥6.1 (2001); ≥5.6 (2005)	≥5.6 or diagnosed with type 2 diabetes	≥5.6 or treatment

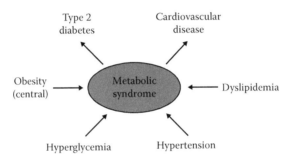

FIGURE 15.1   Scheme of the defining factors of metabolic syndrome and of its major health consequences.

advice is typically part of the strategy for promoting weight loss and for improving the profile of the other components of MetS (Te Morenga and Mann, 2011). Dietary advice is aimed at reducing calorie intake and the intake of less healthy dietary components such as saturated fat, simple sugars and salt and promoting the intake of more healthy components such as mono- and polyunsaturated fatty acids (PUFAs), and unrefined carbohydrates (Te Morenga and Mann, 2011). Amongst the most health promoting nutrients are omega-3 (n-3) PUFAs, particularly those found in seafood (Calder, 2014). This chapter provides an overview of the influence of n-3 PUFAs on the individual components of MetS and in persons with MetS. Prior to discussing these effects of n-3 PUFAs, relevant metabolic, nutritional, and functional aspects of n-3 PUFAs are described.

15.2   OMEGA-3 POLYUNSATURATED FATTY ACIDS

15.2.1   STRUCTURE AND METABOLISM

Omega-3 fatty acids are a family of PUFAs characterized by the position of the double bond closest to the methyl terminus of the hydrocarbon chain being on carbon number three (counting the methyl carbon as number one). Functionally, the most important n-3 fatty acids appear to be

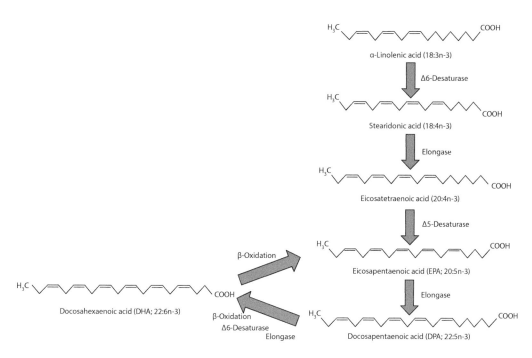

FIGURE 15.2   The pathway of biosynthesis of EPA, DPA, and DHA from α-linolenic acid.

eicosapentaenoic acid (EPA; 20:5n-3) and docosahexaenoic acid (DHA; 22:6n-3) (Calder, 2014), although the role of docosapentaenoic acid (DPA; 22:5n-3) is now also being reported (Kaur et al., 2011). Since they have long hydrocarbon chains, EPA, DPA, and DHA are sometimes termed very long chain n-3 fatty acids. EPA, DPA, and DHA are found in fairly high amounts in seafood, especially fatty fish (sometimes called "oily fish"), in supplements such as fish oils, cod liver oil, and krill oil, in some algal oils, and in a limited, but increasing, number of pharmaceutical-grade preparations. EPA, DPA, and DHA are related metabolically and there is a pathway by which EPA can be synthesized from simpler, plant-derived n-3 fatty acids (Figure 15.2). The initial substrate for this pathway is α-linolenic acid (18:3n-3), an essential fatty acid in animals. The pathway of the conversion of α-linolenic acid to EPA involves three steps, catalyzed in turn by delta-6 desaturase, elongase, and delta-5 desaturase (Figure 15.2). These enzymes are shared with the analogous omega-6 (n-6) fatty acid biosynthetic pathway of the conversion of linoleic acid (18:2n-6) to arachidonic acid (20:4n-6). Many Western diets have a much higher intake of linoleic than α-linolenic acid [EFSA Panel on Dietetic Products, Nutrition, and Allergies (NDA), 2010; Blasbalg et al., 2011] which favors linoleic acid conversion over that of α-linolenic acid. This may be one of the reasons why conversion of α-linolenic acid along this pathway occurs at a low rate (Burdge and Calder, 2006), although this rate may be affected by hormones, sex, genetics, age, and disease (see Calder, 2014 for references). The pathway for conversion of EPA to DHA involves several steps including an elongation to produce DPA and then a further elongation, a desaturation (catalyzed by delta-6 desaturase) and then one round of β-oxidation (Figure 15.2). It is also possible for DHA to be converted back to EPA by β-oxidation, a process sometimes referred to as retroconversion (Conquer and Holub, 1997).

15.2.2 DIETARY SOURCES AND INTAKES

As indicated earlier, seafood and products derived from seafood are good sources of EPA, DPA, and DHA. One typical adult size serving of fatty fish (e.g., mackerel, salmon, tuna, sardines, and herring) is able to provide 1–3 g of EPA + DPA + DHA, while a serving of lean fish (e.g., cod, haddock, and plaice) typically provides 0.1–0.4 g EPA + DPA + DHA. EPA, DPA, and DHA are also found in more modest amounts in animal-derived foods like eggs and meat. The relative distribution of EPA and DHA differs among foods, including fatty fish, such that some foods contain more EPA than DHA, while others contain more DHA than EPA. Because fatty fish are the richest dietary source of very long chain n-3 fatty acids, intake of those fatty acids is heavily influenced by fish consumption. In most Western countries, only a relatively small proportion of the population is regular consumers of fatty fish. Mean intakes of EPA+DPA+DHA among Western adult populations are considered to be around 0.1–0.3 g/day (Meyer et al., 2003; Scientific Advisory Committee on Nutrition/Committee on Toxicity, 2004; Howe et al., 2006; EFSA Panel on Dietetic Products, Nutrition, and Allergies [NDA], 2010; Rahmawaty et al. 2013; Papanikolaou et al., 2014), although those who rarely or never eat fatty fish will have a much lower intake than this.

EPA, DPA, and DHA are present in oils, supplements, and pharmaceutical-grade preparations. These vary according to very long chain n-3 fatty acid content. For example, cod liver oil and standard fish oil supplements contain about 30% of their fatty acids as EPA + DHA (i.e., about 300 mg/g oil), while concentrated n-3 supplements contain 45%–60% of their fatty acids as EPA + DHA, and the pharmaceutical preparation Omacor® (also known as Lovaza®) contains almost 90% EPA + DHA (in the ethyl ester form).

15.2.3 EPA AND DHA CONTENT OF DIFFERENT BODY LIPID POOLS

In common with other fatty acids, EPA and DHA are transported in the bloodstream esterified into more complex lipids like triacylglycerols (aka triglycerides; TGs), phospholipids, and cholesteryl esters as components of lipoproteins and noncovalently bound to albumin in the nonesterified form. EPA and DHA are stored in adipose tissue esterified into TGs and they are found in all cell membranes esterified into phospholipids and related complex lipids. Cell membrane phospholipids and their fatty acid composition are important in determining the physical characteristics of cell membranes (Stubbs and Smith, 1984), the way that membranes change in response to external stimuli (Brenner, 1984), and the functions of membrane-bound proteins like ion channels, receptors, and transporters (Murphy, 1990). The proportional contribution of EPA or DHA to the total fatty acids present within any of the transport, storage, or functional pools differs according to the pool (Browning et al., 2012). Most often, DHA is present in a greater proportion than EPA and within cell membranes EPA and DHA are distributed differently among the different phospholipid components. The typically reported contributions of EPA and DHA to lipids in human liver, skeletal muscle, heart, adipose tissue, and leukocytes are shown in Table 15.2.

Increased intakes of EPA and DHA from fish or from supplements are reflected in increased proportions of both fatty acids in blood lipid, blood cell, and many tissue pools. This has been reported many times for total plasma or serum lipids or for the complex lipid components of plasma or serum (i.e., TGs, phospholipids, and cholesteryl esters) and is also well described for erythrocytes, platelets, and leukocytes (see Calder, 2014 for references). There are also descriptions of increased proportions of EPA and DHA in human tissues, including liver, skeletal muscle, heart, and adipose tissue when their intake is increased (Table 15.2). Where different doses of n-3 PUFAs and/or different durations of intake have been studied, dose- and time-dependent incorporation of both EPA and DHA are seen (von Schacky et al., 1985; Blonk et al., 1990; Harris et al., 1991; Katan et al., 1997; Healy et al., 2000; Yaqoob et al., 2000; Rees et al., 2006; Browning et al., 2012). However, the precise pattern of intake and its time course and dose dependence depend upon the specific location being studied. As a generalization, pools that are turning over rapidly show faster incorporation of EPA and DHA than slower turning over pools. Recently, the time course of incorporation of EPA and DHA into human skeletal muscle (*Vastus lateralis*) was reported for healthy subjects consuming 3.5 g EPA plus 0.9 g DHA/day for 4 weeks (McGlory et al. 2014). The higher status of EPA and DHA achieved through increased intake of EPA and DHA is maintained while the increased

TABLE 15.2

Eicosapentaenoic Acid (EPA) and Docosahexaenoic Acid (DHA) Content of Lipid Pools in Selected Cells and Tissues Before and After Increased Intake of EPA and DHA

Tissue/Cell Type	Lipid Fraction	Without n-3 PUFA Intervention		Details of n-3 PUFA Intervention	After n-3 PUFA Intervention		References
		EPA	DHA		EPA	DHA	
Liver	Total	0.4	6.8	—			Araya et al. (2004)
	Phospholipid	4.8	15.1	—			Elizato et al. (2007)
	Total	1.4	6.3	—			Stephenson et al. (2013)
Adipose tissue	Total	0.2	0.2	13 g/week EPA + DHA for 1 year	0.3	0.4	Browning et al. (2012)
Skeletal muscle	Phospholipid	0.7	1.9	3.4 g/day EPA + DHA for 8 weeks	2.6	4.1	Smith et al. (2011)
	Total	0.6	1.5	4.4 g/day EPA + DHA for 4 weeks	2.4	2.1	McGlory et al. (2014)
Cardiac muscle	Total	0.2	1.5	1 g/day EPA + DHA for 6 months	0.6	2.3	Harris et al. (2004)
	Phospholipid	0.5	4.8	6 g/day EPA + DHA for 33 days	3.0	8.5	Metcalf et al. (2007)
	Phospholipid	0.7	5.7	—			Metcalf et al. (2010)
	Phosphatidylcholine	0.7	3.3	1.7 g/day EPA + DHA for 17 days	1.2	4.5	Saravanan et al. (2010)
Mononuclear cells	Total	0.3	2.8	3.2 g/day EPA + DHA for 12 weeks	3.6	4.9	Yaqoob et al. (2000)
	Total	0.8	1.9	3.3 g/week EPA + DHA for 12 months	0.9	2.3	Browning et al. (2012)
	Total	0.7	1.9	6.6 g/week EPA + DHA for 12 months	2.0	2.6	Browning et al. (2012)
	Total	0.7	1.9	13 g/week EPA + DHA for 1 year	2.3	3.3	Browning et al. (2012)

intake of EPA and DHA is maintained. If, after a period of increased intake of EPA and DHA, intake returns to the earlier lower levels then EPA and DHA status will decline, eventually returning to earlier levels. This is well described for blood lipids, platelets, leukocytes, and erythrocytes (see Calder, 2014 for references).

Since EPA and DHA content in lipid pools is frequently described as a percentage or proportion, the increase in content of these fatty acids is accompanied by a decrease in content (proportion) of other, usually unsaturated, fatty acids. Depending upon the pool, since once again there are differences among pools, these other fatty acids include oleic (18:1n-9), linoleic (18:2n-6), dihomo-γ-linolenic (20:3n-6), and arachidonic (20:4n-6) acids. There are good demonstrations of dose- and time-dependent decreases in the proportion of arachidonic acid in leukocytes and platelets (von Schacky et al., 1985; Healy et al., 2000; Rees et al., 2006; Browning et al., 2012), which might be functionally important with regard to platelet reactivity, blood clotting, and inflammation.

15.2.4 MOLECULAR AND CELLULAR ACTIONS OF EPA AND DHA

Many, though not all, of the functional effects of EPA and DHA relate to their incorporation into cell membrane phospholipids (Calder, 2012, 2013a,b, 2015). Since they are highly unsaturated, EPA and DHA have been shown, in some studies, to decrease membrane order (i.e., increase membrane fluidity) (Stubbs and Smith, 1984; Calder et al., 1994) and they create a specific environment for membrane proteins like receptors, transporters, ion channels, and signaling enzymes that influences the activity of those proteins (Brenner, 1984; Murphy, 1990; Miles and Calder, 1998). Through these actions, EPA and DHA modulate cell responses that are dependent upon membrane proteins. Cell membranes contain microdomains called rafts. These have specific lipid and fatty acid compositions and they act as platforms for receptor action and as sites where intracellular signaling pathways are initiated (Pike, 2003; Yaqoob, 2009; Simons and Gerl, 2010). EPA and DHA modify raft formation in a variety of cell types (Calder and Yaqoob, 2007; Yaqoob, 2009), although the exact effect varies according to cell type. Consequently, intracellular signaling pathways are modulated, leading to altered transcription factor activation and, subsequently, changed patterns of gene expression (Miles and Calder, 1998; Calder, 2012, 2013c). Several transcription factors have been shown to be affected by EPA and DHA including nuclear factor κ B (Novak et al., 2003), peroxisome proliferator-activated receptor-α and γ (Gottlicher et al., 1992; Krey et al., 1997), and the sterol regulatory element-binding proteins (Clarke, 2004; Lapillone et al., 2004; Deckelbaum et al., 2006; Jump, 2008). The effects of n-3 fatty acids on transcription factor activation and gene expression are central to their role in controlling inflammation, fatty acid and triacylglycerol metabolism, and adipocyte differentiation (Calder, 2012).

A second result of an increased amount of EPA and DHA in cell membrane phospholipids, and the associated decreased amount of arachidonic acid, is that they alter availability of substrates for synthesis of bioactive lipid mediators. The major substrate for the biosynthesis of various prostaglandins, thromboxanes, and leukotrienes, together termed eicosanoids, is usually arachidonic acid. These eicosanoids have well-established roles in regulation of inflammation, immunity, platelet aggregation, smooth muscle contraction, and renal function. Eicosanoids are oxidized derivatives of 20-carbon PUFAs and are produced via the cyclooxygenase (prostaglandins and thromboxanes), lipoxygenase (leukotrienes and other products), and/or cytochrome P450 pathways (Calder, 2015). Many disease processes involve excess or inappropriate production of eicosanoids from arachidonic acid. It is well described that increasing the EPA and DHA content of cell membranes results in decreased production of eicosanoids from arachidonic acid (see Calder, 2015 for references), resulting in an impact of EPA and DHA on inflammation, immune function, blood clotting, vasoconstriction, and bone turnover amongst other processes. As well as decreasing production of eicosanoids from arachidonic acid, EPA and DHA are themselves substrates for the synthesis of lipid mediators. Some of these are simply analogs of those produced from arachidonic acid. For example, prostaglandin E_3 produced from EPA is an analog of prostaglandin E_2 produced from arachidonic acid. Frequently, though not always, the EPA-derived mediator has weaker biological activity than the arachidonic acid–derived one (Wada et al., 2007). EPA and DHA are also substrates for more complex biosynthetic pathways that result in generation of a large number of mediators known as resolvins (E-series formed from EPA and D-series formed from DHA), protectins/neuroprotectins (formed from DHA), and maresins (formed from DHA) (Serhan et al., 2008a,b; Bannenberg and Serhan, 2010). It is now known that DPA also gives rise to similar mediators (Dalli et al., 2013). The major role of resolvins, protectins, and maresins appears to be in the resolution of inflammation and modulation of immune function and it seems likely that many of the anti-inflammatory actions of EPA and DHA are mediated through resolvins, protectins, and maresins.

These mechanisms of action of EPA and DHA rely upon incorporation of those fatty acids into cell membrane phospholipids. Extracellular unesterified EPA and DHA can also act directly via G-protein-coupled receptors (GPR) that exhibit some specificity for very long chain n-3 fatty acids over other fatty acids as ligands (Oh et al., 2010). In particular, GPR120, which is highly expressed on inflammatory macrophages and on adipocytes, was shown in cell culture experiments to play a central role in mediating anti-inflammatory effects of DHA on macrophages and insulin-sensitizing effects of DHA on adipocytes (Oh et al., 2010).

Through these mechanisms, EPA and DHA act to modify cell and tissue metabolism and functional responses to various stimuli (electrical, chemical, hormonal, and antigenic) in a way

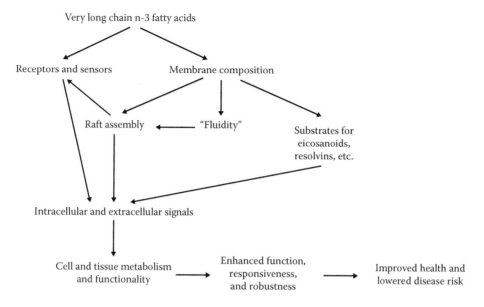

FIGURE 15.3 Overview of the general mechanisms by which n-3 PUFAs enhance cell and tissue metabolic and functional responses and thereby promote health and lowered disease risk.

that appears to benefit cell and tissue function, responsiveness, and robustness to challenge (Figure 15.3). Consequently, increased intake of EPA and DHA improves the disease risk factor profile indicating reduced risk, particularly for cardiometabolic diseases.

15.3 INFLUENCE OF OMEGA-3 FATTY ACIDS ON COMPONENTS OF METABOLIC SYNDROME

15.3.1 OMEGA-3 FATTY ACIDS AND BODY FATNESS

Many studies of supplemental n-3 PUFAs have reported body weight and body mass index as a way of characterizing the study population; the majority of these studies report no change in these measures with n-3 PUFAs. There are fewer reports of waist circumference, waist-to-hip ratio, or body fatness with increased n-3 PUFA intake. Some of the key studies are described in Table 15.3 and this area is discussed fully elsewhere (Buckley and Howe, 2010; Martinez-Victoria and Yago, 2012; Lorente-Cebrian et al., 2013). Most of these studies report no significant effect of n-3 PUFAs on body weight, body fat, or waist circumference (Table 15.3). However, some studies show that combining n-3 PUFAs with exercise or energy restriction is beneficial, with greater effects seen than with exercise or energy restriction alone (Table 15.3). In a study in overweight or obese insulin-resistant women, Krebs et al. (2006) investigated the effects of a low-fat, high-carbohydrate weight loss diet for 5 weeks with supplemental n-3 PUFAs or placebo followed by a gradual return to a maintenance diet over 7 weeks, which was then maintained for 12 weeks. Both groups lost weight (~12%) and body fat with no differences between them. Thorsdottir et al. (2007) combined energy restriction with supplemental n-3 PUFAs (or with lean or fatty fish) for 8 weeks in overweight or obese men and women. Weight loss and a reduction in waist circumference occurred in men consuming n-3 PUFAs. Taken together, these two studies suggest that n-3 PUFAs might aid fat and weight loss with energy restriction in men but not in women. This may relate to the different fat distribution between the sexes. Hill et al. (2007) compared the effects of exercise alone, n-3 PUFAs alone, and the combination of the two in overweight subjects. Body weight was decreased by exercise but not n-3 PUFAs, but the combination of exercise and n-3 PUFAs resulted in greater fat

TABLE 15.3
Selected Intervention Studies Evaluating the Effect of n-3 PUFAs on Body Weight and Fatness in Humans

References	Subjects	n-3 PUFA Dose and Duration	Findings with n-3 PUFAs
Couet et al. (1997)	Healthy (n=6)	1.8 g/day EPA + DHA; 3 weeks	No change in body weight; decreased body fat
Krebs et al. (2006)	Overweight/obese and insulin resistant (n=93)	Initial energy restricted diet (5 weeks) before gradual return to maintenance diet + 4.2 g/day EPA + DHA; 24 weeks	No change in body weight; no change in body fat
Kunesova et al. (2006)	Obese women (n=29)	Energy restricted diet + 2.8 g/day EPA + DHA + exercise; 4 weeks	Decreased body weight; decreased body mass index
Hill et al. (2007)	Overweight (n=65)	2 g/day EPA + DHA ± exercise; 12 weeks	Decreased body fat
Kabir et al. (2007)	Type 2 diabetic women (n=26)	1.8 g/day EPA + DHA; 2 months	No change in body weight; decreased body fat
Thorsdottir et al. (2007)	Overweight or obese (n=278)	Energy restricted diet + 1.3 g/day EPA + DHA; 8 weeks	Decreased body weight in men; decreased waist circumference in men
DeFina et al. (2011)	Overweight or obese (n=128)	3 g/day EPA + DHA + exercise; 24 weeks	No change in body weight; no change in body fat; no change in waist circumference
Munro and Garg (2012)	Obese (n=32)	Energy restricted diet + 2 g/day EPA + DHA; 14 weeks	No change in body weight
Munro and Garg (2013)	Obese (n=35)	Energy restricted diet + 2 g/day EPA + DHA; 12 weeks	No change in body weight; no change in body fat

loss than exercise alone. Kunesova et al. (2006) combined energy restriction and exercise in obese women who also took n-3 PUFAs or placebo. The group consuming n-3 PUFAs had slightly greater weight loss and greater reductions in body mass index and hip circumference. The effects of n-3 PUFAs could have been related to induction of β-oxidation. In summary, there is emerging evidence that n-3 PUFAs may promote loss of body fat and weight reduction, especially when combined with energy restriction, or exercise, or both. Nevertheless, a number of studies do not report weight or fat loss with n-3 PUFAs alone, and there is a need to explore these effects further to be clearer about the role that n-3 PUFAs may have.

15.3.2 OMEGA-3 FATTY ACIDS AND BLOOD PRESSURE

N-3 PUFAs affect many processes related to blood pressure including the production of eicosanoids with vasoactive effects (von Schacky et al., 1985), the secretion of aldosterone (Fischer et al., 2008), the generation of nitric oxide by the endothelium (Das, 2004), vascular reactivity (Engler et al., 2003), and cardiac hemodynamics (Mozaffarian, 2007). Acting through one or more, or perhaps all, of these mechanisms n-3 PUFAs could act to lower blood pressure. Indeed, a large number of studies have examined the effect of supplemental n-3 fatty acids on blood pressure in humans. Several meta-analyses of these studies have been conducted over the years (Appel et al., 1993; Morris et al., 1993; Geleijnse et al., 2002; Balk et al., 2004; Hartweg et al. 2007a), the most recent in 2014 (Miller et al., 2014). The findings of these meta-analyses are summarized in Table 15.4. It is evident that n-3 PUFAs can lower blood pressure in subjects with untreated hypertension and also in other types of subject including healthy normotensives (Table 15.4). The size of the effect in hypertensive subjects

TABLE 15.4
Summary of Meta-Analyses of Studies of the Effect of n-3 PUFAs on Blood Pressure (BP) in Humans

References	Number of Studies Included	Effect on Systolic BP (Δ mmHg [95% Confidence Interval])	Effect on Diastolic BP (Δ mmHg [95% Confidence Interval])	Comments
Appel et al. (1993)	17 (11 in normotensive subjects; 6 in untreated hypertensive subjects)	Normotensives: −1.0 (−2.0 to 0.0) Hypertensives: −5.5 (−8.1 to −2.9)	Normotensives: −0.5 (−1.2 to 0.2) Hypertensives: −3.5 (−5.0 to −2.1)	Doses of EPA + DHA used typically high (>3 g/day in 11 studies); BP reduction greater with higher starting BP
Morris et al. (1993)	31 (8 in healthy subjects; 6 in hypercholesterolemic subjects; 4 in patients with CVD; 13 in untreated hypertensive subjects)	Overall: −3.0 (−4.5 to −1.5) Healthy subjects: No effect Hypertensives: −3.4 Hypercholesterolemic: −4.1 CVD: −6.3	Overall: −1.5 (−2.2 to −0.8) Healthy subjects: No effect Hypertensives: −2.0 Hypercholesterolemic: −1.1 CVD: −2.9	Effect of n-3 PUFAs dose dependent; Both EPA and DHA related to BP lowering
Geleijnse et al. (2002)	36	Overall:−2.1 (−3.2 to −1.0)	Overall: −1.6 (−2.2 to −1.0)	Effect more likely in older or hypertensive subjects
Balk et al. (2004)	6 (in type 2 diabetics)	None	None	
Hartweg et al. (2007a)	5 (in type 2 diabetics)	−1.7 (−5.0 to 1.7)	−1.8 (−3.6 to −0.1)	
Miller et al. (2014)	70	Overall:−1.5 (−2.3 to −0.8) Normotensives:−1.3 (−2.1 to −0.5) Hypertensives:−4.5 (−6.1 to −2.8)	Overall : −1.0 (−1.5 to −0.4) Normotensives: −0.6 (−1.2 to −0.1) Hypertensives: −3.1 (−4.4 to −1.7)	

is 3–6 mmHg for systolic blood pressure and 1–4 mmHg for diastolic blood pressure (Table 15.4). The effect in normotensive subjects is rather smaller than this. Meta-analyses devoted to type 2 diabetics identify only a limited effect of n-3 PUFAs on blood pressure (Balk et al., 2004; Hartweg et al., 2007a) although some individual studies did find a blood pressure lowering effect, so this is an area that needs further exploration. It is important to note that most studies examining the blood pressure lowering effect of n-3 PUFAs have typically used high doses, often more than 3 g EPA + DHA/day. Such doses are difficult to achieve except through use of pharmaceutical preparations, and given that the effect of n-3 PUFAs is likely to be dose dependent (Morris et al., 1993), low doses may have little impact.

15.3.3 OMEGA-3 FATTY ACIDS AND BLOOD TRIGLYCERIDES AND HDL CHOLESTEROL

N-3 PUFAs have a range of molecular and metabolic actions that could influence blood lipid concentrations, particularly fasting TGs (as reviewed by Shearer et al., 2012). One important action is the reduced hepatic assembly and secretion of very-low-density lipoproteins (VLDL), which are the main TG-carrying lipoproteins in the fasting state. This effect comes about through a combination of actions including diversion of hepatic fatty acids toward β-oxidation and away from TG synthesis, inhibition of hepatic TG synthesis and downregulation of synthesis of apolipoprotein B100 required for VLDL assembly (see Shearer et al., 2012 for references). Hence, hepatic output of VLDL is decreased by n-3 PUFAs. There is evidence that n-3 PUFAs also upregulate the expression of lipoprotein lipase in adipose tissue (see Shearer et al., 2012), an effect that would promote TG clearance from the bloodstream. Nonesterified fatty acids (NEFAs) link TG metabolism in adipose tissue and liver. Hydrolysis of TGs stored in adipose tissue releases NEFAs into the circulation which become an important source of fatty acids for hepatic TG synthesis. There is evidence that n-3 PUFAs reduce NEFA output from the adipose tissue acting through metabolic effects, changing hormone sensitivity and reducing local inflammation (see Shearer et al., 2012); the latter serves to promote hydrolysis of stored TGs so liberating NEFAs (so contributing to hepatic TG production) and to prevent clearance of circulating TGs so contributing to hypertriglyceridemia. Finally, n-3 PUFAs promote β-oxidation in skeletal and cardiac muscle (Shearer et al., 2012) drawing circulating NEFAs away from the liver. Acting through one or more, or perhaps all, of these mechanisms n-3 PUFAs could act to lower blood TG concentrations. In turn, this could affect the concentrations of other blood lipids, like high-density lipoproteins (HDL).

A large number of studies have examined the effect of supplemental n-3 fatty acids on fasting blood TG concentrations. Indeed as long ago as 1996, Harris provided an overview of 72 placebo-controlled studies of n-3 PUFAs and fasting plasma TG concentrations in humans. He concluded that n-3 PUFAs lowered TGs by 25% in subjects with starting fasting TGs <2 mmol/L and by 28% in those with starting fasting TGs ≥2 mmol/L (Harris, 1996). Subsequently, several meta-analyses of such studies have been published (Harris 1997; Balk et al., 2006) including some devoted to type 2 diabetics (Montori et al., 2000; Hartweg et al., 2007b, 2008) as summarized in Table 15.5. It is evident that n-3 PUFAs can lower fasting TG concentrations by 25%–30% in persons with either low or high starting TG concentrations and in type 2 diabetics. However, there is evidence that a greater effect is seen with a higher starting TG concentration (Montori et al., 2000; Balk et al., 2004, 2006). Once again, doses of n-3 PUFAs used in many studies of TG lowering have been high, and there is clear evidence that the TG lowering effect of n-3 PUFAs is dose dependent (Roche, 1999; Balk et al., 2004, 2006). Several studies have attempted to establish whether EPA or DHA is responsible for the TG-lowering effect of mixed n-3 PUFA preparations. Mori et al. (2000) reported a 20% reduction in fasting TGs with 4 g/day DHA over 6 weeks and an 18% reduction with 4 g/day EPA in mildly hypertriglyceridemic subjects. Woodman et al. (2002) using the same study design found 19% reduction of fasting TGs with DHA and 15% with EPA in type 2 diabetics. In a study using almost 5 g/day EPA or DHA for 4 weeks in healthy subjects, Buckley et al. (2004) found 22% reduction of fasting TGs with DHA and 15% reduction with EPA. Thus, there is quite consistent

TABLE 15.5

Summary of Meta-Analyses of Studies of the Effect of n-3 PUFAs on Fasting Blood Triglyceride (TG) and High-Density Lipoprotein Cholesterol (HDL-C) Concentrations in Humans

References	Number of Studies Included	Effect on Fasting TG (%Δ [95% Confidence Interval])	Effect on Fasting HDL-C (%Δ [95% Confidence Interval])	Comments
Harris (1997)	36 cross over design studies and 32 parallel design studies	Cross over design with starting TG <2 mmol/L: −25.2 Cross over design with starting TG ≥2 mmol/L: −33.8 Parallel design with starting TG <2 mmol/L: −25.4 Parallel design with starting TG ≥2 mmol/L: −25.2	Cross over design with starting TG <2 mmol/L: 2.9 Cross over design with starting TG ≥2 mmol/L: 1.2 Parallel design with starting TG <2 mmol/L: 2.8 Parallel design with starting TG ≥2 mmol/L: −0.1	Doses of EPA + DHA used typically high (~3–4 g/day); Total cholesterol was little changed; Low-density lipoprotein cholesterol was increased by 4.5% in subjects with TG <2 mmol/L and by 5%–10% in subjects with TG ≥2 mmol/L
Montori et al. (2000)	14 (in diabetics) for TG; 12 (in diabetics) for HDL-C	%Δ not given; −0.56 mmol/L (−0.71 to −0.41); larger effect in hypertriglyceridemic subjects (−0.73 mmol/L (−0.95 to −0.51)); larger effect with higher doses (−0.85 mmol/L (−1.44 to −0.26))	%Δ not given; 0.02 mmol/L (0.01–0.05)	Total cholesterol (13 studies) was not affected (0.01 mmol/L (−0.13 to 0.15); Low-density lipoprotein cholesterol (10 studies) was increased by 0.21 mmol/L (0.02–0.41)
Balk et al. (2006)	17	−27 (−33 to −20)	1.6 (0.8–2.3)	Total cholesterol (19 studies) was not affected (0% change (−1 to 2); Low-density lipoprotein cholesterol (13 studies) was increased by 6% (3–8)
Hartweg et al. (2007b)	18 (in diabetics) for TG; 16 (in diabetics) for HDL-C	−25 (equivalent to −0.45 mmol/L (−0.58 to −0.32))	~2 (equivalent to 0.02 mmol/L (−0.01 to 0.06)	Total cholesterol (17 studies) was not affected (~0% change); Low-density lipoprotein cholesterol (16 studies) was increased by ~3.5% (equivalent to 0.11 mmol/L (0–0.22))
Hartweg et al. (2008)	18 (in diabetics) for TG; 16 (in diabetics) for HDL-C	%Δ not given; −0.45 mmol/L (−0.58 to −0.32)	%Δ not given; 0.02 mmol/L (−0.01 to 0.06)	Total cholesterol (16 studies) was not affected (−0.02 mmol/L (−0.15 to 0.11); Low-density lipoprotein cholesterol (16 studies) was increased by 0.11 mmol/L (0.00–0.22)

evidence that both EPA and DHA lower fasting blood TG concentration but that DHA is a little more effective.

The ability of n-3 PUFAs to lower fasting TG concentrations reflects their impact of fatty acid, TG, and TG-rich lipoprotein metabolism as outlined ealier. Such effects will also modify metabolism of lipoproteins other than those rich in TGs. Consequently, n-3 PUFAs have been reported to also alter the concentrations of cholesterol and cholesterol-carrying lipoproteins including high-density lipoprotein (HDL). The findings of meta-analyses of the effect of n-3 PUFAs on total cholesterol, HDL cholesterol (HDL-C), and low-density lipoprotein cholesterol (LDL-C) are shown in Table 15.5. They reveal a fairly consistent 1%–3% increase in fasting HDL-C concentration. However, there is also a consistent 2.5%–10% elevation in LDL-C concentration. Suzukawa et al. (1995) reported that n-3 PUFAs increased LDL particle size. Mori et al. (2000) found that 4 g/day DHA, but not EPA, elevated LDL-C (by 8%) and that this was associated with a larger LDL particle size. Likewise, Woodman et al. (2003) found that DHA, but not EPA, increased LDL particle size in type 2 diabetics, whereas Neff et al. (2011) reported that DHA increased the concentration of large LDL particles and decreased the concentration of small LDL particles. Because of these observations, it is argued that the potentially deleterious effect of raised LDL-C concentration after increased intake of n-3 PUFAs is negated by the beneficial increase in LDL particle size, since larger particles are less likely to permeate the blood vessel wall and so are considered to be less atherogenic.

15.3.4 Omega-3 Fatty Acids and Blood Glucose

A number of molecular and metabolic actions of n-3 PUFAs may be useful in maintaining and improving glucose homeostasis (see Flachs et al., 2014). N-3 PUFA-mediated improvements in inflammation and effects on insulin signaling pathways in adipose tissue and skeletal muscle enhance insulin sensitivity, thus promoting more efficient glucose removal from the circulation. Coupled with this, lower blood NEFA concentrations that result from improved insulin sensitivity permit more efficient glucose utilization. Hence, n-3 PUFAs would be expected to result in a lower fasting blood glucose concentration. A large number of studies have examined the effect of supplemental n-3 fatty acids on fasting blood glucose concentrations. These studies have been performed in healthy subjects, type 2 diabetics, hyperlipidemics, and patients with cardiovascular disease. Meta-analyses of the effects of supplemental n-3 PUFAs on fasting blood glucose concentration are shown in Table 15.6. None of the meta-analyses identified a significant effect of n-3 PUFAs on fasting blood glucose (or on HbA1c) (Table 15.6). Nevertheless, some individual studies do report a significant elevation in blood glucose, perhaps related to the high doses of n-3 PUFAs used. In their study of 4 g/day EPA or DHA for 6 weeks in mildly hyperlipdemic men, Mori et al. (2000)

TABLE 15.6

Summary of Meta-Analyses of Studies of the Effect of n-3 PUFAs on Fasting Blood Glucose Concentration in Humans

References	Number of Studies Included	Effect on Fasting Glucose (Δ[95% Confidence Interval])	Comments
Montori et al. (2000)	12 (in diabetics)	0.26 mmol/L (−0.08 to 0.60)	HbA1c (11 studies) increased by 0.15% (−0.08 to 0.37)
Balk et al. (2006)	17	3% (−0.2 to 6)	HbA1c (18 studies) increased by 0.1% (−0.01 to 0.20)
Hartweg et al. (2008)	21 (in diabetics)	0.16 mmol/L (−0.13 to 0.46)	HbA1c (15 studies) increased by 0.01% (−0.03 to 0.01)

found that EPA, but not DHA, tended to increase fasting glucose. Woodman et al. (2002) reported elevations of fasting glucose with 4 g/day EPA or DHA in type 2 diabetics (increases of 1.40 and 0.98 mmol/L, respectively).

15.4 TRIALS OF OMEGA-3 FATTY ACIDS IN PEOPLE WITH METABOLIC SYNDROME

The previous section described the findings of studies, or of meta-analyses of studies, in which n-3 PUFAs have been examined for their effects on outcomes that form part of the definition of MetS (body fatness, dyslipidemia, hypertension, and hyperglycemia). A large number of studies have reported on these outcomes, with many reporting favorable effects, particularly with regard to dyslipidemia and hypertension. These studies were conducted in a broad range of population subgroups including healthy subjects, overweight and/or obese subjects, hyperlipidemics, hypertensives, type 2 diabetics, and patients with cardiovascular disease. Many of these studies have not claimed to have been conducted in people with MetS, although it is likely that many subjects included in these studies, and in some cases probably all subjects, had MetS. The findings are suggestive that n-3 PUFAs, at sufficient dose and for sufficient duration, could be very useful for improving the risk factor profile in people with MetS. This, would, in turn, be expected to reduce the risk of developing type 2 diabetes and cardiovascular disease. Some studies have specifically evaluated n-3 PUFAs in people with MetS.

Satoh et al. (2007) randomized obese type 2 diabetics (who met the criteria for MetS) to dietary modification or dietary modification plus 1.8 g/day EPA (as a near-pure ethyl ester) for 3 months. The EPA group showed decreases in fasting TG, total cholesterol, LDL-C, small, dense LDL, and C-reactive protein (CRP) concentrations, but there was no effect on body mass index (BMI), or fasting plasma glucose, HbA1c, insulin, or HDL-C concentrations. In a second study with the same design and performed in obese dyslipidemics who met the criteria for MetS, Satoh et al. (2009) demonstrated the EPA decreased fasting TG and CRP concentrations, but did not affect BMI, waist circumference, blood pressure, or fasting blood glucose, insulin, HbA1c, cholesterol, HDL-C, or LDL-C concentrations. EPA did increase adiponectin concentration and improved arterial stiffness. Simão et al. (2010) conducted a controlled study of n-3 PUFAs (3 g/day EPA + DHA for 3 months) in subjects with MetS. N-3 PUFAs decreased fasting TG concentration but increased fasting blood glucose, total cholesterol, and LDL-C concentrations and worsened insulin resistance. Most recently, Tousoulis et al. (2014) reported the effects of 1.8 g/day EPA + DHA for 12 weeks in subjects with MetS. N-3 PUFAs decreased fasting blood TG, total cholesterol, LDL-C, glucose, and interleukin (IL)-6 concentrations and improved flow-mediated dilation and carotid-femoral pulse wave velocity. HDL-C concentration was not affected. The LIPGENE study, which involved a dose of 1.24 g/day EPA + DHA for 12 weeks, reported a favorable effect on the LDL phenotype with a shift away from small dense LDL (Hartwich et al., 2009) and a decrease in fasting TG concentration (Tierney et al., 2011). However, there was no effect on blood pressure (Gulseth et al., 2010; Tierney at al., 2011), total cholesterol, or LDL-C concentrations (Tierney et al., 2011) or on blood markers of inflammation (Petersson et al., 2010; Tierney et al., 2011).

Taken together, these studies consistently demonstrate that n-3 PUFAs are able to decrease fasting blood TG concentration in people with MetS. However, these studies do not reveal strong or consistent effects of n-3 PUFAs on obesity, blood pressure, or fasting blood glucose in people with MetS. The lack of a blood pressure lowering effect in these studies most likely relates to the low dose of n-3 PUFAs, which is typically less than the doses used in studies revealing a hypotensive effect of n-3 PUFAs. The lack of effect of n-3 PUFAs on obesity and fasting blood glucose is consistent with studies described earlier. Thus, amongst the criteria used to define MetS, n-3 PUFAs (at the doses that have been used) are effective at beneficially modifying one (fasting TGs) but not the others. However, the studies in MetS reveal benefits of n-3 PUFAs on outcomes beyond those that are used within the MetS definition. For example, n-3 PUFAs are reported to beneficially modify LDL phenotype, inflammation, and blood flow in people with MetS. Therefore, n-3 PUFAs may have a range of benefits in people with MetS. However, the potential for n-3 PUFAs to worsen insulin resistance, as reported by Simão et al. (2010), needs further investigation and greater understanding.

15.5 OMEGA-3 FATTY ACIDS, INFLAMMATION, OBESITY, AND METABOLIC SYNDROME

15.5.1 Adipose Tissue as a Source of Inflammatory Mediators

Obesity, particularly abdominal obesity, is a requisite criterion of MetS, and being obese, especially abdominally obese, confers significant cardiometabolic risk on the individual. The reason for this appears to be the combination of inflammation and insulin resistance that accompanies obesity. Obese people have higher blood concentrations of several proinflammatory mediators than seen in normal weight people. Among the inflammatory markers with elevated concentrations are tumor necrosis factor (TNF)-α, IL-6, monocyte chemoattractant protein (MCP)-1, IL-18, and CRP (Müller et al., 2002; Herder et al., 2005, 2006). There is a positive relationship between body mass index and other measures of obesity such as waist circumference and circulating concentrations of CRP and other inflammatory markers (Kim et al., 2006). Thus, inflammation is worse in those who are abdominally obese. A reduction in concentrations of numerous inflammatory molecules has been observed during weight loss programs and with bariatric surgery, clearly demonstrating the relation between excess adipose tissue and inflammation (see Calder et al., 2011 for references).

Adipose tissue itself produces and secretes a broad range of inflammatory mediators including cytokines, chemokines, and acute-phase proteins (Hotamisligil et al., 1993; Trayhurn and Wood, 2004: Calder et al., 2011) and this production and secretion appears to be greater for abdominal adipose tissue. Immune cells, including inflammatory macrophages, accumulate in adipose tissue and this accumulation is enhanced in obesity (Wellen and Hotamisligl, 2003; Tilg and Moschen, 2006). Macrophages are considered to be the major sources of the cytokines and chemokines released from adipose tissue (Figure 15.4), although adipocytes and infiltrating immune cells other than

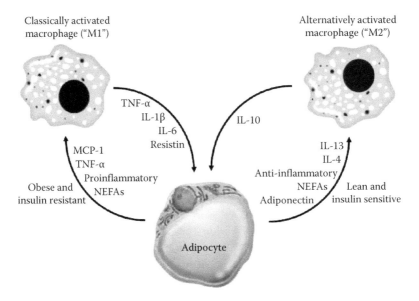

FIGURE 15.4 Interaction between the macrophage and the adipocyte. IL, interleukin; MCO, monocyte chemoattractant protein; NEFAs, nonesterified fatty acids; TNF, tumor necrosis factor.

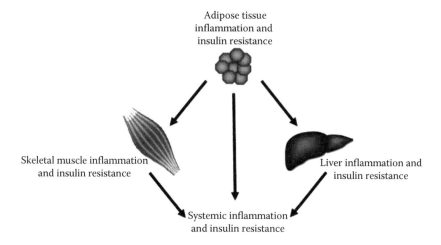

FIGURE 15.5   Central role of adipose tissue inflammation in causing metabolic and functional abnormalities in other tissues.

macrophages (e.g., T cells) are also active in this regard (Trujillo and Scherer, 2006). Inflammatory cytokines play a role in causing insulin resistance because they downregulate factors involved in insulin signaling (de Luca and Olefsky, 2008). In addition to cytokines and chemokines, a number of hormones released from adipose tissue play roles in inflammation. For example, leptin is proinflammatory while adiponectin is anti-inflammatory and insulin sensitizing (Gil-Campos et al., 2004; Stofkova, 2009). Macrophages within adipose tissue are of two distinct phenotypes (Figure 15.4). The M1 macrophage produces high amounts of inflammatory mediators and seems to be associated with obesity and insulin resistance, while the M2 macrophage is anti-inflammatory. Research in mice indicates that excessive weight gain is accompanied by transformation from the M2 to the M1 phenotype (Lumeng et al., 2007).

Inflammatory mediators are probably the link between adipose tissue and obesity and cardio-metabolic risk (Figure 15.5) (Chen, 2006; Matsuzawa, 2006a,b; Malavazos et al., 2005, 2007). In the obese state, local activated macrophages dominate synthesis and secretion, which leads to spillover of inflammatory mediators into the general circulation, resulting in induction of insulin resistance in the main metabolic tissues (Figure 15.5). Hence, adipose tissue inflammation could be a valuable target to reduce cardiometabolic risk in the overweight and obese, including those with MetS.

15.5.2   N-3 PUFAs and Adipose Tissue Inflammation

N-3 PUFAs exert anti-inflammatory effects through several mechanisms (Calder, 2012, 2013a,b, 2015). Thus, they may be useful in controlling or decreasing inflammation within adipose tissue, an effect that could have potential benefit in reducing co-morbidities of obesity and MetS. Despite the long recognition of the anti-inflammatory effects of n-3 PUFAs, there are few studies of n-3 PUFAs and adipose tissue inflammation in humans. Kabir et al. (2007) provided 1.8 g/day EPA + DHA to nonhypertriglyceridemic women with type 2 diabetes for 2 months. Subcutaneous adipocyte diameter was decreased by 6% in the n-3 PUFA group and did not change in the control group. Adipose tissue expression of 12 genes was upregulated with n-3 PUFA treatment and thirteen genes were downregulated. Most of these were genes associated with metabolism, although mRNAs for matrix metalloproteinase 9 and for some macrophage markers were lower with n-3 PUFA treatment. MCP-1 mRNA was not affected by n-3 PUFAs.

Itariu et al. (2012) gave severely obese nondiabetic patients 3.4 g/day EPA+DHA for 8 weeks and measured inflammatory gene expression in visceral and subcutaneous adipose tissue. The n-3 PUFA group showed lower mRNA for MCP-1 and macrophage inhibitory protein-1α in subcutaneous adipose tissue than in the control group and there were trends toward lower IL-6 and higher adiponectin mRNA. Finally, expression of the M1 macrophage marker CD40 was lower in subcutaneous adipose tissue in the n-3 PUFA group. Most recently, Spencer et al. (2013) studied the effect of 3.6 g/day EPA + DHA for 12 weeks in nondiabetic subjects with impaired glucose tolerance, elevated fasting glucose or at least there features of MetS. The n-3 PUFA group showed a reduction in number of macrophages in abdominal adipose tissue and decreased level of mRNA for MCP-1 and for the macrophage marker CD68. There was no effect of n-3 PUFAs on expression of a number of other inflammatory genes including those for several cytokines and chemokines. These three studies report that n-3 PUFAs alter expression of specific inflammatory genes in human adipose tissue, but the exact genes influenced vary among studies and all three studies found that most inflammatory genes were not affected. The differences seen among these studies and the absence of a generalized "anti-inflammatory" effect may reflect: (a) differences in doses of n-3 PUFA used; (b) differences between the adipose depots studied; (c) differences in phenotype of the individuals studied; (d) the short duration of intervention in each of these studies; and (e) differences in, and the generally small, sample size. It may require longer than two or three months for n-3 PUFAs to sufficiently permeate adipose tissue (Katan et al., 1997; Browning et al., 2012) and to induce changes in gene expression and functional activity of adipocytes and macrophages. In contrast to the generally encouraging findings of these three studies, Kratz et al. (2013) saw no effect of increased intake of n-3 PUFAs for 14 weeks on inflammatory gene expression in subcutaneous adipose tissue from overweight to mildly obese men and women. This result again may reflect the relatively short duration of intervention but may also relate to the type of subjects studied who were generally more healthy than those in the other studies. It seems important to conduct larger studies of sufficient duration (perhaps more than 6 months) and to compare effects of n-3 PUFAs in subcutaneous and visceral adipose depots.

15.6   SUMMARY AND CONCLUSIONS

MetS is the combination of abdominal obesity with two out of three of dyslipidemia, hypertension, and hyperglycemia. When their intake is increased, the n-3 PUFAs EPA and DHA are incorporated into cell membranes in metabolic tissues like skeletal and heart muscle and most probably liver also, and they are stored in adipose tissue. A higher EPA and DHA status affects many molecular aspects of cell and tissue function influencing activities from the membrane to the nucleus and altering the profile of lipid mediators produced by inflammatory cells. These molecular changes result in altered cell function and in improved cell and tissue responsiveness, and they impact on metabolic activities, inflammation, and insulin sensitivity. Consequently, n-3 PUFAs have the potential to improve the metabolic and functional abnormalities that contribute to MetS. A large number of human intervention studies have investigated effects of supplemental n-3 PUFAs on outcomes that form part of the definition of MetS (body fatness; dyslipidemia; hypertension; hyperglycemia). Many of these studies report favorable effects of n-3 PUFAs on dyslipidemia, especially on fasting blood TG concentrations, which can be lowered by as much as 20%–30%, and on hypertension. Both EPA and DHA decrease fasting blood TG, although DHA has a stronger effect than EPA. Studies of n-3 PUFAs and blood lipids or blood pressure have often used high doses and effects seen are dose dependent. The LDL-C raising effect of n-3 PUFAs may be negated by an increase in LDL particle size, so producing less atherogenic LDLs. N-3 PUFAs appear not to affect body fatness but, through mechanisms that are not clear, they may enhance the effects of caloric restriction or exercise on body fatness. N-3 PUFAs seem not to lower fasting blood glucose and may even increase it, which would be an undesirable effect. N-3 PUFAs have a number of effects beyond the defining components of MetS such as improving vascular function and blood flow, decreasing inflammation, and increasing LDL particle size. Thus, n-3 PUFAs seem to favorably modify a range of factors involved in future cardiometabolic disease risk, although the potential for elevating blood glucose is a concern that needs to be better understood. Adipose tissue itself may contribute to cardiometabolic disease risk through release of inflammatory mediators that induce systemic inflammation and local and systemic insulin resistance. A small number of recent studies suggest that n-3 PUFAs may decrease inflammation within adipose tissue. However, these studies are limited by short duration and limited sample size and the exact findings are inconsistent. This will be an important area for future research, since modifying adipose tissue inflammation could be a key central mechanism of action of n-3 PUFAs.

In summary, n-3 PUFAs have been consistently demonstrated to improve fasting blood TG concentrations and to favorably modify other lipid-related factors in a variety of subgroups including people with MetS. They have little impact on the other defining features of MetS but they favorably modify several other factors of relevance to MetS and its progression to type 2 diabetes and cardiovascular disease. Effects of n-3 PUFAs on adipose tissue inflammation are of great interest and warrant further research.

REFERENCES

Alberti, K.G., Eckel, R.H., Grundy, S.M. et al. 2009. Harmonizing the metabolic syndrome: A joint interim statement of the International Diabetes Federation Task Force on Epidemiology and Prevention; National Heart, Lung, and Blood Institute; American Heart Association; World Heart Federation; International Atherosclerosis Society; and International Association for the Study of Obesity. *Circulation* 120:1640–1645.

Alberti, K.G., Zimmet, P., Shaw, J., IDF Epidemiology Task Force Consensus Group. 2005. The metabolic syndrome—A new worldwide definition. *Lancet* 366:1059–1062.

Appel, L.J., Miller, E.R. 3rd, Seidler, A.J., Whelton, P.K. 1993. Does supplementation of diet with 'fish oil' reduce blood pressure? A meta-analysis of controlled clinical trials. *Archives of Internal Medicine* 153:1429–1438.

Araya, J., Rodrigo, R., Videla, L.A. et al. 2004. Increase in long-chain polyunsaturated fatty acid n-6/n-3 ratio in relation to hepatic steatosis in patients with non-alcoholic fatty liver disease. *Clinical Science* 106:635–643.

Balk, E., Chung, M., Lichtenstein, A. et al. 2004. Effects of omega-3 fatty acids on cardiovascular risk factors and intermediate markers of cardiovascular disease. *Evidence Report/Technology Assessment (Summary)* 93:1–6.

Balk, E.M., Lichtenstein, A.H., Chung, M., Kupelnick, B., Chew, P., Lau, J. 2006. Effects of omega-3 fatty acids on serum markers of cardiovascular disease risk: A systematic review. *Atherosclerosis* 189:19–30.

Bannenberg, G., Serhan, C.N. 2010. Specialized pro-resolving lipid mediators in the inflammatory response: An update. *Biochimica et Biophysica Acta* 1801:1260–1273.

Blasbalg, T.L., Hibbeln, J.R., Ramsden, C.E., Majchrzak, S.F., Rawlings, R.R. 2011. Changes in consumption of omega-3 and omega-6 fatty acids in the United States during the 20th century. *American Journal of Clinical Nutrition* 93:950–962.

Blonk, M.C., Bilo, H.J., Popp-Snijders, C., Mulder, C., Donker, A.J. 1990. Dose-response effects of fish oil supplementation in healthy volunteers. *American Journal of Clinical Nutrition* 52:120–127.

Brenner, R.R. 1984. Effect of unsaturated fatty acids on membrane structure and enzyme kinetics. *Progress in Lipid Research* 23:69–96.

Browning, L.M., Walker, C.G., Mander, A.P. et al. 2012. Incorporation of eicosapentaenoic and docosahexaenoic acids into lipid pools when given as supplements providing doses equivalent to typical intakes of oily fish. *American Journal of Clinical Nutrition* 96:748–758.

Buckley, J.D., Howe, P.R. 2010. Long-chain omega-3 polyunsaturated fatty acids may be beneficial for reducing obesity-a review. *Nutrients* 2:1212–1230.

Buckley, R., Shewring, B., Turner, R., Yaqoob, P., Minihane, A.M. 2004. Circulating triacylglycerol and apoE levels in response to EPA and docosahexaenoic acid supplementation in adult human subjects. *British Journal of Nutrition* 92:477–483.

Burdge, G.C., Calder, P.C. 2006. Dietary α-linolenic acid and health-related outcomes: A metabolic perspective. *Nutrition Research Reviews* 19:26–52.

Calder, P.C. 2012. Mechanisms of action of (n-3) fatty acids. *Journal of Nutrition* 142:592S–599S.

Calder, P.C. 2013a. Omega-3 polyunsaturated fatty acids and inflammatory processes: Nutrition or pharmacology? *British Journal of Clinical Pharmacology* 75:645–662.

Calder, P.C. 2013b. n-3 Fatty acids, inflammation and immunity: New mechanisms to explain old actions. *Proceedings of the Nutrition Society* 72:326–336.

Calder, P.C. 2013c. Long chain fatty acids and gene expression in inflammation and immunity. *Current Opinion in Clinical Nutrition and Metabolic Care* 16:425–433.

Calder, P.C. 2014. Very long chain omega-3 (n-3) fatty acids and human health. *European Journal of Lipid Science and Technology* 116:1280–1300.

Calder, P.C. 2015. Marine omega-3 fatty acids and inflammatory processes: Effects, mechanisms and clinical relevance. *Biochimica et Biophysica Acta* 1851:469–484.

Calder, P.C., Ahluwalia, N., Brouns, F. et al. 2011. Dietary factors and low-grade inflammation in relation to overweight and obesity. *British Journal of Nutrition* 106(Suppl 3):S5–S78.

Calder, P.C., Yaqoob, P. 2007. Lipid rafts—Composition, characterization and controversies. *Journal of Nutrition* 137:545–547.

Calder, P.C., Yaqoob, P., Harvey, D.J., Watts, A., Newsholme, E.A. 1994. The incorporation of fatty acids by lymphocytes and the effect on fatty acid composition and membrane fluidity. *Biochemical Journal* 300:509–518.

Chen, H. 2006. Cellular inflammatory responses: Novel insights for obesity and insulin resistance. *Pharmacological Research* 53:469–477.

Clarke, S.D. 2004. The multi-dimensional regulation of gene expression by fatty acids: Polyunsaturated fats as nutrient sensors. *Current Opinion in Lipidology* 15:13–18.

Conquer, J.A., Holub, B.J. 1997. Dietary docosahexaenoic acid as a source of eicosapentaenoic acid in vegetarians and omnivores. *Lipids* 32:341–345.

Couet, C., Delarue, J., Ritz, P., Antoine, J.M., Lamisse, F. 1997. Effect of dietary fish oil on body fat mass and basal fat oxidation in healthy adults. *International Journal of Obesity and Related Metabolic Disorders* 21:637–643.

Dalli, J., Colas, R.A., Serhan, C.N. 2013. Novel n-3 immunoresolvents: Structures and roles. *Science Reports* 3:1940.

Das, U.N. 2004. Long-chain polyunsaturated fatty acids interact with nitric oxide, superoxide anion, and transforming growth factor-beta to prevent human essential hypertension. *European Journal of Clinical Nutrition* 58:195–203.

Deckelbaum, R.J., Worgall, T.S., Seo, T. 2006. N-3 fatty acids and gene expression. *American Journal of Clinical Nutrition* 83:1520S–1525S.

DeFina, L.F., Marcoux, L.G., Devers, S.M., Cleaver, J.P., Willis, B.L. 2011. Effects of omega-3 supplementation in combination with diet and exercise on weight loss and body composition. *American Journal of Clinical Nutrition* 93:455–462.

de Luca, C., Olefsky, J.M. 2008. Inflammation and insulin resistance. *FEBS Letters* 582:97–105.

Eckel, R.H., Grundy, S.M., Zimmet, P.Z. 2005. The metabolic syndrome. *Lancet* 365:1415–1428.

EFSA Panel on Dietetic Products, Nutrition, and Allergies (NDA). 2010. Scientific opinion on dietary reference values for fats, including saturated fatty acids, polyunsaturated fatty acids, monounsaturated fatty acids, trans fatty acids, and cholesterol. *EFSA Journal* 8:1461.

Elizondo, A., Araya, J., Rodrigo, R. et al. 2007. Polyunsaturated fatty acid pattern in liver and erythrocyte phospholipids from obese patients. *Obesity* 15:24–31.

Engler, M.M., Engler, M.B., Pierson, D.M., Molteni, L.B., Molteni, A. 2003. Effects of docosahexaenoic acid on vascular pathology and reactivity in hypertension. *Experimental Biology and Medicine* (Maywood) 228:299–307.

Fischer, R., Dechend, R., Qadri, F. et al. 2008. Dietary n-3 polyunsaturated fatty acids and direct renin inhibition improve electrical remodeling in a model of high human renin hypertension. *Hypertension* 51:540–546.

Flachs, P., Rossmeisl, M., Kopecky, J. 2014. The effect of n-3 fatty acids on glucose homeostasis and insulin sensitivity. *Physiological Research* 63(Suppl 1):S93–S118.

Ford, E.S. 2005. Risks for all-cause mortality, cardiovascular disease, and diabetes associated with the metabolic syndrome: A summary of the evidence. *Diabetes Care* 28:1769–1778.

Ford, E.S., Li, C., Sattar, N. 2008. Metabolic syndrome and incident diabetes: Current state of the evidence. *Diabetes Care* 31:1898–1904.

Galassi, A., Reynolds, K., He, J. 2006. Metabolic syndrome and risk of cardiovascular disease: A meta-analysis. *American Journal of Medicine* 119:812–819.

Gami, A.S., Witt, B.J., Howard, D.E. et al. 2007. Metabolic syndrome and risk of incident cardiovascular events and death: A systematic review and meta-analysis of longitudinal studies. *Journal of the American College of Cardiology* 49:403–414.

Geleijnse, J.M., Giltay, E.J., Grobbee, D.E., Donders, A.R., Kok, F.J. 2002. Blood pressure response to fish oil supplementation: Metaregression analysis of randomized trials. *Journal of Hypertension* 20:1493–1499.

Gil-Campos, M., Cañete, R.R., Gil, A. 2004. Adiponectin, the missing link in insulin resistance and obesity. *Clinical Nutrition* 23:963–974.

Gottlicher, M., Widmaek, E., Li, Q., Gustafsson, J.-A. 1992. Fatty acids activate a chimera of the clofibric acid-activated receptor and the glucocorticoid receptor. *Proceedings of the National Academy of Sciences of the United States of America* 89:4653–4657.

Gulseth, H.L., Gjelstad, I.M., Tierney, A.C. et al. 2010. Dietary fat modifications and blood pressure in subjects with the metabolic syndrome in the LIPGENE dietary intervention study. *British Journal of Nutrition* 104:160–163.

Hanefield, M., Schatz, U., Schaper, F. 2011. Treatments for the metabolic syndrome. In *The Metabolic Syndrome*, eds. C.D. Byrne and S.H. Wild, pp. 327–346. Oxford, U.K.: Blackwell Publishing.

Harris, W.S. 1996. n-3 Fatty acids and lipoproteins: Comparison of results from human and animal studies. *Lipids* 31:243–252.

Harris, W.S. 1997. n-3 Fatty acids and serum lipoproteins: Human studies. *American Journal of Clinical Nutrition* 65(5 Suppl):1645S–1654S.

Harris, W.S., Sands, S.A., Windsor, S.L. et al. 2004. Omega-3 fatty acids in cardiac biopsies from heart transplantation patients: Correlation with erythrocytes and response to supplementation. *Circulation* 110:1645–1649.

Harris, W.S., Windsor, S.L., Dujovne, C.A. 1991. Effects of four doses of n-3 fatty acids given to hyperlipidemic patients for six months. *Journal of the American College of Nutrition* 10:220–227.

Hartweg, J., Farmer, A.J., Holman, R.R., Neil, H.A. 2007a. Meta-analysis of the effects of n-3 polyunsaturated fatty acids on haematological and thrombogenic factors in type 2 diabetes. *Diabetologia* 50:250–258.

Hartweg, J., Farmer, A.J., Perera, R., Holman, R.R., Neil, H.A. 2007b. Meta-analysis of the effects of n-3 polyunsaturated fatty acids on lipoproteins and other emerging lipid cardiovascular risk markers in patients with type 2 diabetes. *Diabetologia* 50:1593–1602.

Hartweg, J., Perera, R., Montori, V., Dinneen, S., Neil, H.A., Farmer, A. 2008. Omega-3 polyunsaturated fatty acids (PUFA) for type 2 diabetes mellitus. *Cochrane Database of Systematic Reviews* 1:CD003205.

Hartwich, J., Malec, M.M., Partyka, L. et al. 2009. The effect of the plasma n-3/n-6 polyunsaturated fatty acid ratio on the dietary LDL phenotype transformation—Insights from the LIPGENE study. *Clinical Nutrition* 28:510–515.

Healy, D.A., Wallace, F.A., Miles, E.A., Calder, P.C., Newsholme, P. 2000. The effect of low to moderate amounts of dietary fish oil on neutrophil lipid composition and function. *Lipids* 35:763–768.

Herder, C., Illig, T., Rathmann, W. et al. 2005. Inflammation and type 2 diabetes: Results from KORA Augsburg. *Gesundheitswesen* 67(Suppl 1):S115–S121.

Herder, C., Peltonen, M., Koenig, W. et al. 2006. Systemic immune mediators and lifestyle changes in the prevention of type 2 diabetes: Results from the Finnish Diabetes Prevention Study. *Diabetes* 55:2340–2346.

Hill, A.M., Buckley, J.D., Murphy, K.J., Howe, P.R. 2007. Combining fish-oil supplements with regular aerobic exercise improves body composition and cardiovascular disease risk factors. *American Journal of Clinical Nutrition* 85:1267–1274.

Hotamisligil, G.S., Shargill, N.S., Spiegelman, B.M. 1993. Adipose expression of tumor necrosis factor-alpha: Direct role in obesity-linked insulin resistance. *Science* 259:87–91.

Howe, P., Meyer, B., Record, S., Baghurst, K. 2006. Dietary intake of long-chain omega-3 polyunsaturated fatty acids: Contribution of meat sources. *Nutrition* 22:47–53.

Itariu, B.K., Zeyda, M., Hochbrugger, E.E. et al. 2012. Long-chain n-3 PUFAs reduce adipose tissue and systemic inflammation in severely obese nondiabetic patients: A randomized controlled trial. *American Journal of Clinical Nutrition* 96:1137–1149.

Jump, D.B. 2008. N-3 polyunsaturated fatty acid regulation of hepatic gene transcription. *Current Opinion in Lipidology* 19:242–247.

Kabir, M., Skurnik, G., Naour, N. et al. 2007. Treatment for 2 mo with n 3 polyunsaturated fatty acids reduces adiposity and some atherogenic factors but does not improve insulin sensitivity in women with type 2 diabetes: A randomized controlled study. *American Journal of Clinical Nutrition* 86:1670–1679.

Kim, C.S., Park, H.S., Kawada, T. et al. 2006. Circulating levels of MCP-1 and IL-8 are elevated in human obese subjects and associated with obesity-related parameters. *International Journal of Obesity* 30:1347–1355.

Katan, M.B., Deslypere, J.P., van Birgelen, A.P.J.M., Penders, M., Zegwaars, M. 1997. Kinetics of the incorporation of dietary fatty acids into serum cholesteryl esters, erythrocyte membranes and adipose tissue: An 18 month controlled study. *Journal of Lipid Research* 38:2012–2022.

Kaur, G., Cameron-Smith, D., Garg, M., Sinclair, A.J. 2011. Docosapentaenoic acid (22:5n-3): A review of its biological effects. *Progress in Lipid Research* 50:28–34.

Kratz, M., Kuzma, J.N., Hagman, D.K. et al. 2013. n3 PUFAs do not affect adipose tissue inflammation in overweight to moderately obese men and women. *Journal of Nutrition* 143:1340–1347.

Krebs, J.D., Browning, L.M., McLean, N.K. et al. 2006. Additive benefits of long-chain n-3 polyunsaturated fatty acids and weight-loss in the management of cardiovascular disease risk in overweight hyperinsulinaemic women. *International Journal of Obesity* 30:1535–1544.

Krey, G., Braissant, O., L'Horset, F., Kalkhoven, E., Perroud, M., Parker, M.G., Wahli, W. 1997. Fatty acids, eicosanoids, and hypolipidemic agents identified as ligands of peroxisome proliferator-activated receptors by coactivator-dependent receptor ligand assay. *Molecular Endocrinology* 11:779–791.

Kunesová, M., Braunerová, R., Hlavatý, P. et al. 2006.The influence of n-3 polyunsaturated fatty acids and very low calorie diet during a short-term weight reducing regimen on weight loss and serum fatty acid composition in severely obese women. *Physiological Research* 55:63–72.

Lapillonne, A., Clarke, S.D., Heird, W.C. 2004. Polyunsaturated fatty acids and gene expression. *Current Opinion in Clinical Nutrition and Metabolic Care* 7:151–156.

Li, W., Ma, D., Liu, M. et al. 2008. Association between metabolic syndrome and risk of stroke: A meta-analysis of cohort studies. *Cerebrovascular Disease* 25:539–547.

Lorente-Cebrián, S., Costa, A.G., Navas-Carretero, S., Zabala, M., Martínez, J.A., Moreno-Aliaga, M.J. 2013. Role of omega-3 fatty acids in obesity, metabolic syndrome, and cardiovascular diseases: A review of the evidence. *Journal of Physiological Biochemistry* 69:633–651.

Lumeng, C.N., Bodzin, J.L., Saltiel, A.R. 2007. Obesity induces a phenotypic switch in adipose tissue macrophage polarization. *Journal of Clinical Investigation* 117:175–184.

Malavazos, A.E., Cereda, E., Morricone, L., Coman, C., Corsi, M.M., Ambrosi, B. 2005. Monocyte chemoattractant protein 1: A possible link between visceral adipose tissue-associated inflammation and subclinical echocardiographic abnormalities in uncomplicated obesity. *European Journal of Endocrinology* 153:871–877.

Malavazos, A.E., Corsi, M.M., Ermetici, F., Coman, C., Sardanelli, F., Rossi, A., Morricone, L., Ambrosi, B. 2007. Proinflammatory cytokines and cardiac abnormalities in uncomplicated obesity: Relationship with abdominal fat deposition. *Nutrition, Metabolism and Cardiovascular Diseases* 17:294–302.

Martínez-Victoria, E., Yago, M.D. 2012. Omega 3 polyunsaturated fatty acids and body weight. *British Journal of Nutrition* 107:S107–S116.

Matsuzawa, Y. 2006a. The metabolic syndrome and adipocytokines. *FEBS Letters* 580:2917–2921.

Matsuzawa, Y. 2006b. Therapy insight: Adipocytokines in metabolic syndrome and related cardiovascular disease. Nature Clinical Practice. *Cardiovascular Medicine* 3:35–42.

McGlory, C., Galloway, S.D., Hamilton, D.L. et al. 2014. Temporal changes in human skeletal muscle and blood lipid composition with fish oil supplementation. *Prostaglandins Leukotrienes and Essential Fatty Acids* 90:199–206.

Metcalf, R.G., James, M.J., Gibson, R.A. et al. 2007. Effects of fish-oil supplementation on myocardial fatty acids in humans. *American Journal of Clinical Nutrition* 85:1222–1228.

Metcalf, R.G., Cleland, L.G., Gibson, R.A. et al. 2010. Relation between blood and atrial fatty acids in patients undergoing cardiac bypass surgery. *American Journal of Clinical Nutrition* 91:528–534.

Meyer, B.J., Mann, N.J., Lewis, J.L., Milligan, G.C., Sinclair, A.J., Howe, P.R. 2003. Dietary intakes and food sources of omega-6 and omega-3 polyunsaturated fatty acids. *Lipids* 38:391–398.

Miles, E.A., Calder, P.C. 1998. Modulation of immune function by dietary fatty acids. *Proceedings of the Nutrition Society* 57:277–292.

Miller, P.E., Van Elswyk, M., Alexander, D.D. 2014. Long-chain omega-3 fatty acids eicosapentaenoic acid and docosahexaenoic acid and blood pressure: A meta-analysis of randomized controlled trials. *American Journal of Hypertension* 27:885–896.

Montori, V.M., Farmer, A., Wollan, P.C., Dinneen, S.F. 2000. Fish oil supplementation in type 2 diabetes: A quantitative systematic review. *Diabetes Care* 23:1407–1415.

Mori, T.A., Burke, V., Puddey, I.B. et al. 2000. Purified eicosapentaenoic and docosahexaenoic acids have differential effects on serum lipids and lipoproteins, LDL particle size, glucose, and insulin in mildly hyperlipidemic men. *American Journal of Clinical Nutrition* 71:1085–1094.

Morris, M.C., Sacks, F., Rosner, B. 1993. Does fish oil lower blood pressure? A meta-analysis of controlled trials. *Circulation* 88:523–533.

Mottillo, S., Filion, K.B., Genest, J. et al. 2010. The metabolic syndrome and cardiovascular risk a systematic review and meta-analysis. *Journal of the American College of Cardiology* 56:1113–1132.

Mozaffarian, D. 2007. Fish, n-3 fatty acids, and cardiovascular haemodynamics. *Journal of Cardiovascular Medicine* (Hagerstown) 8(Suppl 1):S23–S26.

Müller, S., Martin, S., Koenig, W. et al. 2002. Impaired glucose tolerance is associated with increased serum concentrations of interleukin 6 and co-regulated acute-phase proteins but not TNF-alpha or its receptors. *Diabetologia* 45:805–812.

Munro, I.A., Garg, M.L. 2012. Dietary supplementation with n-3 PUFA does not promote weight loss when combined with a very-low-energy diet. *British Journal of Nutrition* 108:1466–1474.

Munro, I.A., Garg, M.L. 2013. Dietary supplementation with long chain omega-3 polyunsaturated fatty acids and weight loss in obese adults. *Obesity Research and Clinical Practice* 7:e173–e181.

Murphy, M.G. 1990. Dietary fatty acids and membrane protein function. *Journal of Nutritional Biochemistry* 1:68–79.

National Cholesterol Education Program (NCEP) Expert Panel on Detection, Evaluation and Treatment of High Blood Cholesterol in Adults. 2001. Executive summary of the third report of the National Cholesterol Education Program (NCEP) Expert Panel on Detection, Evaluation and Treatment of High Blood Cholesterol in Adults (Adult Treatment Panel III). *JAMA* 285:2486–2497.

Neff, L.M., Culiner, J., Cunningham-Rundles, S. et al., 2011. Algal docosahexaenoic acid affects plasma lipoprotein particle size distribution in overweight and obese adults. *Journal of Nutrition* 141:207–213.

Novak, T.E., Babcock, T.A., Jho, D.H., Helton, W.S., Espat, N.J. 2003. NF-kappa B inhibition by omega-3 fatty acids modulates LPS-stimulated macrophage TNF-alpha transcription. *American Journal of Physiology* 284: L84–L89.

Oh, D.Y., Talukdar, S., Bae, E.J. et al. 2010. GPR120 is an omega-3 fatty acid receptor mediating potent anti-inflammatory and insulin-sensitizing effects. *Cell* 142:687–698.

Papanikolaou, Y., Brooks, J., Reider, C., Fulgoni, V.L. 3rd. 2014. U.S. adults are not meeting recommended levels for fish and omega-3 fatty acid intake: Results of an analysis using observational data from NHANES 2003–2008. *Nutrition Journal* 13:31.

Petersson, H., Risérus, U., McMonagle, J. et al. 2010. Effects of dietary fat modification on oxidative stress and inflammatory markers in the LIPGENE study. *British Journal of Nutrition* 104:1357–1362.

Pike, L.J. 2003. Lipid rafts: Bringing order to chaos. *Journal of Lipid Research* 44:655–667.

Rahmawaty, S., Charlton, K., Lyons-Wall, P., Meyer, B.J. 2013. Dietary intake and food sources of EPA, DPA and DHA in Australian children. *Lipids* 48:869–877.

Reaven, G.M. 1988. Banting lecture 1988. Role of insulin resistance in human disease. *Diabetes* 37:1595–607.

Rees, D., Miles, E.A., Banerjee, T. et al. 2006. Dose-related effects of eicosapentaenoic acid on innate immune function in healthy humans: A comparison of young and older men. *American Journal of Clinical Nutrition* 83:331–342.

Roche, H.M. 1999. Unsaturated fatty acids. *Proceedings of the Nutrition Society* 58:397–401.

Saravanan, P., Bridgewater, B., West, A.L., O'Neill, S.C., Calder, P.C., Davidson, N.C. 2010. Omega-3 fatty acid supplementation does not reduce risk of atrial fibrillation after coronary artery bypass surgery: A randomized, double-blind, placebo-controlled clinical trial. *Circulation Arrhythmia and Electrophysiology* 3:46–53.

Satoh, N., Shimatsu, A., Kotani, K. et al. 2007. Purified eicosapentaenoic acid reduces small dense LDL, remnant lipoprotein particles, and C-reactive protein in metabolic syndrome. *Diabetes Care* 30:144–146.

Satoh, N., Shimatsu, A., Kotani, K. et al. 2009. Highly purified eicosapentaenoic acid reduces cardio-ankle vascular index in association with decreased serum amyloid A-LDL in metabolic syndrome. *Hypertension Research* 32:1004–1008.

Scientific Advisory Committee on Nutrition/Committee on Toxicity. 2004. *Advice on Fish Consumption: Benefits and Risks.* London, U.K.: TSO.

Serhan, C.N., Chiang, N., van Dyke, T.E. 2008a. Resolving inflammation: Dual anti-inflammatory and pro-resolution lipid mediators. *Nature Reviews Immunology* 8:349–361.

Serhan, C.N., Yacoubian, S., Yang, R. 2008b. Anti-inflammatory and proresolving lipid mediators. *Annual Review of Pathology* 3:279–312.

Shearer, G.C., Savinova, O.V., Harris, W.S.2012. Fish oil—How does it reduce plasma triglycerides? *Biochimica et Biophysica Acta* 1821:843–851.

Simão, A.N., Godeny, P., Lozovoy, M.A., Dichi, J.B., Dichi, I. 2010. Effect of n-3 fatty acids in glycemic and lipid profiles, oxidative stress and total antioxidant capacity in patients with the metabolic syndrome. *Arquivos Brasileiros de Endocrinologia e Metabologia* 54:463–469.

Simons, K., Gerl, M.J. 2010. Revitalizing membrane rafts: New tools and insights. *Nature Reviews Molecular and Cell Biology* 11:688–699.

Smith, G.I., Atherton, P., Reeds, D.N. et al. 2011. Omega-3 polyunsaturated fatty acids augment the muscle protein anabolic response to hyperinsulinaemia-hyperaminoacidaemia in healthy young and middle-aged men and women. *Clinical Science* 121:267–278.

Spencer, M., Finlin, B.S., Unal, R. et al. 2013. Omega-3 fatty acids reduce adipose tissue macrophages in human subjects with insulin resistance. *Diabetes* 62:1709–1717.

Stephenson, J.A., Al-Taan, O., Arshad, A. et al. 2013. Unsaturated fatty acids differ between hepatic colorectal metastases and liver tissue without tumour in humans: Results from a randomised controlled trial of intravenous eicosapentaenoic and docosahexaenoic acids. *Prostaglandins Leukotrienes and Essential Fatty Acids* 88:405–410.

Stofkova, A. 2009. Leptin and adiponectin: From energy and metabolic dysbalance to inflammation and auto-immunity. *Endocrine Regulators* 43:157–168.

Stubbs, C.D., Smith, A.D. 1984. The modification of mammalian membrane polyunsaturated fatty acid composition in relation to membrane fluidity and function. *Biochimica et Biophysica Acta* 779:89–137.

Suzukawa, M., Abbey, M., Howe, P.R., Nestel, P.J. 1995. Effects of fish oil fatty acids on low density lipoprotein size, oxidizability, and uptake by macrophages. *Journal of Lipid Research* 36:473–484.

Te Morenga, L., Mann, J. 2011. Nutrition: Its relevance in development and treatment of the metabolic syndrome. In *The Metabolic Syndrome*, eds. C.D. Byrne and S.H. Wild, pp. 297–326. Oxford, U.K.: Blackwell Publishing.

Thorsdottir, I., Tomasson, H., Gunnarsdottir, I. et al. 2007. Randomized trial of weight-loss-diets for young adults varying in fish and fish oil content. *International Journal of Obesity* 31:1560–1566.

Tierney, A.C., McMonagle, J., Shaw, D.I. et al. 2011. Effects of dietary fat modification on insulin sensitivity and on other risk factors of the metabolic syndrome—LIPGENE: A European randomized dietary intervention study. *International Journal of Obesity* 35:800–809.

Tilg, H., Moschen, A.R. 2006. Adipocytokines: Mediators linking adipose tissue, inflammation and immunity. *Nature Reviews Immunology* 6:772–783.

Tousoulis, D., Plastiras, A., Siasos, G. et al. 2014. Omega-3 PUFAs improved endothelial function and arterial stiffness with a parallel antiinflammatory effect in adults with metabolic syndrome. *Atherosclerosis* 232:10–16.

Trayhurn, P., Wood, I.S. 2004. Adipokines: Inflammation and the pleiotropic role of white adipose tissue. *British Journal of Nutrition* 92:347–355.

Trujillo, M.E., Scherer, P.E. 2006. Adipose tissue-derived factors: Impact on health and disease. *Endocrine Reviews* 27:762–778.

von Schacky, C., Fischer, S., Weber, P.C. 1985. Long term effects of dietary marine omega-3 fatty acids upon plasma and cellular lipids, platelet function, and eicosanoid formation in humans. *Journal of Clinical Investigation* 76:1626–1631.

Wada, M., DeLong, C.J., Hong, Y.H. et al. 2007. Enzymes and receptors of prostaglandin pathways with arachidonic acid-derived versus eicosapentaenoic acid-derived substrates and products. *Journal of Biological Chemistry* 282:22254–22266.

Wellen, K.E., Hotamisligil, G.S. 2003. Obesity-induced inflammatory changes in adipose tissue. *Journal of Clinical Investigation* 112:1785–1788.

Wild, S.H., Byrne, C.D. 2011. The epidemiology of the metabolic syndrome and its association with diabetes, cardiovascular disease and other conditions. In *The Metabolic Syndrome*, eds. C.D. Byrne and S.H. Wild, pp. 1–18. Oxford, U.K.: Blackwell Publishing.

Woodman, R.J., Mori, T.A., Burke, V., Puddey, I.B., Watts, G.F., Beilin, L.J. 2002. Effects of purified eicosapentaenoic and docosahexaenoic acids on glycemic control, blood pressure, and serum lipids in type 2 diabetic patients with treated hypertension. *American Journal of Clinical Nutrition* 76:1007–1015.

Woodman, R.J., Mori, T.A., Burke, V. et al. 2003. Docosahexaenoic acid but not eicosapentaenoic acid increases LDL particle size in treated hypertensive type 2 diabetic patients. *Diabetes Care* 26:253.

Yaqoob, P. 2009. The nutritional significance of lipid rafts. *Annual Review of Nutrition* 29:257–282.

Yaqoob, P., Pala, H.S., Cortina-Borja, M., Newsholme, E.A., Calder, P.C. 2000. Encapsulated fish oil enriched in α-tocopherol alters plasma phospholipid and mononuclear cell fatty acid compositions but not mononuclear cell functions. *European Journal of Clinical Investigations* 30:260–274.

Zimmet, P., Alberti, K.G., Shaw, J. 2001 Global and societal implications of the diabetes epidemic. *Nature* 414:782–787.

16 Whole Grains and Metabolic Syndrome

Anthony Fardet

CONTENTS

16.1 INTRODUCTION

Whole grains are cereal and pseudocereal grains that contain the germ, endosperm, and bran fractions, in contrast to refined grains, which retain only the endosperm. Therefore, the whole-grain concept does not include leguminous seeds, nuts, and seeds. Common whole grains include wheat, maize, oat, brown (medium and long grain) and wild rice, barley—hulled and dehulled (not pearled), spelt (an ancient species of wheat), emmer (awned wheat), einkorn (diploid species of hulled wheat), kamut (Khorasan wheat cultivar), rye, millet, triticale, teff, and sprouted grains as cereals, but also quinoa, amaranth, and buckwheat as pseudocereals. Common whole-grain products include whole-wheat flour, triticale flour, faro, teff flour, rye flour (dark, medium, and light), whole-grain breads (e.g., dark, brown, whole meal, and rye bread), whole-wheat pasta, rolled oats, oat groats, whole-grain breakfast cereals (e.g., muesli), popcorn, cooked porridges (oatmeal or whole wheat), wheat germ, brown rice, bran, cooked grains (e.g., wheat, millet, and roasted buckwheat), and other grain-based foods such as bulgur and couscous (Cleveland et al. 2000).

Today, there are good scientific evidences to say that whole-grain products are protective against weight gain (Kristensen et al. 2011, Mozaffarian et al. 2011), type 2 diabetes (de Munter et al. 2007, Nettleton et al. 2010, Priebe et al. 2008, Schulze et al. 2007, Sun et al. 2010), cardiovascular diseases (CVDs) (Anderson 2003, Anderson et al. 2000, Mellen et al. 2008), and colorectal cancer (Aune et al. 2011). Concerning the metabolic syndrome (MetS), observational studies are less prevalent. MetS includes several impaired physiological mechanisms (obesity, insulin resistance, hyperglycemia, dyslipidemia, and hypertension) that notably aim at identifying subjects at high risk of CVDs since the risk is threefold in such patients (Potenza and Mechanick 2009). In this perspective, it is particularly relevant that whole grains are protective against weight gain, type 2 diabetes, and CVDs.

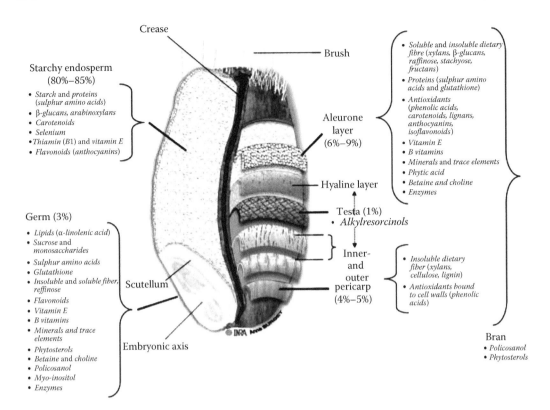

FIGURE 16.1 The three wheat fraction (bran, germ, and endosperm) with their main bioactive compounds: whole-grain wheat has a heterogeneous structure with bioactive compounds unevenly distributed within its different parts. (From Fardet, A., *Nutr. Res. Rev.*, 23, 65, 2010, Cambridge University Press; Adapted from Surget, A. and Barron, C., *Industries des Cereales*, 145, 3, 2005.)

Indeed, the MetS is a cluster of risk factors. Therefore, in addition to studying association of whole grains with MetS prevalence taken as a "whole" syndrome, the effect of whole grains also deserves to be considered as regard with each of these risk factors. Indeed, whole grain contains numerous phytochemicals with numerous protective effects: some of these bioactive compounds may have several protective effects (e.g., anticarcinogenic and anti-inflammatory effects) and several bioactive compounds may act in synergy to protect organism vis-à-vis a single deregulated metabolism (e.g., antioxidants and hypolipidemic) (Fardet 2010). So, the potential protective effect of whole grain should be considered with an integrative and holistic approach, that is, not to associate only one compound with one physiological effect (reductionist approach). This leads us to the concept of the whole-grain package as illustrated in Figure 16.1.

The aim of this chapter is to lay bases for the potential protectiveness of whole grains toward MetS by notably taking into consideration each of its components *via* human observational and interventional studies. Whole grains being rich in fiber, this specific compound will be also considered. First, the definition of whole grain will be defined since, according to the definition considered, the results of observational studies may differ from a significant effect to no effect.

16.2 WHOLE GRAIN DEFINITIONS

De Moura et al. (2009) convincingly demonstrated that according to the definition applied and foods considered as whole-grain products, results from observational studies may completely differ: for example, by taking the U.S. FDA (United States Food and Drug Administration) definition of whole grain, there is not sufficient evidence to support a protective effect of whole grain toward CVDs while taking a broader concept of whole grain allowed demonstrating a protective effect.

The definition of whole grain is somewhat always under debate. To summarize, today, the most widely accepted definition includes cereals and pseudocereals: according to the AACC (The American Association of Cereal Chemists), "Whole grains shall consist of the intact, ground, cracked or flaked caryopsis, whose principal anatomical components - the starchy endosperm, germ and bran - are present in the same relative proportions as they exist in the intact caryopsis" (AACC 1999); according to the Whole Grains Council, "Whole grains or foods made from them contain all the essential parts and naturally-occurring nutrients of the entire grain seed. If the grain has been processed (e.g., cracked, crushed, rolled, extruded, and/or cooked), the food product should deliver approximately the same rich balance of nutrients that are found in the original grain seed" (EUFIC 2009); according to the FDA: "The US FDA published a Draft Guidance on Whole grain Label Statements in 2006 that adopted the international AACC definition and included amaranth, barley, buckwheat, bulgur, maize (including popcorn), millet, quinoa, rice, rye, oats, sorghum, teff, triticale, wheat and wild rice; pearled barley was not included because some outer layers of the bran fraction are removed (FDA 2006). Pseudocereals such as amaranth, buckwheat, and quinoa have similar macronutrient compositions (carbohydrates, proteins, and lipids), and are used in the same traditional ways as cereals (AACC 2006, Jones 2008). The response to the US DFA Draft Guidance by the AACC International recommended that some traditional cereals such as 'lightly pearled barley, grano (lightly pearled wheat), nixtamalized corn and bulgur that has been minimally processed be also classified as whole grains' (AACC 2006), making allowance for small losses of components that occur through traditional processing" (Fardet 2010). The Whole Grain Task Force replaced "as they exist in the intact caryopsis" in the AACC definition by "as found in the least-processed, traditional forms of the edible grain kernels" and completed by adding "as they exist in the intact caryopsis to the extent feasible by the best modern milling technology." This last definition is probably the best adapted to our Western country technologies. However, to the best of our knowledge, there is still no international consensus as to the right proportion of whole grain by dry weight in a product in order for it to be called a whole-grain product (Fardet 2010). However, most research and observational studies estimate the whole-grain intake from products containing at least 25% whole grains or bran by weight, largely below the value of 51% of total weight given by the U.S. FDA (Fardet 2010).

16.3 WHOLE GRAIN VERSUS METABOLIC SYNDROME

16.3.1 Observational Studies

There are no meta-analyses—based on observational and longitudinal studies—that have quantified the effect of whole-grain consumption on MetS prevalence. However, one meta-analysis has investigated the association between adherence to the Mediterranean diet and MetS risk, the Mediterranean diet encouraging daily the consumption of whole grains (Kastorini et al. 2011). Results showed that adherence to the Mediterranean diet was associated with reduced risk of MetS (log hazard ratio: −0.69, 95% confidence interval CI: −1.24 to −1.16) (Kastorini et al. 2011). Although not directly related to MetS prevalence, the recent study by Ye et al. (2012) allows giving relevant information about the association between whole-grain consumption and two parameters of the MetS (i.e., type 2 diabetes and obesity) and CVD, a well-known consequence of MetS. Results showed that compared with never/rare consumers of whole grains, those consuming 48–80 g whole grain/day (3–5 servings/day)—which is the recommended daily amount of whole grain for consumption—had a ~26% lower risk of type 2 diabetes (Relative risk RR = 0.74 [95% CI: 0.69, 0.80], based on 6 prospective cohort studies), a ~21% lower risk of CVD (RR = 0.79 [95% CI: 0.74, 0.85], based on 10 prospective cohort studies), and consistently less weight gain during 8–13 years (1.27 vs. 1.64 kg; P = 0.001, data not pooled). Comparing now the highest and lowest categories of dietary cereal fiber intake, results showed ~13% lower risk of type 2 diabetes (RR=0.87 [95% CI: 0.81, 0.94], based on 10 prospective cohort studies) and ~13% lower risk of CVD (RR=0.80 [95% CI: 0.73, 0.88], based on 10 prospective cohort studies) (Ye et al. 2012).

Considering now observational studies that have investigated the association of whole-grain consumption with MetS, some tendencies emerge. First, except one study, only cross-sectional studies were led, limiting relevance, applicability, and generalization of the results; and, obviously, no causal relations can be unraveled. Nevertheless, all six cross-sectional studies gave significant inverse association between whole-grain products/cereal fiber consumption and MetS prevalence with closed odd ratios (OR) of 0.74 (CI: 0.57–0.97) for cereal fiber (Hosseinpour-Niazi et al. 2011), and 0.46 (0.27–0.79) (Sahyoun et al. 2006), 0.68 (0.60–0.78) (Esmaillzadeh et al. 2005), 0.67 (0.48–0.91) (Mckeown et al., 2004), and 0.87 (0.75–0.99) (Younjhin et al., 2013) for whole grain products with one study showing no significant association (Song et al. 2014). Concerning refined grains, they were either positively (OR=2.16 [1.20–3.87]) (Sahyoun et al. 2006), OR=2.25 (1.80–2.84) (Esmaillzadeh et al. 2005), OR Q5 for women only = 1.72 (1.24–2.40), the effect being likely to be attributed to white rice with OR Q5 = 1.74 (1.23–2.48) (Song et al. 2014) or not (OR=0.76 [0.53–1.09] [Mckeown et al. 2004]) associated with a higher prevalence of the MetS. One study showed no association between whole-grain intake and the prevalence of the MetS in young adults (Yoo et al. 2004).

In the study by McKeown et al. after adjustment for cereal fiber, the significant association was no longer observed with an OR of 0.77 (0.55–1.09; P=0.20), which prompted authors to suggest that the association of whole grain with MetS prevalence may be mainly due to cereal fiber fraction or to factors related to cereal fiber intake (Mckeown et al. 2004). In addition, while cereal fiber is inversely association with MetS prevalence (OR=0.62 [0.45–0.86], P=0.002), total dietary fiber, fiber from fruits, vegetables, and legumes was not. Contrary to the study by McKeown et al., in the study by Hosseinpour-Niazi et al., ORs (highest and lowest quartiles) for MetS prevalence and fiber intake were inversely associated: 0.53 (0.39–0.74; P for trend <0.05) for total dietary fiber, 0.60 (0.43–0.84; P for trend <0.05) for soluble fiber, 0.51 (0.35–0.72; P for trend <0.05) for insoluble fiber, 0.51 for fruit fiber (0.37–0.72; P for trend <0.005), and 0.73 for legume fiber (0.53–0.99; P for trend = 0.043), but not for cereal fiber (Hosseinpour-Niazi et al. 2011). Taking cereal fiber as a continuous variable (per 1 g increment/1000 kcal), the association becomes significant (OR=0.92 [0.84–0.97], P=0.011). So, due to the presence of several hundred of phytochemicals in bound form associated to the fiber fraction in whole-grain cereals (fiber *copassengers*), whether or not the MetS protection by whole grain should be associated with the fiber fraction only remains to be elucidated or confirmed in further longitudinal and interventional studies. In the study by Sahyoun et al., the intake of whole grain was also associated with a lower incidence of cardiovascular mortality, the main consequence of MetS (Sahyoun et al. 2006). In this latter study, the main source of whole-grain foods was whole-wheat breads (53%), then ready-to-eat cold breakfast cereal (19%), and hot breakfast cereal (15%), emphasizing breads and breakfast cereals as good vectors for consuming more whole-grain products.

In the study by Esmaillzadeh et al., subjects in the top quartile of whole-grain consumption consumed 229 g/day (approximately 5.5 servings/day), and whole-grain foods included dark breads (i.e., Sangak—a plain, rectangular, or triangular Iranian whole-wheat sourdough flatbread, Barbari—a Persian flatbread, and Taftoon—a leavened flour bread), barley bread, popcorn, cornflakes (a whole-grain breakfast cereal), wheat germ, and bulgur. Refined grains included white breads (Lavash—soft, thin flatbread, Baguette), iceberg bread, noodle, pasta, rice, toasted bread, milled barley, sweet bread, white flour, starch, and biscuits (Esmaillzadeh et al. 2005), interestingly emphasizing that other vectors than Western breads and breakfast cereals can be favorably used as whole-grain products.

Although not directly studying the association of MetS with particular food groups, the study by Wirfalt reported that food patterns dominated by "fiber bread" provided favorable effects toward some parameters of the MetS (notably central obesity, dyslipidemia, and hyperglycemia), whereas food patterns high in refined bread or in cheese, cake, and alcoholic beverages contributed adverse effects (Wirfalt et al. 2001). Among the six food patterns identified by cluster analysis, the "fiber bread" pattern is among the richer in micronutrients and phytochemicals. Always considering food patterns, Ahn et al. (2013) classified 26,006 subjects (enrolled in the Korean Genome and Epidemiology Study between 2004 and 2006) into four dietary patterns—"white rice" (reference group), "rice with beans," "rice with multigrains," and "mixed" based on their food frequency questionnaire responses—and realized a cross-sectional analysis for men and women (pre- and postmenopausal). No significant effects were observed for men in each dietary pattern, whereas women in the "mixed" group exhibited a borderline but significant lower prevalence of MetS (OR = 0.87 [0.75–0.99]). When stratified according to menopausal status, only postmenopausal women showed a reduced prevalence of MetS in the "rice with multigrains" (OR = 0.85 [0.73–0.98]) and "mixed" (OR = 0.74 [0.62–0.89]) groups. Therefore, the "rice with multigrains" group showed the benefits of whole grain. According to the authors, positive effects are likely to be supplied by cereal fibers and various components of unpolished grains. These results were not confirmed in 5830 males and females aged between 20 and 64 years (2007–2008 KNHNES data, The Korea National Health and Nutrition Examination Survey) classified by quartile of percent energy intake from cooked rice (OR = 1.089 [0.773–1.534]) or cooked rice mixed with multigrains (OR = 0.921 [0.725–1.170]): no association was found with MetS when comparing 0 versus ≥1 serving/day (Son et al. 2013).

To the best of our knowledge, the study by Shi et al. (2012) was the only longitudinal cohort study (Shi et al. 2012). It has been led in 935 Chinese adults upon a follow-up of 5 years. No significant association was found between OR of MetS according to rice intake and staple food patterns (measured by percentage of rice in staple food). Unfortunately, authors did not point out the type of rice consumed: white, brown, or a mix.

16.3.2 Interventional Studies

Beyond observational studies, interventional studies are the best scientific evidence to unravel direct causal effects between a diet or a food and a modified physiological or metabolic effect.

In a recent meta-analysis based on 21 randomized controlled trials, significantly lower concentrations of fasting glucose (differences in fasting glucose: −0.93 mmol/L [95% CI: 1.65, −0.21]), fasting insulin (−0.29 mmol/L [95% CI: −0.59, 0.01]), total (−0.83 mmol/L [95% CI: −1.24, −0.42]) and LDL (−0.72 mmol/L [95% CI: −1.34, −0.11]) (Low-Density Lipoprotein)-cholesterol, lower systolic [−0.06 (−0.21, 0.10)] and diastolic [−0.05 (−0.21, 0.11)] blood pressure, and less weight gain [−0.18 (−0.54, 0.18)] (all are parameters of MetS) after whole-grain interventions compared with controls were observed (Ye et al. 2012). However, heterogeneity was observed between trials (P < 0.05), which remained significant in subgroups after stratification by duration, study quality, and health status.

In 2012, Björck et al. reviewed intervention studies investigating the impact of whole-grain diets on clinical outcomes potentially related to the MetS (i.e., serum lipids, glucose metabolism, BMI and waist-to-hip ratio, blood pressure, C-reactive protein (CRP), plasminogen activator inhibitor-1, IL-6, and TNF-α). Authors made the following conclusions based on 24 studies (1) there are still limited data from interventional studies, notably for emerging risk markers such as oxidative stress and low-grade inflammation; (2) results suggest improved parameters of the MetS by whole-grain cereal products consumption although results are sometimes not consistent from one study to another, probably due to the various status of the subjects (normal, obese, hyperlipidemic, or hypertensive) and the cereal variety used (wheat, barley, rice, etc.) (Björck et al. 2012). Despite these limits, it is interesting to observe that no study reported negative effect of consuming whole-grain cereal products.

Beyond systematic reviews and meta-analyses, a recent interventional study showed, in 50 overweight and obese individuals with increased waist circumference and one or more other MetS criteria, that "replacing refined grains with whole grains within a weight-loss diet does not beneficially affect abdominal adipose tissues loss and has modest effects on markers of MetS, and that whole grains appear to be effective at normalizing blood glucose concentrations, especially in those individuals with prediabetes" (Jackson et al. 2014, p. 577).

16.4 WHOLE GRAIN VERSUS PARAMETERS OF THE METABOLIC SYNDROME TAKEN SEPARATELY

Scientific literature about associations or causal relations of whole-grain food products and the different parameters of the MetS taken separately are more numerous and the objective is not here to review all studies. So, I chose to focus on meta-analyses, considering that study quality analysis has already been realized in these quantitative reviews (i.e., exclusion or not from the final meta-analysis).

16.4.1 LIPID METABOLISM

Meta-analyses about the association between whole-grain products and lipid parameters are rare. Recently, Ye et al. (2012) systematically examine longitudinal studies and randomized controlled trials investigating whole-grain and fiber intake in relation to risk of type 2 diabetes, CVD, weight gain, and metabolic risk factors (see above). Concerning lipids and randomized settings, they found significant lower concentrations of total and LDL cholesterol. The other meta-analysis was realized in 1992 and was based on 10 randomized controlled trials: Ripsin et al. (1992) examined the association between oat products consumption (oatmeal and oat bran) and lipid lowering. They unraveled a summary effect size for change in blood total cholesterol level of −0.13 mmol/L (−5.9 mg/dL) (95% CI: −0.19 to −0.017 mmol/L [−8.4 to −3.3 mg/dL]) for the group consuming oat products compared to controls.

Beyond meta-analyses and taking into consideration recent studies, an interventional study carried out in 200 overweight subjects (30–65 years of age) with two diagnostic criteria for MetS showed that a greater proportion of whole-grain rye intake (issued from a Nordic diet and measured via the plasma alkylresorcinols ratio C17:0/C21:0) is associated with favorable outcomes in blood lipid concentrations (LDL cholesterol, triglycerides, apolipoprotein B, and LDL/HDL ratio) (Magnusdottir et al. 2014). Favorable effect on blood triglycerides was also observed recently in 61 men and women (age range 40–65 years) with the MetS upon a 12-week intervention with a whole-grain-based diet (Giacco et al. 2014).

Now, it is interesting to consider some cereal compounds typical of whole-grain cereals and their association with lipid parameters based on meta-analyses.

First, considering the fiber fraction and based on 67 trials, soluble fiber (2–10 g/day) was associated with small but significant decreases in total cholesterol (−0.045 mmol/L/g soluble fiber [95% CI: −0.054, −0.035]) and LDL cholesterol (−0.057 mmol/L/g [95% CI: −0.070, −0.044]) (Brown et al. 1999). Authors also found a nonlinear dose–response between dose of soluble fiber and mean lipid changes, notably significant nonlinearity with doses >10 g/day for total cholesterol and with doses >8 g/day for LDL cholesterol. But the effect remains small within the practical range of intake: thus, 3 g soluble fiber from oats (three servings of oatmeal, 28 g each) decreased total and LDL cholesterol by approximate only 0.13 mmol/L (Brown et al. 1999). In the end, effects on plasma lipids did not differ whatever the fiber origin, be from oat products, psyllium, or pectin.

When considering β-glucans from oat and barley products, a recent meta-analysis (126 clinical studies were selected) found a significant inverse relation in total cholesterol (−0.60 mmol/L, 95% CI: −0.85 to −0.34), low-density lipoprotein (−0.66 mmol/L, 95% CI: −0.96 to −0.36), and triglyceride/triacylglycerol (−0.04 mmol/L, 95% CI: −0.15 to 0.07) after consumption of β-glucan (Tiwari and Cummins 2011). Using the dose–response model, authors further showed that a 3-g/day dose of oat or barley β-glucans was sufficient to decrease total cholesterol. Their results were in agreement with those published 1 year before: indeed, AbuMweis et al. (2010) also showed based on 11 randomized controlled trials that barley and β-glucan isolated from barley lowered total and LDL cholesterol concentrations by 0.30 mmol/L (95% CI: −0.39 to −0.21, P < 0.00001) and 0.27 mmol/L (95% CI: −0.34 to −0.20, P < 0.00001), respectively, compared with control. No significant effect was observed for HDL (High-Density Lipoprotein)-cholesterol and triacylglycerols. In addition, no dose–response pattern could have been found between doses of β-glucans and total cholesterol lowering, the highest decrease being observed with a consumption of 5.1–7 g/day β-glucans (AbuMweis et al. 2010). Overall, heterogeneity of studies was not significant.

Fructans are another cereal fiber type that can be found in relevant quantity in cereals. For example, in wheat, one can find 0.6–2.3 g fructans/100 g of whole grain, 0.6–4.0 g/100 g of bran and 1.7–2.5 g/100 g of germ (Fardet 2010). Based on nine studies, Wu et al. (2010) demonstrated that "the total cholesterol and triacylglycerol of subjects with hyperlipidemia could be significantly decreased by dietary inulin-type fructans (foods enriched with 17 g of inulin-type fructans per day), whereas the effects were absent in normal subjects."

In the same way, cereals are also a relevant source of phytosterols, well-known lipid lowering compounds. They can be found in whole-grain wheat (up to 0.08% by weight), and its bran (up to 0.16% by weight) and germ (up to 0.43% by weight) fractions (Fardet 2010). I found three quite recent meta-analyses investigating the association between phytosterols consumption and lowering of lipid parameters. The first one by Ting et al. was based on 20 randomized controlled trials (Ting et al. 2009). Considering all subjects (normal and hypercholesterolemic), phytosterols/stanols could significantly decrease LDL cholesterol (mean differences: 0.35 mmol/L, 95% CI: 0.47, 0.22, P < 0.00001), total cholesterol (mean difference: 0.36 mmol/L, 95% CI: 0.46, 0.26, P < 0.00001) and triacylglycerol (mean difference: 0.1 mmol/L, 95% CI: 0.16, 0.03, P = 0.004) in treatment groups compared with control groups. As for fructans, effects were more pronounced in borderline and hypercholesterolemic subjects than in normal subjects (Ting et al. 2009). The second meta-analysis was based on four randomized controlled trials in familial hypercholesterolemic subjects (Moruisi et al. 2006). Phytosterols/stanols (2.3 ± 0.5 g/day) significantly reduced total cholesterol by 0.65 mmol/L (95% CI: −0.88, −0.42 mmol/L, P < 0.00001) and LDL cholesterol by 0.64 mmol/L (95% CI: −0.86, −0.43 mmol/L, P < 0.00001). No effect was observed for triglycerides and HDL cholesterol. The third study by Chen et al. found similar results, that is, weighted estimates of percent change in LDL were −11.0% for plant sterol and stanol esters (3.4 g/day, range 2–9 g/day, 893 patients) versus −2.3% for placebo (769 patients) in 23 eligible studies (Chen et al. 2005).

To conclude with lipid parameters, it is worth mentioning two last meta-analyses about zinc and niacin, two compounds found in whole-grain cereals: 0.8–8.9 mg zinc/100 g of whole-grain wheat and 1.9–11.1 mg niacin/100 g of whole-grain wheat (Fardet 2010). While no overall significant effects of zinc supplementation were observed for plasma cholesterol, LDL cholesterol, HDL cholesterol, or plasma triglyceride concentrations (Foster et al. 2010), each increase of 500 mg extended-release niacin daily (when above 1 g) was associated with greater reduction in LDL in women compared to men (Miller 2004), but the niacin concentrations were largely above normal ranges found in whole grains. In the study by Foster et al. (2010), a secondary analysis in individuals classified as healthy revealed that zinc supplementation is associated with a significant decrease in plasma HDL cholesterol concentrations (−0.10 ± 0.02 mmol/L, P < 0.001), equivalent to a 7% decrease from baseline.

In whole-grain cereals, fructans, β-glucans, phytosterols, zinc, and niacin are generally in lower amounts than those encountered in the meta-analyses previously cited, and therefore cannot probably lead individually to significant decreases in lipid parameters. However, when considered together as a whole package of hypolipidemic phytochemicals, whole grains may well lead to significant lowering of blood total and LDL cholesterol as observed in the meta-analysis by Ye et al. (2012) mentioned above.

16.4.2 BLOOD PRESSURE

Blood pressure is also an important parameter of MetS and its association with whole-grain intake deserve to be discussed, notably on the basis of meta-analyses.

As mentioned earlier in the meta-analysis by Ye et al. (2012) based on randomized controlled trials, whole grain and cereal fiber consumption was associated with reduced systolic and diastolic blood pressure, although the effect was borderline: −0.06 (−0.21, 0.10) mmHg for systolic blood pressure and −0.05 (−0.21, 0.11) mmHg for diastolic blood pressure. I found no meta-analysis quantifying the risk of hypertension in association with whole-grain cereal intake. However, two recent observational studies clearly showed that whole-grain intake was significantly and inversely associated with risk of hypertension (Flint et al. 2009, Wang et al. 2007). Relative risks were 0.81 (95% CI: 0.75–0.87) in the highest compared with the lowest quintile (P for trend <0.0001) in the study by Flint et al. (2009) and 0.89 (0.82, 0.97) in the fifth quintile of whole-grain intake (≥4 whole-grain servings/day vs. <0.5 whole-grain servings/day; P for trend = 0.007) in the study by Wang et al. (2007). In this last study, refined grains were not associated with risk of hypertension. Interestingly, total bran was also inversely associated with hypertension (RR of 0.85, 95% CI: 0.78, 0.92) in the highest compared with the lowest quintile (P for trend = 0.002) (Flint et al. 2009).

When comparing whole-grain species, one observational study in China reported a significant lower prevalence of hypertension in subjects consuming buckwheat seed (a pseudocereal of the Polygonaceae family) as a staple food compared to subjects consuming corn as a staple food (Zhang et al. 2007).

As whole grains are rich sources of fiber, it is important to report the results of the meta-analyses by both Whelton et al. (2005) and Streppel et al. (2005), who showed that increased dietary fiber intake or fiber supplementation may be associated with a significant reduction in blood pressure (both diastolic and systolic) in the range −1.65 to 1.13 mmHg. Whelton et al. (2005) add that "an intervention period of at least 8 weeks may be necessary to achieve the maximum reduction in blood pressure." The mechanism by which fiber may reduce blood pressure still remains uncertain: their effect could be indirect (1) via decreased glycemic response attenuating insulin response that play a role in blood pressure regulation (Landsberg 2001) or (2) via enhanced mineral absorption by fiber (Coudray et al. 2003) which may have an indirect favorable effect on blood pressure.

Whole grains are also a source of other antihypertensive compounds such as potassium (209–635 mg/100 g), magnesium (17–191 mg/100 g), and calcium (7–70 mg/100 g) (Fardet 2010). When taken separately, all meta-analyses showed they are significantly and inversely associated with reduced blood pressure (Bucher et al. 1996, Geleijnse et al. 2003, Imdad et al. 2011, Jee et al. 2002, Kass et al. 2012, van Bommel and Cleophas 2012, van Mierlo et al. 2006, Whelton et al. 1997).

To conclude, as for hypolipidemic compounds, antihypertensive compounds are several and, put together in the whole-grain package, may well contribute to lower hypertension—or at least to maintain a normal tension—in people consuming high amounts of whole grains.

16.4.3 OBESITY AND WEIGHT GAIN

As for hyperlipidemia and hypertension, excess weight or obesity (notably abdominal obesity) is an important feature of the MetS.

As mentioned earlier, increased whole-grain consumption was associated with consistently less weight gain during 8–13 years (1.27 vs. 1.64 kg; P = 0.001) (Ye et al. 2012). Yet, in the previous year, Kristensen et al. (2011) concluded in a systematic review based on 25 randomized controlled trials that "There is little evidence that whole grains are more effective than control in prevention or treatment of overweight and obesity" with the following reserve that "many trials to date have not aimed specifically at assessing effects on body weight and study designs have been variable." Conversely, in three separate cohorts that included 120,877 U.S. women and men, Mozaffarian et al. (2011)

calculated that within each 4-year period, weight change was positively associated with whole-grain consumption (−0.37 [−0.48 to −0.25] lb, P<0.001; with 1 lb=453.6 g) and negatively associated with refined grain consumption (0.39 [0.21–0.58] lb, P<0.001).

The mechanisms behind the effect of whole grain on reduced weight gain may be explained not only by the increased feeling of satiety following increased fiber consumption, especially viscous one (Wanders et al. 2011), but also following the consumption of food products with a preserved intact food structure (Fardet 2010)—as it may be the case with whole-grain cereal products: such an effect has been well demonstrated with intact apple, purée apple, and apple juice (Haber et al. 1977), but also with breads with more dense crumb texture (leaf volume) (Burton and Lightowler 2006).

16.4.4 GLUCOSE METABOLISM AND DIABETES

The last recognized parameter characterizing MetS is increased fasting plasma glucose (≥6.1 mmol/L or 110 mg/dL) or previously diagnosed diabetes—in other words, impaired glucose metabolism.

Again, as mentioned previously in the meta-analysis by Ye et al., compared with never/rare consumers of whole grains, those consuming 48–80 g whole grain/day (3–5 servings/day) had an ~26% lower risk of type 2 diabetes (RR=0.74 [95% CI: 0.69, 0.80]); and weighted mean differences in postintervention circulating concentrations of fasting glucose was significant and equal to −0.93 mmol/L (95% CI: −1.65, −0.21) (Ye et al. 2012).

Contrary to other MetS features, more systematic reviews and meta-analyses were found in relation with whole/refined grain consumption and impaired glucose metabolism. First, Nettleton et al. (2010) recently observed (and confirmed) in over 48,000 European individuals (14 cohorts) a solid association of whole-grain intake with lower fasting glucose and fasting insulin concentrations independent of demographics, other dietary and lifestyle factors, and BMI (regression coefficient per 1-serving greater whole-grain intake [β]: −0 009 mmol/L glucose [95% CI: −0.013 to −0.005], P < 0.0001 and −0.011 pmol/L insulin [−0.015 to −0.007], P=0.0003). Conversely, higher consumption of white rice (i.e., refined cereal) is associated with a significantly increased risk of type 2 diabetes, especially in Asian (Chinese and Japanese) populations where the pooled relative risk was 1.55 (95% CI: 1.20–2.01) comparing the highest with the lowest category of white rice intake (Hu et al. 2012). In Western population, the corresponding RR was 1.12 (0.94–1.33). These results confirmed a previous meta-analysis led by Sun et al. in 2010 in which (1) higher white rice intake (≥5 servings per week vs. <1 per month) was associated with a higher risk of type 2 diabetes with a pooled RR of 1.17 (1.02–1.36) and (2) higher brown rice (i.e., whole-grain cereal) intake (≥2 servings per week vs. <1 per month) was associated with a lower risk of type 2 diabetes with a pooled relative risk of 0.89 (95% CI: 0.81–0.97). Interestingly, authors estimated that substitution of white rice by brown rice was associated with a 16% (95% CI: 9%–21%) lower risk of type 2 diabetes and that equivalent substitution of white rice with whole grains as a group was associated with a 36% (30%–42%) lower diabetes risk. Similar results have been also reported by Priebe et al. (2008) in another meta-analysis where a reduced risk of type 2 diabetes is associated with high intake of whole-grain foods (−27% to −30%) or cereal fiber (−28% to −37%). The meta-analysis by de Munter et al. (2007) supplied additional information in showing that the inverse association between whole-grain intake and risk of type 2 diabetes (0.63 [95% CI: 0.57–0.69]) is stronger for bran (similar association than for whole grain) than for germ (no association). In the end, Murakami et al. (2005), via a systematic review, showed that "the risk of type 2 diabetes was positively associated with the ratio of refined to whole grain and inversely associated with several types of whole-grain products (such as dark bread, whole-grain breakfast cereal, brown rice, wheat germ, bran, and other whole grains in one study)."

Concerning the fiber fraction, in a prospective cohort study of 9,702 men and 15,365 women aged 35–65 years who were observed for incident diabetes from 1994 to 2005, Schulze et al. (2007) showed that higher cereal fiber intake was inversely associated with diabetes risk (RR for extreme quintiles, 0.72 [95% CI: 0.56–0.93]), whereas fruit fiber (0.89 [95% CI: 0.70–1.13]) and vegetable fiber (0.93 [95% CI: 0.74–1.17]) were not significantly associated, emphasizing a possible specific effect of cereal fiber not found in fruits and vegetables. No association was also found with total, insoluble, and soluble fibers, although the association with soluble fibers was almost significant (borderline). Authors then performed a meta-analysis based on six to eight prospective cohort studies including their previously mentioned cohort and found a reduced diabetes risk of 33% with higher cereal fiber intake (RR for extreme categories, 0.67 [95% CI: 0.62–0.72]), but no significant associations for fruit and vegetable fiber (Schulze et al. 2007). In addition to the specific nature or structure of cereal fiber, one may also hypothesize that the compounds associated to fiber fraction in cereal (and not in fruits and vegetables) and called today fiber *copassengers* may also play a role. However, this point has to be confirmed.

When considering other whole-grain compound separately, in their meta-analysis based on six prospective cohort studies, Schulze et al. (2007) found a significant inverse association between magnesium intake and type 2 diabetes risk (RR for extreme categories, 0.77 [95% CI: 0.72–0.84]). More generally, concerning β-glucans, magnesium, iron, and zinc, other observational studies revealed either positive or no significant association with diabetes risk or lower fasting glucose and insulin, but never a negative association (Bao et al. 2012, Dong et al. 2011, Hruby et al. 2013, Jayawardena et al. 2012, Kanoni et al. 2011, Schulze et al. 2007, Tiwari and Cummins 2011).

Therefore, as pointed out for other features of the MetS, whole grains contain a whole set of phytochemicals able to act in synergy for better controlling glycemia and insulinemia, and in the end to protect from MetS development.

16.5 MICROALBUMINURIA AND FIBRINOLYSIS

As a function of research progress, other criteria than those cited previously may be well added for MetS diagnostic in a near future. In effect, increased serum levels of proinflammatory cytokines (IL-6 and TNF-α) and CRP have also been observed in patients with MetS, along with microalbuminuria (which is a good and independent biomarker of CVD risk) and an increase in coagulability (Kozirog et al. 2011, Tsuda 2008). However, the association between whole-grain consumption and both microalbuminuria and fibrinolysis has been apparently little studied and would probably deserve more attention (Pereira et al. 1998, 2000).

16.6 MECHANISMS UNDERLYING METABOLIC SYNDROME PROTECTION BY WHOLE GRAINS

Whole grains contain a whole set of several hundred phytochemicals having all different potential and beneficial effects. In effect, while one compound may exert several physiological effects, such as antioxidative, hypoglycemic, hypotensive, etc., several compounds may associate in a synergetic way to protect the organism from the development of one given deregulated metabolism: for example, at least 21 phytochemicals and groups of phytochemicals may play a direct or indirect role in lowering plasma lipids (Table 16.1). The antioxidant potential, one of the most studied deregulated mechanisms, has been added as a reference in deregulated metabolism and is concerned by at least 22 compounds or groups of compounds found in whole-grain cereals (Table 16.1).

Therefore, to explain each mechanism associated with each cereal compound via a reductionist perspective would not be very new and would need another chapter to be exhaustive.

It is probably more interesting to lay emphasis upon complexity of the potential mechanisms involved. Thus, based on existing knowledge, Figure 16.2 presents the associations between whole-grain compounds, deregulated mechanisms, and chronic diseases. The reality is obviously and probably largely more complex. However, Figure 16.2 allows underlining a beginning of interconnectedness between all mechanisms as unraveled by human studies. Probably those new high-throughput techniques, such as metabolomics and nutrigenomics, would allow going further in explaining more precisely which metabolic networks are stimulated following whole-grain

TABLE 16.1

Whole-Grain Cereal Compounds and Their Potential Physiological Effects as Regards to Deregulated Metabolisms Involved in the Metabolic Syndrome

Phytochemicals	Potential Physiological Properties						
	Antioxidants	Hypolipidemic	Hypoglycemic/ Hypo-insulinemic	Hypotensive/ Vascular System	Antiobesity	Anti-Inflammatory	Anticoagulant
α-linolenic acid	+			+		+	+
Sulfur compounds (e.g., glutathione)		+					
Insoluble fiber					+		
Soluble fiber		+	+		+		
Resistant starch		+	+		+		
Oligosaccharides (e.g., fructans)		+	+		+		
Phytic acid	+	+	+				
Lignins	+	+					
Iron	+	+			+		
Magnesium	+	+	+			+	+
Zinc	+		+		+	+	
Selenium	+		+				+
Calcium				+	+		+
Phosphore	+						
Potassium	+			+			
B vitamins	+	+	+	+			
Vitamin E	+	+		+	+	+	
Carotenoids	+					+	
Phenolic acid	+	+	+		+	+	+
Flavonoids	+	+			+		
Lignans	+	+					
Alkylresorcinols	+	+					
Betaine	+		+	+	+	+	

(Continued)

TABLE 16.1 (*Continued*)

Whole-Grain Cereal Compounds and Their Potential Physiological Effects as Regards to Deregulated Metabolisms Involved in the Metabolic Syndrome

Phytochemicals	Antioxidants	Hypolipidemic	Hypoglycemic/ Hypo-insulinemic	Hypotensive/ Vascular System	Antiobesity	Anti-Inflammatory	Anticoagulant
			Potential Physiological Properties				
Choline	+				+		
Inositols		+					
Policosanol	+	+					+
γ-oryzanol (rice)	+	+	+				+
Avenanthramides (oats)	+			+		+	
Saponins (oat)	+	+	+				
β-glucans (oat and barley)		+	+				
Total:	≥22	≥21	≥14	≥7	≥11	≥9	≥9

Source: Adapted from Fardet, A., *Nutr. Res. Rev.*, 23, 65, 2010.

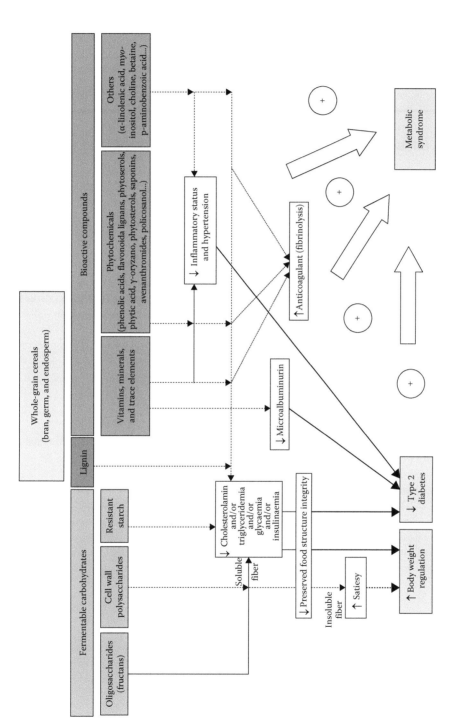

FIGURE 16.2 Associations between whole-grain phytochemicals, deregulated metabolisms, chronic diseases, and MetS. The dotted arrows (⇢) indicate the link between whole-grain bioactive compounds and protective physiological mechanisms, whereas the plain arrows (→) indicate the relationship between physiological mechanisms and health outcomes.

consumption, especially in MetS subjects. At least, this clearly underlined that whole-grain protection against MetS cannot be probably reduced to only the fiber fraction.

Notably, the role of food structure and low degree of starch gelatinization on slow release of carbohydrate has been already thoroughly discussed and commented and it does not need to be confirmed again. Briefly, slower release of glucose from starch in whole-grain food products leads to a more progressive release of glucose into bloodstream and is favorable to control plasma glycemic response, notably for diabetic people. Mechanisms are notably related to limited enzyme accessibility, either by compact structure of partially gelatinized starch, food particle size, or viscous cereal fiber as β-glucans (for more details, see Fardet 2010).

16.7   CONCLUSIONS AND PERSPECTIVES

Whole grains clearly appear as protective against MetS prevalence. It is true that one still lacks longitudinal cohort studies and randomized controlled trials to assess more firmly such a conclusion; but scientific evidence is today quite convincing. Whole grains have all the necessary bioactive compounds to combat each of the deregulated metabolisms involved in the MetS. And the protective effect would be attributable apparently rather to the bran than the germ fraction (de Munter et al. 2007), which lead to suggest that the fiber fraction plays an important role in protection since what differentiate germ from bran is primarily the fiber content: for example, whole-grain wheat, wheat bran, and wheat germ contain ≈13.2, 44.6, and 17.7 g of fiber/100 g by weight, respectively (Fardet 2010). In addition, what authors called whole grains in their study are most of the time whole-grain food products in which the germ fraction is rarely preserved due to its property to rancid upon time.

In addition to the role played by fiber, whole-grain products are also often characterized by a more or less intact food structure that play a significant role in increasing satiety and slowing release of glucose within bloodstream, two important factor to help control weight gain and glucose homeostasis and in the end to prevent from obesity and type 2 diabetes. Cereal technologists should explore more the possibilities of producing new whole-grain cereal food products with a more preserved structure or matrix, as found in muesli.

Otherwise, this review of literature again underlines the important role of grain products in human worldwide nutrition, not only whole-grain cereals, but also leguminous seeds and nuts. Compared to other food groups such as fruits and vegetables, grain products are rich in energy, fiber, and protective bioactive phytochemicals, are generally less expensive, and are easier to store.

However, what is protective against MetS is probably not only one food group such as whole grains but a way of eating or specific dietary patterns. Although they would deserve to be clearly identified, it is very likely that they should include whole grains.

REFERENCES

AACC. 1999. Definition of whole grain. Retrieved March 13, 2009, from http://www.aaccnet.org/definitions/wholegrain.asp.

AACC. 2006. AACC international comments on part III of the draft guidance on whole grain label statements. Retrieved March 13, 2009, from http://www.aaccnet.org/definitions/pdfs/AACCIntlWholeGrainComments.pdf.

AbuMweis, S.S., Jew, S., Ames, N.P. 2010. β-glucan from barley and its lipid-lowering capacity: A meta-analysis of randomized, controlled trials. *European Journal of Clinical Nutrition* 64:1472–1480.

Ahn, Y., Park, S., Kwack, H., Kim, M., Ko, K., Kim, S. 2013. Rice-eating pattern and the risk of metabolic syndrome especially waist circumference in Korean genome and epidemiology study (koges). *BMC Public Health* 13:61.

Anderson, J.W. 2003. Whole grains protect against atherosclerotic cardiovascular disease. *Proceedings of the Nutrition Society* 62:135–142.

Anderson, J.W., Hanna, T.J., Peng, X., Kryscio, R.J. 2000. Whole grain foods and heart disease risk. *Journal of the American College of Nutrition* 19:291S–299S.

Aune, D., Chan, D.S.M., Lau, R., Vieira, R., Greenwood, D.C., Kampman, E. et al. 2011. Dietary fibre, whole grains, and risk of colorectal cancer: Systematic review and dose-response meta-analysis of prospective studies. *BMJ* 343:d6617.

Bao, W., Rong, Y., Rong, S., Liu, L. 2012. Dietary iron intake, body iron stores, and the risk of type 2 diabetes: A systematic review and meta-analysis. *BMC Medicine* 10:119.

Björck, I., Östman, E., Kristensen, M., Anson, N.M., Price, R.K., Haenen, G.R.M.M. et al. 2012. Cereal grains for nutrition and health benefits: Overview of results from in vitro, animal and human studies in the HEALTHGRAIN project. *Trends in Food Science & Technology* 25:87–100.

Brown, L., Rosner, B., Willett, W.W., Sacks, F.M. 1999. Cholesterol-lowering effects of dietary fiber: A meta-analysis. *American Journal of Clinical Nutrition* 69:30–42.

Bucher, H.C., Cook, R.J., Guyatt, G.H., Lang, J.D., Cook, D.J., Hatala, R. et al. 1996. Effects of dietary calcium supplementation on blood pressure - A meta-analysis of randomized controlled trials. *JAMA* 275:1016–1022.

Burton, P., Lightowler, H.J. 2006. Influence of bread volume on glycaemic response and satiety. *British Journal of Nutrition* 96:877–882.

Chen, J.T., Wesley, R., Shamburek, R.D., Pucino, F., Csako, G. 2005. Meta-analysis of natural therapies for hyperlipidemia: Plant sterols and stanols versus policosanol. *Pharmacotherapy* 25:171–183.

Cleveland, L.E., Moshfegh, A.J., Albertson, A.M., Goldman, J.D. 2000. Dietary intake of whole grains. *Journal of the American College of Nutrition* 19:331S–338S.

Coudray, C., Demigne, C., Rayssiguier, Y. 2003. Effects of dietary fibers on magnesium absorption in animals and humans. *Journal of Nutrition* 133:1–4.

De Moura, F.F., Lewis, K.D., Falk, M.C. 2009. Applying the FDA definition of whole grains to the evidence for cardiovascular disease health claims. *Journal of Nutrition* 139:2220S–2226S.

de Munter, J.S., Hu, F.B., Spiegelman, D., Franz, M., van Dam, R.M. 2007. Whole grain, bran, and germ intake and risk of type 2 diabetes: A prospective cohort study and systematic review. *PLoS Medicine* 4:e261.

Dong, J.-Y., Xun, P., He, K., Qin, L.-Q. 2011. Magnesium intake and risk of type 2 diabetes meta-analysis of prospective cohort studies. *Diabetes Care* 34:2116–2122.

Esmaillzadeh, A., Mirmiran, P., Azizi, F. 2005. Whole-grain consumption and the metabolic syndrome: A favorable association in Tehranian adults. *European Journal of Clinical Nutrition* 59:353–362.

EUFIC. 2009. Whole grain fact sheet. Retrieved from http://www.eufic.org/article/en/page/BARCHIVE/expid/Whole-grain-Fact-Sheet/. (Accessed on July 18, 2013.)

Fardet, A. 2010. New hypotheses for the health-protective mechanisms of whole-grain cereals: What is beyond fibre? *Nutrition Research Reviews* 23:65–134.

FDA 2006. Draft guidance for industry and FDA staff: Whole grain label statements. Retrieved from http://www.cfsan.fda.gov/~dms/flgragui.html, (Accessed on July 18, 2013.) Washington, DC.

Flint, A.J., Hu, F.B., Glynn, R.J., Jensen, M.K., Franz, M., Sampson, L. et al. 2009. Whole grains and incident hypertension in men. *American Journal of Clinical Nutrition* 90:493–498.

Foster, M., Petocz, P., Samman, S. 2010. Effects of zinc on plasma lipoprotein cholesterol concentrations in humans: A meta-analysis of randomised controlled trials. *Atherosclerosis* 210:344–352.

Geleijnse, J.M., Kok, F.J., Grobbee, D.E. 2003. Blood pressure response to changes in sodium and potassium intake: A metaregression analysis of randomised trials. *Journal of Human Hypertension* 17:471–480.

Giacco, R., Costabile, G., Della Pepa, G., Anniballi, G., Griffo, E., Mangione, A. et al. 2014. A whole-grain cereal-based diet lowers postprandial plasma insulin and triglyceride levels in individuals with metabolic syndrome. *Nutrition Metabolism and Cardiovascular Diseases* 24:837–844.

Haber, G.B., Heaton, K.W., Murphy, D., Burroughs, L.F. 1977. Depletion and disruption of dietary fibre. Effects on satiety, plasma-glucose, and serum-insulin. *Lancet* 2:679–682.

Hosseinpour-Niazi, S., Mirmiran, P., Sohrab, G., Hosseini-Esfahani, F., Azizi, F. 2011. Inverse association between fruit, legume, and cereal fiber and the risk of metabolic syndrome: Tehran lipid and glucose study. *Diabetes Research and Clinical Practice* 94:276–283.

Hruby, A., Ngwa, J.S., Renstrom, F., Wojczynski, M.K., Ganna, A., Hallmans, G. et al. 2013. Higher magnesium intake is associated with lower fasting glucose and insulin, with no evidence of interaction with select genetic loci, in a meta-analysis of 15 charge consortium studies. *Journal of Nutrition* 143:345–353.

Hu, E.A., Pan, A., Malik, V., Sun, Q. 2012. White rice consumption and risk of type 2 diabetes: Meta-analysis and systematic review. *BMJ* 344:e1454.

Imdad, A., Jabeen, A., Bhutta, Z.A. 2011. Role of calcium supplementation during pregnancy in reducing risk of developing gestational hypertensive disorders: A meta-analysis of studies from developing countries. *BMC Public Health* 11 (Suppl 3):S18.

Jackson, K.H., West, S.G., Vanden Heuvel, J.P., Jonnalagadda, S.S., Ross, A.B., Hill, P.M. 2014. Effects of whole and refined grains in a weight-loss diet on markers of metabolic syndrome in individuals with increased waist circumference: A randomized controlled-feeding trial. *American Journal of Clinical Nutrition* 100:577–586.

Jayawardena, R., Ranasinghe, P., Galappatthy, P., Malkanthi, R.L.D.K., Constantine, G.R., Katulanda, P. 2012. Effects of zinc supplementation on diabetes mellitus: A systematic review and meta-analysis. *Diabetology and Metabolic Syndrome* 19 (4):13.

Jee, S.H., Miller, E.R., Guallar, E., Singh, V.K., Appel, L.J., Klag, M.J. 2002. The effect of magnesium supplementation on blood pressure: A meta-analysis of randomized clinical trials. *American Journal of Hypertension* 15:691–696.

Jones, J.M. 2008. Whole grains—Issues and deliberations from the whole grain task force. *Cereal Foods World* 53:260–264.

Kanoni, S., Nettleton, J.A., Hivert, M.-F., Ye, Z., van Rooij, F.J.A., Shungin, D. et al. 2011. Total zinc intake may modify the glucose-raising effect of a zinc transporter (SLC30A8) variant a 14-cohort meta-analysis. *Diabetes* 60:2407–2416.

Kass, L., Weekes, J., Carpenter, L. 2012. Effect of magnesium supplementation on blood pressure: A meta-analysis. *European Journal of Clinical Nutrition* 66:411–418.

Kastorini, C.M., Milionis, H.J., Esposito, K., Giugliano, D., Goudevenos, J.A., Panagiotakos, D.B. 2011. The effect of Mediterranean diet on metabolic syndrome and its components: A meta-analysis of 50 studies and 534,906 individuals. *Journal of the American College of Cardiology* 57:1299–1313.

Kozirog, M., Poliwczak, A.R., Duchnowicz, P., Koter-Michalak, M., Sikora, J., Broncel, M. 2011. Melatonin treatment improves blood pressure, lipid profile, and parameters of oxidative stress in patients with metabolic syndrome. *Journal of Pineal Research* 50:261–266.

Kristensen, M., Raben, A., Tetens, I. 2011. Whole grains in weight management - A systematic review of randomized human intervention studies. *Annals of Nutrition and Metabolism* 58:35.

Landsberg, L. 2001. Insulin-mediated sympathetic stimulation: Role in the pathogenesis of obesity-related hypertension (or, how insulin affects blood pressure, and why). *Journal of Hypertension* 19:523–528.

Magnusdottir, O.K., Landberg, R., Gunnarsdottir, I., Cloetens, L., Akesson, B., Rosqvist, F. et al. 2014. Whole grain rye intake, reflected by a biomarker, is associated with favorable blood lipid outcomes in subjects with the metabolic syndrome - A randomized study. *PLoS One* 9:e110827–e110827.

McKeown, N.M., Meigs, J.B., Liu, S., Saltzman, E., Wilson, P.W., Jacques, P.F. 2004. Carbohydrate nutrition, insulin resistance, and the prevalence of the metabolic syndrome in the Framingham Offspring Cohort. *Diabetes Care* 27:538–546.

Mellen, P.B., Walsh, T.F., Herrington, D.M. 2008. Whole grain intake and cardiovascular disease: A meta-analysis. *Nutrition, Metabolism and Cardiovascular Diseases* 18:283–290.

Miller, M. 2004. Meta-analysis finds women with dyslipidemia respond as well or better than men to extended-release niacin. *Evidence-Based Cardiovascular Medicine* 8:311–312.

Moruisi, K.G., Oosthuizen, W., Opperman, A.M. 2006. Phytosterols/stanols lower cholesterol concentrations in familial hypercholesterolemic subjects: A systematic review with meta-analysis. *Journal of the American College of Nutrition* 25:41–48.

Mozaffarian, D., Hao, T., Rimm, E.B., Willett, W.C., Hu, F.B. 2011. Changes in diet and lifestyle and long-term weight gain in women and men. *New England Journal of Medicine* 364:2392–2404.

Murakami, K., Okubo, H., Sasaki, S. 2005. Effect of dietary factors on incidence of type 2 diabetes: A systematic review of cohort studies. *Journal of Nutritional Science and Vitaminology* 51:292–310.

Nettleton, J.A., McKeown, N.M., Kanoni, S., Lemaitre, R.N., Hivert, M.-F., Ngwa, J. et al. 2010. Interactions of dietary whole-grain intake with fasting glucose- and insulin-related genetic loci in individuals of European descent a meta-analysis of 14 cohort studies. *Diabetes Care* 33:2684–2691.

Pereira, M.A., Jacobs, D.R., Kroenke, C.H., Slattery, M.L., Van Horn, L., Hilner, J.E. 1998. Whole grain intake, hyperinsulinemia, and microalbuminuria in young adults. *Circulation* 98:374.

Pereira, M.A., Jacobs, D.R., Pins, J.J., Raatz, S.K., Gross, M.D., Slavin, J. et al. 2000. The effect of whole grains on inflammation and fibrinolysis. *Circulation* 101:711.

Potenza, M.V., Mechanick, J.I. 2009. The metabolic syndrome: Definition, global impact, and pathophysiology. *Nutrition in Clinical Practice* 24:560–577.

Priebe, M.G., van Binsbergen, J.J., de Vos, R., Vonk, R.J. 2008. Whole grain foods for the prevention of type 2 diabetes mellitus. *Cochrane Database of Systematic Reviews* 23(1):CD006061.

Ripsin, C.M., Keenan, J.M., Jacobs, D.R., Elmer, P.J., Welch, R.R., Vanhorn, L. et al. 1992. Oat products and lipid lowering - A metaanalysis. *JAMA* 267:3317–3325.

Sahyoun, N.R., Jacques, P.F., Zhang, X.L., Juan, W., McKeown, N.M. 2006. Whole-grain intake is inversely associated with the metabolic syndrome and mortality in older adults. *American Journal of Clinical Nutrition* 83:124–131.

Schulze, M.B., Schulz, M., Heidemann, C., Schienkiewitz, A., Hoffmann, K., Boeing, H. 2007. Fiber and magnesium intake and incidence of type 2 diabetes: A prospective study and meta-analysis. *Archives of Internal Medicine* 167:956–965.

Shi, Z., Taylor, A.W., Hu, G., Gill, T., Wittert, G.A. 2012. Rice intake, weight change and risk of the metabolic syndrome development among Chinese adults: The Jiangsu Nutrition Study (JIN). *Asia Pacific Journal of Clinical Nutrition* 21:35–43.

Son, S., Lee, H., Park, K., Ha, T., Seo, J. 2013. Nutritional evaluation and its relation to the risk of metabolic syndrome according to the consumption of cooked rice and cooked rice with multi-grains in Korean adults: Based on 2007-2008 Korean National Health and Nutrition Examination Survey. *Korean Journal of Community Nutrition* 18:77–87.

Song, S., Lee, J.E., Song, W.O, Paik, H.-Y., Song, Y. 2014. Carbohydrate intake and refined-grain consumption are associated with metabolic syndrome in the Korean adult population. *Journal of the Academy of Nutrition and Dietetics* 114:54–62.

Streppel, M.T., Arends, L.R., van't Veer, P., Grobbee, D.E., Geleijnse, J.M. 2005. Dietary fiber and blood pressure - A meta-analysis of randomized placebo-controlled trials. *Archives of Internal Medicine* 165:150–156.

Sun, Q., Spiegelman, D., van Dam, R.M., Holmes, M.D., Malik, V.S., Willett, W.C. et al. 2010. White rice, brown rice, and risk of type 2 diabetes in us men and women. *Archives of Internal Medicine* 170:961–969.

Surget, A., Barron, C. 2005. Histologie du grain de blé. *Industries des Cereales* 145:3–7.

Ting, W., Jia, F., Yuexin, Y., Lishi, Z., Junhua, H. 2009. The effects of phytosterols/stanols on blood lipid profiles: A systematic review with meta-analysis. *Asia Pacific Journal of Clinical Nutrition* 18:179–186.

Tiwari, U., Cummins, E. 2011. Meta-analysis of the effect of beta-glucan intake on blood cholesterol and glucose levels. *Nutrition* 27:1008–1016.

Tsuda, T. 2008. Regulation of adipocyte function by anthocyanins; possibility of preventing the metabolic syndrome. *Journal of Agricultural and Food Chemistry* 56:642–646.

van Bommel, E., Cleophas, T. 2012. Potassium treatment for hypertension in patients with high salt intake: A meta-analysis. *International Journal of Clinical Pharmacology and Therapeutics* 50:478–482.

van Mierlo, L.A.J., Arends, L.R., Streppel, M.T., Zeegers, M.P.A., Kok, F.J., Grobbee, D.E. et al. 2006. Blood pressure response to calcium supplementation: A meta-analysis of randomized controlled trials. *Journal of Human Hypertension* 20:571–580.

Wanders, A.J., van den Borne, J., de Graaf, C., Hulshof, T., Jonathan, M.C., Kristensen, M. et al. 2011. Effects of dietary fibre on subjective appetite, energy intake and body weight: A systematic review of randomized controlled trials. *Obesity Reviews* 12:724–739.

Wang, L., Gaziano, J.M., Liu, S., Manson, J.E., Buring, J.E., Sesso, H.D. 2007. Whole- and refined-grain intakes and the risk of hypertension in women. *American Journal of Clinical Nutrition* 86:472–479.

Whelton, P.K., He, J., Cutler, J.A., Brancati, F.L., Appel, L.J., Follmann, D. et al. 1997. Effects of oral potassium on blood pressure - Meta-analysis of randomized controlled clinical trials. *JAMA* 277:1624–1632.

Whelton, S.P., Hyre, A.D., Pedersen, B., Yi, Y., Whelton, P.K., He, J. 2005. Effect of dietary fiber intake on blood pressure: A meta-analysis of randomized, controlled clinical trials. *Journal of Hypertension* 23:475–481.

Wirfalt, E., Hedblad, B., Gullberg, B., Mattisson, I., Andren, C., Rosander, U. et al. 2001. Food patterns and components of the metabolic syndrome in men and women: A cross-sectional study within the malmo diet and cancer cohort. *American Journal of Epidemiology* 154:1150–1159.

Wu, T., Yang, Y., Zhang, L., Han, J. 2010. Systematic review of the effects of inulin-type fructans on blood lipid profiles: A meta-analysis. *Journal of Hygiene Research* 39:172–176.

Ye, E.Q., Chacko, S.A., Chou, E.L., Kugizaki, M., Liu, S. 2012. Greater whole-grain intake is associated with lower risk of type 2 diabetes, cardiovascular disease, and weight gain. *The Journal of Nutrition* 142:1304–1313.

Yoo, S., Nicklas, T., Baranowski, T., Zakeri, I.F., Yang, S.J., Srinivasan, S.R. et al. 2004. Comparison of dietary intakes associated with metabolic syndrome risk factors in young adults: The Bogalusa Heart Study. *American Journal of Clinical Nutrition* 80:841–848.

Younjhin, A., Seon-Joo, P., Hye-kyoung, K., Mi Kyung, K., Kwang-Pil, K., Sung Soo, K. 2013. Rice-eating pattern and the risk of metabolic syndrome especially waist circumference in Korean Genome and Epidemiology Study (KoGES). *BMC Public Health* 13:61–61.

Zhang, H.-W., Zhang, Y.-H., Lu, M.-J., Tong, W.-J., Cao, G.-W. 2007. Comparison of hypertension, dyslipidae-mia and hyperglycaemia between buckwheat seed-consuming and non-consuming Mongolian-Chinese populations in inner Mongolia, China. *Clinical and Experimental Pharmacology and Physiology* 34:838–844.

17 Nut Consumption and Metabolic Syndrome

Siew Ling Tey, Alexandra Wynne-Ankaret Hamilton Chisholm, and Rachel Clare Brown

CONTENTS

17.1 INTRODUCTION

Nuts have formed an important part of the human diet since ancient times. They are a source of energy and provide a wide array of essential nutrients (Dreher et al. 1996, Salas-Salvado et al. 2011). It has been known for many years that cardiovascular disease (CVD) rates are lower in vegetarians and other health-conscious populations such as the Seventh Day Adventist and those who follow a Mediterranean diet (Sabate 1999, Estruch et al. 2006). One of the key differences between these diets and the typical Western diet is that nut consumption is twice as high (Sabate 1993, Dreher et al. 1996).

This chapter focuses first on the nutrient composition of nuts that may impart healthful effects (Section 17.2). Second, an overview of major epidemiological studies (Section 17.3.1) and randomized controlled trials (RCTs) (Section 17.3.2) that have investigated the relationship between nut consumption and the risk factors for metabolic syndrome (MetS) in various population groups will be discussed. The methods and findings of the studies that were conducted in participants with MetS will be presented in Section 17.4. Finally, the future directions for research in the nut and MetS area will be discussed (Section 17.5).

17.2   NUTRIENT COMPOSITION OF NUTS

A tree nut is defined as a one-seeded dried fruit or an edible kernel surrounded by a hard shell (Coulston 2003). These include almonds, Brazil nuts, cashews, hazelnuts, pecans, pine nuts, pistachios, macadamias, and walnuts. Most consumers also perceive peanuts as nuts, although they are botanically classed as a legume (Ros 2010). For this chapter, the term *nuts* includes peanuts and all tree nuts, except for chestnuts and coconuts. This is because peanuts have a very similar nutrient profile to other tree nuts, whereas chestnuts and coconuts differ from tree nuts in several ways. Chestnuts are relatively high in carbohydrate (53.2 g/100 g), and coconuts are high in saturated fatty acids (SFA) (29.7 g/100 g). In addition, these two nuts contain high amounts of moisture (49 g/100 g) and very little protein (<7 g/100 g). These attributes make their nutrient profiles different from the other aforementioned nuts (Sathe et al. 2009, Ros 2010).

Tables 17.1 and 17.2 show the macronutrients and selected micronutrients per 100 g and one serving (30 g) of nuts obtained from food composition data. Nuts are one of the most nutritionally dense foods. Most nuts, although relatively high in fat, have a high content of *cis*-unsaturated fatty acids, whereas the SFA content is relatively low (4%–17%). Together, monounsaturated fatty acids (MUFA) and polyunsaturated fatty acids (PUFA) in nuts contribute around 70%–87% of the energy from fat (Table 17.1). Almost one-half of the total fat content of most nuts such as almonds, cashew nuts, hazelnuts, macadamia nuts, peanuts, pecan nuts, and pistachio nuts is MUFA, whereas walnuts contain mostly PUFA. Similar proportions of MUFA and PUFA are found in Brazil nuts and pine nuts (Ros and Mataix 2006). In addition, nuts are very low in carbohydrate while high in protein and dietary fiber, where 100 g of nuts can provide up to 26 g of protein and 8 g of fiber (Brufau et al. 2006, Salas-Salvado et al. 2006, Kendall et al. 2010a).

Nuts are important sources of an array of phytochemicals including phenolics such as flavonoids, phenolic acids, and tannins, as well as lipids including carotenoids and phytosterols (Bolling et al. 2011, Vinson and Cai 2012). The phytosterol content in tree nuts range from 72 to 214 mg/100 g (Table 17.2). Nuts are low in sodium while rich in a wide range of essential micronutrients such as folate, vitamin E, calcium, magnesium, copper, and potassium, which are required in very small amounts yet perform a vital role in maintaining overall good health (Segura et al. 2006, Sathe et al. 2009, Lee et al. 2011). Nut consumption has been consistently reported to improve nutrient intakes and diet quality (Jaceldo-Siegl et al. 2004, King et al. 2008, O'Neil et al. 2010, 2012, Tey et al. 2011).

17.3   NUT CONSUMPTION AND RISK FACTORS FOR CHRONIC DISEASE

Both epidemiological studies and clinical trials have shown that regular nut consumption plays an important protective role in the management of chronic disease (Sabate and Ang 2009, Ros 2010). This section will summarize the findings of several large epidemiological studies and RCTs on frequent nut consumption and risk factors of chronic disease associated with the MetS.

17.3.1   EPIDEMIOLOGICAL STUDIES

17.3.1.1   Cardiovascular Disease

Individuals with MetS have an increased risk of CVD (Mottillo et al. 2010). Four large epidemiological studies conducted in the United States have examined the associations between nut

TABLE 17.1

Average Macronutrient Composition for 100 g and One Serving (30 g) of Raw Nuts

	Energy (kJ)		Total Fat (g)		SFA (g)		MUFA (g)		PUFA (g)		Protein (g)		CHO (g)		Fiber (g)	
	100 g	30 g	100 g	30 g	100 g	30 g	100 g	30 g	100 g	30 g	100 g	30 g	100 g	30 g	100 g	30 g
Almonds	2550	765	55.6	16.7	4.4	1.3	38.0	11.4	10.4	3.1	21.0	6.3	6.4	1.9	7.4	2.2
Brazil nuts	2830	849	68.2	20.5	17.4	5.2	22.4	6.7	25.4	7.6	12.0	3.6	3.8	1.1	4.3	1.3
Cashews	2440	732	49.2	14.8	8.4	2.5	31.1	9.3	7.5	2.3	17.7	5.3	17.8	5.3	5.9	1.8
Hazelnuts	2620	786	59.8	17.9	5.7	1.7	42.4	12.7	8.7	2.6	17.0	5.1	5.2	1.6	7.4	2.2
Macadamias	2990	897	73.7	22.1	11.0	3.3	58.2	17.5	1.3	0.4	8.3	2.5	4.5	1.4	5.3	1.6
Mixed nuts	2520	756	52.5	15.8	7.5	2.3	23.5	7.1	18.0	5.4	22.6	6.8	10.1	3.0	6.0	1.8
Peanuts	2390	717	49.0	14.7	9.2	2.8	23.4	7.0	13.9	4.2	24.3	7.3	8.0	2.4	8.0	2.4
Pecan nuts	2910	873	67.6	20.3	5.4	1.6	42.2	12.7	16.7	5.0	7.8	2.3	13.8	4.1	4.7	1.4
Pine nuts	2520	756	50.7	15.2	7.8	2.3	19.2	5.8	21.5	6.5	24.0	7.2	12.6	3.8	1.9	0.6
Pistachios	2610	783	54.4	16.3	6.9	2.1	36.8	11.0	8.3	2.5	20.6	6.2	13.2	4.0	6.0	1.8
Walnuts	2930	879	64.5	19.4	6.5	2.0	12.4	3.7	42.5	12.8	25.7	7.7	4.0	1.2	5.2	1.6

Source: Lesperance, L., *The Concise New Zealand Food Composition Tables*, 8th edn., New Zealand Institute for Plant & Food Research, Palmerston North, New Zealand, 2009.

CHO, carbohydrate; MUFA, monounsaturated fatty acids; PUFA, polyunsaturated fatty acids; SFA, saturated fatty acids.

TABLE 17.2

Average Phytosterol and Micronutrient Composition for 100 g and One Serving (30 g) of Raw Nuts

	Phytosterol (mg)[a,b]		Vitamin E (mg)[a,c]		Folate (mcg)		Calcium (mg)		Magnesium (mg)[a]		Copper (mg)[a]		Potassium (mg)		Sodium (mg)	
	100 g	30 g	100 g	30 g	100 g	30 g	100 g	30 g	100 g	30 g	100 g	30 g	100 g	30 g	100 g	30 g
AI/RDI[d]	N/A		M, 10		M, 400		M, 1000		M, 400–420		M, 1.7		M, 3800		M, 460–920	
			F, 7		F, 400		F, 1000–1300		F, 310–320		F, 1.2		F, 2800		F, 460–920	
Almonds	141	43	26.2	7.9	96	29	250	75	268	80	1.0	0.3	860	258	6	2
Brazil nuts	N/A	N/A	5.7	1.7	4	1	180	54	376	113	1.7	0.5	760	228	2	1
Cashews	N/A	N/A	0.9	0.3	67	20	34	10	292	88	2.2	0.7	550	165	11	3
Hazelnuts	96	29	15.0	4.5	116	35	179	54	163	49	1.7	0.5	900	270	T	T
Macadamias	116	35	0.5	0.2	16	5	70	21	130	39	0.8	0.2	368	110	5	2
Mixed nuts	N/A	N/A	N/A	N/A	50	15	70	21	225	67	1.3	0.4	597	179	12	4
Peanuts	N/A	N/A	N/A	N/A	110	33	61	18	N/A	N/A	N/A	N/A	680	204	6	2
Pecan nuts	102	31	1.4	0.4	39	12	36	11	121	36	1.2	0.4	392	118	1	0
Pine nuts	141	42	9.3	2.8	54	16	26	8	251	75	1.3	0.4	599	180	4	1
Pistachios	214	64	2.3	0.7	58	17	135	41	121	36	1.3	0.4	1090	327	6	2
Walnuts	72	22	0.7	0.2	83	25	129	39	158	47	1.6	0.5	575	173	1	0

Source: Lesperance, L., *The Concise New Zealand Food Composition Tables*, 8th edn., New Zealand Institute for Plant & Food Research, Palmerston North, New Zealand, 2009.

AI, adequate intake; F, female; M, male; N/A, not available; RDI, recommended dietary intake; T, trace value.

[a] USDA National Nutrient Database for Standard Reference, Release 23 (U.S. Department of Agriculture and Agriculture Research Service 2011).

[b] Phytosterol is calculated as the total amount of stigmasterol, campesterol, and beta-sitosterol.

[c] Vitamin E refers to the α-tocopherol content.

[d] Nutrition Reference Values for Australia and New Zealand (National Health and Medical Research Council 2006). AI (vitamin E, copper, potassium, sodium) and RDI (folate, calcium, magnesium) for adults aged 19–70 years.

consumption and coronary heart disease (CHD) risk. These studies include the Adventist Health Study (Fraser et al. 1992, 1995, Fraser and Shavlik 1997), the Iowa Women's Health Study (IWHS) (Prineas et al. 1993, Kushi et al. 1996, Ellsworth et al. 2001, Blomhoff et al. 2006), the Nurses' Health Study (NHS) (Hu et al. 1998, Li et al. 2009), and the Physicians' Health Study (PHS) (Albert et al. 2002, Djousse et al. 2008). A food frequency questionnaire (FFQ) was used to assess nut consumption, with categories ranging from *never consume* to *consume more than five times per week*, where one time is equivalent to one serving (1 ounce = 28.35 g). Results from these four large U.S. epidemiological studies are remarkably consistent. An inverse, dose–response relationship was found between nut intake and several clinical outcomes, such as CHD, sudden cardiac death, and all-cause mortality in different population groups after 6–22 years of follow-up (Kelly and Sabate 2006, Ros 2010). A pooled analysis of these four cohorts published up until 2006 showed that participants who had the highest nut intake had a 34% (95% CI 23%, 44%) reduction in the risk of CHD incidence and 35% (95% CI 11%, 53%) reduction in the risk of total CHD (Kris-Etherton et al. 2008). For an increase in one serving (~30 g) of nut consumption weekly, there was an average 8.3% reduction in the risk of CHD death (Kelly and Sabate 2006). Similar reductions were seen for the risks of sudden cardiac death and all-cause mortality (Sabate and Ang 2009).

In summary, the results from the epidemiological studies suggest that nuts have a cardioprotective effect. This effect appears to be independent of recognized coronary risk factors, such as participants' age (from young adults to the oldest-old population), sex (men or women), race (non-Hispanic white or Black American), hypertension, smoking status, relative weight and physical activity level, alcohol use, and other nutritional characteristics (Sabate 1999, Fraser 2000, deLorgeril et al. 2001, Sabate and Ang 2009, Sabaté and Wien 2010).

17.3.1.2 Diabetes

Previous research has shown that individuals with MetS have higher risk of developing type 2 diabetes mellitus (Ford et al. 2008). To date, only four epidemiological studies have examined the effects of nut consumption and the risk of type 2 diabetes. Two studies have reported an inverse relationship between nut consumption and type 2 diabetes in women (Jiang et al. 2002, Villegas et al. 2008). The strengths of these two cohorts include repeated dietary measurements and the use of a validated FFQ. On the other hand, a positive association between frequent nut consumption and the risk of diabetes was observed in the IWHS (Parker et al. 2003), whereas no association was found in the PHS (Kochar et al. 2010). The contradictory results observed in these four cohorts could be due to the differences in participants' characteristics such as sex and age, sample size, definition of nuts, frequency of dietary assessments, questionnaire used to confirm diabetes diagnoses, and the level of adjustments in the statistical analyses (Jenkins et al. 2008a, Kendall et al. 2010a,b).

Given the limited epidemiologic studies in this area, further prospective studies of longer duration, using multiple validated dietary assessments, and standardized diagnostic for cases are required to determine the potential role of nut consumption in type 2 diabetes.

17.3.1.3 Hypertension

Elevated blood pressure is one of the major modifiable risk factors of MetS and accounts for 7.6 million premature deaths worldwide (Lawes et al. 2008, World Health Organisation 2004). Compliance with advice to consume nuts has been found to inversely correlate with systolic and diastolic blood pressures (Jenkins et al. 2008b). It is possible that the reduction in blood pressure with frequent nut consumption may result in a lower risk of hypertension, stroke, and atrial fibrillation, which is an important risk factor for stroke (Fuster et al. 2006).

To date, only the PHS and the Seguimiento Universidad de Navarra (SUN) cohorts have examined the association between frequent nut consumption and hypertension (Djousse et al. 2009, Martinez-Lapiscina et al. 2010), stroke (Djousse et al. 2010), and atrial fibrillation (Khawaja et al. 2012).

The current limited epidemiologic evidence suggests a protective effect of nut consumption on the risk of hypertension, especially those with BMI < 25 kg/m^2 (Djousse et al. 2009), but no effect on stroke (Djousse et al. 2010) and atrial fibrillation (Khawaja et al. 2012). It is important to point out that the forms (i.e., fried, grilled, raw, roasted, salted, spiced) and types of nuts consumed, which may influence the risk of hypertension, stroke, and arterial fibrillation, were not examined in either cohort (Casas-Agustench et al. 2011c).

17.3.1.4 Oxidative Stress, Inflammation, and Endothelial Dysfunction

Novel risk factors, including oxidative stress, chronic inflammation, and endothelial dysfunction, play important roles in the development of MetS, CVD, cancer, and diabetes (Brown and Hu 2001, Pradhan and Ridker 2002, Mantovani et al. 2008, Valavanidis et al. 2009, Monteiro and Azevedo 2010, Oliver et al. 2010, Bartunek and Vanderheyden 2012). Several epidemiological studies have examined the association between nut consumption and novel risk factors in different population groups (Jiang et al. 2006, Mantzoros et al. 2006, Salas-Salvado et al. 2008b, Gopinath et al. 2011, O'Neil et al. 2011, 2012). The Multi-Ethnic Study of Atherosclerosis was the first study consisting of an ethnically diverse population that showed significant inverse, dose–response associations between nuts and seed consumption and concentrations of C-reactive protein (CRP), IL-6, and fibrinogen after adjusting for potential confounders (P for trend = 0.003 in all cases). However, these associations were attenuated slightly after additional adjustment for BMI, which is a strong determinant of inflammatory markers (P values range from 0.03 to 0.06). The associations did not change appreciably when nuts, seeds, and peanuts and peanut butter were analyzed separately (Jiang et al. 2006). Two recent National Health and Nutrition Examination Survey (NHANES) studies have shown that tree nut consumers and *out-of-hand* nut consumers (i.e., those nuts consumed solely as nuts and not as part of products) had significantly lower CRP than nonconsumers (O'Neil et al. 2011, 2012). On the other hand, Li et al. (2009) failed to show any association between frequent nut consumption and inflammatory markers such as tumor necrosis factor receptor II, intercellular adhesion molecule 1, E-selectin, CRP, and fibrinogen among 1171 female nurses with type 2 diabetes. The contradictory results could be due to the differences in participant characteristics and the use of different dietary assessment tools (24 h recall vs. FFQ).

To date, only one prospective study has examined the association between frequent nut consumption and inflammatory disease mortality (Gopinath et al. 2011). This prospective study with 15 years follow-up, consisting of 2514 participants, showed that compared with the participants in the lowest tertile of nut consumption, those who were in the second and third tertiles of nut consumption at baseline had a significant respective 51% and 32% reduction in the risk of developing inflammatory disease mortality (Gopinath et al. 2011).

When the results are taken together, the majority of the studies suggest that nut consumption is inversely related to inflammatory markers, cell adhesion molecules, and mortality from inflammatory disease.

17.3.1.5 Body Weight

Obesity especially abdominal adiposity is an important predictor of MetS (Despres and Lemieux 2006). Nuts are high-fat, energy-dense foods, and in theory, frequent consumption of nuts could potentially contribute to a high-energy intake and promote weight gain, which may offset the cardioprotective effects of nuts (St-Onge 2005). However, the PREvención con DIeta MEDiterránea (PREDIMED) study showed each daily serving (30 g) of nuts was associated with a decrease in BMI by 0.78 kg/m^2 and waist circumference by 2.1 cm. The reductions were similar in each gender (Casas-Agustench et al. 2011a). In addition, several cross-sectional studies have consistently demonstrated an inverse or no association between baseline frequency of nut consumption and BMI (Fraser et al. 1992, Hu et al. 1998, Ellsworth et al. 2001, Jiang et al. 2002, 2006, Djousse et al. 2009, Li et al. 2009, Kochar et al. 2010, Khawaja et al. 2012). Also, the NHS and the SUN cohort studies showed that frequent nut consumption was associated with less weight gain (Bes-Rastrollo et al. 2007, 2009, Martinez-Gonzalez and Bes-Rastrollo 2011) and lower risk of becoming overweight or obese (Bes-Rastrollo et al. 2007, Martinez-Gonzalez and Bes-Rastrollo 2011).

17.3.2 RANDOMIZED CONTROLLED TRIALS

Abnormal blood lipid profiles and glycemic control, elevated blood pressure, inflammation and endothelial dysfunction, and central obesity are a constellation of characteristics observed in people with MetS (Alberti et al. 2006). A large multicenter RCT conducted in older participants at high risk of CVD, the PREDIMED study, has shown that a Mediterranean diet supplemented with mixed nuts significantly reduced the incidence of major cardiovascular events (Estruch et al. 2013) and the prevalence of MetS (Salas-Salvado et al. 2008a) compared to those who consumed a low-fat control diet. These reductions could be explained by the significant improvements in blood pressure, blood lipid profiles, insulin resistance (Estruch 2010), inflammatory markers (Urpi-Sarda et al. 2012), and oxidative damage to DNA (Mitjavila et al. 2013). However, it should be noted that it is difficult to interpret the results of the PREDIMED study as the Mediterranean diet with nuts was compared with a low-fat diet. The following section will discuss the findings of RCTs that have compared the effects of nut-enriched diets with either comparable control diets or participant's habitual diets on components associated with the MetS.

17.3.2.1 Blood Lipids and Lipoproteins

Numerous RCTs have investigated the effects of nut consumption on blood lipids and lipoproteins (Kris-Etherton et al. 2008). In line with the findings from epidemiological studies, RCTs have shown that nuts lowered total cholesterol (TC) and low-density lipoprotein cholesterol (LDL-C) concentrations in a dose-dependent manner (Jenkins et al. 2002, 2011, Sabate et al. 2003, Gebauer et al. 2008). These studies also reported that the incorporation of nuts into a Step I diet (Sabate et al. 2003, Gebauer et al. 2008), Step II diet (Jenkins et al. 2002), or a diet recommended by the National Cholesterol Education Program Adult Treatment Panel III and the American Diabetes Association (Jenkins et al. 2011) produced further improvements in lipid profiles, compared with the recommended control diets without nuts.

A pooled analysis consisting of 25 intervention trials among 583 participants showed a greater improvement in blood lipids with nut consumption among participants with high baseline LDL-C (>3.37 mmol/L) and lower BMI (<25 kg/m^2), and this effect was independent of the nut type consumed (Sabate et al. 2010). The pooled analysis estimated an average reduction of 0.28 mmol/L (5.1%) in TC and 0.26 mmol/L (7.4%) in LDL-C, while no significant effects were found on high-density lipoprotein cholesterol (HDL-C) and triglycerides (TAG) with a consumption of 67 g of nuts daily. Consistent with this finding, a meta-analysis of five RCTs with almonds (25–168 g/day) (Phung et al. 2009) and a meta-analysis of 13 feeding studies with walnuts (30–108 g/day) (Banel and Hu 2009) reported significant reductions of TC (0.18–0.27 mmol/L) and LDL-C (0.15–0.24 mmol/L) following a nut-enriched diet, without altering HDL-C and TAG compared to a control diet or participants' baseline diet.

The primary mechanism that may likely explain the improvement in blood lipid profiles following nut consumption is the increase in MUFA and PUFA intakes while with a decrease in SFA intake (Ros and Mataix 2006, Berryman et al. 2011). However, the observed reductions in cholesterol concentrations with nut consumption are greater than those predicted by the equations based on the fatty acid exchange alone, suggesting that other nutrients and bioactive compounds in nuts such as phytosterols, arginine, fiber, and vitamin E might also contribute to the hypocholesterolemic effect (Kris-Etherton 1999, Kris-Etherton et al. 2000, Berryman et al. 2011, Bolling et al. 2011).

In summary, although the clinical trials presented here differ in the degree of dietary control, participant characteristics, comparison diets, study design, sample size, duration of the intervention, as well as the amount or type of nuts consumed, collectively the trials have convincingly found that the inclusion of nuts in the diet results in significant reductions in TC and LDL-C and have minor influence on HDL-C and TAG.

17.3.2.2 Glycemic Control

Recent evidence suggests that the high amounts of unsaturated fatty acids in nuts may improve beta cell efficiency by increasing the secretion of glucagon-like peptide-1, which plays an important role in the regulation of postprandial glucose clearance and insulin sensitivity (Casas-Agustench et al. 2010). Several small short-term clinical trials have investigated the effects of chronic nut consumption on glycemic control. Overall, these studies have produced equivocal results with the majority of them reporting no effect on blood glucose, insulin, and HbA1c in different population groups. A small number of studies reported significant improvements in blood glucose (Li et al. 2011), insulin (Tapsell et al. 2009, Wien et al. 2010, Li et al. 2011), or HbA1c (Cohen and Johnston 2011, Jenkins et al. 2011) concentrations after consuming a nut-enriched diet. On the other hand, one study showed a significant increase in blood insulin after the consumption of a walnut-enriched diet among people with type 2 diabetes (Ma et al. 2010). It should be noted that most of these studies might be underpowered and had a relatively short intervention period (Jenkins et al. 2008a, Kendall et al. 2010b). Future studies with appropriate sample size calculation and longer duration are warranted to draw definitive conclusions on the effects of nuts on glycemic control and potential mechanisms for this.

17.3.2.3 Blood Pressure

Unprocessed raw nuts are low in sodium while high in unsaturated fatty acids, potassium, calcium, and magnesium. These dietary components may have a beneficial effect on blood pressure (Casas-Agustench et al. 2011c). Several RCTs have investigated the effects of nut consumption on systolic and diastolic blood pressures (Casas-Agustench et al. 2011c). Most of these small-sized clinical trials performed to date have found no effect of nut consumption on blood pressure. Only three studies showed that blood pressure was significantly lower following a nut-enriched diet, when compared with an average American diet (West et al. 2010), a complex-carbohydrate low-calorie diet (Wien et al. 2003), and a low-SFA and low-cholesterol control diet (Jenkins et al. 2011). One study reported a significantly higher systolic and diastolic blood pressures after 8 weeks of consuming an ad libitum diet enriched with 56 g of walnuts, compared with an ad libitum diet without nuts in 24 type 2 diabetic patients (Ma et al. 2010). It is not clear whether there is a difference in the response to nut consumption on blood pressure between persons with diabetes and healthy or hypercholesterolemic participants. When taken together, there is no apparent effect of nut consumption on blood pressure. Future research should be adequately powered and use a more comprehensive measure for blood pressure (i.e., ambulatory blood pressure) in order to determine whether there is a true blood pressure–lowering effect with nut consumption (Casas-Agustench et al. 2011c).

17.3.2.4 Oxidative Stress, Inflammation, and Endothelial Dysfunction

As previously mentioned, oxidative stress, inflammation, and endothelial dysfunction are more prevalent in people with MetS. Recent reviews suggest that the bioactive antioxidants and dietary polyphenols in nuts may work synergistically to protect against oxidative stress and inflammation (Blomhoff et al. 2006, López-Uriarte et al. 2009, Bolling et al. 2011, Vinson and Cai 2012). Additionally, the enrichment of the diet with unsaturated fatty acids, arginine, and antioxidant vitamins following nut intake may reduce inflammation and cell adhesion molecule expression and improve endothelial function (Brown and Hu 2001, Faxon et al. 2004, Giugliano et al. 2006, Calder et al. 2011). Thus, a diet high in nuts may exert additional health benefits beyond the cholesterol-lowering effect.

The predominant fatty acids found in most nuts are MUFA, which is not an oxidation substrate. On the other hand, walnuts are rich in PUFA, which are the most vulnerable to LDL-oxidation due to their double bonds. Previous research suggests that the large amounts of antioxidants and phytochemicals in walnuts may counteract the pro-oxidant effect of PUFA and prevent oxidation from occurring (López-Uriarte et al. 2009, Ros 2009, McKay et al. 2010). Clinical trials show that a nut-enriched diet improves antioxidant activity and biomarkers of antioxidant status (Ros et al. 2004, Jambazian et al. 2005, Kocyigit et al. 2006, Li et al. 2007, 2011, Thomson et al. 2008, Kay et al. 2010, Nouran et al. 2010, Wien et al. 2010). Most of the results suggest diets high in MUFA-rich nuts such as almonds (Jenkins et al. 2002, 2008c, Jia et al. 2006, Li et al. 2007), peanuts (Hargrove et al. 2001), pecans (Haddad et al. 2006), and pistachios (Kocyigit et al. 2006, Kay et al. 2010) improve biomarkers of oxidative stress. On the other hand, the consumption of PUFA-rich walnuts has no apparent effect on these biomarkers (Zambon and Sabate 2000, Iwamoto et al. 2002, Ros et al. 2004, Spaccarotella et al. 2008, Damasceno et al. 2011). It should be noted that it is difficult to draw definitive conclusions on the effects of regular nut consumption on oxidative stress due to differences in methods and the relatively small number of studies using the same biomarker (López-Uriarte et al. 2009, Bullo et al. 2011).

Clinical trials that have investigated the effects of nut consumption on inflammatory markers suggest that the consumption of 27–100 g/day of nuts over 4–12 weeks may elicit an anti-inflammatory effect, when there is also modification of the background diet (e.g., Mediterranean diet or a diet low in SFA) (Ros et al. 2004, Zhao et al. 2004, Rajaram et al. 2010, Sari et al. 2010, Jenkins et al. 2011, Liu et al. 2013). However, these studies have not isolated nut-specific effects. Currently, there is a gap in knowledge regarding the true anti-inflammatory effect of nut consumption without changing the background diet.

There is some evidence to indicate that chronic walnut consumption favorably affects endothelial function (Ros et al. 2004, Zhao et al. 2004, Perez-Martinez et al. 2007, Ma et al. 2010, West et al. 2010). Furthermore, incorporating MUFA-rich almonds into a Step I diet has also improved endothelial function (Rajaram et al. 2010). It is important to point out that the majority of these studies were conducted in a tightly controlled feeding situation and included modification of the background diet as well as advice to consume nuts. This makes it difficult to evaluate the effects of nuts per se. There is a need for further investigations using the simple inclusion of nuts into the habitual diet to provide conclusive answers on the independent effect of nut consumption on endothelial function.

17.3.2.5 Body Weight

Nuts are high in fat and are energy dense, and thus frequent nut consumption may promote weight gain. To date, only five studies involving the regular consumption of nuts have included body weight as a primary outcome: two on almonds (Fraser et al. 2002, Hollis and Mattes 2007), one on hazelnuts (Tey et al. 2011), one on peanuts (Alper and Mattes 2002), and one on walnuts (Sabate et al. 2005). The findings from these five studies provide evidence that adding 28–89 g/day of nuts to habitual diets for 8–26 weeks resulted in either no weight change or less weight gain than predicted from the additional calories provided by the nuts. The potential mechanisms for this include dietary compensation, an increase in resting metabolic rate, and malabsorption of lipids from nuts, which leads to a reduction in metabolizable energy (Mattes et al. 2008, Mattes and Dreher 2010, Baer et al. 2012, Novotny et al. 2012). Nevertheless, one should be mindful that nuts are energy dense and should be consumed in place of other less healthful foods as part of a cardioprotective diet.

17.4 NUT CONSUMPTION AND METS

As previously discussed, frequent nut consumption may improve the risk factors for chronic disease. This section will describe the epidemiological studies and RCTs that have looked at the effects of nut consumption on MetS.

17.4.1　Epidemiological Studies

A cross-sectional study consisting of 13,292 adults who took part in the 1999–2004 NHANES found that tree nut consumers and *out-of-hand* nut consumers (i.e., excluding those who consumed nuts as part of other food products) had superior diet quality and significantly lower prevalence of several risk factors for MetS such as systolic blood pressure, hypertension, low HDL-C, overweight or obesity, abdominal obesity, body weight, BMI, waist circumference, and elevated fasting blood glucose than non-nut consumers (all $P < 0.05$) (O'Neil et al. 2011, 2012). Similarly, the PREDIMED study recently reported significant inverse associations between baseline nut consumption and risk of MetS and abdominal obesity in 7210 older participants at high risk of CHD (both P for trend < 0.001) (Ibarrola-Jurado et al. 2013).

To date, only one cohort study has examined the association between nut consumption and incidence of MetS (Fernandez-Montero et al. 2012). The SUN study is a prospective cohort study with Spanish university graduates. After 6 years of follow-up, 567 new cases of MetS were observed among 9887 participants. Compared to participants who never or almost never consumed nuts, those who consumed ≥2 servings of nuts per week had a significant 27% (95% CI 1%, 46%) reduction in the risk of developing MetS, after adjusting for potential confounders. This inverse association between frequent nut consumption and MetS was evident among females (P for trend = 0.001), whereas no association was observed among males (P for trend = 0.58). In addition, frequent nut consumption was inversely correlated with the risk of having waist circumference ≥80 cm (P for trend < 0.001) and fasting glucose ≥ 5.55 mmol/L (P for trend = 0.004) among females. It is not known whether these findings obtained from highly educated, relatively young cohort at low risk for MetS can be replicated in other population groups. Further studies are warranted to confirm this.

17.4.2　Randomized Controlled Trials among Individuals with MetS

Five randomized studies have examined the effects of nut consumption on the components of MetS among people with this disorder. Table 17.3 shows the characteristics of these studies. Of the five studies, two were conducted in China, and one each in South Africa, Spain, and the United States. These studies have generated 12 publications in total, which focus on different outcome measurements. Four studies were conducted using a randomized parallel design with the number of participants ranging from 22 to 95 per treatment (Mukuddem-Petersen et al. 2007, Lopez-Uriarte et al. 2010, Wu et al. 2010, Wang et al. 2012). The other study was conducted using a randomized, double-blinded, placebo-controlled crossover design with a relatively small sample size ($n = 15$) and short intervention period (4 days) (Brennan et al. 2010). Due to the short duration, the findings of this study will be discussed but not included in Tables 17.4 through 17.7 (Brennan et al. 2010). Only one study has reported power calculations, and hence, the other four studies might not have adequate power to detect a clinically meaningful difference in the primary outcome. Two studies were carried out in tightly controlled metabolic feeding trials (Mukuddem-Petersen et al. 2007, Brennan et al. 2010), and the other three instructed participants to follow the American Heart Association recommendations, as well as advised to consume nuts (Lopez-Uriarte et al. 2010, Wu et al. 2010, Wang et al. 2012). The types of nuts used in these trials include mixed nuts ($n = 1$), pistachios ($n = 1$), walnuts ($n = 2$), and cashews and walnuts ($n = 1$). The dose of nuts used in these studies ranges from 30 to 115 g/day, with an intervention period between 4 days and 12 weeks.

17.4.2.1　Blood Lipids and Lipoproteins

Table 17.4 shows the effects of nut consumption on blood lipids and lipoproteins among individuals with MetS. All five studies reported no significant differences in the changes of blood lipid profiles after regular consumption of a nut-enriched diet compared to a control diet

TABLE 17.3

Characteristics of Randomized Controlled Trials Conducted among Individuals with MetS

Author (Year)	No. of Participants, Power Calculation, Mean BMI, Country	Study Design	Duration	Treatments
Pieters et al. (2005), Schutte et al. (2006), Davis et al. (2007), Mukuddem-Petersen et al. (2007)	64 (29 M, 35 F); Power calculation: 22 per group; Mean BMI = 35 kg/m^2; South Africa	Randomized Parallel Three arms Controlled feeding	8 weeks	1. Control (No nuts) 2. Unsalted cashews (20% TE: 66–115 g/day) 3. Walnuts (20% TE: 60–100 g/day)
Brennan et al. (2010), Aronis et al. (2012)	15 (9 M, 6 F); Power calculation: NR; Obese, Mean BMI = 36.6 kg/m^2; USA	Randomized Double blinded Crossover Two arms Controlled feeding	4 days	1. Placebo shake (Safflower oil: 32 g/day) 2. Walnut shake (Walnuts: 48 g/day)
Lopez-Uriarte et al. (2010), Casas-Agustench et al. (2011b), Tulipani et al. (2011), Tulipani et al. (2012)	50 (28 M, 22 F); Power calculation: NR; Mean BMI: Control = 30.0; Nut = 31.6 kg/m^2; Spain	Randomized Parallel Two arms	12 weeks	1. Control (AHA guidelines) 2. AHA guidelines + mixed raw nuts (7.5 g/day almonds, 7.5 g/day hazelnuts, 15 g/day walnuts)
Wu et al. (2010)	283 (158 M, 125 F); Power calculation: NR; Mean BMI = 25 kg/m^2; China	Randomized Parallel Three arms	12 weeks	1. Lifestyle counseling + control (AHA guidelines) 2. Lifestyle counseling + flaxseed (30 g/day) 3. Lifestyle counseling + walnuts (30 g/day)
Wang et al. (2012)	90 (41 M, 49 F); Power calculation: NR; Mean BMI = 28 kg/m^2; China	Randomized Parallel Three arms	12 weeks	1. AHA step I diet + control (no nuts) 2. AHA step I diet + pistachios (42 g/day) 3. AHA step I diet + pistachios (70 g/day)

AHA, American Heart Association; BMI, body mass index; NR, Not reported; % TE, Percent of total energy intake.

(Mukuddem-Petersen et al. 2007, Brennan et al. 2010, Wu et al. 2010, Casas-Agustench et al. 2011b). It is noteworthy that the mean BMIs of these study populations were higher than normal, ranging from 25 to 36.6 kg/m^2 (Table 17.3). Previous studies that were conducted in participants with BMI ≥ 25 kg/m^2 (Wien et al. 2003, Tapsell et al. 2009, Li et al. 2010), prediabetes (Wien et al. 2010), or type 2 diabetes (Lovejoy et al. 2002, Ma et al. 2010, Cohen and Johnston 2011) also failed to show an improvement in blood lipid profiles with a nut-enriched diet in comparison with the control diet. The decreased lipid response to nut-enriched diets in participants with higher BMIs and insulin resistance could be explained by elevated endogenous cholesterol synthesis, decreased LDL-C receptors, and reduced intestinal cholesterol absorption (Simonen et al. 2000, 2002, Flock and Kris-Etherton 2011, Paramsothy et al. 2011). It has been reported that greater flux of cholesterol through the liver will downregulate LDL receptors making them less responsive to the effects of dietary fatty acids. Hence, the hypocholesterolemic properties of the unsaturated fatty acids found in nuts would be less pronounced. In addition, a reduction in intestinal cholesterol absorption in the obese and insulin-resistant participants could negate the cholesterol-lowering potential of the plant sterols present in nuts (Ros et al. 2010, Sabate et al. 2010).

TABLE 17.4
Dietary Intervention Trials Investigating the Effects of Nut Consumption on Blood Lipids and Lipoproteins ($n = 4$)[a]

Author (Year)	Treatment	TC (mmol/L)	LDL-C (mmol/L)	HDL-C (mmol/L)	TAG (mmol/L)	Between Treatments
Mukuddem-	*Baseline*	*4.90*[c]	*3.21*[c]	*0.85*	*1.86*	Compared to the control
Petersen	1. Control	5.39	3.36	0.91	1.96	diet, both nut intervention
et al. (2007)	Change[b]	+0.07	+0.19	+0.06[a]	+0.11	diets had no significant
	Baseline	*4.49*[c]	*2.64*[c]	*1.02*	*1.81*	effect on blood lipids (all
	2. Cashews	4.51	2.84	1.01	1.64	$P \geq 0.11$).
	Change[b]	+0.07	+0.12	−0.01	−0.16	
	Baseline	*4.80*[c]	*2.99*[c]	*0.94*	*1.90*	
	3. Walnuts	4.72	3.19	0.91	1.86	
	Change[b]	−0.03	+0.18	−0.03	−0.04	
Wu et al.	*Baseline*	*6.10*	*4.30*	*1.40*	*1.94*[c]	There were no significant
(2010)	1. Control	5.63	3.93	1.28	1.90	differences in blood
	Change[b]	−0.47*	−0.37*	−0.12*	−0.04	lipids between the groups
	Baseline	*6.00*	*4.20*	*1.40*	*1.89*[c]	(all $P > 0.05$).
	2. Flaxseed	5.44	3.76	1.25	1.82	
	Change[b]	−0.56*	−0.44*	−0.15*	−0.07	
	Baseline	*5.80*	*4.10*	*1.30*	*1.99*[c]	
	3. Walnuts	5.45	3.83	1.21	1.92	
	Change[b]	−0.35*	−0.27*	−0.09*	−0.07	
Casas-	*Baseline*	*5.82*	*3.79*	*1.12*	*1.69*	There were no significant
Agustench	1. Control	5.34	3.43	1.10	1.62	differences in changes
et al. (2011b)	Change[b]	−0.48*	−0.36*	−0.02	−0.07	between the groups in
	Baseline	*5.38*	*3.45*	*1.17*	*1.53*	blood lipid profile (all
	2. Mixed nuts	5.22	3.32	1.15	1.51	$P \geq 0.071$).
	Change[b]	−0.16	−0.13	−0.02	−0.02	
Wang et al.	*Baseline*	*5.01*	*2.70*	*NR*	*2.09*	There were no significant
(2012)	1. Control	5.15	2.99	NR	1.88	differences in blood
	Change[b]	+0.14	+0.29*	NS	−0.21	lipids between the groups
	Baseline	*5.29*	*3.08*	*NR*	*2.47*	(all $P > 0.05$).
	2. Pistachio, 42 g	5.20	3.10	NR	2.14	
	Change[b]	−0.09	+0.02	NS	−0.33*	
	Baseline	*5.29*	*3.00*	*NR*	*2.19*	
	3. Pistachio, 70 g	5.41	3.30	NR	2.05	
	Change[b]	+0.12	+0.30**	NS	−0.14	

HDL-C, high-density lipoprotein cholesterol; LDL-C, low-density lipoprotein cholesterol; NR, not reported; NS, nonsignificant; TAG, triacylglycerol; TC, total cholesterol.

[a] SI conversion factors: To convert mmol/L TC, LDL-C, HDL-C to mg/dL, multiply mmol/L by 38.67. To convert mmol/L TAG to mg/dL, multiply mmol/L by 88.57.

[b] Change (within group) = Posttreatment value − pretreatment value (baseline).

[c] Data were reported as median. Analysis was performed either using nonparametric tests or log-transformed values.

*$P < 0.05$; **$P < 0.01$. Significant difference between pretreatment value and posttreatment value.

TABLE 17.5

Dietary Intervention Trials Investigating the Effects of Nut Consumption on Markers of Glycemic Control (*n* = 4)

Author (Year)	Treatment	Glucose (mmol/L)	Insulin	Between Treatments
Mukuddem-Petersen et al. (2007)	*Baseline*	*4.55*[b]	*NE*	Plasma glucose concentrations at the end of the study was significantly higher in the cashew nut group compared to the control group (*P* = 0.04).
	1. Control	4.55	NE	
	Change[a]	−0.75	NE	
	Baseline	*4.70*[b]	*NE*	
	2. Cashews	5.30	NE	
	Change[a]	+0.70*	NE	
	Baseline	*4.50*[b]	*NE*	
	3. Walnuts	4.70	NE	
	Change[a]	+0.40	NE	
Wu et al. (2010)	*Baseline*	*6.3*	*52.4*[c]	There were no significant differences in blood glucose and insulin concentrations between the control group and the walnut group (both *P* > 0.05).
	1. Control	5.86	56.5	
	Change[a]	−0.44*	+4.1	
	Baseline	*6.3*	*47.1*[c]	
	2. Flaxseed	5.73	46.6	
	Change[a]	−0.57*	−0.5	
	Baseline	*6.1*	*47.5*[c]	
	3. Walnuts	5.70	51.2	
	Change[a]	−0.40*	+3.7	
Casas-Agustench et al. (2011b)	*Baseline*	*5.82*	*6.01*[d]	The mixed-nut diet decreased fasting insulin concentrations (*P* = 0.013) and HOMA-IR (*P* = 0.013) when compared with the control diet.
	1. Control	5.78	6.54	
	Change[a]	−0.04	+0.53	
	Baseline	*5.82*	*8.01*[d]	
	2. Mixed nuts	5.76	5.94	
	Change[a]	−0.06	−2.07*	
Wang et al. (2012)	*Baseline*	*5.27*	*16.7*[e]	There were no significant differences in blood glucose and insulin concentrations between the groups (both *P* > 0.05).
	1. Control	5.57	18.7	
	Change[a]	+0.30*	+2.0	
	Baseline	*5.30*	*14.1*[e]	
	2. Pistachio, 42 g	5.41	14.4	
	Change[a]	+0.11	+0.3	
	Baseline	*5.18*	*17.1*[e]	
	3. Pistachio, 70 g	5.20	14.7	
	Change[a]	+0.02	−2.4	

NE, not evaluated.

[a] Change (within group) = Posttreatment value − pretreatment value (baseline).

[b] Data were reported as median. Analysis was performed either using nonparametric tests or log-transformed values.

[c] Insulin reported as pmol/L.

[d] Insulin reported as μU/mL. To convert μU/mL insulin to pmol/L, multiply μU/mL by 6.945.

[e] Insulin reported as μU/L.

*$P < 0.05$. Significant difference between pretreatment value and posttreatment value.

TABLE 17.6

Dietary Intervention Trials Investigating the Effects of Nut Consumption on Diastolic and Systolic Blood Pressure ($n = 4$)

Author (Year)	Treatment	Systolic (mm/Hg)	Diastolic (mm/Hg)	Between Treatments
Mukuddem-Petersen	*Baseline*	*131*	*79.2*	There were no significant
et al. (2007)	1. Control	133	79.6	differences in the changes
	Change[a]	+2	+0.5	of systolic and diastolic
	Baseline	*131*	*77.0*	blood pressures from
	2. Cashews	128	76.0	baseline to the end of the
	Change[a]	−2	−0.6	study between the groups
	Baseline	*128*	*78.7*	(both $P \geq 0.22$).
	3. Walnuts	130	79.1	
	Change[a]	+2	+1.2	
Wu et al. (2010)	*Baseline*	*133.7*	*85.4*	There were no significant
	1. Control	126.7	81.0	differences in blood
	Change[a]	−7.0*	−4.4*	pressure between the
	Baseline	*133.0*	*85.6*	control group and the
	2. Flaxseed	124.2	80.6	walnut group (both
	Change[a]	−8.8*	−5.0*	$P > 0.05$).
	Baseline	*135.0*	*86.5*	
	3. Walnuts	126.8	82.3	
	Change[a]	−8.2*	−4.2*	
Casas-Agustench et al.	*Baseline*	*137*	*82*	There were no differences
(2011b)	1. Control	127	78	in changes between
	Change[a]	−10*	−4*	groups in systolic
	Baseline	*145*	*86*	($P = 0.238$) and diastolic
	2. Mixed nuts	139	83	($P = 0.466$) blood
	Change[a]	−6*	−3*	pressures.
Wang et al. (2012)	*Baseline*	*128.5*	*79.3*	There were no significant
	1. Control	NR	NR	differences in systolic and
	Change[a]	NS	NS	diastolic blood pressures
	Baseline	*129.1*	*81.1*	between the groups (both
	2. Pistachio, 42 g	NR	NR	$P > 0.05$).
	Change[a]	NS	NS	
	Baseline	*128.7*	*81.7*	
	3. Pistachio, 70 g	NR	NR	
	Change[a]	NS	NS	

NR, not reported; NS, not significant.

[a] Change (within group) = Posttreatment value – pretreatment value (baseline)

*$P < 0.05$. Significant difference between pretreatment value and posttreatment value.

17.4.2.2   Glycemic Control

Table 17.5 shows the findings of the studies that have investigated the effects of regular nut consumption on blood glucose, insulin, fructosamine (short-term marker of glycemic control), and HbA1c (long-term marker of glycemic control) in individuals with MetS. Overall, these studies have produced mixed results. Most studies showed no significant between-group differences in the changes of blood glucose (Brennan et al. 2010, Wu et al. 2010, Casas-Agustench et al. 2011b), insulin (Brennan et al. 2010), fructosamine (Mukuddem-Petersen et al. 2007), and HbA1c (Wu et al. 2010). One study showed a significantly higher blood glucose concentration after consuming

TABLE 17.7
Dietary Intervention Trials Investigating the Effects of Nut Consumption on Body Weight and Waist Circumference ($n = 4$)

Author (Year)	Treatment	Body Weight (kg)	Waist Circumference (cm)	Between Treatments
Schutte et al.	*Baseline*	*106*	*108.3*	There were no differences in
(2006),	1. Control	105	107.7	the change in body weight
Mukuddem-	*Change*[a]	−0.51	−0.41	($P = 0.78$) and waist
Petersen	*Baseline*	*99.2*	*104.7*	circumference ($P = 0.38$)
et al. (2007)	2. Cashews	99.1	105.2	between the groups. N.B.
	Change[a]	−0.17	+0.52	Participants' energy
	Baseline	*106.0*	*109.3*	intakes were adjusted in
	3. Walnuts	106.0	108.6	order to maintain their
	Change[a]	−0.22	−0.82	body weight during the
				intervention.
Wu et al.	*Baseline*	*70.6*	*89.7*	The changes of body weight
(2010)	1. Control	69.8	88.5	and waist circumference
	Change[a]	−0.82*	−1.2*	from baseline to week 12
	Baseline	*69.7*	*88.7*	were not significantly
	2. Flaxseed	68.5	87.2	different between the
	Change[a]	−1.18*	−1.5*	control group and the
	Baseline	*72.2*	*90.0*	walnut group (both
	3. Walnuts	71.3	88.8	$P > 0.05$).
	Change[a]	−0.92*	−1.2*	
Casas-	*Baseline*	*79.9*	*101.3*	There were no significant
Agustench	1. Control	78.4	98.6	differences in the changes
et al. (2011b)	*Change*[a]	−1.5*	−2.7*	of body weight ($P = 0.363$)
	Baseline	*86.4*	*105.6*	and waist circumference
	2. Mixed nuts	84.2	101.8	($P = 0.678$) between the
	Change[a]	−2.2*	−3.8*	groups.
Wang et al.	*Baseline*	*28.0*[b]	*0.92*[c]	There were no significant
(2012)	1. Control	NR	0.92	between-group differences
	Change[a]	NS	0.0	in body weight and waist
	Baseline	*28.1*[b]	*0.93*[c]	circumference (both
	2. Pistachio, 42 g	NR	0.92	$P > 0.05$).
	Change[a]	NS	−0.01	
	Baseline	*28.0*[b]	*0.92*[c]	
	3. Pistachio, 70 g	NR	0.93	
	Change[a]	NS	+0.01	

NR, not reported; NS, not significant.

[a] Change (within group) = Posttreatment value − pretreatment value (baseline).

[b] Reported as BMI.

[c] Reported as waist-to-hip ratio.

*$P < 0.05$. Significant difference between pretreatment value and posttreatment value.

66–115 g/day of cashew nuts for 8 weeks (Mukuddem-Petersen et al. 2007), whereas another study reported significantly lower fasting insulin and Homeostasis Model Assessment (HOMA)-insulin resistance after consuming 30 g/day of mixed nuts for 12 weeks compared to the control diet (Casas-Agustench et al. 2011b). The contradictory results could be due to the differences in the dose and types of nuts, level of dietary control, and diet composition.

17.4.2.3 Blood Pressure

Table 17.6 shows the effects of nut consumption on blood pressure among people with MetS. These studies demonstrated that regular consumption of a nut-enriched diet did not have an apparent effect on either systolic or diastolic blood pressure compared to a control diet among individuals with MetS (Mukuddem-Petersen et al. 2007, Wu et al. 2010, Casas-Agustench et al. 2011b). Baroreflex sensitivity plays a key role in the regulation of blood pressure, and MetS is associated with decreased baroreflex sensitivity. Schutte et al. (2006) performed the first study to investigate the effects of cashew nut or walnut consumption (20% of total energy intake from nuts) on baroreflex sensitivity. There was a significant increase in baroreflex sensitivity after consuming a diet high in cashew nuts, whereas a significant decrease in baroreflex sensitivity was found following a walnut-enriched diet (Schutte et al. 2006). The detrimental effect associated with walnut consumption could be due to the exceptionally high PUFA and total fat intake during the walnut intervention period, that is, PUFA and total fat contributed to 21% and 41% of the total energy in the analyzed diet, respectively (Laaksonen 2006). Several reviews suggest that a nut-enriched diet improves risk factors of chronic disease when the total fat intake comprises less than 35% of the total energy intake (Mukuddem-Petersen et al. 2005, Laaksonen 2006).

17.4.2.4 Body Weight

Table 17.7 illustrates the effects of nut consumption on body weight and waist circumference among individuals with MetS. Despite the energy-dense and high-fat nature of nuts, all the studies show that regular nut consumption does not adversely affect body weight and waist circumference (Mukuddem-Petersen et al. 2007, Wu et al. 2010, Casas-Agustench et al. 2011b, Wang et al. 2012) (Table 17.7). In addition, Wu et al. (2010) reported a significant higher reversion rate of central obesity in those consuming walnuts compared to a control group (16.0 vs. 6.3; $P < 0.05$). The potential mechanisms for this include the high satiating value of nuts, energy malabsorption as a result of excretion of fat in the stools, and increase in resting energy expenditure. Brennan et al. (2010) investigated the effects of a walnut shake or a placebo shake consumption on satiety over a 4-day period. The reported satiety level was significantly higher following the consumption of a walnut shake at breakfast on day 3 and day 4 when compared with the placebo shake. However, the gut hormones known to influence satiety were not statistically significantly different between the walnut and placebo groups (Brennan et al. 2010). Casas-Agustench et al. (2011b) reported a significant higher stool fat in the nut group compared to the control group, indicating that some of the fat in nuts were not available for digestion and metabolism. On the other hand, two studies reported no significant differences in resting energy expenditure between the nut-enriched and control diets (Brennan et al. 2010, Casas-Agustench et al. 2011b). Therefore, it appears that the increase in satiety and stool fat could be the main reasons that protect nuts against weight gain among individuals with MetS.

17.4.2.5 Other Health Outcomes

Several studies have also examined the effects of nut consumption on other outcomes that are associated with MetS including impaired antioxidant status, oxidative stress, inflammation, endothelial function, and hemostatic abnormalities among individuals with MetS. Pieters et al. (2005) reported that the consumption of a diet high in cashews or walnuts for 8 weeks did not significantly improve any of the hemostatic variables including fibrinogen, von Willebrand factor antigen (vWF_{ag}), tissue plasminogen activator activity (tPA_{act}), plasminogen activator inhibitor 1 activity ($PAI-1_{act}$), factor VII coagulant activity (FVIIc), and thrombin activatable fibrinolysis inhibitor. Similarly, other studies have also failed to show a beneficial effect of nut consumption on antioxidant status (Davis et al. 2007, Lopez-Uriarte et al. 2010), oxidative stress (Brennan et al. 2010, Lopez-Uriarte et al. 2010), inflammation (Mukuddem-Petersen et al. 2007, Casas-Agustench et al. 2011b, Aronis et al. 2012), and endothelial function (Lopez-Uriarte et al. 2010, Aronis et al. 2012). However, a study using mixed nuts reported a significant decrease in DNA damage, as evaluated by urinary 8-oxo-7,8-di-hydro-20-deoxyguanosine, following a 12-week mixed-nut-enriched diet, compared to a control heart-healthy diet (Lopez-Uriarte et al. 2010). In addition, this study used an innovative nontargeted metabolomics method to measure all endogenous and exogenous metabolites in the urine and reported a significant increase in serotonin, urolithins, and unsaturated fatty acids in the nut group (Tulipani et al. 2011, 2012). The decrease in DNA damage and the increase in urinary metabolites may play a role in the cardioprotective benefits observed with regular nut consumption. In addition, Wu et al. (2010) reported that participants who consumed walnuts for 12 weeks had a significantly lower mean number of MetS components compared to the control group.

17.4.2.6 Summary

To date, the research investigating the effects of nut consumption on the MetS has produced disappointing results. When the results are taken together, it appears that regular nut consumption has minimal influence on individual MetS components such as dyslipidemia, hyperglycemia, and blood pressure among individuals with MetS. Nonetheless, contrary to popular perception (Pawlak et al. 2009), moderate nut consumption does not compromise body weight. It is also important to note that incorporating nuts into the usual diet significantly improves diet quality, which may lead to positive effects on health outcomes over a longer period.

17.5 FUTURE DIRECTIONS

This chapter has revealed several areas that could be addressed in future research, in order to gain a better understanding on the role of nuts in modulating the components of MetS among individuals with MetS:

- Nut studies that were conducted in individuals with MetS employed relatively short intervention periods, ranging from 4 days to 12 weeks. Thus, long-term interventions (e.g., 12 months) are warranted to show whether nut consumption could improve the MetS components.
- Only one out of five studies among people with MetS reported a sample size calculation. Future research that aims to investigate the effects of nut consumption on the components of MetS should ensure sufficient power.
- The health effects of nut consumption should be examined in participants with a range of BMI, including both lean and overweight individuals with MetS. In addition, it would be interesting to investigate the independent effects of nuts on the risk factors for MetS.
- Most nut studies carried out to date have used whole unsalted raw nuts. It would therefore be interesting to determine whether the health effects observed with raw nut consumption can be generalized to nuts with different physical forms (i.e., may differ in bioaccessibility) or preparation methods (i.e., roasting vs. frying; dry vs. oil/honey roasted; low vs. high temperature; low vs. high sodium content). In addition, future research is needed to determine the type and the dose of nuts required to improve dyslipidemia, hyperglycemia, and ambulatory blood pressure without compromising body weight.
- Further research is warranted to elucidate the underlying mechanisms and the potential role of nuts in ameliorating MetS components.

REFERENCES

Albert, C.M., J.M. Gaziano, W.C. Willett, and J.E. Manson. 2002. Nut consumption and decreased risk of sudden cardiac death in the Physicians' Health Study. *Arch Intern Med* 162:1382–1387.
Alberti, K.G., P. Zimmet, and J. Shaw. 2006. MetS—A new world-wide definition. A consensus statement from the International Diabetes Federation. *Diabet Med* 23:469–480.

Alper, C.M. and R.D. Mattes. 2002. Effects of chronic peanut consumption on energy balance and hedonics. *Int J Obes Relat Metab Disord* 26:1129–1137.

Aronis, K.N., M.T. Vamvini, J.P. Chamberland et al. 2012. Short-term walnut consumption increases circulating total adiponectin and apolipoprotein A concentrations, but does not affect markers of inflammation or vascular injury in obese humans with the MetS: Data from a double-blinded, randomized, placebo-controlled study. *Metabolism* 61:577–582.

Baer, D.J., S.K. Gebauer, and J.A. Novotny. 2012. Measured energy value of pistachios in the human diet. *Br J Nutr* 107:120–125.

Banel, D.K. and F.B. Hu. 2009. Effects of walnut consumption on blood lipids and other cardiovascular risk factors: A meta-analysis and systematic review. *Am J Clin Nutr* 90:56–63.

Bartunek, J. and M. Vanderheyden. 2012. Inflammation and related biomarkers in cardiovascular disease. *Biomark Med* 6:1–3.

Berryman, C.E., A.G. Preston, W. Karmally, R.J. Deckelbaum, and P.M. Kris-Etherton. 2011. Effects of almond consumption on the reduction of LDL-cholesterol: A discussion of potential mechanisms and future research directions. *Nutr Rev* 69:171–185.

Bes-Rastrollo, M., J. Sabate, E. Gomez-Gracia, A. Alonso, J.A. Martinez, and M.A. Martinez-Gonzalez. 2007. Nut consumption and weight gain in a Mediterranean cohort: The SUN Study. *Obesity* 15:107–116.

Bes-Rastrollo, M., N.M. Wedick, M.A. Martinez-Gonzalez, T.Y. Li, L. Sampson, and F.B. Hu. 2009. Prospective study of nut consumption, long-term weight change, and obesity risk in women. *Am J Clin Nutr* 89:1913–1919.

Blomhoff, R., M.H. Carlsen, L.F. Andersen, and D.R. Jacobs. 2006. Health benefits of nuts: Potential role of antioxidants. *Br J Nutr* 96:S52–S60.

Bolling, B.W., C.Y. Chen, D.L. McKay, and J.B. Blumberg. 2011. Tree nut phytochemicals: Composition, antioxidant capacity, bioactivity, impact factors. A systematic review of almonds, Brazils, cashews, hazelnuts, macadamias, pecans, pine nuts, pistachios and walnuts. *Nutr Res Rev* 24:244–275.

Brennan, A.M., L.L. Sweeney, X. Liu, and C.S. Mantzoros. 2010. Walnut consumption increases satiation but has no effect on insulin resistance or the metabolic profile over a 4-day period. *Obesity* 18:1176–1182.

Brown, A.A. and F.B. Hu. 2001. Dietary modulation of endothelial function: Implications for cardiovascular disease. *Am J Clin Nutr* 73:673–686.

Brufau, G., J. Boatella, and M. Rafecas. 2006. Nuts: Source of energy and macronutrients. *Br J Nutr* 96:S24–S28.

Bullo, M., R. Lamuela-Raventos, and J. Salas-Salvado. 2011. Mediterranean diet and oxidation: Nuts and olive oil as important sources of fat and antioxidants. *Curr Top Med Chem* 11:1797–1810.

Calder, P.C., N. Ahluwalia, F. Brouns et al. 2011. Dietary factors and low-grade inflammation in relation to overweight and obesity. *Br J Nutr* 106:S5–S78.

Casas-Agustench, P., M. Bullo, E. Ros, J. Basora, and J. Salas-Salvado. 2011a. Cross-sectional association of nut intake with adiposity in a Mediterranean population. *Nutr Metab Cardiovasc Dis* 21:518–525.

Casas-Agustench, P., M. Bullo, and J. Salas-Salvado. 2010. Nuts, inflammation and insulin resistance. *Asia Pac J Clin Nutr* 19:124–130.

Casas-Agustench, P., P. López-Uriarte, M. Bulló, E. Ros, J.J. Cabré-Vila, and J. Salas-Salvadó. 2011b. Effects of one serving of mixed nuts on serum lipids, insulin resistance and inflammatory markers in patients with the MetS. *Nutr Metab Cardiovasc Dis* 21:126–135.

Casas-Agustench, P., P. López-Uriarte, E. Ros, M. Bulló, and J. Salas-Salvadó. 2011c. Nuts, hypertension and endothelial function. *Nutr Metab Cardiovasc Dis* 21:S21–S33.

Cohen, A.E. and C.S. Johnston. 2011. Almond ingestion at mealtime reduces postprandial glycemia and chronic ingestion reduces hemoglobin A1c in individuals with well-controlled type 2 diabetes mellitus. *Metabolism* 60:1312–1317.

Coulston, A.M. 2003. Do nuts have a place in a healthful diet? *Nutr Today* 38:95–99.

Damasceno, N.R.T., A. Perez-Heras, M. Serra et al. 2011. Crossover study of diets enriched with virgin olive oil, walnuts or almonds. Effects on lipids and other cardiovascular risk markers. *Nutr Metab Cardiovasc Dis* 21:S14–S20.

Davis, L., W. Stonehouse, T. Loots du et al. 2007. The effects of high walnut and cashew nut diets on the anti-oxidant status of subjects with MetS. *Eur J Nutr* 46:155–164.

de Lorgeril, M., P. Salen, F. Laporte, F. Boucher, and J. de Leiris. 2001. Potential use of nuts for the prevention and treatment of coronary heart disease: From natural to functional foods. *Nutr Metab Cardiovasc Dis* 11:362–371.

Despres, J.-P. and I. Lemieux. 2006. Abdominal obesity and MetS. *Nature* 444:881–887.

Djousse, L., J.M. Gaziano, C.S. Kase, and T. Kurth. 2010. Nut consumption and risk of stroke in US male physicians. *Clin Nutr* 29:605–609.

Djousse, L., T. Rudich, and J.M. Gaziano. 2008. Nut consumption and risk of heart failure in the Physicians' Health Study I. *Am J Clin Nutr* 88:930–933.

Djousse, L., T. Rudich, and J.M. Gaziano. 2009. Nut consumption and risk of hypertension in US male physicians. *Clin Nutr* 28:10–14.

Dreher, M.L., C.V. Maher, and P. Kearney. 1996. The traditional and emerging role of nuts in healthful diets. *Nutr Rev* 54:241–245.

Ellsworth, J., L. Kushi, and A. Folsom. 2001. Frequent nut intake and risk of death from coronary heart disease and all causes in postmenopausal women: The Iowa Women's Health Study. *Nutr Metab Cardiovasc Dis* 11:372–377.

Estruch, R. 2010. Anti-inflammatory effects of the Mediterranean diet: The experience of the PREDIMED study. *Proc Nutr Soc* 69:333–340.

Estruch, R., M.A. Martinez-Gonzalez, D. Corella et al. 2006. Effects of a Mediterranean-style diet on cardiovascular risk factors: A randomized trial. *Ann Intern Med* 145:1–11.

Estruch, R., E. Ros, J. Salas-Salvado et al. 2013. Primary prevention of cardiovascular disease with a Mediterranean diet. *N Engl J Med* 368:1279–1290.

Faxon, D.P., V. Fuster, P. Libby et al. 2004. Atherosclerotic vascular disease conference: Writing group III: Pathophysiology. *Circulation* 109:2617–2625.

Fernandez-Montero, A., M. Bes-Rastrollo, J.J. Beunza et al. 2013. Nut consumption and incidence of MetS after 6-year follow-up: The SUN (Seguimiento Universidad de Navarra, University of Navarra Follow-up) cohort. *Public Health Nutr* 16:2064–2072.

Flock, M.R. and P.M. Kris-Etherton. 2011. Dietary guidelines for Americans 2010: Implications for cardiovascular disease. *Curr Atheroscler Rep* 13:499–507.

Ford, E.S., C. Li, and N. Sattar. 2008. MetS and incident diabetes: Current state of the evidence. *Diabetes Care* 31:1898–1904.

Fraser, G.E. 2000. Nut consumption, lipids, and risk of a coronary event. *Asia Pac J Clin Nutr* 9:S28–S32.

Fraser, G.E., H.W. Bennett, K.B. Jaceldo, and J. Sabate. 2002. Effect on body weight of a free 76 kilojoule (320 calorie) daily supplement of almonds for six months. *J Am Coll Nutr* 21:275–283.

Fraser, G.E., K.D. Lindsted, and W.L. Beeson. 1995. Effect of risk factor values on lifetime risk of and age at first coronary event. The Adventist Health Study. *Am J Epidemiol* 142:746–758.

Fraser, G.E., J. Sabate, W.L. Beeson, and T.M. Strahan. 1992. A possible protective effect of nut consumption on risk of coronary heart disease. The Adventist Health Study. *Arch Intern Med* 152:1416–1424.

Fraser, G.E. and D.J. Shavlik. 1997. Risk factors for all-cause and coronary heart disease mortality in the oldest-old. The Adventist Health Study. *Arch Intern Med* 157:2249–2258.

Fuster, V., L.E. Ryden, D.S. Cannom et al. 2006. ACC/AHA/ESC 2006 guidelines for the management of patients with atrial fibrillation—Executive summary: A report of the American College of Cardiology/American Heart Association Task Force on practice guidelines and the European society of cardiology committee for practice guidelines (writing committee to revise the 2001 guidelines for the management of patients with atrial fibrillation) developed in collaboration with the European Heart Rhythm Association and the Heart Rhythm Society. *J Am Coll Cardiol* 48:854–906.

Gebauer, S.K., S.G. West, C.D. Kay, P. Alaupovic, D. Bagshaw, and P.M. Kris-Etherton. 2008. Effects of pistachios on cardiovascular disease risk factors and potential mechanisms of action: A dose-response study. *Am J Clin Nutr* 88:651–659.

Giugliano, D., A. Ceriello, and K. Esposito. 2006. The effects of diet on inflammation: Emphasis on the MetS. *J Am Coll Cardiol* 48:677–685.

Gopinath, B., A.E. Buyken, V.M. Flood, M. Empson, E. Rochtchina, and P. Mitchell. 2011. Consumption of polyunsaturated fatty acids, fish, and nuts and risk of inflammatory disease mortality. *Am J Clin Nutr* 93:1073–1079.

Haddad, E., P. Jambazian, M. Karunia, J. Tanzman, and J. Sabaté. 2006. A pecan-enriched diet increases [gamma]-tocopherol/cholesterol and decreases thiobarbituric acid reactive substances in plasma of adults. *Nutr Res* 26:397–402.

Hargrove, R.L., T.D. Etherton, T.A. Pearson, E.H. Harrison, and P.M. Kris-Etherton. 2001. Low fat and high monounsaturated fat diets decrease human low density lipoprotein oxidative susceptibility in vitro. *J Nutr* 131:1758–1763.

Hollis, J. and R. Mattes. 2007. Effect of chronic consumption of almonds on body weight in healthy humans. *Br J Nutr* 98:651–656.

Hu, F.B., M.J. Stampfer, J.E. Manson et al. 1998. Frequent nut consumption and risk of coronary heart disease in women: Prospective cohort study. *BMJ* 317:1341–1345.

Ibarrola-Jurado, N., M. Bullo, M. Guasch-Ferre et al. 2013. Cross-sectional assessment of nut consumption and obesity, MetS and other cardiometabolic risk factors: The PREDIMED study. *PLoS ONE* 8:e57367.

Iwamoto, M., K. Imaizumi, M. Sato et al. 2002. Serum lipid profiles in Japanese women and men during consumption of walnuts. *Eur J Clin Nutr* 56:629–637.

Jaceldo-Siegl, K., S. Joan, S. Rajaram, and G.E. Fraser. 2004. Long-term almond supplementation without advice on food replacement induces favourable nutrient modifications to the habitual diets of free-living individuals. *Br J Nutr* 92:533–540.

Jambazian, P.R., E. Haddad, S. Rajaram, J. Tanzman, and J. Sabaté. 2005. Almonds in the diet simultaneously improve plasma [alpha]-tocopherol concentrations and reduce plasma lipids. *J Am Diet Assoc* 105:449–454.

Jenkins, D.J.A., F.B. Hu, L.C. Tapsell, A.R. Josse, and C.W.C. Kendall. 2008a. Possible benefit of nuts in type 2 diabetes. *J Nutr* 138:S1752–S1756.

Jenkins, D.J.A., C.W.C. Kendall, M.S. Banach et al. 2011. Nuts as a replacement for carbohydrates in the diabetic diet. *Diabetes Care* 34:1706–1711.

Jenkins, D.J.A., C.W.C. Kendall, D.A. Faulkner et al. 2008b. Long-term effects of a plant-based dietary portfolio of cholesterol-lowering foods on blood pressure. *Eur J Clin Nutr* 62:781–788.

Jenkins, D.J.A., C.W.C. Kendall, A. Marchie et al. 2002. Dose response of almonds on coronary heart disease risk factors: Blood lipids, oxidized low-density lipoproteins, lipoprotein(a), homocysteine, and pulmonary nitric oxide: A randomized, controlled, crossover trial. *Circulation* 106:1327–1332.

Jenkins, D.J.A., C.W.C. Kendall, A. Marchie et al. 2008c. Almonds reduce biomarkers of lipid peroxidation in older hyperlipidemic subjects. *J Nutr* 138:908–913.

Jia, X., N. Li, W. Zhang et al. 2006. A pilot study on the effects of almond consumption on DNA damage and oxidative stress in smokers. *Nutr Cancer* 54:179–183.

Jiang, R., D.R. Jacobs, Jr., E. Mayer-Davis et al. 2006. Nut and seed consumption and inflammatory markers in the Multi-Ethnic Study of Atherosclerosis. *Am J Epidemiol* 163:222–231.

Jiang, R., J.E. Manson, M.J. Stampfer, S. Liu, W.C. Willett, and F.B. Hu. 2002. Nut and peanut butter consumption and risk of type 2 diabetes in women. *JAMA* 288:2554–2560.

Kay, C.D., S.K. Gebauer, S.G. West, and P.M. Kris-Etherton. 2010. Pistachios increase serum antioxidants and lower serum oxidized-LDL in hypercholesterolemic adults. *J Nutr* 140:1093–1098.

Kelly, J.H. and J. Sabate. 2006. Nuts and coronary heart disease: An epidemiological perspective. *Br J Nutr* 96:S61–S67.

Kendall, C.W., A. Esfahani, J. Truan, K. Srichaikul, and D.J. Jenkins. 2010a. Health benefits of nuts in prevention and management of diabetes. *Asia Pac J Clin Nutr* 19:110–116.

Kendall, C.W.C., A.R. Josse, A. Esfahani, and D.J.A. Jenkins. 2010b. Nuts, MetS and diabetes. *Br J Nutr* 104:465–473.

Khawaja, O.A., J.M. Gaziano, and L. Djousse. 2012. Nut consumption and risk of atrial fibrillation in the Physicians' Health Study. *Nutr J* 11:17.

King, J.C., J. Blumberg, L. Ingwersen, M. Jenab, and K.L. Tucker. 2008. Tree nuts and peanuts as components of a healthy diet. *J Nutr* 138:S1736–S1740.

Kochar, J., J.M. Gaziano, and L. Djousse. 2010. Nut consumption and risk of type II diabetes in the Physicians' Health Study. *Eur J Clin Nutr* 64:75–79.

Kocyigit, A., A.A. Koylu, and H. Keles. 2006. Effects of pistachio nuts consumption on plasma lipid profile and oxidative status in healthy volunteers. *Nutr Metab Cardiovasc Dis* 16:202–209.

Kris-Etherton, P.M. 1999. Monounsaturated fatty acids and risk of cardiovascular disease. *Circulation* 100:1253–1258.

Kris-Etherton, P.M., F.B. Hu, E. Ros, and J. Sabate. 2008. The role of tree nuts and peanuts in the prevention of coronary heart disease: Multiple potential mechanisms. *J Nutr* 138:1746S–1751S.

Kris-Etherton, P.M., G. Zhao, C.L. Pelkman, V.K. Fishell, and S.M. Coval. 2000. Beneficial effects of a diet high in monounsaturated fatty acids on risk factors for cardiovascular disease. *Nutr Clin Care* 3:153–162.

Kushi, L.H., A.R. Folsom, R.J. Prineas, P.J. Mink, Y. Wu, and R.M. Bostick. 1996. Dietary antioxidant vitamins and death from coronary heart disease in postmenopausal women. *N Engl J Med* 334:1156–1162.

Laaksonen, D.E. 2006. High dietary nut intake: Too much of a good thing? *Am J Hypertens* 19:637–638.

Lawes, C.M.M., S.V. Hoorn, and A. Rodgers. 2008. Global burden of blood-pressure-related disease, 2001. *Lancet* 371:1513–1518.

Lee, J.H., C.J. Lavie, J.H. O'Keefe, and R. Milani. 2011. Nuts and seeds in cardiovascular health. In: Preddy, V.R., R.R. Watson, and V.B. Patel, eds., *Nuts and Seeds in Health and Disease Prevention*. San Diego, CA: Academic Press.

Lesperance, L. 2009. *The Concise New Zealand Food Composition Tables*, 8th edn. Palmerston North, New Zealand: New Zealand Institute for Plant & Food Research.

Li, N., X. Jia, C.Y. Chen et al. 2007. Almond consumption reduces oxidative DNA damage and lipid peroxidation in male smokers. *J Nutr* 137:2717–2722.

Li, S.-C., Y.-H. Liu, J.-F. Liu, W.-H. Chang, C.-M. Chen, and C.Y.O. Chen. 2011. Almond consumption improved glycemic control and lipid profiles in patients with type 2 diabetes mellitus. *Metabolism* 60:474–479.

Li, T.Y., A.M. Brennan, N.M. Wedick, C. Mantzoros, N. Rifai, and F.B. Hu. 2009. Regular consumption of nuts is associated with a lower risk of cardiovascular disease in women with type 2 diabetes. *J Nutr* 139:1333–1338.

Li, Z., R. Song, C. Nguyen et al. 2010. Pistachio nuts reduce triglycerides and body weight by comparison to refined carbohydrate snack in obese subjects on a 12-week weight loss program. *J Am Coll Nutr* 29:198–203.

Liu, J.-F., Y.-H. Liu, C.-M. Chen, W.-H. Chang, and C.Y.O. Chen. 2013. The effect of almonds on inflammation and oxidative stress in Chinese patients with type 2 diabetes mellitus: A randomized crossover controlled feeding trial. *Eur J Nutr* 52:927–935.

López-Uriarte, P., M. Bulló, P. Casas-Agustench, N. Babio, and J. Salas-Salvadó. 2009. Nuts and oxidation: A systematic review. *Nutr Rev* 67:497–508.

Lopez-Uriarte, P., R. Nogues, G. Saez et al. 2010. Effect of nut consumption on oxidative stress and the endothelial function in MetS. *Clin Nutr* 29:373–380.

Lovejoy, J.C., M.M. Most, M. Lefevre, F.L. Greenway, and J.C. Rood. 2002. Effect of diets enriched in almonds on insulin action and serum lipids in adults with normal glucose tolerance or type 2 diabetes. *Am J Clin Nutr* 76:1000–1006.

Ma, Y., V.Y. Njike, J. Millet et al. 2010. Effects of walnut consumption on endothelial function in type 2 diabetic subjects: A randomized controlled crossover trial. *Diabetes Care* 33:227–232.

Mantovani, A., P. Allavena, A. Sica, and F. Balkwill. 2008. Cancer-related inflammation. *Nature* 454:436–444.

Mantzoros, C.S., C.J. Williams, J.E. Manson, J.B. Meigs, and F.B. Hu. 2006. Adherence to the Mediterranean dietary pattern is positively associated with plasma adiponectin concentrations in diabetic women. *Am J Clin Nutr* 84:328–335.

Martinez-Gonzalez, M.A. and M. Bes-Rastrollo. 2011. Nut consumption, weight gain and obesity: Epidemiological evidence. *Nutr Metab Cardiovasc Dis* 21:S40–S45.

Martinez-Lapiscina, E.H., A.M. Pimenta, J.J. Beunza, M. Bes-Rastrollo, J.A. Martinez, and M.A. Martinez-Gonzalez. 2010. Nut consumption and incidence of hypertension: The SUN prospective cohort. *Nutr Metab Cardiovasc Dis* 20:359–365.

Mattes, R.D. and M.L. Dreher. 2010. Nuts and healthy body weight maintenance mechanisms. *Asia Pac J Clin Nutr* 19:137–141.

Mattes, R.D., P.M. Kris-Etherton, and G.D. Foster. 2008. Impact of peanuts and tree nuts on body weight and healthy weight loss in adults. *J Nutr* 138:S1741–S1745.

McKay, D.L., C.Y. Chen, K.J. Yeum, N.R. Matthan, A.H. Lichtenstein, and J.B. Blumberg. 2010. Chronic and acute effects of walnuts on antioxidant capacity and nutritional status in humans: A randomized, crossover pilot study. *Nutr J* 9:21.

Mitjavila, M.T., M. Fandos, J. Salas-Salvado et al. 2013. The Mediterranean diet improves the systemic lipid and DNA oxidative damage in MetS individuals. A randomized, controlled, trial. *Clin Nutr* 32:172–178.

Monteiro, R. and I. Azevedo. 2010. Chronic inflammation in obesity and the MetS. *Mediators Inflamm* 2010:289645.

Mottillo, S., K.B. Filion, J. Genest et al. 2010. The MetS and cardiovascular risk: A systematic review and meta-analysis. *J Am Coll Cardiol* 56:1113–1132.

Mukuddem-Petersen, J., W. Oosthuizen, and J.C. Jerling. 2005. A systematic review of the effects of nuts on blood lipid profiles in humans. *J Nutr* 135:2082–2089.

Mukuddem-Petersen, J., W. Stonehouse, J.C. Jerling, S.M. Hanekom, and Z. White. 2007. Effects of a high walnut and high cashew nut diet on selected markers of the MetS: A controlled feeding trial. *Br J Nutr* 97:1144–1153.

National Health and Medical Research Council. 2006. Nutrient reference values for Australia and New Zealand: Executive summary. Canberra, Australian Capital Territory, Australia: NHMRC.

Nouran, M.G., M. Kimiagar, A. Abadi, M. Mirzazadeh, and G. Harrison. 2010. Peanut consumption and cardiovascular risk. *Public Health Nutr* 13:1581–1586.

Novotny, J.A., S.K. Gebauer, and D.J. Baer. 2012. Discrepancy between the Atwater factor predicted and empirically measured energy values of almonds in human diets. *Am J Clin Nutr* 96:296–301.

Oliver, E., F. McGillicuddy, C. Phillips, S. Toomey, and H.M. Roche. 2010. The role of inflammation and macrophage accumulation in the development of obesity-induced type 2 diabetes mellitus and the possible therapeutic effects of long-chain n-3 PUFA. *Proc Nutr Soc* 69:232–243.

O'Neil, C.E., D.R. Keast, V.L. Fulgoni, and T.A. Nicklas. 2010. Tree nut consumption improves nutrient intake and diet quality in US adults: An analysis of National Health and Nutrition Examination Survey (NHANES) 1999–2004. *Asia Pac J Clin Nutr* 19:142–150.

O'Neil, C.E., D.R. Keast, T.A. Nicklas, and V.L. Fulgoni. 2011. Nut consumption is associated with decreased health risk factors for cardiovascular disease and MetS in U.S. adults: NHANES 1999–2004. *J Am Coll Nutr* 30:502–510.

O'Neil, C.E., D.R. Keast, T.A. Nicklas, and V.L. Fulgoni. 2012. Out-of-hand nut consumption is associated with improved nutrient intake and health risk markers in US children and adults: National Health and Nutrition Examination Survey 1999–2004. *Nutr Res* 32:185–194.

Paramsothy, P., R.H. Knopp, S.E. Kahn et al. 2011. Plasma sterol evidence for decreased absorption and increased synthesis of cholesterol in insulin resistance and obesity. *Am J Clin Nutr* 94:1182–1188.

Parker, E.D., L.J. Harnack, and A.R. Folsom. 2003. Nut consumption and risk of type 2 diabetes. *JAMA* 290:38–39.

Pawlak, R., S. Colby, and J. Herring. 2009. Beliefs, benefits, barriers, attitude, intake and knowledge about peanuts and tree nuts among WIC participants in eastern North Carolina. *Nutr Res Pract* 3:220–225.

Perez-Martinez, P., J. Lopez-Miranda, L. Blanco-Colio et al. 2007. The chronic intake of a Mediterranean diet enriched in virgin olive oil, decreases nuclear transcription factor kappaB activation in peripheral blood mononuclear cells from healthy men. *Atherosclerosis* 194:e141–e146.

Phung, O.J., S.S. Makanji, C.M. White, and C.I. Coleman. 2009. Almonds have a neutral effect on serum lipid profiles: A meta-analysis of randomized trials. *J Am Diet Assoc* 109:865–873.

Pieters, M., W. Oosthuizen, J.C. Jerling, D.T. Loots, J. Mukuddem-Petersen, and S.M. Hanekom. 2005. Clustering of haemostatic variables and the effect of high cashew and walnut diets on these variables in MetS patients. *Blood Coagul Fibrinolysis* 16:429–437.

Pradhan, A.D. and P.M. Ridker. 2002. Do atherosclerosis and type 2 diabetes share a common inflammatory basis? *Eur Heart J* 23:831–834.

Prineas, R.J., L.H. Kushi, A.R. Folsom, R.M. Bostick, and Y. Wu. 1993. Walnuts and serum lipids. *N Engl J Med* 329:359.

Rajaram, S., K.M. Connell, and J. Sabate. 2010. Effect of almond-enriched high-monounsaturated fat diet on selected markers of inflammation: A randomised, controlled, crossover study. *Br J Nutr* 103:907–912.

Ros, E. 2009. Nuts and novel biomarkers of cardiovascular disease. *Am J Clin Nutr* 89:1649S–1656S.

Ros, E. 2010. Health benefits of nut consumption. *Nutrients* 2:652–682.

Ros, E. and J. Mataix. 2006. Fatty acid composition of nuts—Implications for cardiovascular health. *Br J Nutr* 96:S29–S35.

Ros, E., I. Nunez, A. Perez-Heras et al. 2004. A walnut diet improves endothelial function in hypercholesterolemic subjects: A randomized crossover trial. *Circulation* 109:1609–1614.

Ros, E., L.C. Tapsell, and J. Sabate. 2010. Nuts and berries for heart health. *Curr Atheroscler Rep* 12:397–406.

Sabate, J. 1993. Does nut consumption protect against ischaemic heart disease. *Eur J Clin Nutr* 47 S71–S75.

Sabate, J. 1999. Nut consumption, vegetarian diets, ischemic heart disease risk, and all-cause mortality: Evidence from epidemiologic studies. *Am J Clin Nutr* 70:S500–S503.

Sabate, J. and Y. Ang. 2009. Nuts and health outcomes: New epidemiologic evidence. *Am J Clin Nutr* 89:1643S–1648S.

Sabate, J., Z. Cordero-MacIntyre, G. Siapco, S. Torabian, and E. Haddad. 2005. Does regular walnut consumption lead to weight gain? *Br J Nutr* 94:859–864.

Sabate, J., E. Haddad, J.S. Tanzman, P. Jambazian, and S. Rajaram. 2003. Serum lipid response to the graduated enrichment of a Step I diet with almonds: A randomized feeding trial. *Am J Clin Nutr* 77:1379–1384.

Sabate, J., K. Oda, and E. Ros. 2010. Nut consumption and blood lipid levels: A pooled analysis of 25 intervention trials. *Arch Intern Med* 170:821–827.

Sabaté, J. and M. Wien. 2010. Nuts, blood lipids and cardiovascular disease. *Asia Pac J Clin Nutr* 19:131–136.

Salas-Salvado, J., M. Bullo, A. Perez-Heras, and E. Ros. 2006. Dietary fibre, nuts and cardiovascular diseases. *Br J Nutr* 96:S45–S51.

Salas-Salvado, J., P. Casas-Agustench, and A. Salas-Huetos. 2011. Cultural and historical aspects of Mediterranean nuts with emphasis on their attributed healthy and nutritional properties. *Nutr Metab Cardiovasc Dis* 21:S1–S6.

Salas-Salvado, J., J. Fernandez-Ballart, E. Ros et al. 2008a. Effect of a Mediterranean diet supplemented with nuts on MetS status: One-year results of the PREDIMED randomized trial. *Arch Intern Med* 168:2449–2458.

Salas-Salvado, J., A. Garcia-Arellano, R. Estruch et al. 2008b. Components of the Mediterranean-type food pattern and serum inflammatory markers among patients at high risk for cardiovascular disease. *Eur J Clin Nutr* 62:651–659.

Sari, I., Y. Baltaci, C. Bagci et al. 2010. Effect of pistachio diet on lipid parameters, endothelial function, inflammation, and oxidative status: A prospective study. *Nutrition* 26:399–404.

Sathe, S.K., E.K. Monaghan, H.H. Kshirsagar, and M. Venkatachalam. 2009. Chemical composition of edible nut seeds and its implications in human health. In Alasalvar, C. and F. Shahidi, eds., *Tree Nuts: Composition, Phytochemicals, and Health Effects*. Boca Raton, FL: Taylor & Francis Group.

Schutte, A.E., J.M. Van Rooyen, H.W. Huisman et al. 2006. Modulation of baroreflex sensitivity by walnuts versus cashew nuts in subjects with MetS. *Am J Hypertens* 19:629–636.

Segura, R., C. Javierre, M.A. Lizarraga, and E. Ros. 2006. Other relevant components of nuts: Phytosterols, folate and minerals. *Br J Nutr* 96:S36–S44.

Simonen, P., H. Gylling, A.N. Howard, and T.A. Miettinen. 2000. Introducing a new component of the MetS: Low cholesterol absorption. *Am J Clin Nutr* 72:82–88.

Simonen, P.P., H. Gylling, and T.A. Miettinen. 2002. Body weight modulates cholesterol metabolism in non-insulin dependent type 2 diabetics. *Obes Res* 10:328–335.

Spaccarotella, K., P. Kris-Etherton, W. Stone et al. 2008. The effect of walnut intake on factors related to prostate and vascular health in older men. *Nutr J* 7:13.

St-Onge, M.-P. 2005. Dietary fats, teas, dairy, and nuts: Potential functional foods for weight control? *Am J Clin Nutr* 81:7–15.

Tapsell, L.C., M.J. Batterham, G. Teuss et al. 2009. Long-term effects of increased dietary polyunsaturated fat from walnuts on metabolic parameters in type II diabetes. *Eur J Clin Nutr* 63:1008–1015.

Tey, S.L., R. Brown, A. Gray, A. Chisholm, and C. Delahunty. 2011. Nuts improve diet quality compared to other energy-dense snacks while maintaining body weight. *J Nutr Metab* 2011:357350.

Thomson, C.D., A. Chisholm, S.K. McLachlan, and J.M. Campbell. 2008. Brazil nuts: An effective way to improve selenium status. *Am J Clin Nutr* 87:379–384.

Tulipani, S., R. Llorach, O. Jauregui et al. 2011. Metabolomics unveils urinary changes in subjects with MetS following 12-week nut consumption. *J Proteome Res* 10:5047–5058.

Tulipani, S., M. Urpi-Sarda, R. Garcia-Villalba et al. 2012. Urolithins are the main urinary microbial-derived phenolic metabolites discriminating a moderate consumption of nuts in free-living subjects with diagnosed MetS. *J Agric Food Chem* 60:8930–8940.

Urpi-Sarda, M., R. Casas, G. Chiva-Blanch et al. 2012. Virgin olive oil and nuts as key foods of the Mediterranean diet effects on inflammatory biomarkers related to atherosclerosis. *Pharmacol Res* 65:577–583.

U.S. Department of Agriculture, and Agriculture Research Service. 2011. USDA national nutrient database for standard reference 2010 [cited September 28, 2011]. Available from Nutrient Data Laboratory: http://www.nal.usda.gov/fnic/foodcomp/search/.

Valavanidis, A., T. Vlachogianni, and C. Fiotakis. 2009. 8-Hydroxy-2′-deoxyguanosine (8-OHdG): A critical biomarker of oxidative stress and carcinogenesis. *J Environ Sci Health C Environ Carcinog Ecotoxicol Rev* 27:120–139.

Villegas, R., Y.-T. Gao, G. Yang et al. 2008. Legume and soy food intake and the incidence of type 2 diabetes in the Shanghai Women's Health Study. *Am J Clin Nutr* 87:162–167.

Vinson, J.A. and Y. Cai. 2012. Nuts, especially walnuts, have both antioxidant quantity and efficacy and exhibit significant potential health benefits. *Food Funct* 3:134–140.

Wang, X., Z. Li, Y. Liu, X. Lv, and W. Yang. 2012. Effects of pistachios on body weight in Chinese subjects with MetS. *Nutr J* 11:20.

West, S.G., A.L. Krick, L.C. Klein et al. 2010. Effects of diets high in walnuts and flax oil on hemodynamic responses to stress and vascular endothelial function. *J Am Coll Nutr* 29:595–603.

Wien, M., D. Bleich, M. Raghuwanshi et al. 2010. Almond consumption and cardiovascular risk factors in adults with prediabetes. *J Am Coll Nutr* 29:189–197.

Wien, M.A., J.M. Sabaté, D.N. Iklé, S.E. Cole, and F.R. Kandeel. 2003. Almonds vs complex carbohydrates in a weight reduction program. *Int J Obes Relat Metab Disord* 27:1365–1372.

World Health Organisation. 2004. The atlas of heart disease and stroke 2004 [cited January 15, 2008]. Available from: http://www.who.int/cardiovascular_diseases/resources/altas/en.

Wu, H., A. Pan, Z. Yu et al. 2010. Lifestyle counseling and supplementation with flaxseed or walnuts influence the management of MetS. *J Nutr* 140:1937–1942.

Zambon, D. and J. Sabate. 2000. Substituting walnuts for monounsaturated fat improves the serum lipid profile of hypercholesterolemic men and woman. A randomized crossover trial. *Ann Intern Med* 132:538–546.

Zhao, G., T.D. Etherton, K.R. Martin, S.G. West, P.J. Gillies, and P.M. Kris-Etherton. 2004. Dietary {alpha}-linolenic acid reduces inflammatory and lipid cardiovascular risk factors in hypercholesterolemic men and women. *J Nutr* 134:2991–2997.

18 Eggs Effects on HDL-C Metabolism, Inflammation, and Insulin Resistance

Christopher N. Blesso, Catherine J. Andersen, and Maria Luz Fernandez

CONTENTS

18.1 INTRODUCTION

Metabolic syndrome is a cluster of abnormalities characterized by central adiposity, hypertension, dyslipidemias, high fasting plasma glucose, insulin resistance, and low-grade inflammation (Cornier et al. 2008). There are a number of dietary treatments that can reduce one or more of these metabolic problems, including low-carbohydrate diets (Al-Sarraj et al. 2009), the Mediterranean diet (Jones et al. 2011), or weight loss interventions (Elizondo-Montemayor et al. 2013). Some dietary components have also been shown to target specific metabolic abnormalities; for example, grapes reduce blood pressure (Barona et al. 2012), fatty fish reduces plasma triglycerides and inflammatory markers (Klemsdal et al. 2010), and moderate wine consumption has been shown to increase plasma HDL-cholesterol (HDL-C) (Koppes et al. 2005). The focus of this chapter will be the effects of eggs in improving dyslipidemias and increasing reverse cholesterol transport (RCT), as well as reducing inflammation and insulin resistance across populations, with an emphasis on individuals with metabolic syndrome.

Data from epidemiological studies and clinical interventions indicate that concerns regarding egg intake and risk for coronary heart disease (CHD) are unfounded (Fernandez 2012). Not only do eggs not increase CHD risk, but they have been shown to consistently increase HDL-cholesterol (HDL-C) even in the absence of increments in LDL-cholesterol (LDL-C) (Mutungi et al. 2008; Blesso et al. 2013a). Eggs have also been reported to reduce inflammatory markers including C-reactive protein (CRP) (Ratliff et al. 2008), serum amyloid A (SAA), and tumor necrosis factor-α (TNF-α) (Blesso et al. 2013b), in addition to improving insulin sensitivity in the context of a low-carbohydrate diet (Blesso et al. 2013a). Moreover, eggs attenuate the formation of the more atherogenic lipoproteins including small LDL-C, large VLDL, and medium HDL-C (Herron et al. 2004; Mutungi et al. 2010; Blesso et al. 2013a).

18.2   EGGS AND DYSLIPIDEMIA

The lack of association between eggs and risk of cardiovascular disease (CVD) has been clearly demonstrated in several epidemiological studies (Hu et al. 1999; Nakamura et al. 2006; Qureshi et al. 2007). Clinical studies have also shown that only 25%–30% of the population experiences an increase in blood cholesterol following a cholesterol challenge (Fernandez 2006). Studies in children (Ballesteros et al. 2004), young adults (Herron et al. 2002, 2003), and older individuals (Greene et al. 2005) have shown that for those who respond to a dietary cholesterol challenge, there is an increase in both LDL-C and HDL-C; therefore, the ratio LDL-C/HDL-C, a major determinant of heart disease risk (Fernandez and Webb 2008), is maintained. Furthermore, in cases of weight loss (Mutungi et al. 2008; Blesso et al. 2013a), the LDL-C/HDL-C ratio is improved. In addition to these specific effects on plasma lipids, eggs appear to substantially affect lipoprotein metabolism, as addressed in the following paragraphs.

18.2.1   Effects on HDL-cholesterol

Therapies aimed at increasing plasma HDL-C may be beneficial to prevent cardiovascular events. Plasma HDL-C levels have been found to be inversely associated with the risk of CVD (Linsel-Nitschke and Tall 2005). Based on data from large prospective cohort studies, it can be estimated that for every 1 mg/dL (0.0259 mmol/L) increase in HDL-C, there is a 2%–3% reduction in CVD risk (Gordon et al. 1989). Lifestyle factors that influence HDL-C levels include physical activity, obesity, smoking, and diet (Weissglas-Volkov and Pajukanta 2010). Weight loss is generally associated with small increases in HDL-C (Dattilo and Kris-Etherton 1992). Only a few dietary modifications consistently increase plasma HDL-C in research studies. Replacing dietary carbohydrate intake with fat (Mensink et al. 2003) and ingesting alcohol (Rimm et al. 1999) have been shown to modestly increase plasma HDL-C. Daily egg intake has also been shown to increase plasma HDL-C under both weight maintenance (Fernandez 2012) (Table 18.1) and weight loss (Harman et al. 2008; Pearce et al. 2011) conditions (Table 18.2).

The contents of eggs that are responsible for influencing HDL-C have not been examined; however, there are a number of bioactive components that may be involved. Compared with other foods, egg yolk is a rich source of phosphatidylcholine (PC) and other phospholipids (Kovacs-Nolan et al. 2005). Dietary phospholipid intake has been associated with increases in HDL-C in animal and human studies (Burgess et al. 1982; O'Brien and Corragan 1998). Interestingly, dietary PC has been observed to preferentially incorporate into HDL-C particles (Zierenberg and Grundy 1985), and HDL-phospholipid is shown to increase after egg yolk ingestion (Dubois et al. 1994). This may alter HDL-C function, as phospholipid enrichment improves the cholesterol-accepting capacity of the particle (Yancey et al. 2000). Thus, egg phospholipid may enhance the ability of HDL-C particles to mobilize cholesterol from cell membranes by aqueous diffusion, as well as efflux pathways associated with ATP-binding cassette transporter G1 (ABCG1) and scavenger receptor class B1 (SR-B1) activities.

Eggs also contain dietary cholesterol, which has been shown to raise HDL-C levels in animal models and humans (Clarke et al. 1997; Escola-Gil et al. 2011). Increases in RCT have been seen with high dietary cholesterol intakes in animals (Escola-Gil et al. 2011). A meta-analysis was conducted to quantitatively assess the effect of dietary cholesterol intake on plasma HDL-C. McNamara (2000) reviewed the effects of egg feeding on plasma cholesterol in 167 crossover designed studies ($n = 3519$) published between 1960 and 1999. Studies using dietary cholesterol challenges greater than 1200 mg/day were excluded from the analyses due to known reductions in cholesterol absorption efficiency at extreme intakes. The plasma cholesterol response to an additional 100 mg of dietary cholesterol/day was predicted to increase plasma HDL-C by 0.44 mg/dL.

Importantly, there seems to be a significant heterogeneity in the plasma cholesterol response to egg feeding. The response of plasma HDL-C with egg feeding is likely influenced by the metabolic

TABLE 18.1

Crossover Design Studies – Weight Maintenance

Intervention	Population	Study Design	Dietary Treatment	Δ HDL-C: Egg vs. No Egg
Herron et al. 2002	Pre-menopausal women (aged 18-49 y , n = 51)	30-day; *ad libitum* diet	3 eggs per day vs. egg substitute	Caucasians: +6.3% Hispanics: +3.9%
Herron et al. 2003	Men (aged 18–57 y, n = 40)	30-day; *ad libitum* diet	3 eggs per day vs. egg substitute	Hyper-responders : +8.4% Hypo-responders: −0.8%
Knopp et al. 2003	Men and women (n = 197)	4-week; *ad libitum* diet	4 eggs per day vs. egg substitute	Lean insulin-sensitive: +8.8% Obese insulin-resistant: +3.6%
Ballesteros et al. 2004	Children (aged 8–12 y, n = 54)	30-day; *ad libitum* diet	2 eggs per day vs. egg substitute	Hyper-responders : +9.8% Hypo-responders: +4.9%
Greene et al. 2005	Elderly men and women (aged ≥ 60 y, n = 42)	30-day; *ad libitum* diet	3 eggs per day vs. egg substitute	Men: +10.0% Women: +2.6%
Vishwanathan et al. 2009	Statin-taking elderly (aged ≥ 60 y, n = 28)	5-week; *ad libitum* diet	2 or 4 eggs per day vs. egg exclusion	2 eggs per day: +5.4% 4 eggs per day: +5.4%

TABLE 18.2

Parallel Design Studies - Weight Loss

Intervention	Population	Study Design	Dietary Treatment	Δ HDL-C from Baseline
Harman et al. 2008	Men and women (aged 18–55 y)	12-week; energy-restricted diet	2 eggs per day (n = 24)	+13.4%
Mutungi et al. 2008	Overweight men (aged 40–70 y)	12-week; carbohydrate-restricted diet	3 eggs per day (n = 15)	+19.5%
Pearce et al. 2011	Type 2 diabetic men and women (aged 20–75 y)	12-week; energy-restricted diet	2 eggs per day (n = 31)	+2.5%
Blesso et al. 2012	Men and women with metabolic syndrome (aged 30–70 y)	12-week; carbohydrate-restricted diet	3 eggs per day (n = 20)	+19.1%

status of the individual. Both obesity (Miettinen and Gylling 2000; Simonen et al. 2000) and insulin resistance (Pihlajamaki et al. 2004) are associated with reduced dietary cholesterol absorption efficiency compared to healthy, normal weight controls. Several recent studies reporting effects of egg feeding on plasma HDL-C in those that are overweight and/or insulin-resistant will be discussed briefly.

Knopp et al. (2003) studied the effect of metabolic status on the lipoprotein response to egg feeding. Lean insulin-sensitive (LIS, $n = 66$), lean insulin-resistant (LIR, $n = 76$), and obese insulin-resistant (OIR, $n = 59$) participants consumed 0, 2, and 4 egg yolks/day for 4 weeks as equal-weight egg mixtures (using egg yolk and yolk-free egg substitute). In the LIS group, there was a significant 8.8% increase in plasma HDL-C with the 4 egg yolks/day diet compared to 0 yolk/day. The response was significantly greater for plasma HDL-C for the LIS group compared to the OIR group, whose HDL-C increased by an average of 3.6%. Though not significant, plasma cholesterol responses were attenuated in the LIR group compared to the LIS group. Notably, the LIR and OIR groups had greater percent increases in HDL-C compared to LDL-C increases. Overall, insulin-resistant subjects were less sensitive to the LDL-C raising effects of egg feeding. This study suggests that those who are insulin resistant may have more favorable lipoprotein responses to egg feeding than those who are insulin sensitive, with greater relative increases in HDL-C than LDL-C.

Mutungi et al. (2008) examined the combined effect of egg feeding (3 eggs/day) and carbohydrate-restriction (<20% of energy) on plasma lipoprotein responses. Twenty-eight overweight men (BMI = 25–37 kg/m^2) participated in a 12-week parallel study, either consuming 3 eggs ($n = 15$) or yolk-free egg substitute ($n = 13$) per day. In both groups, there were significant reductions in weight and waist circumference. In the whole egg group, plasma HDL-C significantly increased by 12 mg/dL, with no change observed in the egg substitute group. Results from this study support the concept that daily egg ingestion, in the context of a weight loss diet, can markedly improve plasma HDL-C in overweight men.

Recently, we investigated the effects of daily egg intake, in combination with carbohydrate restriction, on plasma lipids in adult men and women with metabolic syndrome (Blesso et al. 2013a). Thirty-seven participants with MetS were instructed to follow a carbohydrate-restricted diet (<30% energy) and randomly assigned to consume either 3 eggs ($n = 20$) or yolk-free egg substitute ($n = 17$) per day for 12 weeks. Both groups exhibited modest reductions in weight after 12 weeks (~4%). Those consuming whole eggs had a greater percent increase in plasma HDL-C than those consuming egg substitute (19.1% vs. 9.9%). Importantly, this robust increase in HDL-C was observed in the absence of any changes in LDL-C, thus reducing the LDL-C/HDL-C ratio.

Overall, there is a multitude of evidence suggesting that daily egg intake increases plasma HDL-C concentrations. However, the mechanisms behind such effects are not well understood and warrant further study.

18.2.2 Effects on Atherogenic Lipoproteins

The relationships between standard blood lipid measures, such as LDL-C and HDL-C, and CVD are well established. However, despite their strengths in disease prediction, individuals with similar blood lipid values can often have very different relative risks for CVD. In these circumstances, examining the lipoprotein particle profile may be warranted (Davidson et al. 2011). Nuclear magnetic resonance (NMR) spectroscopy enables the characterization of lipoprotein subclasses that may differ in their atherogenicity, thereby offering a tool to identify residual CVD risk among individuals with similar blood lipid values. Distinct lipoprotein subclasses, measured by NMR analysis, have been shown to be markers of CVD severity (Freedman et al. 1998), and predictive of risk for future CVD (Otvos et al. 2006; El Harchaoui et al. 2009; Mora et al. 2009; Arsenault et al. 2010) and type 2 diabetes (Festa et al. 2005; Hodge et al. 2009). These associations are often independent of other common risk factors such as age and standard blood lipid measures. For example, a greater concentration of large HDL-C in plasma is strongly associated with reduced risk for CVD, while smaller HDL-C subclasses are less robust in their association (Freedman et al. 1998; Davidson et al. 2011). Furthermore, small LDL-C particles are strongly associated with increased CVD risk, while larger LDL-C particles are generally not associated with CVD (Mora et al. 2009).

In healthy populations, daily egg intake consistently shifts the proportion of small LDL-C and small HDL-C subclasses toward larger, more buoyant particles (Fernandez 2006). Daily egg intake has been demonstrated to increase LDL-C size and the number of large LDL-C, shown by both gel electrophoresis (Ballesteros et al. 2004) and NMR methods (Mutungi et al. 2010). Daily egg intake has also been shown to increase lecithin-cholesterol acyltransferase (LCAT) activity, potentially improving RCT (Herron et al. 2004; Mutungi et al. 2010). LCAT is critically important in facilitating HDL-C particle stability and HDL-C maturation (Rousset et al. 2011). Increases in LCAT activity with egg intake may enhance HDL-C maturation and explain the shift toward larger HDL-C subclasses.

We recently examined the lipoprotein particle profile response to 12 weeks of daily egg ingestion, in combination with weight loss, in adults with metabolic syndrome (Blesso et al. 2013a). Lipoprotein particle number and size were assessed at baseline and at the end of the 12-week diet study. Importantly, consuming 3 eggs/day did not increase atherogenic lipoproteins present in MetS, but actually shifted the lipoprotein particle profile to a healthier phenotype. Compared to consuming a yolk-free egg substitute, daily egg intake resulted in many putative improvements in plasma lipoprotein metabolism, including larger HDL-C and LDL-C particle size, greater reductions in total VLDL and medium VLDL particles, and greater increases in large HDL-C particles and LCAT activity. Increases in HDL-C size and large HDL-C were strongly correlated with increases in plasma HDL-C, consistent with what has been observed in other studies using NMR (Freedman et al. 1998; Mora et al. 2009). It is worth mentioning that in the presence of MetS, not only did eggs improve HDL-C characteristics, but appeared to strongly affect VLDL metabolism—something that has not been observed in healthy populations. If confirmed with larger studies, this effect of egg intake may be significant, as the total number of plasma VLDL particles and the medium VLDL subclass are linked to increased incidence of CVD (Knopp et al. 2003) and type 2 diabetes (Hodge et al. 2009).

Along with exhibiting a greater amount of atherogenic lipoproteins in plasma, MetS is associated with reduced plasma carotenoid concentrations (Kritchevsky et al. 2000; Suzuki et al. 2011). Carotenoids are lipid-soluble pigments that display antioxidant and anti-inflammatory activities (Sies and Stahl 1995; Kim et al. 2012). Lipoproteins are the major carriers of carotenoids in circulation, with apolar (carotenes) and polar (xanthophylls) carotenoids primarily transported on LDL-C and HDL-C particles, respectively (Clevidence and Bieri 1993). Observational studies have linked low serum carotenoid concentrations with increased risks for cancer (Toniolo et al. 2001), CHD (Morris et al. 1994), and all-cause mortality (Shardell et al. 2011).

Daily egg consumption has been shown to increase plasma lutein concentrations by approximately 20%–65% from baseline, depending on the study design and population of interest (Goodrow et al. 2006; Greene et al. 2006; Herron et al. 2006; Vishwanathan et al. 2009). Plasma zeaxanthin is also commonly increased with egg ingestion, with increases of approximately 10%–40% from baseline observed in most studies (Goodrow et al. 2006; Greene et al. 2006; Herron et al. 2006). These observations are consistent with the additional lutein and zeaxanthin consumed in the diet provided by egg yolk. In adults with MetS (Blesso et al. 2013c), consuming 3 eggs/day resulted in 21% increases in plasma lutein, 48% increases in zeaxanthin, and 24% increases in β-carotene compared to baseline. Furthermore, there was a significant enrichment of HDL-C and LDL-C in both lutein and zeaxanthin after 12 weeks of egg intake. Benefits on carotenoid status were due to additional yolk consumption, as plasma and lipoprotein lutein and zeaxanthin actually decreased over time for participants consuming yolk-free egg substitute.

While several recent studies clearly demonstrate a dramatic shift in atherogenic lipoprotein profiles with egg feeding, how these changes ultimately affect long-term cardiovascular outcomes has not been established. Future research is warranted to examine if egg feeding improves or impairs more sophisticated biomarkers of lipoprotein metabolism and function.

18.2.3 EFFECTS ON REVERSE CHOLESTEROL TRANSPORT

Numerous therapeutic strategies aimed at reducing CVD risk have targeted RCT—one primary mechanism by which HDL-C protects against atherosclerosis development (von Eckardstein et al. 2001). RCT is the process of retrieving cellular cholesterol from peripheral tissues for excretion from the body via the liver and bile, in addition to nonbiliary excretion via the transintestinal cholesterol efflux (TICE) pathway (Rader et al. 2009; Temel and Brown 2012). Overall, RCT is a dynamic process that can be regulated at the level of cellular cholesterol efflux to HDL-C, cholesteryl ester transfer protein (CETP)-mediated lipid exchange between HDL-C and apoB-containing lipoproteins, hepatic/intestinal cholesterol uptake, and ultimately, cholesterol excretion from the body (Rader et al. 2009). Macrophage-specific RCT is particularly essential in reducing atherosclerotic burden, as lipid-laden macrophage foam cells within the arterial wall are considered the hallmark of atherosclerosis (Libby et al. 1996; deGoma et al. 2008). Numerous studies have investigated the effects of egg intake on various parameters of RCT (Ginsberg et al. 1994; Blanco-Molina et al. 1998; Mutungi et al. 2008; Yang et al. 2012; Andersen et al. 2013a; Blesso et al. 2013a). Together, findings from these studies suggest that egg intake favorably promotes RCT and may therefore reduce the risk and severity of atherosclerosis.

The initial step of RCT involves the efflux of cellular cholesterol to HDL-C (deGoma et al. 2008). HDL-mediated cholesterol efflux is dependent on the quality of HDL-C as a lipid acceptor, as well as the capacity of cholesterol-loaded cells to facilitate efflux to this lipoprotein via the transporters ABCA1 and ABCG1, plus the binding of HDL-C to SR-BI (Rosenson et al. 2012). In healthy men, consumption of 2 eggs/day during a 24-day National Education Program Step I diet (<30% fat, <10% saturated fat) increased cholesterol efflux from rat Fu5AH hepatoma cells to subject serum when compared to an egg-free diet. Conversely, egg intake had no effect on cholesterol efflux during consumption of an oleic acid–rich diet (22% of energy) (Blanco–Molina et al. 1998). Furthermore, the effects of egg intake appear to be a result of habitual consumption, as a single-dose egg meal does not appear to affect postprandial cholesterol efflux in healthy men (Ginsberg et al. 1994). Murine macrophage-like J774 cells incubated with postprandial serum following consumption of 1, 2, or 4 eggs had no effect on cellular total, free, or esterified cholesterol. However, cellular free cholesterol was slightly higher when combining all egg groups and comparing to the 0-egg meal (Ginsberg et al. 1994).

Increases in serum cholesterol efflux capacity following habitual egg feeding have also been demonstrated in subjects with MetS. We have recently reported that intake of 3 eggs/day for 12 weeks during moderate-carbohydrate restriction (<30% of energy) increases the cholesterol-accepting capacity of serum from RAW 264.7 macrophage foam cells in MetS, whereas consumption of a yolk-free egg substitute has no effect (Andersen et al. 2013a). This observation corresponded to modulation of HDL-C lipid composition, where egg feeding promoted enrichment of HDL-phosphatidylethanolamine and relative reductions in HDL-triglyceride. Furthermore, HDL-C became more enriched in sphingomyelin molecular species present in whole egg, suggesting that the dietary phospholipids provided by egg may be directly incorporated into HDL-C particles (Andersen et al. 2013a). These findings complement the increasing body of research that demonstrates that the modulation of HDL-C phospholipid content can differentially alter the capacity of HDL-C to accept cellular cholesterol (Fournier et al. 1996, 1997; Davit-Sparaul et al. 1999; Tchoua et al. 2010).

Aside from improving the capacity of HDL-C to accept foam cell lipids, egg feeding may also affect the expression of lipid transporters (Andersen et al. 2013a). Consumption of 3 eggs/day as part of a 12-week moderate carbohydrate-restricted diet increased the mRNA expression of ABCA1 (+127%) in peripheral blood mononuclear cells (PBMCs) from subjects with metabolic syndrome. Increases in PBMC ABCA1 mRNA expression were dependent on the intake of egg yolk, as no changes in ABCA1 expression were observed in subjects consuming a yolk-free egg substitute (Andersen et al. 2013a).

Egg intake has additionally been shown to alter the activity of proteins involved in HDL-C metabolism and RCT, including LCAT and CETP. Intake of 3 eggs/day during carbohydrate restriction has been shown to increase LCAT activity in overweight men (Mutungi et al. 2010), as well as men and women with metabolic syndrome (Blesso et al. 2013a). While it remains controversial as to whether increased LCAT activity is beneficial, some studies suggest that LCAT promotes RCT and reduces atherosclerosis (Rader et al. 2009). In addition, CETP activity was shown to be 6%

higher in healthy male subjects following a 24-day diet of 4 eggs when compared to intake of 0, 1, or 2 eggs/day (combined) (Ginsberg et al. 1994). Although high CETP activity has been implicated in the development of atherosclerosis due to the transfer of HDL-cholesterol to apoB-containing lipoproteins, CETP has also been shown to be important for macrophage RCT and HDL-derived cholesterol excretion in human and animal models (Schwartz et al. 2004; Tanigawa et al. 2007).

Egg feeding has additionally been shown to promote sterol excretion—potentially due to a combination of decreased absorption and increased RCT (Yang et al. 2012). In Sprague Dawley rats, egg-enriched diets increased fecal neutral sterol and bile acid concentrations, as well as hepatic mRNA expression of LDL-receptor, cholesterol 7α-hydroxylase, and LCAT when compared to egg-free control. Furthermore, egg feeding blunted increases in plasma total and LDL-C and liver triglyceride and cholesterol levels that were observed in a pure cholesterol-fed group, while also promoting greater increases in plasma HDL-C. These observations corresponded to decreased apolipoprotein (apo) B and increased apoA-I (Yang et al. 2012). Overall, findings from the studies presented earlier suggest that egg intake favorably promotes RCT, and may therefore reduce CVD risk.

18.3 EGGS AND INFLAMMATION

Chronic low-grade, systemic inflammation is commonly associated with obesity-related metabolic disturbances, including CVD, type 2 diabetes, and metabolic syndrome. Obesity promotes the release of inflammatory markers from metabolically stressed tissues (e.g., adipose, liver, and skeletal muscle), which may further perpetuate the development of insulin resistance and dyslipidemias (Pradhan 2007; Guilherme et al. 2008).

Eggs contain a number of dietary factors with the potential to promote pro- and anti-inflammatory pathways. Egg white–derived hen egg lysozyme has been shown to reduce intestinal inflammation in an experimental model of colitis (Lee et al. 2009), whereas egg yolk serves as a rich, bioavailable source of antioxidant carotenoids lutein and zeaxanthin (Chung et al. 2004). Eggs are also a good source of bioactive phospholipids—particularly PC (Weihrauch and Son 1983; Coh et al. 2010). While PC is known to have anti-inflammatory properties (Eros et al. 2009; Treede et al. 2009; Tokes et al. 2011), it has also been shown to promote gut microflora-mediated production of trimethylamine-*N*-oxide—a PC metabolite associated with an increased risk of adverse cardiovascular events (Tang et al. 2013). Egg yolk is also a rich source of cholesterol, which can be cytotoxic in high doses (Goodrow and Nicolosi 2007).

Multiple studies have demonstrated that habitual egg consumption can alter markers of inflammation, with effects varying across populations and metabolic disease status. In a subset of older adults (over 60 years old) taking cholesterol-lowering medication, consumption of 2 or 4 eggs/day for 4 weeks did not alter CRP (Goodrow and Nicolosi 2007)—an acute phase protein that is a strong predictor of CVD risk (Ridker et al. 2000). However, in overweight men consuming an *ad libitum* carbohydrate-restricted diet for 12 weeks, the addition of 3 eggs/day resulted in decreases in plasma CRP (Ratliff et al. 2008). Beneficial reductions in CRP were not observed in overweight men consuming an equivalent amount of yolk-free egg substitute, although pro-inflammatory monocyte chemoattractant protein-1 (MCP-1) was reduced in this group. Both egg and egg substitute groups displayed increases in adiponectin—an adipose-derived protein with anti-inflammatory and insulin-sensitizing properties (Wiecek et al. 2007); however, changes in the whole egg group (+21%) were greater than those in the egg substitute group (+7%). Daily consumption of whole egg and egg substitute during carbohydrate restriction had no effect on plasma levels of other inflammatory markers in this population, including pro-inflammatory soluble vascular cell adhesion molecule-1 (sVCAM-1), soluble intracellular adhesion molecule-1 (sICAM-1), TNFα, and interleukin (IL)-8 (Ratliff et al. 2008). These data suggest that whole egg and egg white intake during carbohydrate restriction promotes reductions in systemic inflammation, with whole egg intake conferring a slightly greater benefit.

Egg consumption has similarly led to improvements in circulating plasma inflammatory markers in men and women classified with metabolic syndrome (Blesso et al. 2013b). While consuming a moderate carbohydrate-restricted diet, the addition of 3 eggs/day led to decreases in plasma TNFα and SAA, whereas no changes were observed in metabolic syndrome subjects consuming a yolk-free egg substitute. Differing from the results observed in overweight men, no changes in CRP or adiponectin were observed in either egg group in the metabolic syndrome population, nor were changes observed in sVCAM-1, sICAM-1, IL-6, or anti-inflammatory IL-10 (Blesso et al. 2013b).

While numerous studies have demonstrated beneficial effects of eggs on markers of inflammation, additional evidence suggests that the degree of insulin sensitivity is an important factor in determining the response to egg feeding. Tannock et al. (2005) found that consumption of 4 eggs/day for 4 weeks increased CRP and SAA in lean insulin-sensitive subjects following an American Heart Association–National cholesterol education program step 1 diet, whereas no changes in these inflammatory markers were observed in lean or obese insulin-resistant subjects. These observations may be due to the fact that lean and obese insulin-resistant patients have a diminished capacity to absorb cholesterol (Berglund and Hyson 2003; Paramsothy et al. 2011), which may promote tissue inflammation if compensatory mechanisms to mitigate cholesterol-mediated cytotoxicity are inadequate (Subramanian and Chait 2009).

In addition to systemic markers of inflammation, recent data suggest that egg intake increases pro-inflammatory gene expression in PBMC. In MetS subjects consuming a carbohydrate-restricted diet, intake of 3 eggs/day increased PBMC mRNA expression of toll-like receptor-4 (TLR4), a cell-surface receptor capable of mediating pro-inflammatory signaling cascades in response to lipopolysaccharide and fatty acid ligation (Coenen et al. 2009). Changes in TLR4 mRNA positively correlated with nuclear factor κ B (NF-κB) p65 subunit's DNA-binding activity, suggesting that this pro-inflammatory transcription factor may become activated in response to egg intake. However, egg consumption did not affect mRNA expression of other NF-κB target genes, such as the pro-inflammatory TNF-α, IL-6, and IL-1β (Andersen et al. 2013b).

Egg intake may increase inflammatory gene expression in PBMC by promoting cellular cholesterol loading, which can enhance leukocyte-mediated inflammatory responses (Surls et al. 2012). The relationship between cellular cholesterol flux and inflammatory potential may have profound effects on both atherosclerosis development and immunity (Yvan-Charvet et al. 2008; Surls et al. 2012). Evidence of egg-induced leukocyte cholesterol loading is further supported by the upregulation of ABCA1 mRNA expression in PBMC from MetS subjects (Fournier et al. 1997), which potentially serves as a mechanism to reduce cellular cholesterol content, thereby suppressing cellular inflammatory potential (Yin et al. 2010). While these findings highlight an intriguing physiological response to egg consumption, the extent by which egg intake influences leukocyte inflammation in relation to immune response and metabolic disease outcomes remains to be determined. Increased PBMC inflammatory gene expression following habitual egg intake appears to be in contrast with the documented improvements in plasma inflammation markers—suggesting the impact of eggs on whole body inflammation is complex.

18.4   EGGS AND INSULIN RESISTANCE

Numerous prospective cohort studies have found no significant association between egg consumption and risk for CVD in healthy populations (Hu et al. 1999; Nakamura et al. 2006; Qureshi et al. 2007). In contrast, some epidemiological evidence suggests that those with type 2 diabetes may not benefit from egg consumption (Djousse and Gaziano 2008). However, data regarding fasting insulin, fasting glucose, or other measurements that may explain the findings are often not available. While epidemiological studies can be informative of nutrient-disease associations, randomized controlled clinical trials must eventually be performed to confirm true cause-and-effect relationships between variables.

In clinical intervention studies, we have not noted any detrimental effects of egg intake on plasma glucose or insulin, regardless of whether acute or long-term responses are examined. Egg-based meals often result in lower postprandial glucose and insulin responses compared with other foods (Ratliff et al. 2010). Furthermore, egg protein may have unique properties, as replacement of ham protein with egg protein was shown to significantly diminish postprandial insulin response (Villaume et al. 1986).

Ratliff et al. (2010) performed an acute crossover feeding study to examine the effects of isocaloric egg- vs. bagel-based breakfasts on postprandial plasma glucose and insulin excursions. The egg breakfast consisted of 3 eggs and 1.5 pieces of white toast, while the bagel-based breakfast consisted of 1 white bagel, 1/2 tbsp. of low-fat cream cheese, and 6 oz low-fat yogurt. Participants had significantly lower area under the curve (AUC) values for plasma glucose and insulin after consuming the egg breakfast compared to the bagel-based breakfast.

Insulin resistance is a common facet of MetS and may be the underlying factor responsible for most cases (Grundy et al. 2004). We examined the effect of consuming 3 whole eggs/day versus yolk-free egg substitute for 12 weeks on fasted plasma glucose, insulin, and insulin resistance in participants with metabolic syndrome (Blesso et al. 2013a). After 12 weeks, no detrimental effects of egg yolk consumption on risk factors for type 2 diabetes were observed. In contrast, improvements in plasma insulin and insulin resistance (measured by the homeostatic model assessment, HOMA-IR) over time in participants consuming 3 whole eggs/day were seen, while this was not as apparent in participants consuming yolk-free egg substitute.

A recent study in type 2 diabetics by Pearce et al. (2011) showed that a diet, containing 2 eggs/day combined with weight loss, did not result in any difference in glycemic control compared to an egg-free isocaloric control diet. Compared to baseline, both diets significantly improved fasting blood glucose, insulin, insulin resistance determined by HOMA-IR, hemoglobin A1c, and a 2 h glucose tolerance test after 12 weeks.

Overall, there appears to be some relationship between egg consumption and diabetes based on observational studies; however, clinical trials have not demonstrated any detrimental effect of egg intake on traditional risk factors for diabetes. In fact, there appears to be improvements in glucose–insulin homeostasis in the recent clinical studies mentioned earlier. Improvements in systemic inflammation with habitual egg intake may be related to the observed effects on insulin resistance. Larger studies of longer duration are needed to clarify any relationship between egg consumption and insulin resistance.

18.5 CONCLUSIONS

A summary of the existing literature on the effects of eggs on lipoprotein metabolism, inflammation, and insulin resistance has been presented in this chapter. An overview of the effects of eggs on MetS parameters is presented in Figure 18.1. It is clear that eggs improve dyslipidemias, as has been documented by their consistent effect in raising HDL-C under different circumstances including weight loss (Mutungi et al. 2008; Blesso et al. 2013b) or weight maintenance (Herron et al. 2002, 2003; Ballesteros et al. 2004; Greene et al. 2005). Eggs also favor the formation of less atherogenic lipoproteins by inducing production of large LDL-C (Mutungi et al. 2010; Blesso et al. 2013a) and HDL-C particles (Greene et al. 2006; Blesso et al. 2013b). An increase in RCT has been shown by egg intake, which might explain the observed raises in HDL-C (Andersen et al. 2013a). Eggs also have been shown to decrease insulin resistance (Ratliff et al. 2010; Blesso et al. 2013a) and inflammatory markers (Goodrow and Nicolosi 2007; Andersen et al. 2013b; Blesso et al. 2013b), as well as improve plasma antioxidant status via highly bioavailable lutein and zeaxanthin (Chung et al. 2004; Blesso et al. 2013c). We conclude that a number of different populations varying in age (Ballesterols et al. 2004; Greene et al. 2005; Herron et al. 2006), weight status (Herron et al. 2002; Mutungi et al. 2008), or presenting increased risk for diabetes or insulin resistance (Blesso et al. 2013a) may benefit from egg consumption.

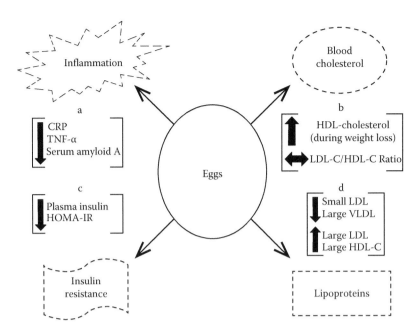

FIGURE 18.1 From clinical interventions, eggs have been shown to decrease inflammation by lowering CRP (Goodrow and Nicolosi 2007; Ratliff et al. 2008; Blesso et al. 2012b), TNF-α (Blesso et al. 2013b), and SAA (panel a); affect plasma cholesterol by increasing HDL-C during weight loss (Harman et al. 2008; Mutungi et al. 2008; Pearce et al. 2011; Blesso et al. 2013b), and maintain the LDL-C/HDL-C ratio during weight maintenance studies (Herron et al. 2002; Knopp et al. 2003; Ballesteros et al. 2004; Vishwanathan et al. 2009) (panel b); lower insulin resistance by lowering plasma insulin (Villaume et al. 1986; Ratliff et al. 2010; Blesso et al. 2013a), and HOMA-IR (Blesso et al. 2013a) (panel c); and decrease atherogenic lipoproteins in plasma by lowering small LDL-C and large VLDL (Mutungi et al. 2010; Blesso et al. 2013a) and increasing large LDL-C and large HDL-C (Mutungi et al. 2010; Blesso et al. 2013a) (panel d).

REFERENCES

Al-Sarraj, T., Saadi, H., Calle, M.C. et al. 2009. Carbohydrate restriction as a first-line dietary intervention therapy effectively reduces the biomarkers of metabolic syndrome in Emirati adults. *J Nutr* 139:1667–1676.

Andersen, C.J., Blesso, C.N., Lee, J.Y. et al. 2013a. Egg consumption modulates HDL composition and increases the cholesterol accepting capacity of serum in metabolic syndrome. *Lipids* 48:557–567.

Andersen, C.J., Blesso, C.N., Lee, J.Y. et al. 2013b. Egg intake increases peripheral blood mononuclear cell expression of ATP-binding cassette transporter A1 in parallel with toll-like receptor 4 as a potential mechanism to reduce cellular inflammation in metabolic syndrome. *FASEB* 27:846.7.

Arsenault, B.J., Lemieux, I., Despres, J.P. et al. 2010. Comparison between gradient gel electrophoresis and nuclear magnetic resonance spectroscopy in estimating coronary heart disease risk associated with LDL and HDL particle size. *Clin Chem* 56:789–798.

Ballesteros, M.N., Cabrera, R.M., Saucedo, M.S. et al. 2004. Dietary cholesterol does not increase biomarkers for chronic disease in a pediatric population from northern Mexico. *Am J Clin Nutr* 80:855–861.

Barona, J., Aristizabal, J., Blesso, C.N. et al. 2012. Grape polyphenols reduce blood pressure and increase flow-mediated vasodilation in men with metabolic syndrome. *J Nutr* 142:1626–1632.

Berglund, L., Hyson D. 2003. Cholesterol absorption and the metabolic syndrome: A new look at an old area. *Arterioscler Thromb Vasc Biol* 23:1314–1316.

Blanco-Molina, A., Castro, G., Martín-Escalante, D. et al. 1998. Effects of different dietary cholesterol concentrations on lipoprotein plasma concentrations and on cholesterol efflux from Fu5AH cells. *Am J Clin Nutr* 68:1028–1033.

Blesso, C.N., Andersen, C., Barona, J. et al. 2013a. Whole egg consumption improves lipoprotein profiles and insulin sensitivity to a greater extent than yolk-free egg substitute in individuals with metabolic syndrome. *Metabolism* 62:400–410.

Blesso, C.N., Andersen, C.J., Barona, J. et al. 2013b. Effects of carbohydrate restriction and dietary cholesterol provided by eggs on clinical risk factors in metabolic syndrome. *J Clin Lipidology* 7:463–471.

Blesso, C.N., Andersen, C., Bolling, B. et al. 2013c. Egg intake improves carotenoid status by increasing HDL-cholesterol in adults with metabolic syndrome. *Food Function* 4:213–221.

Burgess, J.W., Neville, T.A., Rouillard, P. et al. 1982. Phosphatidylinositol increases HDL-C levels in humans. *J Lipid Res* 46:350–355.

Chung, H.Y., Rasmussen, H.M., Johnson, E.J. 2004. Lutein bioavailability is higher from lutein-enriched eggs than from supplements and spinach in men. *J Nutr* 134:1887–1893.

Clarke, R., Frost, C., Collins, R. et al. 1997. Dietary lipids and blood cholesterol: Quantitative meta-analysis of metabolic ward studies. *BMJ* 314:112–117.

Clevidence, B.A., Bieri, J.G. 1993. Association of carotenoids with human plasma lipoproteins. *Methods Enzymol* 214:33–46.

Coenen, K.R., Gruen, M.L., Lee-Young, R.S. 2009. Impact of macrophage toll-like receptor 4 deficiency on macrophage infiltration into adipose tissue and the artery wall in mice. *Diabetologia* 52:318–328.

Coh, J.S., Kamili, A., Wat, E. 2010. Dietary phospholipids and intestinal cholesterol absorption. *Nutrients* 2:116–127.

Cornier, M.A., Dabela, D., Hernandez, T.L. et al. 2008. The metabolic syndrome. *Endocrine Rev* 29:777–782.

Dattilo, A.M., Kris-Etherton, P. 1992. Effects of weight reduction on blood lipids and lipoproteins: A meta-analysis. *Am J Clin Nutr* 56:320–328.

Davidson, M.H., Ballantyne, C.M., Jacobson, T.A. et al. 2011. Clinical utility of inflammatory markers and advanced lipoprotein testing: Advice from an expert panel of lipid specialists. *J Clin Lipidology* 5:338–367.

Davit-Spraul, A., Atger, V., Pourci, M.L. 1999. Cholesterol efflux from Fu5AH cells to the serum of patients with Alagille syndrome. Importance of the HDL-phospholipids/free cholesterol ratio and of the HDL size distribution. *J Lipid Res* 40:328–335.

deGoma, E.M., deGoma, R.L., Rader, D.J. 2008. Beyond high-density lipoprotein cholesterol levels evaluating high-density lipoprotein function as influenced by novel therapeutic approaches. *J Am Coll Cardiol* 51:2199–2211.

Djousse, L., Gaziano, J.M. 2008. Egg consumption in relation to cardiovascular disease and mortality: The Physicians' Health Study. *Am J Clin Nutr* 87:964–969.

Dubois, C., Armand, M., Mekki, N. 1994. Effects of increasing amounts of dietary cholesterol on postprandial lipemia and lipoproteins in human subjects. *J Lipid Res* 35:1993–2007.

El Harchaoui, K., Arsenault, B.J., Franssen, R. 2009. High-density lipoprotein particle size and concentration and coronary risk. *Ann Intern Med* 150:84–93.

Elizondo-Montemayor, L., Gutierrez, N.G., Moreno, D.M. et al. 2013. School-based individualized lifestyle interventions decreases obesity and the metabolic syndrome in Mexican children. *J Hum Nutr Diet* 26:82–89. doi 10.111/jhn.12070.

Eros, G., Ibrahim, S., Siebert, N. et al. 2009. Oral phosphatidylcholine pretreatment alleviates the signs of experimental rheumatoid arthritis. *Arthritis Res Ther* 11:R43.

Escola-Gil, J.C., Llaverias, G., Julve, J. et al. 2011. The cholesterol content of Western diets plays a major role in the paradoxical increase in high-density lipoprotein cholesterol and upregulates the macrophage reverse cholesterol transport pathway. *Arterioscler Thromb Vasc Biol* 31:2493–2499.

Fernandez, M.L. 2006. Dietary cholesterol provided by eggs and plasma lipoproteins in healthy populations. *Curr Opin Clin Nutr Metab Care* 9:8–12.

Fernandez, M.L. 2012. Rethinking dietary cholesterol. *Curr. Opin Med Nutr Metab Care* 15:17–21.

Fernandez, M.L., Webb, D. 2008. The LDL to HDL-cholesterol ratio as a valuable tool to evaluate coronary heart disease risk. The impact of dietary cholesterol. *J Am Coll Nutr* 27:1–5.

Festa, A., Williams, K., Hanley, A.J. et al. 2005. Nuclear magnetic resonance lipoprotein abnormalities in prediabetic subjects in the Insulin Resistance Atherosclerosis Study. *Circulation* 111:3465–3472.

Fournier, N., de la Llera-Moya, M., Burkey, B.F. et al. 1996. Role of HDL phospholipid in efflux of cell cholesterol to whole serum: Studies with human apoA-I transgenic rats. *J Lipid Res* 37:1704–1711.

Fournier, N., Paul, J.L., Atger, V. et al. 1997. HDL phospholipid content and composition as a major factor determining cholesterol efflux capacity from Fu5AH cells to human serum. *Arterioscler Thromb Vasc Biol* 17:2685–2691.

Freedman, D.S., Otvos, J.D., Jeyarajah, E.J. et al. 1998. Relation of lipoprotein subclasses as measured by proton nuclear magnetic resonance spectroscopy to coronary artery disease. *Arterioscler Thromb Vasc Biol* 18:1046–1053.

Ginsberg, H.N., Karmally, W., Siddiqui, M. et al. 1994. A dose-response study of the effects of dietary cholesterol on fasting and postprandial lipid and lipoprotein metabolism in healthy young men. *Arterioscler Thromb* 14:576–586.

Goodrow, E.F., Nicolosi, R. 2007. C-reactive protein (CRP) levels are not affected in participants consuming the equivalent of 2 and 4 egg yolks/day while on cholesterol-lowering medication. *FASEB* 21:847.4.

Goodrow, E.F., Wilson, T.A., Houde, S.C. et al. 2006. Consumption of one egg per day increases serum lutein and zeaxanthin concentrations in older adults without altering serum lipid and lipoprotein cholesterol concentrations. *J Nutr* 136:2519–2524.

Gordon, D.J., Probstfield, J.L., Garrison, R.J. et al. 1989. High-density lipoprotein cholesterol and cardiovascular disease. Four prospective American studies. *Circulation* 79:8–15.

Greene, C.M., Waters, D., Clark, R.M. et al. 2006. Plasma LDL and HDL characteristics and carotenoid content are positively influenced by egg consumption in an elderly population. *Nutr Met* 3:6.

Greene, C.M., Zern, T.L., Wood, R.J. et al. 2005. Maintenance of the LDL cholesterol: HDL-cholesterol ratio in an elderly population given a dietary cholesterol challenge. *J Nutr* 135:2793–2798.

Grundy, S.M., Brewer, H.B. Jr., Cleeman, J.I. et al. 2004. Definition of metabolic syndrome: Report of the National Heart, Lung, and Blood Institute/American Heart Association conference on scientific issues related to definition. *Arterioscler Thromb Vasc Biol* 24:e13–e18.

Guilherme, A., Virbasius, J.V., Puri, V. et al. 2008. Adipocyte dysfunctions linking obesity to insulin resistance and type 2 diabetes. *Nat Rev Mol Cell Biol* 9:367–377.

Harman, N.L., Leeds, A.R., Griffin, B.A. 2008. Increased dietary cholesterol does not increase plasma low density lipoprotein when accompanied by an energy-restricted diet and weight loss. *Eur J Nutr* 47:287–293.

Herron, K.L., Lofgren, I.E., Sharma, M. et al. 2004. A high intake of dietary cholesterol does not result in more atherogenic LDL particles in men and women independent of response classification. *Metab Clin Exp* 53:823–830.

Herron, K.L., McGrane, M.M., Lofgren, I.E. et al. 2006. ABCG5 polymorphism contributes to the individual response to dietary cholesterol and to carotenoids present in eggs. *J Nutr* 136:1161–1165.

Herron, K.L., Vega-Lopez, S., Conde, K. et al. 2002. Pre-menopausal women classified as hypo-or hyper-responders, do not alter their LDL/HDL ratio following a high dietary cholesterol challenge. *J Am Coll Nutr* 21:250–258.

Herron, K.L., Vega-Lopez, S., Ramjiganesh, T. et al. 2003. Men classified as hypo- or hyper-responders to dietary cholesterol feeding exhibit differences in lipoprotein metabolism. *J Nutr* 133:1036–1042.

Hodge, A.M., Jenkins, A.J., English, D.R. et al. 2009. NMR-determined lipoprotein subclass profile predicts type 2 diabetes. *Diabetes Res Clin Pract* 83:132–139.

Hu, F.B., Stampfer, M.J., Rimm, E.B. et al. 1999. A prospective study of egg consumption and risk of cardiovascular disease in men and women. *JAMA* 281:1387–1394.

Jones, J.L., Fernandez, M.L., McIntosh, M. et al. 2011. A Mediterranean-style low-glycemic-load diet improves variables of metabolic syndrome in women, and addition of a phytochemical-rich medical food enhances benefits on lipoprotein metabolism. *J Clin Lipidol* 5:188–196.

Kim, J.E., Leite, J.O., DeOgburn, R. et al. 2012. A lutein-enriched diet prevents cholesterol accumulation and decreases oxidized LDL and inflammatory cytokines in the aorta of guinea pigs. *J Nutr* 141:1458–1463.

Klemsdal, T.O., Holme, I., Nerland, H. et al. 2010. Effects of a low glycemic load diet versus a low-fat diet in subjects with and without the metabolic syndrome. *Nutr Metab Cardiovasc Dis* 20:195–201.

Knopp, R.H., Retzlaff, B., Fish, B. et al. 2003. Effects of insulin resistance and obesity on lipoproteins and sensitivity to egg feeding. *Arterioscler Thromb Vasc Biol* 23:1437–1443.

Koppes, L.L., Twisk, J.W., Van Mechelen, W. et al. 2005. Cross-sectional and longitudinal relationships between alcohol consumption and lipids, blood pressure and body weight indices. *J Stud Alcohol* 66:713–721.

Kovacs-Nolan, J., Phillips, M., Mine, Y. 2005. Advances in the value of eggs and egg components for human health. *J Agric Food Chem* 53:8421–8431.

Kritchevsky, S.B., Bush, A.J., Pahor, M. et al. 2000. Serum carotenoids and markers of inflammation in non-smokers. *Am J Epidemiol* 152:1065–1071.

Lee, M., Kovak-Nolas, J., Yang, C. 2009. Hen egg lysozyme attenuates inflammation and modulates local gene expression in a porcine model of dextran sodium sulfate (DSS)-induced colitis. *J Agric Food Chem* 57:2233–2240.

Libby, P., Geng, Y.J., Aikawa, M. et al. 1996. Macrophages and atherosclerotic plaque stability. *Curr Opin Lipidol* 7:330–335.

Linsel-Nitschke, P., Tall, A.R. 2005. HDL as a target in the treatment of atherosclerotic cardiovascular disease. Nature reviews. *Drug Discov* 4:193–205.

McNamara, D.J. 2000. The impact of egg limitations on coronary heart disease risk: Do the numbers add up? *J Am Coll Nutr* 19:540S–548S.

Mensink, R.P., Zock, P.L., Kester, A.D. et al. 2003. Effects of dietary fatty acids and carbohydrates on the ratio of serum total to HDL-cholesterol and on serum lipids and apolipoproteins: A meta-analysis of 60 controlled trials. *Am J Clin Nutr* 77:1146–1155.

Miettinen, T.A., Gylling, H. 2000. Cholesterol absorption efficiency and sterol metabolism in obesity. *Atherosclerosis* 153:241–248.

Mora, S., Otvos, J.D., Rifai, N. et al. 2009. Lipoprotein particle profiles by nuclear magnetic resonance compared with standard lipids and apolipoproteins in predicting incident cardiovascular disease in women. *Circulation* 119:931–939.

Morris, D.L., Kritchevsky, S.B., Davis, C.E. 1994. Serum carotenoids and coronary heart disease. The Lipid Research Clinics Coronary Primary Prevention Trial and Follow-up Study. *JAMA* 272:1439–1441.

Mutungi. G., Ratliff, J., Puglisi, M. et al. 2008. Dietary cholesterol from eggs increases HDL-cholesterol in overweight men consuming a carbohydrate restricted diet. *J Nutr* 138:272–276.

Mutungi, G., Waters, D., Ratliff, J. et al. 2010. Eggs distinctly modulate plasma carotenoid and lipoprotein subclasses in adult men following a carbohydrate restricted diet. *J Nutr Biochem* 21:261–267.

Nakamura, Y., Iso, H., Kita, Y. et al. 2006. Egg consumption, serum total cholesterol concentrations and coronary heart disease incidence: Japan Public Health Center-based prospective study. *Br J Nutr* 96:921–928.

O'Brien, B.C., Corrigan, S.M. 1988. Influence of dietary soybean and egg lecithins on lipid responses in cholesterol-fed guinea pigs. *Lipids* 23:647–660.

Otvos, J.D., Collins, D., Freedman, D.S. 2006. Low-density lipoprotein and high-density lipoprotein particle subclasses predict coronary events and are favorably changed by gemfibrozil therapy in the Veterans Affairs High-Density Lipoprotein Intervention Trial. *Circulation* 113:1556–1563.

Paramsothy, P., Knopp, R.H., Kahn, S.E. 2011. Plasma sterol evidence for decreased absorption and increased synthesis of cholesterol in insulin resistance and obesity. *Am J Clin Nutr* 94:1182–1188.

Pearce, K.L., Clifton, P.M., Noakes, M. 2011. Egg consumption as part of an energy-restricted high-protein diet improves blood lipid and blood glucose profiles in individuals with type 2 diabetes. *Br J Nutr* 105:584–592.

Pihlajamaki, J., Gylling, H., Miettinen, T.A. et al. 2004. Insulin resistance is associated with increased cholesterol synthesis and decreased cholesterol absorption in normoglycemic men. *J Lipid Res* 45:507–512.

Pradhan, A. 2007. Obesity, metabolic syndrome, and type 2 diabetes: Inflammatory basis of glucose metabolic disorders. *Nutr Rev* 65:S152–S156.

Qureshi, A.I., Suri, F.K., Ahmed, S. et al. 2007. Regular egg consumption does not increase the risk of stroke and cardiovascular diseases. *Med Sci Monit* 13:CR1–CR18.

Rader, D.J., Alexander, E.T., Weibel, G.L. 2009. The role of reverse cholesterol transport in animals and humans and relationship to atherosclerosis. *J Lipid Res* 50(Suppl):S189–S194.

Ratliff, J., Leite, J.O., de Ogburn, R. et al. 2010. Consuming eggs for breakfast influences plasma glucose and ghrelin, while reducing energy intake during the next 24 hours in adult men. *Nutr Res* 30:96–103.

Ratliff, J., Mutungi, G., Puglisi, M. et al. 2008. Eggs modulate the inflammatory response to carbohydrate restricted diets in overweight men. *Nutr Metab (Lond)* 5:6.

Ridker, P.M., Hennekens, C.H., Buring, J.E. et al. 2000. C-reactive protein and other markers of inflammation in the prediction of cardiovascular disease in women. *N Engl J Med* 342:836–843.

Rimm, E.B., Williams, P., Fosher, K. et al. 1999. Moderate alcohol intake and lower risk of coronary heart disease: Meta-analysis of effects on lipids and haemostatic factors. *BMJ* 1999 319:1523–1528.

Rosenson, R.S., Brewer, H.B. Jr, Davidson, W.S. et al. 2012. Cholesterol efflux and atheroprotection: Advancing the concept of reverse cholesterol transport. *Circulation* 125:1905–1919.

Rousset, X., Shamburek, R., Vaisman, B. et al. 2011. Lecithin cholesterol acyltransferase: An anti- or pro-atherogenic factor? *Curr Atheroscler Rep* 13:249–256.

Schwartz, C.C., VandenBroek, J.M., Cooper, P.S. 2004. Lipoprotein cholesteryl ester production, transfer, and output in vivo in humans. *J Lipid Res* 45:1594–1607.

Shardell, M.D., Alley, D.E., Hicks, G.E. et al. 2011. Low-serum carotenoid concentrations and carotenoid interactions predict mortality in US adults: The Third National Health and Nutrition Examination Survey. *Nutr Res* 31:178–189.

Sies, H., Stahl, W. 1995. Vitamins E and C, beta-carotene, and other carotenoids as antioxidants. *Am J Clin Nutr* 62(6 Suppl):1315S–1321S.

Simonen, P., Gylling, H., Howard, A.N. et al. 2000. Introducing a new component of the metabolic syndrome: Low cholesterol absorption. *Am J Clin Nutr* 72:82–88.

Subramanian, S., Chait, A. 2009. The effect of dietary cholesterol on macrophage accumulation in adipose tissue: Implications for systemic inflammation and atherosclerosis. *Curr Opin Lipidol* 20:39–44.

Surls, J., Nazarov-Stoica, C., Kehl, M. et al. 2012. Increased membrane cholesterol in lymphocytes diverts T-cells toward an inflammatory response. *PLoS One* 7:e38733.

Suzuki, K., Ito, Y., Inoue, Y. et al. 2011. Inverse association of serum carotenoids with prevalence of metabolic syndrome among Japanese. *Clin Nutr* 30:369–375.

Tang, W.H., Wang, Z., Leison, F.S. 2013. Intestinal microbial metabolism of phosphatidylcholine and cardiovascular risk. *N Engl J Med* 368:1575–1584.

Tanigawa, H., Billheimer, J.T., Tohyama, J. et al. 2007. Expression of cholesteryl ester transfer protein in mice promotes macrophage reverse cholesterol transport. *Circulation* 116:1267–1273.

Tannock, L.R., O'Brien, K.D., Knopp, R.H. et al. 2005. Cholesterol feeding increases C-reactive protein and serum amyloid A levels in lean insulin-sensitive subjects. *Circulation* 111:3058–3062.

Tchoua, U., Gillard, B.K., Pownall, H.J. 2010. HDL superphospholipidation enhances key steps in reverse cholesterol transport. *Atherosclerosis* 209:430–435.

Temel, R.E., Brown, J. M. 2012. Biliary and nonbiliary contributions to reverse cholesterol transport. *Curr Opin Lipidol* 230:85–90.

Tokes, T., Eros, G., Bebes, A. et al. 2011. Protective effects of a phosphatidylcholine-enriched diet in lipopolysaccharide-induced experimental neuroinflammation in the rat. *Shock* 36:458–465.

Toniolo, P., Van Kappel, A.L., Akhmedkhanov, A. et al. 2001. Serum carotenoids and breast cancer. *Am J Epidemiol* 153:1142–1147.

Treede, I., Braun, A., Jeliaskova, P. et al. 2009. TNF-alpha-induced up-regulation of pro-inflammatory cytokines is reduced by phosphatidylcholine in intestinal epithelial cells. *BMC Gastroenterol* 9:53.

Villaume, C., Beck, B., Rohr, R. et al. 1986. Effect of exchange of ham for boiled egg on plasma glucose and insulin responses to breakfast in normal subjects. *Diabetes Care* 9:46–49.

Vishwanathan, R., Goodrow-Kotyla, E.F., Wooten, B.R. et al. 2009. Consumption of 2 and 4 egg yolks/d for 5 wk increases macular pigment concentrations in older adults with low macular pigment taking cholesterol-lowering statins. *Am J Clin Nutr* 90:1272–1279.

von Eckardstein, A., Nofer, J.R., Assmann, G. et al. 2001. High density lipoproteins and arteriosclerosis. Role of cholesterol efflux and reverse cholesterol transport. *Arterioscler Thromb Vasc Biol* 21:13–27.

Weihrauch, J., Son, Y.-S. 1983. The phospholipid content of foods. *J Am Oil Chem Soc* 60:1971–1978.

Weissglas-Volkov, D., Pajukanta, P. 2010. Genetic causes of high and low serum HDL-cholesterol. *J Lipid Res* 51:2032–2057.

Wiecek, A., Adamczak, M., Chudek, A. 2007. Adiponectin—An adipokine with unique metabolic properties. *Nephrol Dial Transplant* 22:981–988.

Yancey, P.G., de la Llera-Moya, M., Swarnakar, S. et al. 2000. High density lipoprotein phospholipid composition is a major determinant of the bi-directional flux and net movement of cellular free cholesterol mediated by scavenger receptor BI. *J Biol Chem* 275:36596–36604.

Yang, F., Ma, M., Xu, J. et al. 2012. An egg-enriched diet attenuates plasma lipids and mediates cholesterol metabolism of high-cholesterol fed rats. *Lipids* 47:269–277.

Yin, K., Liao, D.F. Tang, C.K. 2010. ATP-binding membrane cassette transporter A1 (ABCA1): A possible link between inflammation and reverse cholesterol transport. *Mol Med* 16:438–449.

Yvan-Charvet, L., Welch, C., Pagler, T.A. et al. 2008. Increased inflammatory gene expression in ABC transporter-deficient macrophages: Free cholesterol accumulation, increased signaling via toll-like receptors, and neutrophil infiltration of atherosclerotic lesions. *Circulation* 118:1837–1847.

Zierenberg, O., Grundy, S.M. 1985. Intestinal absorption of polyenephosphatidylcholine in man. *J Lipid Res* 23:1136–1142.

19 Milk, Dairy Products, and Metabolic Syndrome

Bruna Miglioranza Scavuzzi, Fabiola Malaga Barreto, and Lucia Helena da Silva Miglioranza

CONTENTS

19.1 INTRODUCTION

Dietary guidelines recommend the intake of dairy products as part of a healthy diet. The recommendation is usually two or three servings of these products daily within a balanced diet (WHO European Region CINDI Dietary Guide 2000; Dietary Guidelines for Americans 2010). Dairy consumption is associated with a reduced risk of low bone mass, stroke, and some cancers (Weaver 2010; Dougkas et al. 2011; Da Silva et al. 2014). Nonetheless, the health effects of dairy are still controversial (Melnik 2009; Beavers et al. 2010).

Milk products are an important source of calcium, vitamin D, magnesium, phosphorus, potassium, riboflavin, protein, and carbohydrates. Obtaining adequate intakes of calcium, potassium, and magnesium, without milk in the diet, requires effort (Weaver 2010).

Milk also contains nutrients such as fatty acids and a vast number of bioactive components that have a beneficial effect on human health. These components may play an important role in the metabolic health and are known to have an effect on the satiety response, regulation of insulinemia levels and blood pressure, uptake of free radicals, and alteration of the lipid profile (Korhonen and Pihlanto 2007; Pfeuffer and Schrezenmeir 2007; van Meijl et al. 2008; Dougkas et al. 2011; Ricci-Cabello et al. 2012).

According to observational and interventional studies, consumption of milk and dairy products may be associated with a decrease of the metabolic syndrome (MetS) by affecting one or several risk factors. The effects of dairy intake on the components of MetS may be influenced by age, gender, ethnicity, degree of obesity, and type of dairy product (Scholz-Ahrens and Schrezenmeir 2006; Abreu et al. 2012; Da Silva et al. 2014).

As aforementioned, the type of dairy product may also exert distinct effects on the MetS components. Abreu et al. (2012) observed that only milk intake produced an inverse relationship with cardiometabolic risk factors in Portuguese adolescents. The authors did not find an association between total dairy, yogurt and cheese consumption and cardiometabolic risk factors within the studied group.

Also regarding the different types of dairy products, fat in milk, butter, and cheese reportedly affect blood lipids differently due to matrix effects. Van Meijl and Mensink (2010) and Tholstrup et al. (2004) could not confirm different effects of fat in milk and butter, but found a moderately lower LDL-cholesterol concentration after a cheese diet compared with a butter diet.

Gagliardi et al. (2010) compared effects of margarines and butter consumption on lipid profiles in subjects with MetS and did not find differences among individuals of both groups. They investigated plasma lipids, apolipoproteins, and inflammatory and endothelial dysfunction markers (CRP, IL-6, CD40L, or E-selectin), small dense LDL-cholesterol concentrations and in vitro radioactive lipid transfer from cholesterol-rich emulsions to HDL. The evaluation consisted of 53 MetS subjects, average age of 54, during 5 weeks receiving isocaloric servings of butter, no-trans-fat margarine or plant sterol margarine.

The purported physiological and molecular mechanisms underlying the impact of dairy constituents on the different risk factors of MetS are not completely understood, but reportedly include increased lipolysis, reduced lipogenesis, reduced fatty acid absorption, and augmented satiety. A high intake of dairy protein reduces spontaneous food intake and may be one important mechanism that leads to the lower rates of obesity (Astrup et al. 2010).

Crichton et al. (2011) performed a systematic search for studies that assessed dairy intake in relation to MetS. According to the collected data, dairy intake was inversely associated with incidence or prevalence of MetS in 7 out of 13 published cross-sectional (10) and cohort (3) studies. Three studies found no association between dairy and MetS. Three studies reported mixed relationships between specific dairy foods and MetS.

Da Silva et al. (2014) reviewed 26 studies associating dairy product intake and their effect on the risk factors of the MetS. According to the authors, 15 of the studies showed a beneficial effect on at least one of the five MetS risk factors, 10 studies showed no effect and there was only one negative effect report related to the lipid profile.

Thus, this chapter gathers recent and relevant literature found in at least 130 databases included in the virtual library *Portal CAPES Consortia* (Higher Education Personnel Improvement Coordination-Brazil) published from 1990 to 2013, involving the consumption of milk and dairy products and the prevalence or incidence of metabolic syndrome. The selection strategy consisted of three search words: *milk*, *dairy products*, and *metabolic syndrome*. There were no restriction groups, but searches have focused on texts written in English.

19.2   MILK, DAIRY, AND METABOLIC SYNDROME

Patients are mostly classified as having MetS according to three or more of the following Adult Treatment Panel (ATP) III criteria (1) waist circumference 102 cm in men and 88 cm in women; (2) triglycerides ≥ 1.7 mmol/L; (3) HDL-cholesterol < 1.0 mmol/L (men) or <1.3 mmol/L (women); (4) blood pressure ≥ 130/85 mmHg or antihypertensive medication use, and (5) glucose ≥ 5.6 mmol/L or antidiabetes medication use (or physician diagnosis for Atherosclerosis Risk in Communities, [ARIC]). According to International Diabetes Federation (IDF) definition, abdominal adiposity (waist circumference ≥ 94 cm [men] or ≥80 cm [women]), and two or more risk factors cited from numbers 2 to 5 are used (Wildman et al. 2011).

An important study among current investigations, the Coronary Artery Risk Development in Young Adults (CARDIA) study, examined associations between dairy intake and incidence of MetS in white and African American adults during a 10-year follow-up trial. Pereira et al. (2002) found an inverse association of dairy consumption with obesity, abnormal glucose homeostasis, elevated blood pressure, and dyslipidemia in overweight individuals and a significantly lower incidence of MetS within overweight subjects with higher dairy consumption. The associations were comparable between genders and ethnicities.

Since most studies evaluate the association of dairy with only certain components of the MetS, this chapter is divided into the different risk factors for better comprehension.

19.3 MILK OR DAIRY PRODUCTS, AND OBESITY

Observational studies mainly from Western populations suggest that dairy product consumption is inversely associated with adiposity. In a non-Western setting, milk and other dairy product consumption was not associated with adiposity, suggesting that any observed antiobesogenic effects in Western settings may be due to socially pattern confounding by socioeconomic position (Lin et al. 2012). In the Hong Kong study, only 65.7% regularly consumed milk and 72.4% other dairy products. Milk and other dairy product consumption was positively associated with socioeconomic position but not with body mass index (BMI), z-score, or (waist–hip ratio) WHR with or without adjustment for sex, mother's birthplace, parental education, and physical activity and other food consumption (Table 19.1).

Thereby, what does the current literature demonstrate about the impact of dairy on human obesity?

Skinner et al. (2003) proposed the incorporation of low-fat calcium rich foods such as skim milk and yogurt in the diets of children. This incorporation aimed to reduce body fat gain given the associations between body fat and calcium intake and polyunsaturated fatty acid intake. They found that calcium intake is negatively related to children's body fat indexes.

Zemel et al. (2004) demonstrated that increased calcitriol produced in response to low-calcium diets stimulates adipocyte Ca^{2+} influx and, consequently, promotes adiposity. Therefore, suppressing calcitriol levels by increasing dietary calcium could be an attractive target for obesity intervention.

Besides calcium, trace elements and minerals may also influence the pathogenesis of obesity, mainly through their involvement in peroxidation and inflammation (Bouglé et al. 2009).

Apart from all the discussion about the impact of dairy products consumption and the current obesity crisis in many populations, particularly among children and adolescents, some studies point to other dietary changes that are relevant. Between 1965 and 1996, milk intake decreased by 36%, while the percentage of the consumption of soft drinks and noncitrus juices dramatically increased (Cavadini et al. 2000). Regular sugar-sweetened beverage consumption, between meals, may put some young children at a greater risk for overweight (Dubois et al. 2007). Furthermore, population groups in North America who have preserved traditional lifestyles with substantial embedded physical activity have reduced the prevalence of obesity (Bassett 2008).

19.4 MILK OR DAIRY PRODUCTS AND INFLAMMATORY AND OXIDATIVE STRESS MARKERS

Free radicals and reactive metabolites, also known as reactive oxygen species (ROS), are products of normal cell metabolism and are generated mainly by the mitochondrial respiratory chain. When there is an imbalance between the production of these reactive species and their elimination by antioxidant mechanisms, an excessive accumulation of ROS occurs, leading to oxidative stress. Chronic inflammation may be a result of continued oxidative stress (Reuter et al. 2010).

Scientists consider low-grade systemic inflammation as a key etiologic factor in the development and progression of MetS (MetS) and cardiovascular diseases (Labonté et al. 2013). Elevated plasma concentrations of C-reactive protein (CRP) and of the proinflammatory cytokines TNF-α and IL-6 can be associated with an increased risk of cardiovascular disease (Koenig et al. 1999; Ridker et al. 2002; Ballantyne et al. 2004).

The crossover study of Zemel et al. (2010) compared dairy- with soy-supplemented eucaloric diets. They demonstrated that the dairy-supplemented diet resulted in significant suppression of oxidative stress, lower inflammatory markers, and increase in the anti-inflammatory adipokine adiponectin, whereas the soy exerted no significant effect. They concluded that an increase in dairy food intake produces significant and substantial suppression of the oxidative and inflammatory stress associated with overweight and obesity.

TABLE 19.1
Human Studies Considering Milk or Dairy Products and Obesity

Authors	Study	Population	Conclusion
Rosell et al. (2004)	A cross-sectional study to evaluate the association between abdominal obesity (AD) and the intake of dairy fat and calcium using information from dietary data and the relative contents of the fatty acids 14:0, 15:0, and 17:0 in serum phospholipids (PLs) and adipose tissue (AT), which are suggested biological markers for dairy fat intake.	301 healthy 63-year-old men, born in Sweden, with a body mass index BMI ≥ 20 and ≥ 35 and between March 2000 and October 2001.	The data gave some indications of an inverse association between SAD[a] and the intake of calcium. However, if there is a true inverse association between the intake of dairy fat and SAD, it remains to explain why this association was not seen in the non-URs[b].
Loos et al. (2004)	The authors used cross-sectional data from the men and women who participated in the HERITAGE Family Study.	362 men (109 blacks and 253 whites) and 462 women (201 blacks and 261 whites) aged 17–65.	Calcium intake was inversely associated with measures of adiposity in black men and white women.
Azadbakht et al. (2005a)	A cross-sectional study to evaluate the relationship between dairy consumption and metabolic syndrome in Tehranian adults.	827 subjects (357 men and 470 women) aged 18–74 years.	The subjects who consumed more dairy products had a lower BMI and lower odds of having enlarged waist circumference.
Dixon et al. (2005)	A cross-sectional study to evaluate the association between calcium and dairy intake and measures of obesity in hyper- and normocholesterolemic children using information from dietary data regarding relative weight and adiposity.	342 nonobese children aged 4 to 10 years.	Calcium intake was inversely associated with measures of obesity in 7- to 10-year-old non-HC children, but not with HC children or in the 4- to 6-year-old non-HC children.
Snijder et al. (2008)	The authors used cross-sectional data from the men and women who participated in the Hoorn Study.	1896 subjects (852 men and 1044 women) aged 50–75 years.	Dairy consumption was not associated with lower weight values.
St-Onge et al. (2009)	A randomized trial to compare weight loss and improvements in metabolic risk factors between groups of high and low dairy consumption during a 16-week healthy eating diet.	45 overweight children (9 boys/36 girls) aged 8–10 years.	The group with high-milk consumption (4 servings/day) in conjunction with a healthy diet did not have a greater weight loss.
Kwon et al. (2010)	The authors used cross-sectional data from men and women who participated in the KNHANES III.[c]	4890 Korean subjects (2052 men and 2838 women).	Dairy consumption was not associated with lower weight values. However, the study suggests that increased frequency of milk intake had an inverse relationship with MS among overweight adults.

(Continued)

TABLE 19.1 (*Continued*)
Human Studies Considering Milk or Dairy Products and Obesity

Authors	Study	Population	Conclusion
Lin et al. (2011)	Multivariable linear regression to examine the association of the frequency of milk or other dairy product consumption with clinically measured BMI z-scores at about 13 years.	Large (n = 7488), population-representative Chinese birth cohort/88% of all births in Hong Kong (April/May, 1997).	In a non-Western setting, milk and other dairy product consumption was not associated with adiposity.
Stancliffe et al. (2011)	Randomized parallel-group design to determine the early (7 days) and sustained (4 and 12 weeks) effects of adequate-dairy compared with low-dairy diets.	40 overweight or obese subjects with MetS (19 men and 21 women) 18–74 years.	The group with adequate dairy intake presented significant reduction of waist circumference and trunk fat.
Abreu, et al. (2012)	A cross-sectional analysis for assessment of the association between dairy products intake and AO among Azorean adolescents.	903 adolescents (370 boys) aged 15–16 years.	The authors found a protective association between dairy products intake and AO only in boys.
Holmberg and Thelin (2013)	A male cohort study with two surveys 12 years apart to examine associations between dairy fat intake and development of central obesity.	1589 men (farmers and nonfarmers) aged 40–60 years, from nine municipalities selected from different parts of Sweden representing the rural areas in the country.	A high intake of dairy fat was associated with a lower risk of central obesity, and a low dairy fat intake was associated with a higher risk of central obesity.
Jones et al. (2013)	Randomized design to determine if a dietary pattern high in dairy and calcium improves weight loss and subjective appetite to a greater extent than a low-dairy and low-calcium diet during energy restriction.	Overweight and obese subjects with MetS (aged 20–60 years).	A dairy and calcium-rich diet was not associated with greater weight loss than control.
Barreto et al. (2014)	A 90-day randomized trial to evaluate the influence of *L. plantarum* fermented milk on the parameters of MetS and cardiovascular risks.	24 postmenopausal women with mean age of 63 years.	Fermented and nonfermented milk consumption was not associated with lower weight values.

[a] SAD, sagittal abdominal obesity.
[b] Non-URs: Underreporters (URs) and the validation of the food record were identified according to the Goldberg cutoff, which compares the reported energy intake (EI) with the energy expenditure (EE), both expressed as multiples of the basal metabolic rate (BMR).
[c] KNHANES III: Third Korea National Health and Nutrition Examination Survey.

On the other hand, Nestel et al. (2012) investigated the hypothesis that full-fat dairy foods could influence circulating inflammatory and atherogenic biomarkers according to fermentation status. They concluded that single high-fat meals containing sequentially four different full-fat dairy foods did not increase eight circulating biomarkers related to inflammation or atherogenesis. The biomarkers investigated were interleukin (IL)-6, IL-1 [beta], tumor necrosis factor alpha, high-sensitive C-reactive protein, and the atherogenesis-related markers monocyte chemo attractant protein-1, macrophage inflammatory protein-1[alpha], intercellular adhesion molecule-1, and vascular cell adhesion molecule-1 (Table 19.2).

19.5 MILK, DAIRY PRODUCTS, AND GLUCOSE HOMEOSTASIS

Pereira et al. (2002) reported abnormal glucose homeostasis as a fasting plasma insulin and glucose of at least 20 µU/mL and 110 mg/dL, respectively, or the use of medications to control blood glucose. Matthews et al. (1985) described a mathematical relation (homeostasis model assessment, HOMA-IR) between fasting plasma glucose and insulin to predict insulin resistance. Lower HOMA-IR values represent higher insulin sensitivity and higher values correspond to lower insulin sensitivity; the later finding is known as insulin resistance (IR). IR and hyperinsulinemia contribute to the pathogenesis of diabetes (Reaven 1988; Di Filippo et al. 2007).

Akter et al. (2013) investigated the hypothesis that dairy intake was inversely associated with insulin resistance (IR). The insulin resistance markers tested were fasting serum insulin, fasting plasma glucose, and the homeostatic model assessment of IR (HOMA-IR). The authors found that the full-fat dairy products were inversely associated with fasting plasma insulin and HOMA-IR. Furthermore, subjects who consumed dairy, at least once per day, had significantly lower mean values for fasting insulin and HOMA-IR than those who consumed dairy in smaller frequencies. However, the authors found that full-fat dairy and low-fat dairy consumption were not significantly associated with any IR markers.

Although the mechanisms underlying the effects of dairy on insulin resistance and type 2 diabetes (T2D) are not completely understood, there is evidence that specific milk components, such as calcium and magnesium, are involved in those mechanisms.

To evaluate the role of calcium in the mechanism of insulin resistance, Liu et al. (2005) examined the associations between intake of dairy foods, calcium supplementation, and the incidence of the metabolic syndrome. The authors found an inverse association between calcium and dairy intake and insulin sensitivity.

Ma et al. (2006) investigated the association of dairy, magnesium, and calcium intake with insulin sensitivity during a 5-year follow-up examination program in 1036 nondiabetics patients. The authors suggested that magnesium and calcium intake specifically, but not dairy intake, were associated with insulin sensitivity.

Although type 2 diabetes is a complication and not a risk factor for MetS, studies regarding the relationship between dairy intake and T2D were included in the summary table, since abnormal glucose homeostasis is a major risk factor for T2D (Table 19.3).

19.6 MILK, DAIRY PRODUCTS, AND HYPERTENSION

McGrane et al. (2011) conducted a systematic review on 13 studies published from July 2009 and December 2010, associating dairy consumption, blood pressure, and hypertension. The literature consulted included nine randomized controlled trials, and three prospective cohort studies (Table 19.4). The authors concluded that there was evidence that dairy intake could improve blood pressure and decrease hypertension risk.

Wang et al. (2008) studied the relation between dairy intake, calcium, vitamin D, and hypertension in middle-aged and older women. The prospective cohort studied 28,886 American women

TABLE 19.2

Human Studies Considering Milk or Dairy Products and Inflammatory and Oxidative Stress Markers

Authors	Study	Population	Conclusion
Wennersberg et al. (2009)	Randomized, parallel-group intervention study (6 months).	121 middle-aged (30–65 years) overweight subjects (80 women and 41 men) with at least two traits of MetS.	There were no significant differences in markers of inflammation, adiponectin, or oxidative stress in the milk and the control groups.
Sofi et al. (2010)	A 10-week crossover design study to evaluate the effects of Pecorino cheese (naturally rich in *cis*-9, *trans*-11 conjugated linoleic acid) on inflammatory, lipid, and hemorheological variables.	Ten subjects with an average age of 51.5 (4 men and 6 women). Exclusion criteria were previous vascular and inflammatory diseases.	There was a significant reduction in inflammatory parameters such as interleukin-6, interleukin-8, and tumor necrosis factor-α.
van Meijl et al. (2010)	A crossover design to study the effects of low-fat dairy consumption on inflammatory markers and adhesion molecules.	35 overweight or obese healthy subjects (10 men and 25 women) 18–70 years.	The authors found no effects on the markers of chronic inflammation.
Pal et al. (2010)	A 12-week randomized, single-blind, parallel design to evaluate the chronic effects of whey proteins on blood pressure, vascular function, and inflammatory markers.	70 overweight and obese subjects (10 men and 60 women) aged 18–65.	No significant changes in inflammatory markers.
Stancliffe et al. (2011)	Randomized parallel-group design to determine the early (7 days) and sustained (4 and 12 weeks) effects of adequate-dairy compared with low-dairy diets.	40 overweight or obese subjects with MetS (19 men and 21 women) 18–74 years.	The group with adequate dairy intake presented suppression of inflammatory markers: decreases in tumor necrosis factor-α, interleukin-6, and monocyte chemoattractant protein-1 and an increase in adiponectin.
Sofi et al. (2011)	Cross-sectional analyses to determine if overweight status modified the associations between dairy fatty acids (pentadecanoic acid ([15:0]) and heptadecanoic acid ([17:0])) represented in serum PLs and markers of inflammation and oxidative stress.	305 adolescents (mean age: 15 years) with normal weight (n = 192) and overweight (n = 113).	PL dairy fatty acids were inversely associated with three inflammatory and oxidative stress markers[a] in overweight, but not in normal weight adolescents. Higher level of PL dairy fatty acids was associated with lower IL-6 among all adolescents.
Crichton et al. (2012)	A 12-month crossover trial to evaluate the relation of dairy consumption and cardiometabolic health.	36 overweight subjects aged 18–71 years. The exclusion criteria were as follows: subjects weighing more than 135 kg, current smokers, pregnant women, individuals diagnosed with diabetes, CVD, liver disease, renal disease, or stage 2 hypertension (>160/100 mmHg).	There were no significant changes in high sensitivity C-reactive protein.

(Continued)

TABLE 19.2 (*Continued*)

Human Studies Considering Milk or Dairy Products and Inflammatory and Oxidative Stress Markers

Authors	Study	Population	Conclusion
Labonté et al. (2013)	Eight trials comprising controlled nutritional intervention assessing the impact of dairy product consumption (i.e., milk, yogurt, and/or cheese) on biomarkers of inflammation (limited to randomized controlled trials in humans, PubMed, April 2012).	Overweight and obese subjects (aged ≥ 18 years).	Dairy product consumption does not exert adverse effects on biomarkers of inflammation.
Barreto et al. (2014)	A 90-day randomized trial to evaluate the influence of *L. plantarum* fermented milk on the parameters of MetS and cardiovascular risks.	24 postmenopausal women with a mean age of 63 years.	Significant reduction in IL-6 in fermented and nonfermented milk groups.

[a] C-reactive protein, 15-keto-dihydro-PGF2α and 8-iso-PGF2α.

during a 10-year follow-up program. The authors concluded that low-fat dairy products, calcium, and vitamin D were inversely associated with risk of hypertension in women over the age of 45.

The inverse relation between milk and blood pressure is attributed to several micronutrients. Milk-derived peptides can reportedly cause a significant reduction in hypertension through an inhibitory effect on angiotensin I-converting enzyme. There is also evidence that other dairy nutrients, such as calcium, vitamin D, and magnesium, have an effect on blood pressure reduction (Ascherio et al. 1996; Takano 1998; FitzGerald and Meisel 2000; Liu et al. 2006; Wang et al. 2008; Xu et al. 2008) (Table 19.4).

19.7 MILK, DAIRY PRODUCTS, AND PLASMA LIPID PROFILE

One of the recommendations for healthy diets is to replace high-fat dairy with low-fat dairy (U.S. Department of Agriculture and US Department of Health and Human Services 2010). However, a literature review by German and colleagues (2009) indicated that the influence of dairy products, such as cheese and yogurt, is not consistently related to increases in LDL-cholesterol; and dairy protein could have a protective effect on risk of cardiovascular disease (Kubena 2011).

Although high intakes of saturated fat have been associated with cardiovascular diseases, and milk fat is rich in saturated fat, especially in myristic (14:0), palmitic (16:0), and stearic (18:0) acids, some reports have not confirmed such association; for instance, Warensjö et al. (2010) investigated the association between the serum milk fat biomarkers pentadecanoic acid (15:0), heptadecanoic acid (17:0), or their sum (15:0+17:0) and a first myocardial infarction (MI). They concluded that milk fat biomarkers were associated with a lower risk of developing a first MI, especially in women, and this was partly confirmed in analysis of fermented milk and cheese intake.

The possibility raised in the previously mentioned studies must have led Lorenzen and Astrup (2011) to investigate if the calcium (Ca) content of dairy products influences the effect of dairy fat on the lipid profile. They observed, in a randomized cross-over design study, that dairy Ca seems to partly counteract the raising effect of dairy fat on total and LDL-cholesterol, without reducing HDL-cholesterol. However, the results from intervention studies examining the effect of Ca (dairy or supplementary) on the lipid profile were inconsistent (Denke et al. 1993; Karanja et al. 1994; Shahkhalili et al. 2001; Reid 2004; Zemel et al. 2004; Thompson et al. 2005) (Table 19.5).

TABLE 19.3

Human Studies Considering Milk or Dairy Products and Glucose Homeostasis

Authors	Study	Population	Conclusion
Choi et al. (2005)	A 12-year follow-up study to examine the relation between dairy intake and incident cases of T2D.	41,254 men (40–75 years) with no history of diabetes, cardiovascular disease, and cancer at baseline.	Each serving-per-day increase in dairy intake was associated with a 9% lower risk of T2D. The significant inverse association was primarily limited to low-fat dairy consumption.
Liu et al. (2006)	A 10-year prospective study of the WHS[a] to examine the associations between intake of dairy foods and calcium and incidence of T2D in women.	37,183 women with no history of diabetes, cardiovascular disease, and cancer at baseline.	Each serving-per-day increase in dairy intake was associated with a 4% lower risk of developing T2D. The inverse relation of dairy to T2D was mainly attributed to low-fat dairy intake.
Drouillet et al. (2007)	A 9-year follow-up study from DESIR[b] to investigate the relationship between the intake of dietary calcium and parameters of the insulin resistance syndrome.	4,372 adults (2,235 men and 2,137 women) aged from 30 to 65 years, with no baseline diabetes or taking medications with a source of calcium.	A beneficial association between dietary calcium and insulin levels was observed only in women.
St-Onge et al. (2009)	A randomized trial to compare weight loss and improvements in metabolic risk factors between groups of high and low dairy consumption during a 16-week healthy eating diet.	45 overweight children (9 boys/36 girls) aged 8–10 years.	The group with high-milk consumption (4 servings/day) in conjunction with a healthy diet had ameliorated insulin action when compared with the group of low-milk consumption.
Malik et al. (2011)	A study of the NHS II[c] to evaluate the relation between dairy consumption during adolescence and risk of T2D in adulthood.	37,038 women completed a questionnaire about their diet during high school (HS-FFQ) at age 34–53. The women were followed from the time of return of the questionnaire (1998) until 2005.	The authors suggested that higher dairy product intake during adolescence may be associated with a lower risk of developing T2D in adulthood.

(Continued)

TABLE 19.3 (Continued)
Human Studies Considering Milk or Dairy Products and Glucose Homeostasis

Authors	Study	Population	Conclusion
Louie et al. (2013)	A 10-year Blue Mountains Eye Study[d] to investigate if regular dairy consumption is protective against MetS and T2D.	1,824 subjects (age over 49 years).	There was no association between regular fat dairy consumption and the incidence of T2D.
Crichton et al. (2012)	A 12-month crossover trial to evaluate the relation of dairy consumption and cardiometabolic health.	36 overweight subjects aged from 18 to 71 years.	There were no significant changes in fasting blood glucose.
Rideout et al. (2013)	A randomized crossover trial to evaluate the influence of 6 months of dairy consumption on metabolic parameters.	23 healthy subjects (age 18–75 years) without dietary energy restriction.	There was a beneficial association between high dairy intake (four servings per day) and plasma insulin and insulin resistance.
Struijk et al. (2013)	A 5-year study from Inter99[e] to investigate the relationship between the intake of dairy, measures of glucose metabolism, and the risk of developing T2D.	5,953 adults (30–60 years) with no baseline diabetes or cardiovascular diseases.	There was no significant association between total dairy intake and T2D incidence. However, the authors found a small inverse association between cheese and fermented dairy and measures of glycemia.
Akter et al. (2013)	A cross-sectional study to investigate if higher dairy consumption was associated with lower insulin resistance.	469 subjects (286 men/210 women) aged from 20 to 68 years with no history of diabetes, cardiovascular diseases, or cancer.	The results suggested that intake of full-fat dairy products could be associated with lower IR among Japanese adults.
Barreto et al. (2014)	A 90-day randomized trial to evaluate the influence of *L. plantarum* fermented milk on the parameters of MetS and cardiovascular risks.	24 postmenopausal women with mean age of 63 years.	Significant reduction in glucose levels in the fermented milk group.

[a] WHS, Women's Health Study: A randomized, double-blind, placebo-controlled trial to test the efficacy of low-dose aspirin and vitamin E in the primary prevention of cardiovascular disease and cancer among female health professionals.

[b] DESIR: Data from the Epidemiological Study on the Insulin Resistance Syndrome, a cohort study.

[c] NHS II: Nurses' Health Study II is a prospective cohort of 116,671 female registered nurses aged 24–42 years at study initiation in 1989.

[d] Blue Mountains Eye Study: A population-based cohort study of common eye diseases and other health conditions in residents of the Blue Mountains area.

[e] Inter99: It is a Danish population–based life style intervention study to evaluate the effect of lifestyle intervention on the incidence of ischaemic heart disease.

TABLE 19.4

Human Studies Considering Milk or Dairy Products and Hypertension

Authors	Study	Population	Conclusion
Azadbakht et al. (2005b)	A randomized controlled trial to determine the effects of the DASH[a] eating plan on metabolic risks in patients with MetS.	116 subjects (34 men and 82 women) with the MetS.	The DASH diet resulted in lower systolic blood pressure and diastolic blood pressure.
Liu et al. (2006)	A 10-year prospective study of the WHS[b]	37,183 women with no history of diabetes, cardiovascular disease, and cancer at baseline.	There was an inverse association between calcium intake and blood pressure.
Drouillet et al. (2007)	A 9-year follow-up study from DESIR[c].	4,372 adults (2,235 men/2,137 women) aged from 30 to 65 years, with no baseline diabetes or taking medications with a source of calcium.	Mean systolic and diastolic blood pressures decreased in women. Only mean diastolic blood pressure decreased in men.
Snijder et al. (2008)	A cross-sectional data from men and women who participated in the Hoorn Study.	1,896 subjects (852 men/1,044 women) aged from 50 to 75 years.	A higher dairy consumption was associated with lower blood pressure.
Engberink et al. (2009)	A 6-years of follow-up from the Rotterdam Study[d] to verify if the incidence of hypertension was associated with intake of dairy products.	2,245 Dutch subjects over 55 years.	Intake of low-fat dairy products may contribute to the prevention of hypertension at an older age.
Pal et al. (2010)	A 12-week randomized, single-blind, parallel design to evaluate the chronic effects of whey proteins on blood pressure, vascular function, and inflammatory markers.	70 overweight and obese subjects (10 men/60 women) aged from 18 to 65.	Systolic and diastolic blood pressure decreased significantly.
van Meijl et al. (2010)	A crossover design to study the effects of low-fat dairy consumption on inflammatory markers and adhesion molecules.	35 overweight or obese healthy subjects (10 men/25 women) 18–70 years.	There was a reduction in systolic blood pressure.

(Continued)

TABLE 19.4 (*Continued*)
Human Studies Considering Milk or Dairy Products and Hypertension

Authors	Study	Population	Conclusion
Ivey et al. (2011)	3-year prospective, randomized, controlled trial to investigate the association between yogurt, milk, and cheese consumption and common carotid artery intima–media thickness and cardiovascular disease risk factors.	1,080 white women over 70 years.	There were no significant changes in blood pressure.
Crichton et al. (2012)	A 12-month crossover trial to evaluate the relation of dairy consumption and cardiometabolic health.	36 overweight subjects aged from 18 to 71 years.	There were no significant changes in systolic and diastolic blood pressures.
Barreto et al. (2014)	A 90-day randomized trial to evaluate the influence of *L. plantarum* fermented milk on the parameters of MetS and cardiovascular risks.	24 postmenopausal women with a mean age of 63 years.	Fermented and nonfermented milk consumption was not associated with lower blood pressure.

[a] DASH, Dietary Approaches to Stop Hypertension. An eating plan consisting of reduced calories and increased consumption of fruit, vegetables, low-fat dairy, and whole grains and lower in saturated fat, total fat, and cholesterol and restricted to 2400 mg Na.

[b] WHS, Women's Health Study: A randomized, double-blind, placebo-controlled trial to test the efficacy of low-dose aspirin and vitamin E in the primary prevention of cardiovascular disease and cancer among female health professionals.

[c] DESIR: Data from the Epidemiological Study on the Insulin Resistance Syndrome, a cohort study.

[d] Rotterdam Study: A population-based cohort study of the occurrence and progression of chronic diseases and their risk factors in people over the age of 55.

TABLE 19.5

Human Studies Considering Milk or Dairy Products and Plasma Lipid Profile

Authors	Study	Population	Conclusion
Sjogren et al. (2004)	A cross-sectional study to investigate the relations between LDL profile and dietary fatty acids.	291 healthy men (62–64 years).	Higher dairy intake was associated with a less atherogenic LDL-profile.
Azadbakht et al. (2005b)	A randomized controlled trial to determine the effects of the DASH[a] eating plan on metabolic risks.	116 subjects (34 men/82 women) with the metabolic syndrome.	The DASH diet resulted in higher HDL–cholesterol and lower triglycerides.
Sofi et al. (2010)	A 10-week crossover design study to evaluate the effects of Pecorino cheese consumption on inflammatory, lipid, and hemorheological variables.	10 subjects with an average age of 51.5 (4 men/6 women). Exclusion criteria were: vascular and inflammatory diseases.	There were no significant effects on lipid profiles.
Drouillet et al. (2007)	A 9-year follow-up study from DESIR[b] to investigate the relationship between the intake of calcium and parameters of the insulin resistance syndrome.	4372 adults (2235 men/2137 women) aged 30–65 years, with no baseline diabetes or taking medications with a source of calcium.	Increase in HDL–cholesterol in women only.
van Meijl et al. (2010)	A crossover design to study the effects of low-fat dairy consumption on inflammatory markers and adhesion molecules.	35 overweight or obese healthy subjects (10 men and 25 women) 18–70 years.	Low-fat dairy consumption decreased HDL–cholesterol and apo A-1 concentrations. Serum total cholesterol, LDL-cholesterol, apo B, triacylglycerols, and nonesterified fatty acids were unchanged.
Ivey et al. (2011)	3-year prospective, randomized, controlled trial to investigate the association between yogurt, milk, and cheese consumption and common carotid artery intima media thickness and cardiovascular disease risk factors.	1080 white women over the age of 70.	Only yogurt consumption increased HDL–cholesterol concentrations. There were no significant changes in LDL-cholesterol or triglyceride.
Palacios et al. (2011)	A 21-week randomized clinical trial to determine if dairy or calcium supplementation alters body composition or serum lipids.	30 obese Puerto Rican adults, aged from 21 to 50 years.	There were no significant effects on lipid profiles.
Crichton et al. (2012)	A 12-month crossover trial to evaluate the relation of dairy consumption and cardiometabolic health.	36 overweight subjects aged from 18 to 71 years.	There were no significant changes in total, HDL, or LDL-cholesterol and triglycerides.
Barreto et al. (2014)	A 90-day randomized trial to evaluate the influence of *L. plantarum* fermented milk on the parameters of MetS and cardiovascular risks.	24 postmenopausal women with mean age of 63 years.	Significant reduction in total cholesterol in fermented and nonfermented milk groups.

[a] DASH, Dietary Approaches to Stop Hypertension. An eating plan consisted of reduced calories and increased consumption of fruit, vegetables, low-fat dairy, and whole grains and lower in saturated fat, total fat, and cholesterol and restricted to 2400 mg.

[b] DESIR: Data from the Epidemiological Study on the Insulin Resistance Syndrome, a cohort study.

19.8 CONCLUSION

Most part of the literature found on our extensive database search indicated a favorable association of dairy consumption over at least one risk factor of the MetS. Thirty-one studies found positive effect of milk or dairy consumption on different MetS parameters and 20 did not find association among dairy consumption and any MetS risk factor. Only one study with a negative association between dairy and a risk factor of MetS was found, associating low-fat milk consumption with a decrease in HDL.

However, the effects of dairy products on metabolic health need to be further studied in more controlled trials to conclude with certainty that milk products have a protective effect on MetS patients. The Dietary Guidelines for Americans placed dairy in the "Foods to Increase" category, since Americans consume only about half of the recommended servings.

REFERENCES

Abreu, S., Santos, R., Moreira, C. et al. 2012. Association between dairy product intake and abdominal obesity in Azorean adolescents. *Eur J Clin Nutr* 66(7): 830–835.

Akter, S., Kurotani, K., Nanri, A. et al. 2013. Dairy consumption is associated with decreased insulin resistance among the Japanese. *Nutr Res* 33: 286–292.

Ascherio, A., Hennekens, C., Willett, W.C. et al. 1996. Prospective study of nutritional factors, blood pressure, and hypertension among US women. *Hypertension* 27: 1065–1072.

Astrup, A., Chaput, J.P., Gilbert, J.A., Lorenzen, J.K. 2010. Dairy beverages and energy balance. *Physiol Behav* 100(1): 67–75.

Azadbakht, L., Mirmiran, P., Esmaillzadeh, A., Azizi, F. 2005a. Dairy consumption is inversely associated with the prevalence of the metabolic syndrome in Tehranian adults. *Am J Clin Nutr* 82: 523–530.

Azadbakht, L., Mirmiran, P., Esmaillzadeh, A., Azizi, T., Azizi, F. 2005b. Beneficial effects of a dietary approaches to stop hypertension eating plan on features of the metabolic syndrome. *Diabetes Care* 28(12): 2823–2831.

Ballantyne, C.M., Hoogeveen, R.C., Bang, H. et al. 2004. Lipoprotein-associated phospholipase A2, high-sensitivity C-reactive protein, and risk for incident coronary heart disease in middle-aged men and women in the Atherosclerosis Risk in Communities (ARIC) study. *Circulation* 109: 837–842.

Barreto, F.M., Simão, A.N.C., Morimoto, H.K., Lozovoy, M.A.B., Dichi, I., Miglioranza, L.H.S. 2014. Beneficial effects of *Lactobacillus plantarum* on glycemia and homocysteine levels is postmenopausal women with metabolic syndrome: A pilot study. *Nutrition.* 30(7-8):939–942.

Bassett, D.R. 2008. Physical activity of Canadian and American children: A focus on youth in Amish, Mennonite, and modern cultures. *Appl Physiol Nutr Metab* 33: 831–835.

Beavers, K.M., Serra, M.C., Beavers, D.P., Hudson, G.M., Willoughby, D.S. 2010. The lipid-lowering effects of 4 weeks of daily soymilk or dairy milk ingestion in a postmenopausal female population. *J Med Food* 13(3): 650–656.

Bouglé, D., Bouhallab, S., Bureau, F., Zunquin, G. 2009. Effects of trace elements and calcium on diabetes and obesity, and their complications: Protective effect of dairy products—A mini-review. *Dairy Sci Technol* 89: 213–218.

Cavadini, C., Siega-Riz, A.M., Popkin, B.M. 2000. US adolescent food intake trends for 1965 to 1996. *Arch Dis Child* 83: 18–24.

Choi, H.K., Willett, W.C., Stampfer, M.J., Rimm, E., Hu, F.B. 2005. Dairy consumption and risk of type 2 diabetes mellitus in men: A prospective study. *Arch Intern Med* 165(9): 997–1003.

Crichton, G.E., Bryan, J., Buckley, J., Murphy, K.J. 2011. Dairy consumption and metabolic syndrome: A systematic review of findings and methodological issues. *Obes Rev* 12: e190–e201.

Crichton, G.E., Howe, P.R.C., Buckley, J.D., Coates, A.M., Murphy, K.J. 2012. Dairy consumption and cardiometabolic health: Outcomes of a 12-month crossover trial. *Nutr Metab (Lond)* 9: 19.

Da Silva, M.S., Rudkowska, I. 2014. Dairy products on metabolic health: Current research and clinical implications. *Maturitas* 77(3): 221–228.

Denke, M.A., Fox, M.M., Schulte, M.C. 1993. Short-term dietary calcium fortification increases fecal saturated fat content and reduces serum lipids in men. *J Nutr* 123: 1047–1053.

Di Filippo, C., Verza, M., Coppola, L, Rossi, F, D'Amico, M., Marfella, R. 2007. Insulin resistance and postprandial hyperglycemia the bad companions in natural history of diabetes: Effects on health of vascular tree. *Curr Diabetes Rev* 3: 268–273.

Dixon, L.B., Pellizzon, M.A., Jawad, A.F., Tershakovec, A.M. 2005. Calcium and dairy intake and measures of obesity in hyper and normocholesterolemic children. *Obes Res* 13(10): 1727–1738.

Dougkas, A., Reynolds, C.K., Givens, I.D., Elwood, P.C., Minihane, A.M. 2011. Associations between dairy consumption and body weight: A review of the evidence and underlying mechanisms. *Nutr Res Rev* 24(1): 72–95.

Drouillet, P., Balkau, B., Charles, M.A. et al. 2007. Calcium consumption and insulin resistance syndrome parameters, Data from the Epidemiological Study on the Insulin Resistance Syndrome (DESIR). *Nutr Metabol Cardiovasc Dis* 17: 486–492.

Dubois, L., Farmer, A., Girard, M., Peterson, K. 2007. Regular sugar-sweetened beverage consumption between meals increases risk of overweight among preschool-aged children. *J Am Diet Assoc* 107(6): 924–934.

Engberink, M.F., Hendriksen, M.A.H., Schouten, E.G. et al. 2009. Inverse association between dairy intake and hypertension: The Rotterdam Study. *Am J Clin Nutr* 89(6): 1877–1883.

FAO-Food and Agriculture Organization of the United Nations. 2010. Fats and fatty acids in human nutrition: Report of an expert consultation. Food and Nutrition Paper, 91. FAO, Rome, Italy, 170pp.

FitzGerald, R.J., Meisel, H. 2000. Milk protein-derived peptide inhibitors of angiotensin-I-converting enzyme. *Br J Nutr* 84(Suppl 1): S33–S37.

Gagliardi, A.C., Maranhão, R.C., de Sousa, H.P., Schaefer, E.J., Santos, R.D. 2010. Effects of margarines and butter consumption on lipid profiles, inflammation markers and lipid transfer to HDL particles in free-living subjects with the metabolic syndrome. *Eur J Clin Nutr* 64(10):1141–1149.

German, J.B., Gibson, R.A., Krauss, R.M. et al. 2009. A reappraisal of the impact of dairy foods and milk fat on cardiovascular risk. *Eur J Nutr* 48(4): 191–203.

Holmberg, S., Thelin, A. 2013. High dairy fat intake related to less central obesity: A male cohort study with 12 years' follow-up. *Scan J Primary Health Care* 31(2): 89–94.

Ivey, K.L., Lewis, J.R., Hodgson, J.M. et al. 2011. Association between yogurt, milk, and cheese consumption and common carotid artery intima-media thickness and cardiovascular disease risk factors in elderly women. *Am J Clin Nutr* 94(1): 234–239.

Jones, K.W., Eller, L.K., Reimer, R.A. et al. 2013. Effect of a dairy and calcium rich diet on weight loss and appetite during energy restriction in overweight and obese adults: A randomized trial. *Eur J Clin Nutr* 67(4): 371–376.

Karanja, N., Morris, C.D., Rufolo, P., Snyder, G., Illingworth, D.R., McCarron, D.A. 1994. Impact of increasing calcium in the diet on nutrient consumption, plasma lipids, and lipoproteins in humans. *Am J Clin Nutr* 59(4): 900–907.

Koenig, W., Sund, M., Fröhlich, M. et al. 1999. C-reactive protein, a sensitive marker of inflammation, predicts future risk of coronary heart disease in initially healthy middle-aged men—Results from the MONICA (Monitoring Trends and Determinants in Cardiovascular Disease) Augsburg Cohort Study, 1984 to 1992. *Circulation* 99(2): 237–242.

Korhonen, H., Pihlanto, A. 2007. Technological options for the production of health-promoting proteins and peptides derived from milk and colostrum. *Curr Pharm Des* 13(8): 829–843.

Kubena, K.S. 2011. Metabolic syndrome in adolescents: Issues and opportunities. *J Am Diet Assoc* 111(11): 1674–1679.

Labonté, M.È., Couture, P., Richard, C., Desroches, S., Lamarche, B. 2013. Impact of dairy products on bio-markers of inflammation: A systematic review of randomized controlled nutritional intervention studies in overweight and obese adults. *Am J Clin Nutr* 97(4): 706–717.

Lin, S.L., Tarrant, M., Hui, L.L. et al. 2012. The role of milk and dairy products in childhood obesity: Evidence from the Hong Kong's "children of 1997" birth cohort. *PLoS ONE* 7(12):e52575.

Liu, S., Song, Y., Ford, E.S., Manson, J.E., Buring, J.E., Ridker, P.M. 2005. Dietary calcium, vitamin D, and the prevalence of metabolic syndrome in middle-aged and older U.S. women. *Diabetes Care* 28(12): 2926–2932.

Liu, S., Choi, H.K., Ford, E. et al. 2006. A prospective study of dairy intake and the risk of type 2 diabetes in women. *Diabetes Care* 29(7): 1579–1584.

Lorenzen, J.K., Astrup, A. 2011. Dairy calcium intake modifies responsiveness of fat metabolism and blood lipids to a high-fat diet. *Br J Nutr* 105(12): 1823–1831.

Louie, J.C., Flood, V.M., Rangan, A.M. et al. 2013. Higher regular fat dairy consumption is associated with lower incidence of metabolic syndrome but not type 2 diabetes. *Nutr Metabol Cardiovasc Dis* 23(9): 816–821.

Ma, B., Lawson, A.B., Liese, A.D., Bell, R.A., Mayer-Davis, E.J. 2006. Dairy, magnesium, and calcium intake in relation to insulin sensitivity: Approaches to modeling a dose-dependent association. *Am J Epidemiol* 164(5): 449–458.

Malik, V.S., Sun, Q., van Dam, R.M. et al. 2011. Adolescent dairy product consumption and risk of type 2 diabetes in middle-aged women. *Am J Clin Nutr* 94(3): 854–861.

Matthews, D.R., Hosker, J.P., Rudenski, A.S., Naylor, B.A., Treacher, D.F., Turner, R.C. 1985. Homeostasis model assessment: Insulin resistance and beta-cell function from fasting plasma glucose and insulin concentrations in man. *Diabetologia* 28(7): 412–419.

McGrane, M.M., Essery, E., Obbagy, J. et al. 2011. Dairy consumption, blood pressure, and risk of hypertension: An evidence-based review of recent literature. *Curr Cardiovasc Risk Rep* 5(4): 287–298.

Melnik, B.C. 2009. Milk—The promoter of chronic Western diseases. *Medical Hypotheses* 72(6): 631–639.

Nestel, P.J., Pally, S., MacIntosh, G.L. et al. 2012. Circulating inflammatory and atherogenic biomarkers are not increased following single meals of dairy foods. *Eur J Clin Nutr* 66(1): 25–31.

Pal, S., Ellis, V. 2010. The chronic effects of whey proteins on blood pressure, vascular function, and inflammatory markers in overweight individuals. *Obesity* 18(7): 1354–1359.

Palacios, C., Bertrán, J.J., Ríos, R.E., Soltero, S. 2011. No effects of low and high consumption of dairy products and calcium supplements on body composition and serum lipids in Puerto Rican obese adults. *Nutrition* 27(5): 520–525.

Pereira, M.A., Jacobs, D.R. Jr., Van Horn, L., Slattery, M.L., Kartashov, A.I., Ludwig, D.S. 2002. Dairy consumption, obesity, and the insulin resistance syndrome in young adults. The CARDIA study. *JAMA* 287(16): 2081–2089.

Pfeuffer, M., Schrezenmeir, J. 2007. Milk and the metabolic syndrome. *Obes Rev* 8(2): 109–118.

Reaven, G.M. 1988. Role of insulin resistance in human disease. *Diabetes* 37(12): 1595–1607.

Reid, I.R. 2004. Effects of calcium supplementation on circulating lipids: Potential pharmacoeconomic implications. *Drugs Aging* 21(1): 7–17.

Reuter, S., Gupta, S.C., Chaturvedi, M.M., Aggarwal, B.B. 2010. Oxidative stress, inflammation and cancer: How are they linked? *Free Rad Biol Med* 49(11): 1603–1616.

Ricci-Cabello, I., Herrera, M.O., Artacho, R. 2012. Possible role of milk-derived bioactive peptides in the treatment and prevention of metabolic syndrome. *Nutr Rev* 70(4): 241–255.

Rideout, T.C, Marinangeli, C.P.F., Martin, H., Browne, R.W., Rempel, C.B. 2013. Consumption of low-fat dairy foods for 6 months improves insulin resistance without adversely affecting lipids or bodyweight in healthy adults: A randomized free-living cross-over study. *Nutr J* 12: 56.

Ridker, P.M., Rifai, N., Rose, L., Buring, J.E., Cook, N.R. 2002. Comparison of C-reactive protein and low-density lipoprotein cholesterol levels in the prediction of first cardiovascular events. *N Engl J Med* 347: 1557–1565.

Rosell, M., Johansson, G., Berglund, L., Vessby, B., de Faire, U., Hellénius, M.-L. 2004. Associations between the intake of dairy fat and calcium and abdominal obesity. *Intern J Obes* 28: 1427–1434.

Scholz-Ahrens, K.E., Schrezenmeir, J. 2006. Milk minerals and the metabolic syndrome. *Intern Dairy J* 16(11): 1399–1407.

Shahkhalili, Y., Murset, C., Meirim, I. et al. 2001. Calcium supplementation of chocolate: Effect on cocoa butter digestibility and blood lipids in humans. *Am J Clin Nutr* 73(2): 246–252.

Sjogren, P., Rosell, M., Skoglund-Andersson, C. et al. 2004. Milk-derived fatty acids are associated with a more favorable LDL particle size distribution in healthy men. *J Nutr* 134(7): 1729–1735.

Skinner, J.D., Bounds, W., Carruth, B.R., Ziegler, P. 2003. Longitudinal calcium intake is negatively related to children's body fat indexes. *J Am Diet Assoc* 103(12): 1626–1631.

Snijder, M.B., van Dam, R.M., Stehouwer, C.D., Hiddink, G.J., Heine, R.J., Dekker, J.M. 2008. A prospective study of dairy consumption in relation to changes in metabolic risk factors: The Hoorn Study. *Obesity (Silver Spring)* 16(3): 706–709.

Snijder, M.B., van der Heijden, A.A., van Dam, R.M. et al. 2007. Is higher dairy consumption associated with lower body weight and fewer metabolic disturbances? The Hoorn Study. *Am J Clin Nutr* 85(4): 989–995.

Sofi, F., Buccioni, A., Cesari, F. et al. 2010. Effects of a dairy product (pecorino cheese) naturally rich in cis-9, trans-11 conjugated linoleic acid on lipid, inflammatory and haemorheological variables: A dietary intervention study. *Nutr Metabol Cardiovasc Dis* 20(2): 117–124.

Stancliffe, R.A., Thorpe, T., Zemel, M.B. 2011. Dairy attenuates oxidative inflammatory stress in metabolic syndrome. *Am J Clin Nutr* 94(2): 422–430.

St-Onge, M.-P., Goree, L.L.T., Gower, B. 2009. High-milk supplementation with healthy diet counseling does not affect weight loss but ameliorates insulin action compared with low-milk supplementation in overweight children. *J Nutr* 139(5): 933–938.

Struijk, E.A., Heraclides, A., Witte, D.R. et al. 2013. Dairy product intake in relation to glucose regulation índices and risk of type 2 diabetes. *Nutr Metabol Cardiovasc Dis* 23(9): 822–828.

Takano, T. 1998. Milk derived peptides and hypertension reduction. *Intern Dairy J* 8(5–6): 375–381.

Tholstrup, T., Hoy, C.E., Andersen, L.N., Christensen, R.D., Sandström, B. 2004. Does fat in milk, butter and cheese affect blood lipids and cholesterol differently? *J Am Coll Nutr* 23(2): 169–176.

Thompson, W.G., Rostad, H.N., Janzow, D.J. Slezak, J.M., Morris, K.L., Zemel, M.B. 2005. Effect of energy-reduced diets high in dairy products and fiber on weight loss in obese adults. *Obes Res* 13(8): 1344–1353.

U.S. Department of Agriculture; U.S. Department of Health and Human Services. 2010. *Dietary Guidelines for Americans, 2010*, 7th edn. Washington, DC: U.S. Government Printing Office.

van Meijl, L.E.C., Mensink, R.P. 2010. Effects of low-fat dairy consumption on markers of low-grade systemic inflammation and endothelial function in overweight and obese subjects: An intervention study. *Br J Nutr* 104(10): 1523–1527.

van Meijl, L.E.C., Vrolix, R., Mensink, R.P. 2008. Dairy product consumption and the metabolic syndrome. *Nutr Res Rev* 21(2): 148–157.

Wang, L., Manson, J.E., Buring, J.E., Lee, I.M., Sesso, H.D. 2008. Dietary intake of dairy products, calcium, and vitamin D and the risk of hypertension in middle-aged and older women. *Hypertension* 51(4): 1073–1079.

Wang, H., Steffen, L.M., Vessby, B. et al. 2011. Obesity modifies the relations between serum markers of dairy fats and inflammation and oxidative stress among adolescents. *Obesity* (*Silver Spring*) 19(12): 2404–2410.

Warensjö, E., Jansson, J.-H., Cederholm, T. et al. 2010. Biomarkers of milk fat and the risk of myocardial infarction in men and women: A prospective, matched case-control study. *Am J Clin Nutr* 92(1): 194–202.

Weaver, C.M. 2010. Role of dairy beverages in the diet. *Physiol Behav* 100(1): 63–66.

Wennersberg, M.H., Smedman, A., Turpeinen, A.M. et al. 2009. Dairy products and metabolic effects in overweight men and women: Results from a 6-mo intervention study. *Am J Clin Nutr* 90(4): 960–968.

Wildman, R.P., Aileen, P., McGinn, A.P., Kim, M. et al. 2011. Empirical derivation to improve the definition of the Metabolic Syndrome in the evaluation of cardiovascular disease risk. *Diabetes Care* 34(3): 746–748.

World Health Organisation European Region. 2000. *CINDI dietary guide*. Copenhagen, Denmark: WHO, Europe.

Xu, J.Y., Qin, L.Q., Wang, P.Y., Li, W., Chang, C. 2008. Effect of milk tripeptides on blood pressure: A meta-analysis of randomized controlled trials. *Nutrition* 24(10): 933–940.

Zemel, M.B., Sun, X., Sobhani, T., Wilson, B. 2010. Effects of dairy compared with soy on oxidative and inflammatory stress in overweight and obese subjects. *Am J Clin Nutr* 91(1): 16–22.

Zemel, M.B. 2004. Role of calcium and dairy products in energy partitioning and weight management. *Am J Clin Nutr* 79(5):907S–912S.

Zemel, M.B., Thompson, W., Milstead, A., Morris, K., Campbell, P. 2004. Calcium and dairy acceleration of weight and fat loss during energy restriction in obese adults. *Obes Res* 12(4): 582–590.

20 Berries in the Nutritional Management of Metabolic Syndrome

Arpita Basu and Timothy J. Lyons

CONTENTS

20.1 INTRODUCTION

Berry fruits, a rich source of micronutrients and several bioactive phytochemicals, have been recognized among all fruits and vegetables for their distinct cardiovascular health benefits (Neto 2007; Basu et al. 2010a,b). Strawberries are among the most popular fresh fruits produced and consumed in the United States, followed by blueberries, whereas cranberries as juice and juice blends are also popular sources of phytochemicals in the U.S. diet (Neto 2007; Boriss et al. 2010). The antioxidant properties of these berry fruits have been well documented in various in vitro, animal, and human studies, although the observed cardiovascular effects have been explained by mechanisms beyond antioxidant activity (Scalbert et al. 2005). In comparative analyses of commonly consumed polyphenol-rich beverages in the United States, blueberry juice and cranberry juice were listed among the top 10 beverages of high antioxidant potency measured as the sum of four assays (1,1-diphenyl-2-picrylhydrazyl radical, oxygen radical absorbance capacity, Trolox equivalent antioxidant capacity, and ferric reducing ability of plasma); strawberries were not included as a popular beverage in this study (Seeram et al. 2008). In another paper comparing the antioxidant properties of fresh fruits as determined by cellular antioxidant activity (CAA), blueberries were shown to have the highest CAA values, whereas apples and strawberries were the largest contributors of CAA to the U.S. diet (Wolfe et al. 2008). In a recently reported study identifying food sources and supplements of antioxidant activity in the U.S. diet, blueberries, strawberries, and cranberry juice drink were among the top major food items consumed by U.S. adults (Yang et al. 2011).

The objective of this review is to discuss the key findings from human interventional studies, including those reported by our group, along with pertinent mechanistic data that substantiate the emerging roles of strawberries, blueberries, and cranberries in metabolic syndrome (MetS).

20.2 STRAWBERRIES AND METABOLIC SYNDROME

Strawberries (*Fragaria* × *ananassa*) are a rich source of polyphenols, ellagitannins, vitamin C, folic acid, potassium, and fiber. Approximately 40 phenolic compounds have been identified in strawberries, among which vitamin C, ellagitannins, and anthocyanins were shown to be the most significant

345

contributors to electrochemical responses, a marker of antioxidant capacity (Aaby et al. 2007). The effects of strawberries in lowering lipids, lipid oxidation, and postprandial hyperglycemia, hyperlipidemia, and inflammatory responses have been documented in human interventional studies in healthy subjects or in those with cardiovascular disease (CVD) risks, such as the MetS.

Fresh strawberry intervention in healthy subjects (240–300 g) has been shown to increase postprandial serum antioxidant capacity and vitamin C (Cao et al. 1998; Prior et al. 2007), and strawberry jam (20 g) or mixed-berry puree (150 g) supplementation in healthy subjects has also been shown to attenuate postprandial hyperglycemia when compared to the controls receiving a matched glucose load (Kurotobi et al. 2010; Törrönen et al. 2010). In a similar postprandial study in hyperlipidemic adults, Burton-Freeman and colleagues demonstrated significant attenuation of postprandial lipemia and lipid oxidation by freeze-dried strawberry intervention (10 g/day ~ 100 g fresh strawberries) following a high-fat meal challenge (Burton-Freeman et al. 2010). Postprandial (fed state) hyperglycemia and lipemia have been shown to be exaggerated in the presence of visceral obesity, dyslipidemia, and impaired glucose metabolism, which constitute the key features of MetS, compared with healthy subjects (Kolovou et al. 2005; Tushuizen et al. 2010). Thus, these effects of strawberries in improving postprandial metabolism might have significant implications in the management of MetS.

Few long-term feeding studies have been reported on the effects of strawberries in obese adults with MetS. Thus, our group tested the hypothesis that freeze-dried strawberries (50 g/day, equivalent to ~ 500 g fresh strawberries) will improve features of MetS and associated lipid oxidation and inflammation in obese adults. Our key findings demonstrate a significant reduction in total and low-density lipoprotein (LDL)-cholesterol, small LDL particles, serum malondialdehyde, and adhesion molecules in strawberry-supplemented groups versus controls (Basu et al. 2009, 2010d,e). In fact, ours was the first study to show such lipid-lowering effects of strawberries in selected subjects with at least three features of MetS, in comparison to previous studies showing a decrease in lipid oxidation or an increase in high-density lipoprotein (HDL) following strawberry (454 g) or mixed-berry intervention (two portions including 100 g strawberry puree), respectively, in adults with CVD risk factors (Erlund et al. 2008; Jenkins et al. 2008). Malondialdehyde, a naturally occurring product of lipid peroxidation, has been recognized as influencing the expression of various effector molecules of the immune system, promoting the recruitment of the cells of the innate and adaptive immune systems into the vessel wall. This aids in the development of atherosclerotic lesions (Basu et al. 2009). Adhesion molecules further assist in the recruitment of monocytes and their migration into the subendothelial space, which are key events in the progression of atherosclerotic lesions (Basu et al. 2010). Thus, these preliminary clinical data suggest the potential antiatherosclerotic effects of strawberry consumption, especially in MetS.

Mechanistic studies in cells and in animal models of obesity and diabetes have demonstrated the following treatment effects of strawberry fruits, extracts, or purified anthocyanins: upregulation of endothelial nitric oxide synthase (eNOS) (Lazzè et al. 2006); inhibition of glucose uptake and transport and normalization of blood glucose levels (Roy et al. 2008; Manzano and Williamson 2010); inhibition of carbohydrate and lipid digestive enzymes, especially α-glucosidase and α-amylase, and pancreatic lipase activity (McDougall et al. 2005, 2008); and also inhibition of angiotensin I-converting enzyme (ACE) (Cheplick et al. 2010), which may be linked to the therapeutic management of hyperglycemia and hypertension, key features of MetS. Thus, these clinical and mechanistic findings warrant further investigation, but provide promising data for selecting fresh or frozen strawberries in the dietary management of MetS.

20.3 BLUEBERRIES AND METABOLIC SYNDROME

Highbush (*Vaccinium corymbosum*) and lowbush (*Vaccinium angustifolium* Aiton.) blueberries have been associated with several cardiovascular health benefits. Anthocyanins have been shown to be the main contributors to the antioxidant capacity of blueberries (Borges et al. 2010).

Chromatographic profiling has further shown that anthocyanins comprise approximately 35%–74% total phenolic compounds in blueberries, followed by hydroxycinnamic acid derivatives, flavonols, and flavan-3-ols (Gavrilova et al. 2011). In addition, blueberries are significant sources of folic acid, vitamin C, and fiber, which may act in concert with the blueberry polyphenols in exerting the observed cardiovascular health effects.

Similar to the postprandial effects observed with strawberries (Burton-Freeman et al. 2010), freeze-dried blueberries (100 g) have also been shown to counterbalance the oxidative stress responses to a fast-food-style meal challenge in healthy adults (Kay and Holub 2002). Thus, with the exaggerated postprandial responses in the MetS taken into consideration (Kolovou et al. 2005; Tushuizen et al. 2010), blueberries may also have significant implications in attenuating such responses when consumed concomitantly with high-fat meals. Few studies have examined the cardiovascular effects of blueberries in long-term feeding studies. A 3-week feeding study in smokers has shown the antioxidant effects of blueberries (250 g) in decreasing lipid hydroperoxides versus controls (McAnulty et al. 2005). Because smoking is also associated with elevated lipid oxidation and inflammation occur in the MetS (Padmavathi et al. 2010), blueberry supplementation may be an effective therapy for oxidative stress in smokers. In recent years, two reported human studies have demonstrated the antihypertensive and insulin-sensitizing effects of freeze-dried blueberries in obese adults with MetS and in obese insulin-resistant adults, respectively. In the first study reported by our group, 50 g of freeze-dried blueberries (~350 g fresh blueberries) supplemented for 8 weeks caused a significant reduction in systolic and diastolic blood pressures and markers of lipid oxidation, specifically oxidized LDL and malondialdehyde, versus controls (Basu et al. 2010b). In the second study, a 6-week treatment with 45 g of freeze-dried blueberries (~315 g fresh blueberries) caused a significant improvement in insulin sensitivity, as assessed by the high-dose hyperinsulinemic–euglycemic clamp in obese adults (Stull et al. 2010). These data show the potential of blueberries, at achievable dietary doses, in improving hypertension and insulin resistance associated with MetS, and warrant further investigation in larger studies.

Mechanistic studies in animal models of hypertension further explain the antihypertensive effects of blueberries. Dietary supplementation of 3% freeze-dried blueberries for 8 weeks was shown to decrease systolic blood pressure in spontaneously hypertensive stroke-prone (SHRSP) rats versus controls (Shaughnessy et al. 2009). In addition, the study also showed a decrease in markers of renal oxidative stress in blueberry-fed rats versus controls, indicating protection against renal oxidative damage by blueberries. In another animal model of spontaneously hypertensive rats, 8% wild blueberry supplementation significantly improved vasoconstriction and endothelial dysfunction (Kristo et al. 2010). Blueberries have also been shown to lower plasma ACE activity in SHRSP rats, suggesting another mechanism by which they might be effective in the management of the early stages of hypertension (Wiseman et al. 2011). In addition to decreasing elevated blood pressure, blueberries have also been demonstrated to decrease atherosclerotic lesions and upregulate aortic expression of antioxidant enzymes in apolipoprotein E-deficient mice (Wu et al. 2010). In vitro studies have also reported blueberries to inhibit α-amylase and α-glucosidase activities with implications in the management of hyperglycemia (Johnson et al. 2011). Thus, these mechanistic findings deserve clinical translation in obesity and MetS to identify optimal dosing and duration of blueberry intervention, and to define the risk factors or pathological stage of CVD expected to be modulated by blueberries.

20.4 CRANBERRIES AND METABOLIC SYNDROME

Cranberries (*Vaccinium macrocarpon*) are native to North America and are a rich source of phenolic acids (benzoic, hydroxycinnamic, and ellagic acids) and flavonoids (anthocyanins, flavonols, and flavan-3-ols) (Neto 2007). Comparative analyses of phenolic antioxidants among different cranberry products show the following order of antioxidant content: frozen > 100% juice > dried > 27% juice > sauce > jellied sauce (Vinson et al. 2008). On the basis of these data, dried cranberries and 27% cranberry juice, commonly consumed in the United States, are significant dietary sources of polyphenols.

Several human studies have reported the antioxidant, anti-inflammatory, and HDL-raising effects of cranberry juice in healthy or obese adults (Ruel et al. 2005, 2006, 2008). Cranberries have also been tested in patients with type 2 diabetes and have been shown to lower lipid profiles and postprandial hyperglycemia versus controls. In 2008, Lee et al. reported a significant decrease in total and LDL cholesterol, as well as the total/HDL cholesterol ratio following a 12-week administration of cranberry extracts (1500 mg/day), although blood glucose remained unaffected (Lee et al. 2008). Wilson et al. also reported a postprandial study comparing the effects of sweetened or low-calorie dried cranberries (40 g), raw cranberries (55 g), and white bread (57 g) in glycemic response in patients with type 2 diabetes. The study revealed significantly lower postprandial insulin and glucose following low-calorie dried cranberries or raw cranberry intervention compared to regular sweetened cranberries or white bread (control) (Wilson et al. 2010). Thus, the selection of low-calorie dried cranberries may provide a palatable source of polyphenols and fiber and also aid in producing favorable glycemic response in type 2 diabetes. Our group has previously reported an 8-week double-blind randomized controlled trial in which low-calorie cranberry juice (27% juice, 480 mL/day) caused a significant increase in plasma antioxidant capacity and decreased plasma-oxidized LDL and malondialdehyde in obese adults with MetS, when compared to those consuming the placebo juice (Basu et al. 2011a). Our findings have been further substantiated by a more recently reported study showing the effects of reduced-energy cranberry juice in increasing adiponectin and decreasing oxidative stress biomarkers in participants with the MetS (Simão et al. 2013). Thus, our study findings, in combination with others, provide evidence on the role of specific cranberry products, such as low-calorie cranberry juice or dried cranberries, in attenuating dyslipidemia, hyperglycemia, and biomarkers of atherosclerosis associated with MetS. The role of cranberry extracts needs to be further examined for safety and efficacy in larger trials on MetS or type 2 diabetes.

Mechanistic studies in animal models have also reported the vasodilatory effects of cranberry juice via induction of eNOS (Maher et al. 2000), decrease in total and LDL cholesterol in an animal model of familial hypercholesterolemia via inhibiting enzymes involved in lipid and lipoprotein metabolism (Reed 2002), and protection against chemotherapy-induced cardiac toxicity in rats via antioxidant activity (Elberry et al. 2010). These data need confirmation to define in more detail the cardiovascular benefits of cranberry supplementation in MetS.

20.5 CONCLUSIONS AND PERSPECTIVES

Dietary berries rich in polyphenolic compounds, especially flavonoids, vitamins, and fiber, constitute an important food group in the nutritional management of the MetS. In this regard, strawberries, blueberries, and cranberries deserve special attention as these are commonly consumed berries in the human diet and have been identified as having several roles in ameliorating features of the MetS. Fresh, frozen, and freeze-dried berries and low-calorie berry juices have been shown to improve metabolic profiles, decreasing total and LDL cholesterol, increasing HDL cholesterol, decreasing biomarkers of oxidative stress and inflammation, and increasing plasma antioxidant capacity in human feeding studies. These observations in human studies have also been supported by mechanistic evidence on the role of berries in inhibiting enzymes of carbohydrate and fat digestion, as well as enzymes involved in lipid and lipoprotein metabolism, and upregulating antioxidant enzymes and the activity of the vasodilator eNOS, mostly in animal models of the MetS. These findings deserve further investigation in larger studies in populations with significant CVD risk factors and concomitant low habitual fruit and vegetable consumption.

Future studies must examine the effects of berry supplementation in the context of weight loss diets and how these outcomes may be modulated by the presence of other dietary bioactive compounds in foods and beverages. Future investigation must also involve the form and optimal doses of berries associated with attenuating the features of the MetS. Overall, on the basis of the current findings, the inclusion of commonly available fresh or frozen dietary strawberries and blueberries, and low-calorie berry juices may act as preventative as well as therapeutic strategies in the MetS.

REFERENCES

Aaby, K., Ekeberg, D., and Skrede, G. 2007. Characterization of phenolic compounds in strawberry (*Fragaria* × *ananassa*) fruits by different HPLC detectors and contribution of individual compounds to total antioxidant capacity. *Journal of Agricultural and Food Chemistry* 55: 4395–4406.

Basu, A., Betts, N.M., Ortiz, J., Simmons, B., Wu, M., and Lyons, T.J. 2011. Low-energy cranberry juice decreases lipid oxidation and increases plasma antioxidant capacity in women with metabolic syndrome. *Nutrition Research* 31: 190–196.

Basu, A., Du, M., Leyva, M.J. et al. 2010. Blueberries decrease cardiovascular risk factors in obese men and women with metabolic syndrome. *Journal of Nutrition* 140: 1582–1587.

Basu, A., Fu, D.X., Wilkinson, M. et al. 2010. Strawberries decrease atherosclerotic markers in subjects with metabolic syndrome. *Nutrition Research* 30: 462–469.

Basu, A., Rhone, M., and Lyons, T.J. 2010. Berries: Emerging impact on cardiovascular health. *Nutrition Reviews* 68: 168–177.

Basu, A., Wilkinson, M., Penugonda, K., Simmons, B., Betts, N.M., and Lyons, T.J. 2009. Freeze-dried strawberry powder improves lipid profile and lipid peroxidation in women with metabolic syndrome: Baseline and post intervention effects. *Nutrition Journal* 8: 43.

Borges, G., Degeneve, A., Mullen, W., and Crozier, A. 2010. Identification of flavonoid and phenolic antioxidants in black currants, blueberries, raspberries, red currants, and cranberries. *Journal of Agricultural and Food Chemistry* 58: 3901–3909.

Boriss, H., Brunke, H., and Kreith, M. 2010. Commodity strawberry profile. In: *Agricultural Marketing Resource Center.* Iowa State University, Ames, IA, pp. 1–13.

Burton-Freeman, B., Linares, A., Hyson, D., and Kappagoda, T. 2010. Strawberry modulates LDL oxidation and postprandial lipemia in response to high-fat meal in overweight hyperlipidemic men and women. *Journal of the American College of Nutrition* 29: 46–54.

Cao, G., Russell, R.M., Lischner, N., and Prior, R.L. 1998. Serum antioxidant capacity is increased by consumption of strawberries, spinach, red wine or vitamin c in elderly women. *Journal of Nutrition* 128: 2383–2390.

Cheplick, S., Kwon, Y.I., Bhowmik, P., and Shetty, K. 2010. Phenolic-linked variation in strawberry cultivars for potential dietary management of hyperglycemia and related complications of hypertension. *Bioresource Technology* 101: 404–413.

Elberry, A.A., Abdel-Naim, A.B., Abdel-Sattar, E.A. et al. 2010. Cranberry (*Vaccinium macrocarpon*) protects against doxorubicin-induced cardiotoxicity in rats. *Food and Chemical Toxicology* 48: 1178–1184.

Erlund, I., Koli, R., Alfthan, G. et al. 2008. Favorable effects of berry consumption on platelet function, blood pressure, and HDL cholesterol. *American Journal of Clinical Nutrition* 87: 323–333.

Gavrilova, V., Kajdzanoska, M., Gjamovski, V., and Stefova, M. 2011. Separation, characterization and quantification of phenolic compounds in blueberries and red and black currants by HPLC-DAD-ESI-MSn. *Journal of Agricultural and Food Chemistry* 59: 4009–4018.

Jenkins, D.J., Nguyen, T.H., Kendall, C.W. et al. 2008. The effect of strawberries in a cholesterol-lowering dietary portfolio. *Metabolism* 57: 1636–1644.

Johnson, M.H., Lucius, A., Meyer, T., and de Mejia, E.G. 2011. Cultivar evaluation and effect of fermentation on antioxidant capacity and in vitro inhibition of α-amylase and α-glucosidase by highbush blueberry (*Vaccinium corymbosum*). *Journal of Agricultural and Food Chemistry* 59: 8923–8930.

Kay, C.D. and Holub, B.J. 2002. The effect of wild blueberry (*Vaccinium angustifolium*) consumption on postprandial serum antioxidant status in human subjects. *British Journal of Nutrition* 88: 389–398.

Kolovou, G.D., Anagnostopoulou, K.K., Pavlidis, A.N. et al. 2005. Postprandial lipemia in men with metabolic syndrome, hypertensives and healthy subjects. *Lipids in Health and Disease* 4: 21.

Kristo, A.S., Kalea, A.Z., Schuschke, D.A., and Klimis-Zacas, D.J. 2010. A wild blueberry-enriched diet (*Vaccinium angustifolium*) improves vascular tone in the adult spontaneously hypertensive rat. *Journal of Agricultural and Food Chemistry* 58: 11600–11605.

Kurotobi, T., Fukuhara, K., Inage, H., and Kimura, S. 2010. Glycemic index and postprandial blood glucose response to Japanese strawberry jam in normal adults. *Journal of Nutritional Science and Vitaminology (Tokyo)* 56: 198–202.

Lazzè, M.C., Pizzala, R., Perucca, P. et al. 2006. Anthocyanidins decrease endothelin-1 production and increase endothelial nitric oxide synthase in human endothelial cells. *Molecular Nutrition and Food Research* 50: 44–51.

Lee, I.T., Chan, Y.C., Lin, C.W., Lee, W.J., and Sheu, W.H. 2008. Effect of cranberry extracts on lipid profiles in subjects with Type 2 diabetes. *Diabetic Medicine* 25: 1473–1477.

Maher, M.A., Mataczynski, H., Stefaniak, H.M., and Wilson, T. 2000. Cranberry juice induces nitric oxide-dependent vasodilation in vitro and its infusion transiently reduces blood pressure in anesthetized rats. *Journal of Medicinal Food* 3: 141–147.

Manzano, S. and Williamson, G. 2010. Polyphenols and phenolic acids from strawberry and apple decrease glucose uptake and transport by human intestinal caco-2 cells. *Molecular Nutrition and Food Research* 54: 1773–1780.

McAnulty, S.R., McAnulty, L.S., Morrow, J.D. et al. 2005. Effect of daily fruit ingestion on angiotensin converting enzyme activity, blood pressure, and oxidative stress in chronic smokers. *Free Radical Research* 39: 1241–1248.

McDougall, G.J., Kulkarni, N.N., and Stewart, D. 2008. Current developments on the inhibitory effects of berry polyphenols on digestive enzymes. *Biofactors* 34: 73–80.

McDougall, G.J., Shpiro, F., Dobson, P., Smith, P., Blake, A., and Stewart, D. 2005. Different polyphenolic components of soft fruits inhibit alpha-amylase and alpha-glucosidase. *Journal of Agricultural and Food Chemistry* 53: 2760–2766.

Neto, C.C. 2007. Cranberry and blueberry: Evidence for protective effects against cancer and vascular diseases. *Molecular Nutrition and Food Research* 51: 652–664.

Padmavathi, P., Reddy, V.D., Kavitha, G., Paramahamsa, M., and Varadacharyulu, N. 2010. Chronic cigarette smoking alters erythrocyte membrane lipid composition and properties in male human volunteers. *Nitric Oxide* 23: 181–186.

Prior, R.L., Gu, L., Wu, X. et al. 2007. Plasma antioxidant capacity changes following a meal as a measure of the ability of a food to alter in vivo antioxidant status. *Journal of the American College of Nutrition* 26: 170–181.

Reed, J. 2002. Cranberry flavonoids, atherosclerosis and cardiovascular health. *Critical Reviews in Food Science and Nutrition* 42: 301–316.

Roy, M., Sen, S., and Chakraborti, A.S. 2008. Action of pelargonidin on hyperglycemia and oxidative damage in diabetic rats: Implication for glycation-induced hemoglobin modification. *Life Sciences* 82: 1102–1110.

Ruel, G., Pomerleau, S., Couture, P., Lamarche, B., and Couillard, C. 2005. Changes in plasma antioxidant capacity and oxidized low-density lipoprotein levels in men after short-term cranberry juice consumption. *Metabolism* 54: 856–861.

Ruel, G., Pomerleau, S., Couture, P., Lemieux, S., Lamarche, B., and Couillard, C. 2006. Favourable impact of low-calorie cranberry juice consumption on plasma HDL-cholesterol concentrations in men. *British Journal of Nutrition* 96: 357–364.

Ruel, G., Pomerleau, S., Couture, P., Lemieux, S., Lamarche, B., and Couillard, C. 2008. Low-calorie cranberry juice supplementation reduces plasma oxidized LDL and cell adhesion molecule concentrations in men. *British Journal of Nutrition* 99: 352–359.

Scalbert, A., Johnson, I.T., and Saltmarsh, M. 2005. Polyphenols: Antioxidants and beyond. *American Journal of Clinical Nutrition* 81: 215S–217S.

Seeram, N.P., Aviram, M., Zhang, Y. et al. 2008. Comparison of antioxidant potency of commonly consumed polyphenol-rich beverages in the United States. *Journal of Agricultural and Food Chemistry* 56: 1415–1422.

Shaughnessy, K.S., Boswall, I.A., Scanlan, A.P., Gottschall-Pass, K.T., and Sweeney, M.I. 2009. Diets containing blueberry extract lower blood pressure in spontaneously hypertensive stroke-prone rats. *Nutrition Research* 29: 130–138.

Simão, T.N., Lozovoy, M.A., Simão, A.N. et al. 2013. Reduced-energy cranberry juice increases folic acid and adiponectin and reduces homocysteine and oxidative stress in patients with the metabolic syndrome. *British Journal of Nutrition* 110: 1885–1894.

Stull, A.J., Cash, K.C., Johnson, W.D., Champagne, C.M., and Cefalu, W.T. 2010. Bioactives in blueberries improve insulin sensitivity in obese, insulin-resistant men and women. *Journal of Nutrition* 140: 1764–1768.

Törrönen, R., Sarkkinen, E., Tapola, N., Hautaniemi, E., Kilpi, K., and Niskanen, L. 2010. Berries modify the postprandial plasma glucose response to sucrose in healthy subjects. *British Journal of Nutrition* 103: 1094–1097.

Tushuizen, M.E., Pouwels, P.J., Bontemps, S. et al. 2010. Postprandial lipid and apolipoprotein responses following three consecutive meals associate with liver fat content in type 2 diabetes and the metabolic syndrome. *Atherosclerosis* 211: 308–314.

Vinson, J.A., Bose, P., Proch, J., Al Kharrat, H., and Samman, N. 2008. Cranberries and cranberry products: Powerful in vitro, ex vivo, and in vivo sources of antioxidants. *Journal of Agricultural and Food Chemistry* 56: 5884–5891.

Wilson, T., Luebke, J.L., Morcomb, E.F. et al. 2010. Glycemic responses to sweetened dried and raw cranberries in humans with type 2 diabetes. *Journal of Food Science* 75: H218–H223.

Wiseman, W., Egan, J.M., Slemmer, J.E. et al. 2011. Feeding blueberry diets inhibits angiotensin II-converting enzyme (ACE) activity in spontaneously hypertensive stroke-prone rats. *Canadian Journal of Physiology and Pharmacology* 89: 67–71.

Wolfe, K.L., Kang, X., He, X., Dong, M., Zhang, Q., and Liu, R.H. 2008. Cellular antioxidant activity of common fruits. *Journal of Agricultural and Food Chemistry* 56: 8418–8426.

Wu, X., Kang, J., Xie, C. et al. 2010. Dietary blueberries attenuate atherosclerosis in apolipoprotein E-deficient mice by upregulating antioxidant enzyme expression. *Journal of Nutrition* 140: 1628–1632.

Yang, M., Chung, S.J., Chung, C.E. et al. 2011. Estimation of total antioxidant capacity from diet and supplements in US adults. *British Journal of Nutrition* 106: 254–263.

21 Effects of Tea Consumption on Metabolic Syndrome

Chung S. Yang, Jungil Hong, and William Feng

CONTENTS

21.1 INTRODUCTION

Tea, made of the leaves of the plant *Camellia sinensis*, Theaceae, has been used for medicinal purposes in ancient days and is now a popular beverage worldwide. Depending on the processing of the tea leaves, tea is classified into three major types: green tea, black tea, and oolong tea, which account for 20%, 78%, and 2% of the world's tea production, respectively. Green tea is mainly produced and consumed in Asian countries such as China and Japan. Black tea is produced in South Asia, South America, and Africa and consumed worldwide. Oolong tea is mainly produced and consumed in southeast China, Taiwan, and Japan (Balentine et al. 1997; Sang et al. 2011).

In recent years, tea has been studied for its potential beneficial health effects. These include the reduction of body weight, alleviation of metabolic syndrome (MetS), and prevention of cardiovascular diseases (CVDs), cancer, and neurodegenerative diseases. Most of these beneficial effects are believed to be due to the polyphenols in tea, although caffeine also contributes to some of the effects. Overweight, obesity, and diabetes are emerging as major health issues worldwide, and MetS is an early manifestation of type 2 diabetes and a key risk factor for CVDs. If tea could prevent, delay, or alleviate MetS, the public health implications would be substantial. Because of this, there is immense public interest on this topic.

This chapter intends to critically review the effects of tea consumption on MetS, to elucidate the possible mechanisms involved, and to evaluate the human relevance of the published results. It also discusses other health effects of tea consumption as well as the possible side effects due to the consumption of excessive amount of tea extracts, mainly as dietary supplements. We will use the information from recently published reviews and meta-analysis to help assess the relative strengths of the existing data. We hope this chapter will enhance the overall understanding of the health effects of tea consumption and suggest directions for future research.

21.2 CHEMISTRY OF TEA CONSTITUENTS AND THEIR BIOAVAILABILITIES

In the manufacturing of green tea, tea leaves are steamed, rolled, and dried, which inactivates enzymes. The drying of the tea leaves helps to stabilize the tea constituents. Green tea possesses characteristic

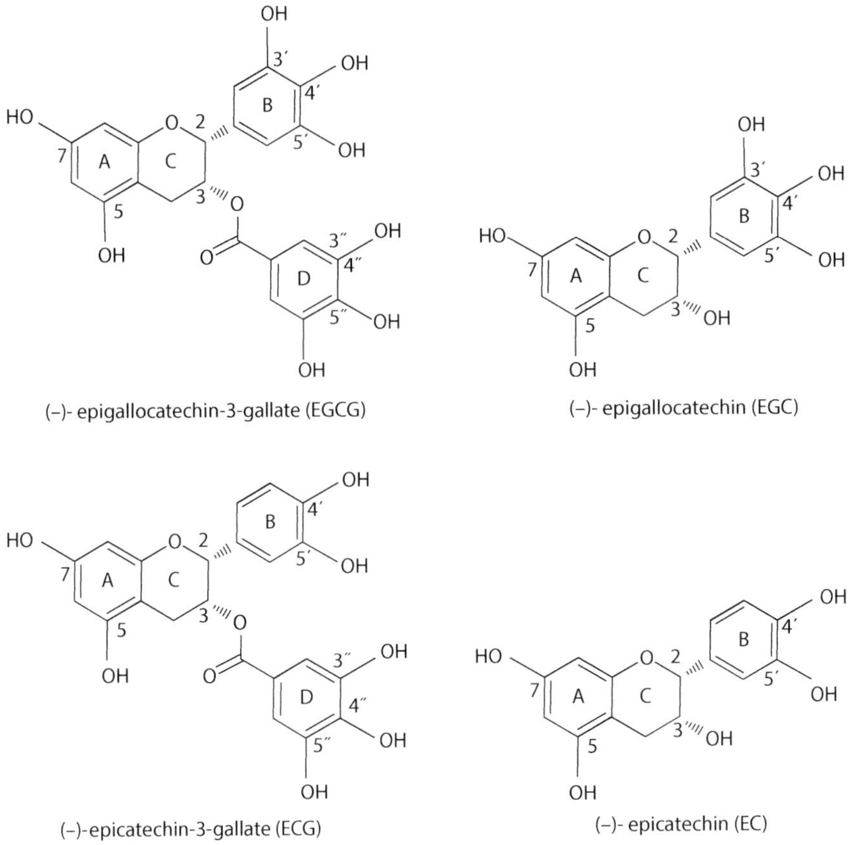

FIGURE 21.1 Structures of tea catechins.

polyphenolic compounds known as catechins, which include (–)-epigallocatechingallate (EGCG), (–)-epigallocatechin (EGC), (–)-epicatechingallate (ECG), and (–)-epicatechin (EC) (Figure 21.1). Catechins account for about 30%–42% of the dry weight of brewed green tea, and EGCG is the major form of tea catechins. Tea leaves also contain lower quantities of other polyphenols, such as quercetin, kaempferol, and myricetin as well as alkaloids, such as caffeine and theobromine. A typical brewed green tea beverage (e.g., 2.5 g tea leaves in 250 mL of hot water) contains 240–320 mg of catechins, of which 60%–65% is EGCG, and 20–50 mg of caffeine (Balentine et al. 1997; Sang et al. 2011). In the manufacturing of black tea, the tea leaves are withered and crushed to cause the release of polyphenol oxidase, which catalyzes the oxidation of catechins in a process commonly referred to as *fermentation*. The oxidized catechins are dimerized and polymerized to form theaflavins and thearubigins, which contribute to the orange, red-brown color and characteristic taste of black tea (Balentine et al. 1997; Sang et al. 2011). Theaflavins are produced from the dimerization of two catechin molecules. Thearubigins are heterogeneous polymers of tea catechins, but their structures are poorly understood (Sang et al. 2011). In brewed black tea, caffeine, catechins, theaflavins, and thearubigins each account for 3%–6%, 3%–10%, 2%–6%, and >20% of the dry weight, respectively. Oolong tea is manufactured by crushing only the rims of the leaves and limiting fermentation to a short period to produce characteristic flavor and taste of the tea. Oolong tea contains catechins, theaflavins, and thearubigins as well as some characteristic components such as epigallocatechin esters, theasinensins, dimericcatechins, and dimericproanthocyanidins (Sang et al. 2011).

Tea catechins and other tea polyphenols are strong antioxidants, efficiently scavenging free radicals. Tea polyphenols also have high affinities to bind metals, preventing metal ion–induced formation of reactive oxygen species (ROS) (Balentine et al. 1997; Sang et al. 2011). The phenolic groups in catechins can be donors for hydrogen bonding. Hydrogen bonding of a catechin molecule to water forms a large hydration shell. This hydrogen bonding capacity also enables tea polyphenols to bind strongly to proteins, lipids, and nucleic acids. EGCG has been shown to bind strongly to 67 kDa laminin receptor, Bcl-2 proteins, and prolyl cis/trans isomerase, and these proteins have been proposed to be the targets of EGCG for anticancer activities (reviewed in Yang et al. 2009). Possessing a greater number of phenolic groups, black tea polyphenols may bind to biomolecules and biomembranes with an affinity even higher than EGCG.

The bioavailability of tea polyphenols follows the Lipinski's rule of 5 (Lipinski et al. 2001) and is dependent on the molecular size, apparent size (due to the formation of a hydration shell), and polarity (reviewed in Yang et al. 2008; Chow and Hakim 2011). For example, the bioavailabilities of EC and catechin (molecular weight 290 and 5 phenolic groups) are much higher than EGCG (molecular weight 458 and 8 phenolic groups). In humans, following the oral administration of the equivalent of two or three cups of green tea, the peak plasma levels of tea catechins (including the conjugated forms) were usually 0.2–0.3 μM (Yang et al. 2008). The plasma concentrations of EGC were usually higher, even though green tea contains less EGC than EGCG. With high pharmacological oral doses of EGCG, peak plasma concentrations of 2–9 and 7.5 μM were reported in mice and humans, respectively (Yang et al. 2008). Active efflux has been shown to limit the bioavailabilities of many polyphenolic compounds. The multidrug resistance-associated protein-2, located on the apical surface of the intestine and liver, mediates the transport of some polyphenolic compounds to the lumen and bile, respectively (Jemnitz et al. 2010). EGCG and its metabolites are predominantly effluxed from the enterocytes into the intestinal lumen, or effluxed from the liver to the bile and excreted in the feces, with little or none of these compounds in the urine (Sang et al. 2011). Theaflavins, because of their higher molecular weights and larger number of phenolic groups, have extremely low bioavailabilities when administered orally (Sang et al. 2011).

EGCG and other tea catechins undergo extensive biotransformations (reviewed in Yang et al. 2008). Because of the catechol structure, EGCG and other catechins are readily methylated by catechol-O-methyltransferase. Catechins are also glucuronidated by UDP-glucuronosyltransferases and sulfated by sulfotransferases. Multiple methylation and conjugation reactions can occur on the same molecule (Sang et al. 2011). Tea catechins can be degraded in the intestinal tract by microorganisms. We have observed the formations of ring fission metabolites 5-(3′,4′,5′-trihydroxyphenyl)-γ-valerolactone (M4), 5-(3′,4′-dihydroxyphenyl)-γ-valerolactone (M6), and 5-(3′,5′-dihydroxyphenyl)-γ-valerolactone (M6′) in human urine and plasma samples due to the ingestion of tea (Li et al. 2000). These compounds can undergo further degradation to phenylacetic and phenylpropionic acids in the intestine and are excreted in the feces and urine.

21.3 LABORATORY STUDIES ON EFFECTS OF TEA ON BODY WEIGHT AND METABOLIC SYNDROME

MetS is a complex of symptoms that include elevated waist circumference and two or more of the following: elevated serum triglyceride, dysglycemia, elevated blood pressure, and reduced high-density lipoprotein–associated cholesterol (Ford 2005). Overweight, obesity, and type 2 diabetes are emerging as major health issues in the United States and many other countries. Therefore, beneficial effects of tea consumption on weight reduction and MetS could have huge public health implications.

The effects of tea and tea polyphenols on body weight and MetS have been studied extensively in animal models. This topic was reviewed recently by Sae-tan et al. (2011). In the 12 publications reviewed concerning body weight reduction, 10 studies showed that the consumption of green tea extracts or EGCG significantly reduced the gaining of body weight and/or adipose tissue weight (Sae-tan et al. 2011). Of the 11 papers reviewed concerning the effects of tea catechin consumption on blood glucose and insulin, all demonstrated beneficial effects in the reduction of blood glucose or insulin levels as well as in the increase of insulin sensitivity or glucose tolerance (Sae-tan et al. 2011). These studies used rodents on high-fat diets or genetically obese/diabetic animal models. For example, in mice fed with a high-fat (60% of the calories) diet, we found that dietary EGCG treatment (3.2 g/kg diet) for 16 weeks significantly reduced body weight gain, percent body fat, and visceral fat weight compared to mice without EGCG treatment (Bose et al. 2008). EGCG treatment also attenuated insulin resistance, plasma cholesterol, and monocyte chemoattractant protein concentrations in mice on the high-fat diet (Basu et al. 2011). These results were also reproduced in a second study using a high-fat/Western-style diet (60% of the calories from fat with low levels of calcium, vitamin D, folic acid, choline bitartrate, and fiber) (Chen et al. 2011). In both studies, EGCG (0.32%) effectively prevented the development of liver steatosis.

As for the mechanisms for weight reduction, there is strong evidence to suggest that tea catechins decreased lipid absorption as reflected in the increased level of fecal lipids (Bose et al. 2008; Chen et al. 2011; Sae-tan et al. 2011). Tea polyphenols can directly bind to lipids and/or change the physicochemical properties of the lipid emulsion to decrease lipid absorption. In a study to investigate the absorption of ^{13}C-enriched dietary triglycerides from corn oil in mice supplemented with 0.25% and 0.50% EGCG, increased ^{13}C levels in the feces of EGCG-treated mice were found, confirming the previously reported phenomenon of EGCG inhibiting lipid absorption (Friedrich et al. 2012). In addition, EGCG treatment also raised the fecal nitrogen content (Friedrich et al. 2012). This finding suggests that in addition to impeding lipid absorption, EGCG also plays a role in inhibiting protein absorption. The finding that EGCG dose dependently decreased food digestibility and increased the fecal mass further supports this idea (Friedrich et al. 2012). There are also reports indicating that dietary supplementation of catechins in rats reduced the activities of enzymes of fatty acid synthesis, such as fatty acid synthase (FAS). Dietary tea catechin treatment in mice has also been shown to activate adenosine monophosphate-activated kinase (AMPK)α to inhibit gluconeogenesis in hepatocytes while simultaneously promoting β-oxidation and other fatty acid degradation enzymes of the liver (Murase et al. 2009). In an experiment with indirect calorimetry to measure oxygen consumption and respiratory quotients for mice exposed to EGCG, a single dosage of EGCG (200 mg/kg body weight) was shown to significantly increase oxygen consumption and fat oxidation in mice during the first 3 h following administration, signifying that EGCG promoted the breakdown of fatty acids for use as an energy source (Murase et al. 2009). Modulation of gene expression, such as peroxisome proliferator-activated receptor (PPAR)γ, FAS, lipases, and uncoupling protein-2 in liver and white adipose tissue by tea catechins, has also been reported (reviewed in Sae-tan et al. 2011).

Obese and insulin-resistant beagle dogs have been used to study the beneficial effect of green tea in alleviating MetS. When the dogs were treated with oral doses of green tea extract (80 mg/kg daily) just before the daily meal for 12 weeks, insulin sensitivity index was markedly increased, and the homeostasis model for insulin resistance was decreased by 20% (Serisier et al. 2008). Tea extract treatment also upregulated mRNA levels of PPARγ, lipoprotein lipase, adiponectin, or glucose transporter (GLUT)-4 in visceral and subcutaneous adipose tissues. The treatment also upregulated PPARα and lipoprotein lipase in the skeletal muscle and induced GLUT4 translocation into the plasma membrane in muscle cells (Serisier et al. 2008). In studies with rats on high-fructose diet, green tea administration for 6 weeks increased GLUT4 and increased insulin receptor substrate (IRS) mRNA levels in the liver and muscle (Cao et al. 2007). In insulin-resistant rats, treatment with green tea polyphenols significantly decreased blood glucose, insulin, triglycerides, total cholesterol, low-density lipoprotein (LDL) cholesterol, and free fatty acids (Qin et al. 2010). It also increased the cardiac mRNA levels of IRS1, IRS2, GLUT1, GLUT4, and glycogen synthase-1 and decreased proinflammatory cytokines (Qin et al. 2010).

Oxidative stress in adipocytes has also been shown to hinder insulin signaling by activating the c-Jun N-terminal kinase (JNK) pathway (Yan et al. 2012). Green tea catechins (150 mg/kg/day) have been shown to reduce JNK phosphorylation in subcutaneous and visceral white adipose tissue and subsequently increase insulin sensitivity by enhancing GLUT4 translocation (Yan et al. 2012). Interestingly, gallated tea catechins such as EGCG (10 mg/kg, i.v.) have shown inhibitory effects on glucose absorption in intestinal cells due to the competitive inhibition of Na-glucose cotransporter-1, while nongallated tea catechins have demonstrated the reversal of this action (Park et al. 2009).

Since diet-induced liver steatosis is becoming a common disease, its possible prevention by tea consumption warrants more investigation in humans. For example, EGCG treatment reduced the incidence of hepatic steatosis, liver size (48% decrease), liver triglycerides (52% decrease), and plasma alanine aminotransferase concentration (67% decrease) in mice fed with the high-fat/Western-style diet (Bose et al. 2008; Chen et al. 2011). Histological analysis of liver samples revealed decreased lipid accumulation in hepatocytes in mice treated with EGCG (Bose et al. 2008; Chen et al. 2011), and this finding may have a potential for practical applications. Tea catechins have been reported to also reduce hepatic steatosis and liver toxicity in rodents treated with ethanol, tamoxifen, or endotoxins and with liver ischemia/reperfusion injury (reviewed in Sae-tan et al. 2011).

21.4 HUMAN STUDIES ON WEIGHT REDUCTION AND ALLEVIATION OF METABOLIC SYNDROME

Results from both epidemiological studies and short-term randomized controlled trials (RCTs) suggest that the consumption of green tea and green tea polyphenol extracts is associated with lower prevalence of clinical features of MetS. The effects of tea consumption on body weight have been studied in many small RCTs during the past decade. Systematic reviews and meta-analysis were conducted by Hursel et al. (2009) and Phung et al. (2010) covering a total of 26 RCTs (Hursel et al. 2009; Phung et al. 2010). Most of these studies used green tea or green tea extracts with caffeine, in studies for 8–12 weeks, in normal weight or overweight subjects. As compared to the caffeine-free controls, most studies demonstrated an effect of lowering body weight, but not waist circumference or waist-to-hip ratio. Several intervention studies have also indicated that green tea drinking had beneficial effects on body composition (reviewed in Rains et al. 2011). A randomized placebo-controlled trial with moderately overweight Chinese subjects showed that daily consumption of 458–886 mg of green tea catechins (<200 mg caffeine) for 90 days reduced total body fat and percent body fat (Wang et al. 2010). In a study on the effect of ingestion of catechin-rich beverages (583 mg daily) in type 2 diabetics over a 12-week period, participants of the experimental group were shown to experience a substantially greater decrease in waist circumference and increase in adiponectin levels as compared to the control group (Nagao et al. 2009). A study with obese patients (body mass index (BMI) ≥ 30 kg/m^2) also demonstrated that 3 months of green tea extract supplementation (379 mg green tea extract and 208 mg of EGCG per day) resulted in decreases in BMI and waist circumference (Suliburska et al. 2012). Improvement of lipid profiles including decreases in levels of total cholesterol, LDL cholesterol, and triglycerides was also observed in this study. A recent metabolomic study with healthy male subjects demonstrated that daily green tea extract supplementation (1200 mg catechins and 240 mg caffeine daily) for 7 days increased metabolite concentrations related to lipolysis (glycerol), fat oxidation(3-β-hydroxybutyrate), and citric acid cycle (citrate) under resting conditions without enhancing adrenergic stimulation (Hodgson et al. 2013). The role of caffeine in these studies was inconsistent among the different studies: some studies suggested that the weight reduction effect was due to caffeine, while others suggested that the effect was due to a combined effect of caffeine and tea catechins. A meta-analysis of metabolic studies showed that both catechin–caffeine mixture and caffeine alone dose dependently stimulated daily energy expenditure, but only the catechin–caffeine combination significantly increased fat oxidation (Hursel et al. 2011).

Two recent clinical studies indicated that green tea supplementation alleviated antioxidant biomarkers and regulated the mineral status in the serum of patients with MetS and/or obesity (Suliburska et al. 2012; Basu et al. 2013). Basu et al. reported that subjects with MetS taking green tea beverage (four cups/day, equivalent to 928 mg of total catechins) or green tea extract capsules (870 mg of total catechins per day) for 8 weeks increased plasma antioxidant capacity and whole blood glutathione, and reduced plasma iron without affecting the serum levels of carotenoids and tocopherols or activities of glutathione peroxidase and catalase (Basu et al. 2013). A study by Suliburska et al. also indicated that, in obese patients, green tea capsules for 3 months increased the serum levels of total antioxidants, zinc, and magnesium but decreased the serum iron concentration (Suliburska et al. 2012). Even shorter-term intake of green tea (up to 900 mg polyphenol equivalent for 5 days) by obese adults at risk for insulin resistance may have beneficial effects in lowering the level of fibrinogen, an acute-phase protein involved in blood clot formation; however, there were no significant effects observed in improving biomarkers of glucose regulation, metabolic homeostasis, oxidative stress, or inflammation (Stote et al. 2012).

Several other human studies have also provided evidence that tea drinking could ameliorate features of MetS and the subsequent risk for type 2 diabetes. An age- and gender-matched study of 35 subjects with obesity and MetS indicated that consumption of green tea beverage (four cups daily) or green tea extracts for 8 weeks significantly decreased body weight, LDL cholesterol, as well as markers of oxidative stress (Basu et al. 2010). The treatments, however, did not significantly alter other features of MetS or biomarkers of inflammation (Basu et al. 2011). An intervention study using green tea capsules for 2 months (400 and 800 mg EGCG as PPE daily) with postmenopausal women showed decreased levels of LDL cholesterol, serum glucose, as well as insulin in groups taking green tea catechins (Wu et al. 2012). Two recent epidemiological studies also support the beneficial effects of green tea consumption on MetS (Chang et al. 2012; Vernarelli and Lambert 2013). One study, on elderly male Taiwanese dwelling in a rural community, indicated that tea drinking, especially for individuals who had drank 240 mL or more tea daily, was inversely associated with incidence of MetS (Chang et al. 2012). The second, a cross-sectional study of U.S. adults, showed that hot tea (but not iced tea) intake was inversely associated with obesity and biomarkers of MetS and CVDs (Vernarelli and Lambert 2013). These results are exciting and need confirmation from additional studies.

There is evidence from some, but not all, human studies that tea consumption is associated with a reduced risk of type 2 diabetes. A meta-analysis based on seven studies ($n = 286,701$ total participants) reported that individuals who drank more than three to four cups of tea per day had lower risks of type 2 diabetes than those consuming no tea (Huxley et al. 2009). A retrospective cohort study of 17,413 Japanese adults aged 40–65 years indicated that consumption of more than six cups of green tea daily (but not oolong or black teas) lowered the risk of diabetes by 33% (Iso et al. 2006). A prospective cross-sectional study with U.S. women aged 45 years and older also showed that the consumption of more than four cups of tea per day was associated with a 30% lower risk of developing type 2 diabetes, whereas the intake of total flavonoids or flavonoid-rich foods was not associated with reduced risk (Song et al. 2005). The effect of caffeine in these epidemiological studies is unclear. Not all epidemiological studies, however, have shown positive results. For example, a recent cross-sectional study that enrolled 554 Japanese adults indicated that there is no correlation between green tea consumption and the prevalence of MetS or any of its components, explaining consumption of coarse tea by Japanese that contains relatively less EGCG as one of the possible reasons for the result (Takami et al. 2013). Several clinical intervention studies have yielded inconclusive results on insulin resistance and blood glucose control, but there are reported changes in certain biomarkers such as an increase in the level of ghrelin (hunger-stimulating peptide), a reduction of hemoglobin A1C, an increase in satiety, and a decrease in diastolic blood pressure (Fukino et al. 2008; Brown et al. 2009; Josic et al. 2010; Hsu et al. 2011).

21.5 RELATIONSHIP TO OTHER DISEASES

The alleviation of MetS by tea logically leads to the reduction of the incidence of type 2 diabetes as reviewed earlier. The lowering of blood lipids and blood pressure by tea is also expected to reduce the risks for CVDs and this has been reported (reviewed in Deka and Vita 2011; Di Castelnuovo et al. 2012). The strongest evidence for the reduction of CVD risk by the consumption of green tea is provided by large cohort studies in Japan. In the Ohsaki National Health Insurance Cohort Study ($n = 40,530$), death due to CVDs was decreased by tea consumption dose dependently from daily consumption of 1 to >5 cups of tea (Kuriyama et al. 2006). In a recent study with 76,979 Japanese adults, the consumption of green tea was also associated with decreased CVD mortality, but daily consumption of >6 cups of tea was needed to manifest the effect (Mineharu et al. 2011). A case-control study in China also showed a correlation between the consumption of green or oolong tea and a decreased risk of ischemic stroke (Liang et al. 2009).

Many, but not all, studies in the United States and Europe demonstrated an inverse association between black tea consumption and CVD risk (Deka and Vita 2011). For example, in the Determinants of Myocardial Infarction Onset Study, black tea consumption (>2 cups daily) was associated with reduced CVD mortality and lower prevalence of ventricular arrhythmia for myocardial infarction during a follow-up for 3.8 years (Mukamal et al. 2006). In a Dutch cohort study involving 37,514 healthy men and women followed for 13 years, consumption of black tea (three to six cups daily) was associated with a decreased risk for CVD mortality (de Koning Gans et al. 2010). In this study, however, tea consumption was also associated with a healthy lifestyle. Apparently, lifestyle and socioeconomic status have confounded the results of many studies (Deka and Vita 2011). The quantity and types of tea consumed are also key factors in affecting the results of these studies. For example, in the Women's Health Study (Sesso et al. 2003), the level of tea consumption was rather low (only a small percentage of women drank more than four cups of black tea per day), and only a trend in the prevention of CVD was observed. In previous meta-analysis, green and black tea drinkers were shown to have lower incidences of myocardial infarction and ischemic stroke (Peters et al. 2001; Arab et al. 2009). However, in a recent meta-analysis of 13 articles investigating the effects of tea consumption on the risk of coronary artery diseases, the consumption of green tea, but not black tea, was found to be beneficial (Wang et al. 2011).

Beneficial effects of tea catechins in preventing hypertension and improving endothelial functions have also been reported. Treatment of rats with green tea extracts (0.6% in drinking water) for 14 days reduced angiotensin II–induced systolic and diastolic blood pressure; this activity may be associated with the inhibition of angiotensin II–induced cardiac NAD(P)H oxidase, which may play a key role in the induction of endothelial oxidative stress (Papparella et al. 2008). In spontaneously hypertensive rats, EGCG treatment significantly decreased systolic blood pressure, decreased myocardial infarct size, and enhanced nitric oxide signaling (Potenza et al. 2007). Tea catechins may suppress caveolin-1, a negative regulator of eNOS (Li et al. 2009), and activate AMPK that leads to activation of PI3K/AKT and eNOS phosphorylation (Zang et al. 2006). Interestingly, EGCG (5 μM) was shown to suppress diabetic vascular inflammation in human critic endothelial cells, while other tea catechins (EC, EGC, and ECG) were ineffective (Babu et al. 2012). While moderate doses of EGCG have yielded beneficial effects, high doses (1% in diet) have been shown to promote, rather than attenuate, vascular inflammation in hyperglycemic mice (Pae et al. 2012).

21.6 MECHANISTIC CONSIDERATIONS

As summarized in Figure 21.2, the prevention of obesity is most likely due to lowering the absorption and digestion of lipids, proteins, and carbohydrates by tea polyphenols. These actions would also alleviate dyslipidemia and dysglycemia. Increasing the rate of fatty acid metabolism by caffeine

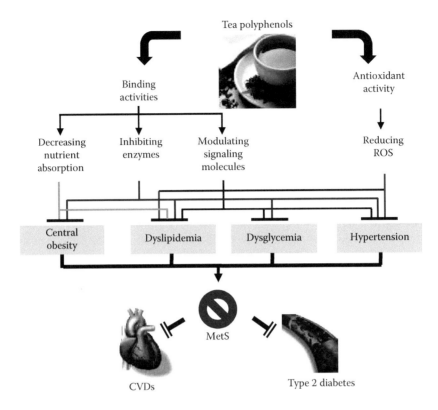

FIGURE 21.2 Proposed mechanisms by which tea polyphenols prevent chronic diseases. ROS, reactive oxygen species; MetS, metabolic syndrome; CVDs, cardiovascular diseases.

and catechins would be an additional mechanism for body weight reduction. These effects would logically result in the alleviation of MetS. The decreased absorption of nutrients could be due to the direct binding activities of tea polyphenols or their alteration of the lipid emulsion in the intestine. Inhibition of carbohydrate digestive enzymes and other enzymes by tea polyphenols has been demonstrated in vitro, and such effect needs to be demonstrated in vivo. It is intriguing that tea polyphenols have been reported to increase the expression or activities of enzymes involved in fatty acid oxidation, but to decrease the levels of enzymes in fatty acid synthesis as well as to alter the expressions or translocations of glucose transporters and IRS. It remains to be determined whether these activities are exerted by tea catechins indirectly through body weight reduction and affecting key metabolic regulators, such as AMPK, or due to direct binding of tea catechins to specific regulators or regulatory elements of genes.

A major mechanism for the lowering of CVD risk is likely due to the cholesterol-lowering effect of green and black tea consumption, which was observed in many observational and intervention studies (Hooper et al. 2008; Deka and Vita 2011). The action could be mainly due to the lowering of the absorption of cholesterol and other lipids by tea polyphenols, as discussed earlier. Specific actions on the inhibition of cholesterol synthesis by EGCG have been proposed, and this topic remains to be further studied. As reviewed by Deka and Vita (2011), a large number of studies showed that green and black tea consumption improves endothelium-dependent vasodilation in individuals with or without atherosclerosis. These beneficial effects may prevent the development or decrease the progression of atherosclerosis, which is a strong risk factor for CVDs.

The antioxidant activities of tea and tea polyphenols have been studied extensively both in vitro and in vivo. A recent meta-analysis of 31 intervention studies on this topic concluded that there was limited evidence that regular consumption of green tea increased plasma antioxidant capacity and reduced LDL oxidation (Ellinger et al. 2011). In recent studies in subjects with MetS or obesity (Suliburska et al. 2012; Basu et al. 2013), however, green tea supplementation has been shown to increase the antioxidant capacity in vivo. It appears that the antioxidant effect of tea is more apparent in animals and humans under higher oxidative stress.

21.7 CONCLUDING REMARKS

As discussed earlier, the beneficial health effects of tea consumption in the alleviation of MetS have been demonstrated by many laboratory studies and epidemiological studies. Whereas many of the effects of green tea are strong and consistent, results on the effects of black tea are inconsistent. The very low or no bioavailability of black tea polyphenols may be a factor that weakens the effects of black tea. Tea polyphenols that are not absorbed into the blood may exert their effects in the gastrointestinal tract, for example, in decreasing lipid and protein absorption. This is probably why black tea is also effective in lowering body weight, body fat, and cholesterol levels.

The intestinal microbiota may degrade tea polyphenols, as have been shown for tea catechins (Li et al. 2000). Some of the metabolites may have interesting biological activities. The microbial degradation of black tea polyphenols has not been sufficiently studied, and more research is needed. The effects of tea consumption on intestinal microorganisms have been studied in past years, and more comprehensive research on the microbiota using newer molecular approaches would provide more information.

In animal studies, conditions are usually optimized to demonstrate the hypothesized effects, and the doses of tea preparations used are usually higher than the levels of human consumption. In human studies, the lack of beneficial effects of tea consumption observed in some studies could be due to the relatively low quantities of tea consumed. Whether we should recommend increased tea consumption to obtain a health benefit is an open question. As a beverage, tea is considered safe, and there are no reports of toxicity from consumption. However, stomach irritation may occur in some individuals due to tea drinking, especially with an empty stomach. Approaches of incorporating green tea powder to food items may be explored to increase the intake of tea polyphenols and fiber.

Ingestion of large amounts of tea, especially as dietary supplement, may cause nutritional and other problems because tea polyphenols may decrease the absorption of nutrients, including minerals and fat-soluble vitamins. Many individuals are taking green tea extracts as dietary supplements for weight reduction. In fact, green tea extracts are the principal ingredients in many weight reduction dietary supplements. Some of the recommended daily doses can reach 1 g or higher. Many cases of hepatotoxicity due to the consumption of green tea extract–based dietary supplements have been reported (reviewed in Mazzanti et al. 2009). The U.S. Pharmacopeia reviewed 216 green tea extract case reports, including 34 reports of liver damage (Sarma et al. 2008). Thus, caution should be applied in the use of high doses of tea extracts for disease prevention.

From a public health perspective, the doses that are required to produce a beneficial effect, such as four cups or more of tea daily for body weight reduction and alleviation of MetS, may be achieved by some individuals but not by others. For the protection against MetS, the effects of lower levels of tea consumption (one to three cups per day) may be subtle. However, in comparison to other beverages, such as sugared or nonsugared soft drinks or ready-made iced tea drinks, freshly brewed green or black tea, consumed without added sugar or cream, appears to be a healthier beverage. In order to obtain a better understanding of the health effects of tea consumption, more research is needed.

ACKNOWLEDGMENTS

This work was supported by NIH grants CA122474 and CA133021.

REFERENCES

Arab, L., W. Liu, and D. Elashoff. 2009. Green and black tea consumption and risk of stroke: A meta-analysis. *Stroke* 40:1786–1792.

Babu, P. V., H. Si, and D. Liu. 2012. Epigallocatechin gallate reduces vascular inflammation in db/db mice possibly through an NF-kappaB-mediated mechanism. *Mol Nutr Food Res* 56:1424–1432.

Balentine, D. A., S. A. Wiseman, and L. C. Bouwens. 1997. The chemistry of tea flavonoids. *Crit Rev Food Sci Nutr* 37:693–704.

Basu, A., N. M. Betts, A. Mulugeta, C. Tong, E. Newman, and T. J. Lyons. 2013. Green tea supplementation increases glutathione and plasma antioxidant capacity in adults with the metabolic syndrome. *Nutr Res* 33:180–187.

Basu, A., M. Du, K. Sanchez et al. 2011. Green tea minimally affects biomarkers of inflammation in obese subjects with metabolic syndrome. *Nutrition* 27:206–213.

Basu, A., K. Sanchez, M. J. Leyva et al. 2010. Green tea supplementation affects body weight, lipids, and lipid peroxidation in obese subjects with metabolic syndrome. *J Am Coll Nutr* 29:31–40.

Bose, M., J. D. Lambert, J. Ju, K. R. Reuhl, S. A. Shapses, and C. S. Yang. 2008. The major green tea polyphenol, (–)-epigallocatechin-3-gallate, inhibits obesity, metabolic syndrome, and fatty liver disease in high-fat-fed mice. *J Nutr* 138:1677–1683.

Brown, A. L., J. Lane, J. Coverly et al. 2009. Effects of dietary supplementation with the green tea polyphenol epigallocatechin-3-gallate on insulin resistance and associated metabolic risk factors: Randomized controlled trial. *Br J Nutr* 101:886–894.

Cao, H., I. Hininger-Favier, M. A. Kelly et al. 2007. Green tea polyphenol extract regulates the expression of genes involved in glucose uptake and insulin signaling in rats fed a high fructose diet. *J Agric Food Chem* 55:6372–6378.

Chang, C. S., Y. F. Chang, P. Y. Liu, C. Y. Chen, Y. S. Tsai, and C. H. Wu. 2012. Smoking, habitual tea drinking and metabolic syndrome in elderly men living in rural community: The Tianliao old people (TOP) study 02. *PloS One* 7:e38874.

Chen, Y. K., C. Cheung, K. R. Reuhl et al. 2011. Effects of green tea polyphenol (–)-epigallocatechin-3-gallate on newly developed high-fat/Western-style diet-induced obesity and metabolic syndrome in mice. *J Agric Food Chem* 59:11862–11871.

Chow, H. H. and I. A. Hakim. 2011. Pharmacokinetic and chemoprevention studies on tea in humans. *Pharmacol Res* 64:105–112.

de Koning Gans, J. M., C. S. Uiterwaal, Y. T. van der Schouw et al. 2010. Tea and coffee consumption and cardiovascular morbidity and mortality. *Arterioscler Thromb Vasc Biol* 30:1665–1671.

Deka, A. and J. A. Vita. 2011. Tea and cardiovascular disease. *Pharmacol Res* 64:136–145.

Di Castelnuovo, A., R. di Giuseppe, L. Iacoviello, and G. de Gaetano. 2012. Consumption of cocoa, tea and coffee and risk of cardiovascular disease. *Eur J Intern Med* 23:15–25.

Ellinger, S., N. Muller, P. Stehle, and G. Ulrich-Merzenich. 2011. Consumption of green tea or green tea products: Is there an evidence for antioxidant effects from controlled interventional studies? *Phytomedicine* 18:903–915.

Ford, E. S. 2005. Prevalence of the metabolic syndrome defined by the International Diabetes Federation among adults in the U.S. *Diabetes Care* 28:2745–2749.

Friedrich, M., K. J. Petzke, D. Raederstorff, S. Wolfram, and S. Klaus. 2012. Acute effects of epigallocatechin gallate from green tea on oxidation and tissue incorporation of dietary lipids in mice fed a high-fat diet. *Int J Obes (Lond)* 36:735–743.

Fukino, Y., A. Ikeda, K. Maruyama, N. Aoki, T. Okubo, and H. Iso. 2008. Randomized controlled trial for an effect of green tea-extract powder supplementation on glucose abnormalities. *Eur J Clin Nutr* 62:953–960.

Hodgson, A. B., R. K. Randell, N. Boon et al. 2013. Metabolic response to green tea extract during rest and moderate-intensity exercise. *J Nutr Biochem* 24:325–334.

Hooper, L., P. A. Kroon, E. B. Rimm et al. 2008. Flavonoids, flavonoid-rich foods, and cardiovascular risk: A meta-analysis of randomized controlled trials. *Am J Clin Nutr* 88:38–50.

Hsu, C. H., Y. L. Liao, S. C. Lin, T. H. Tsai, C. J. Huang, and P. Chou. 2011. Does supplementation with green tea extract improve insulin resistance in obese type 2 diabetics? A randomized, double-blind, and placebo-controlled clinical trial. *Altern Med Rev* 16:157–163.

Hursel, R., W. Viechtbauer, A. G. Dulloo et al. 2011. The effects of catechin rich teas and caffeine on energy expenditure and fat oxidation: A meta-analysis. *Obes Rev* 12:e573–e581.

Hursel, R., W. Viechtbauer, and M. S. Westerterp-Plantenga. 2009. The effects of green tea on weight loss and weight maintenance: A meta-analysis. *Int J Obes (Lond)* 33:956–961.

Huxley, R., C. M. Lee, F. Barzi et al. 2009. Coffee, decaffeinated coffee, and tea consumption in relation to incident type 2 diabetes mellitus: A systematic review with meta-analysis. *Arch Intern Med* 169:2053–2063.

Iso, H., C. Date, K. Wakai, M. Fukui, and A. Tamakoshi. 2006. The relationship between green tea and total caffeine intake and risk for self-reported type 2 diabetes among Japanese adults. *Ann Intern Med* 144:554–562.

Jemnitz, K., K. Heredi-Szabo, J. Janossy, E. Ioja, L. Vereczkey, and P. Krajcsi. 2010. ABCC2/Abcc2: A multi-specific transporter with dominant excretory functions. *Drug Metab Rev* 42:402–436.

Josic, J., A. T. Olsson, J. Wickeberg, S. Lindstedt, and J. Hlebowicz. 2010. Does green tea affect postprandial glucose, insulin and satiety in healthy subjects: A randomized controlled tria. *Nutr J* 30:63.

Kuriyama, S., T. Shimazu, K. Ohmori et al. 2006. Green tea consumption and mortality due to cardiovascular disease, cancer, and all causes in Japan: The Ohsaki study. *JAMA* 296:1255–1265.

Li, C., M. J. Lee, S. Sheng et al. 2000. Structural identification of two metabolites of catechins and their kinetics in human urine and blood after tea ingestion. *Chem Res Toxicol* 13:177–184.

Li, Y., C. Ying, X. Zuo et al. 2009. Green tea polyphenols down-regulate caveolin-1 expression via ERK1/2 and p38MAPK in endothelial cells. *J Nutr Biochem* 20:1021–1027.

Liang, W., A. H. Lee, C. W. Binns, R. Huang, D. Hu, and Q. Zhou. 2009. Tea consumption and ischemic stroke risk: A case-control study in southern China. *Stroke* 40:2480–2485.

Lipinski, C. A., F. Lombardo, B. W. Dominy, and P. J. Feeney. 2001. Experimental and computational approaches to estimate solubility and permeability in drug discovery and development settings. *Adv Drug Deliv Rev* 46:3–26.

Mazzanti, G., F. Menniti-Ippolito, P. A. Moro et al. 2009. Hepatotoxicity from green tea: A review of the literature and two unpublished cases. *Eur J Clin Pharmacol* 65:331–341.

Mineharu, Y., A. Koizumi, Y. Wada et al. 2011. Coffee, green tea, black tea and oolong tea consumption and risk of mortality from cardiovascular disease in Japanese men and women. *J Epidemiol Community Health* 65:230–240.

Mukamal, K. J., M. Alert, M. Maclure, J. E. Muller, and M. A. Mittleman. 2006. Tea consumption and infarct-related ventricular arrhythmias: The determinants of myocardial infarction onset study. *J Am Coll Nutr* 25:472–479.

Murase, T., K. Misawa, S. Haramizu, and T. Hase. 2009. Catechin-induced activation of the LKB1/AMP-activated protein kinase pathway. *Biochem Pharmacol* 78:78–84.

Nagao, T., S. Meguro, T. Hase et al. 2009. A catechin-rich beverage improves obesity and blood glucose control in patients with type 2 diabetes. *Obesity (Silver Spring)* 17:310–317.

Pae, M., Z. Ren, M. Meydani et al. 2012. Dietary supplementation with high dose of epigallocatechin-3-gallate promotes inflammatory response in mice. *J Nutr Biochem* 23:526–531.

Papparella, I., G. Ceolotto, D. Montemurro et al. 2008. Green tea attenuates angiotensin II-induced cardiac hypertrophy in rats by modulating reactive oxygen species production and the Src/epidermal growth factor receptor/Akt signaling pathway. *J Nutr* 138:1596–1601.

Park, J. H., J. Y. Jin, W. K. Baek et al. 2009. Ambivalent role of gallated catechins in glucose tolerance in humans: A novel insight into non-absorbable gallated catechin-derived inhibitors of glucose absorption. *J Physiol Pharmacol* 60:101–109.

Peters, U., C. Poole, and L. Arab. 2001. Does tea affect cardiovascular disease? A meta-analysis. *Am J Epidemiol* 154:495–503.

Phung, O. J., W. L. Baker, L. J. Matthews, M. Lanosa, A. Thorne, and C. I. Coleman. 2010. Effect of green tea catechins with or without caffeine on anthropometric measures: A systematic review and meta-analysis. *Am J Clin Nutr* 91:73–81.

Potenza, M. A., F. L. Marasciulo, M. Tarquinio et al. 2007. EGCG, a green tea polyphenol, improves endothelial function and insulin sensitivity, reduces blood pressure, and protects against myocardial I/R injury in SHR. *Am J Physiol Endocrinol Metab* 292:E1378–E1387.

Qin, B., M. M. Polansky, D. Harry, and R. A. Anderson. 2010. Green tea polyphenols improve cardiac muscle mRNA and protein levels of signal pathways related to insulin and lipid metabolism and inflammation in insulin-resistant rats. *Mol Nutr Food Res* 54:S14–S23.

Rains, T. M., S. Agarwal, and K. C. Maki. 2011. Antiobesity effects of green tea catechins: A mechanistic review. *J Nutr Biochem* 22:1–7.

Sae-tan, S., K. A. Grove, and J. D. Lambert. 2011. Weight control and prevention of metabolic syndrome by green tea. *Pharmacol Res* 64:146–154.

Sang, S., J. D. Lambert, C. T. Ho, and C. S. Yang. 2011. The chemistry and biotransformation of tea constituents. *Pharmacol Res* 64:87–99.

Sarma, D. N., M. L. Barrett, M. L. Chavez et al. 2008. Safety of green tea extracts: A systematic review by the US Pharmacopeia. *Drug Safety* 31:469–484.

Serisier, S., V. Leray, W. Poudroux, T. Magot, K. Ouguerram, and P. Nguyen. 2008. Effects of green tea on insulin sensitivity, lipid profile and expression of PPARalpha and PPARgamma and their target genes in obese dogs. *Br J Nutr* 99:1208–1216.

Sesso, H. D., J. M. Gaziano, S. Liu, and J. E. Buring. 2003. Flavonoid intake and the risk of cardiovascular disease in women. *Am J Clin Nutr* 77:1400–1408.

Song, Y., J. E. Manson, J. E. Buring, H. D. Sesso, and S. Liu. 2005. Associations of dietary flavonoids with risk of type 2 diabetes, and markers of insulin resistance and systemic inflammation in women: A prospective study and cross-sectional analysis. *J Am Coll Nutr* 24:376–384.

Stote, K. S., B. A. Clevidence, J. A. Novotny, T. Henderson, S. V. Radecki, and D. J. Baer. 2012. Effect of cocoa and green tea on biomarkers of glucose regulation, oxidative stress, inflammation and hemostasis in obese adults at risk for insulin resistance. *Eur J Clin Nutr* 66:1153–1159.

Suliburska, J., P. Bogdanski, M. Szulinska, M. Stepien, D. Pupek-Musialik, and A. Jablecka. 2012. Effects of green tea supplementation on elements, total antioxidants, lipids, and glucose values in the serum of obese patients. *Biol Trace Elem Res* 149:315–322.

Takami, H., M. Nakamoto, H. Uemura et al. 2013. Inverse correlation between coffee consumption and prevalence of metabolic syndrome: Baseline survey of the Japan Multi-Institutional Collaborative Cohort (J-MICC) study in Tokushima, Japan. *J Epidemiol* 23:12–20.

Vernarelli, J. A. and J. D. Lambert. 2013. Tea consumption is inversely associated with weight status and other markers for metabolic syndrome in US adults. *Eur J Nutr* 52:1039–1048.

Wang, H., Y. Wen, Y. Du et al. 2010. Effects of catechin enriched green tea on body composition. *Obesity (Silver Spring)* 18:773–779.

Wang, Z. M., B. Zhou, Y. S. Wang et al. 2011. Black and green tea consumption and the risk of coronary artery disease: A meta-analysis. *Am J Clin Nutr* 93:506–515.

Wu, A. H., D. Spicer, F. Z. Stanczyk, C. C. Tseng, C. S. Yang, and M. C. Pike. 2012. Effect of 2-month controlled green tea intervention on lipoprotein cholesterol, glucose, and hormone levels in healthy postmenopausal women. *Cancer Prev Res (Phila)* 5:393–402.

Yan, J., Y. Zhao, S. Suo, Y. Liu, and B. Zhao. 2012. Green tea catechins ameliorate adipose insulin resistance by improving oxidative stress. *Free Radic Biol Med* 52:1648–1657.

Yang, C. S., S. Sang, J. D. Lambert, and M. J. Lee. 2008. Bioavailability issues in studying the health effects of plant polyphenolic compounds. *Mol Nutr Food Res* 52:S139–S151.

Yang, C. S., X. Wang, G. Lu, and S. C. Picinich. 2009. Cancer prevention by tea: Animal studies, molecular mechanisms and human relevance. *Nat Rev Cancer* 9:429–439.

Zang, M., S. Xu, K. A. Maitland-Toolan et al. 2006. Polyphenols stimulate AMP-activated protein kinase, lower lipids, and inhibit accelerated atherosclerosis in diabetic LDL receptor-deficient mice. *Diabetes* 55:2180–2191.

22 Coffee and Metabolic Syndrome

Bruna Miglioranza Scavuzzi, Sílvia Justina Papini, and Édison Miglioranza

CONTENTS

22.1 INTRODUCTION

Coffee is the most valuable agricultural commodity and the second most consumed beverage in the world, behind only plain water (LaComb et al. 2011). It is estimated that more than a billion people around the globe drink coffee daily. The Scandinavian countries have the largest per capita coffee consumption, and the United States has the largest coffee consuming market, where 51% of the population over 20 years consumes approximately 1.5 cups of coffee daily (LaComb et al. 2011). The average size of a coffee cup is about 8 oz or 237 mL. Therefore, due to the widespread consumption of coffee, it is important to know the possible health effects of the beverage.

Coffee is a complex mixture of over 850 volatile and 700 soluble chemical compounds (Padmapriya et al. 2013). The major components in coffee are caffeine, cafestol and kahweol, and chlorogenic acids. Caffeine is a purine alkaloid that has been associated with an increase of metabolic rate and elevation of blood pressure (Higdon and Frei 2006). Cafestol and kahweol are diterpenes that have been linked to anticarcinogenic effects and reports of higher LDL levels in unfiltered coffee (Cavin et al. 2002; Higdon and Frei 2006; Lima et al. 2010). Chlorogenic acids are phenolic compounds that have been associated with anti-inflammatory, antihypertensive, and antidiabetic properties (Farah et al. 2008).

Besides the major components, coffee is also a source of minerals such as potassium, magnesium, manganese, phosphorous, zinc, and chromium (K, Mg, Mn, P, Zn, and Cr, respectively) and vitamins such as niacin and riboflavin (Dórea and Costa 2005; USDA 2014).

The *Coffea* genus contains 103 species (Davis et al. 2006). Of all the species, only two have relevant economic importance: *Coffea arabica* L. and *Coffea canephora* Pierre ex Froehner, marketed as arabica and robusta, respectively. In 2013, the arabica was responsible for 58% and robusta for 42% of global production (USDA 2013). The arabica is the most appreciated in the international market since it produces a milder, fruitier, and acidulous drink. Robusta is considered neutral, weak-flavored, and may have excessive bitterness (Bertrand et al. 2003). There are genetic variations between the two species that result in various concentrations of chemical compounds (Ky et al. 2001).

Lacomb et al. (2011) worked with 38 genotypes of each species (76 total genotypes) and found that the *C. arabica* species has 1.2% of caffeine and 4.1% of chlorogenic acids (CGA), while the *C. canephora* has 2.5% of caffeine and 11.3% CGA (Ky et al. 2001). Therefore, the health effects may vary significantly according to the species of coffee.

Other factors than diverse composition due to genetic differences, the type of brewing and the extent of roasting may also affect the chemical composition of the coffee beverage. Urgert et al. (1995), for example, found that instant, dip-filtered and percolated brews practically did not have cafestol and kahweol. Suzuki et al. (2002) suggested that the hydroxyhydroquinone produced while roasting inhibits the blood pressure lowering effect of chlorogenic acid.

Although coffee was once associated with an unhealthy lifestyle, recent evidences of an inverse association between coffee intake and the risk of type 2 diabetes (T2D) have emerged. Therefore, the potential health effects of coffee on T2D and the metabolic syndrome (MetS) are being debated once again (Schwarz et al. 1994; van Dam and Feskens 2002).

Patients are mostly classified as having MetS according to three or more of the following Adult Treatment Panel (ATP) III criteria: (1) waist circumference ≥ 102 cm in men and ≥88 cm in women, (2) triglycerides ≥ 1.7 mmol/L, (3) HDL cholesterol < 1.0 mmol/L (men) or <1.3 mmol/L (women), (4) blood pressure ≥ 130/85 mmHg or antihypertensive medication use, and (5) glucose ≥ 5.6 mmol/L or antidiabetes medication use (or physician diagnosis for Atherosclerosis Risk in Communities, ARIC). According to International Diabetes Federation (IDF) definition, the presence of abdominal adiposity is mandatory [waist circumference ≥ 94 cm (men) or ≥ 80 cm (women)], and two or more risk factors aforementioned in ATP criteria (Wildman et al. 2011).

Hino et al. (2007) studied the influence of coffee and green tea intake on the components of the MetS in 1902 Japanese over the age of 40. The authors found an inverse and significant association between coffee and every risk factor of the MetS except for HDL cholesterol levels.

Driessen et al. (2009) studied the effects of long-term coffee consumption between the age of 27 and 36 years on the prevalence of the MetS in 368 subjects from the Amsterdam Growth and Health Longitudinal Study. The authors found no association between coffee consumption and the components of the MetS.

Few studies have investigated the influence of coffee on every component of the MetS. Thus, this chapter gathers recent and relevant literature found in at least 130 databases included in the virtual library *Portal CAPES Consortia* (Higher Education Personnel Improvement Coordination–Brazil) published from 1990 to 2014, involving the consumption of coffee and the components of the metabolic syndrome. There were no restriction groups, but searches have focused on texts written in English.

22.2 COFFEE AND OBESITY

Lopes-Garcia et al. (2008) estimated that one cup of coffee has approximately 137 mg of caffeine. Caffeine has been associated with increased thermogenesis, lipogenesis, and energy expenditure (EE) for decades. Acheson et al. (1980) studied changes in metabolic rate after the consumption of coffee in normal and obese individuals and demonstrated a significant thermogenic effect after the ingestion of caffeine. The authors also noticed that fat oxidation was greater in normal-weight individuals than obese subjects. Dulloo et al. (1989) found a significant increase in daily EE of 150 kcal in the lean subjects and 79 kcal in the postobese subjects. Therefore, the expected long-term effect of caffeine intake would be weight reduction.

Besides caffeine, other compounds present in coffee may also have weight loss potential. Greenberg et al. (2005) found an inverse association between coffee consumption (both caffeinated and decaffeinated) with weight loss among subjects under the age of 60. For subjects over the age of 60, only ground-decaffeinated coffee was associated with weight change.

However, the use of high-caloric additions, such as sugar and creamers, may jeopardize the weight loss potential of the beverage. Shields et al. (2004) studied the energy contribution of gourmet coffee beverages to overall dietary intake in college women, and found that regular consumers of those beverages ingested an extra 206 kcal and 32 g of sugar than nonconsumers. The authors concluded that the habit could potentially affect weight status over time. Yannakoulia et al. (2010) noticed a socializing behavior associated to coffee in elderly Mediterranean subjects and reported an increased intake of high calorie foods such as buns and cakes (Table 22.1).

22.3 COFFEE AND INFLAMMATORY AND OXIDATIVE STRESS MARKERS

Free radicals and reactive metabolites, also known as reactive oxygen species (ROS), are products of normal cell metabolism and generated mainly by the mitochondrial respiratory chain. When there is an imbalance between the production of these reactive species and their elimination by antioxidant mechanisms, an excessive accumulation of ROS occurs, leading to oxidative stress. Chronic inflammation may be a result of continued oxidative stress (Reuter et al. 2010).

Scientists consider low-grade systemic inflammation as a key etiologic factor in the development and progression of MetS and cardiovascular diseases (Labonté et al. 2013). Elevated plasma concentrations of C-reactive protein (CRP) and the proinflammatory cytokines tumor necrosis factor α (TNF-α) and interleukin 6 (IL-6) can be associated with an increased risk of cardiovascular disease (Koenig et al. 1999; Ridker et al. 2002; Ballantyne et al. 2004).

Coffee is a major source of antioxidants in the diet, most of which are from the hydroxycinnamic acids family (caffeic, chlorogenic, coumaric, ferulic, and sinapic) (Manach et al. 2004; Svilaas et al. 2004; Dórea and Costa 2005). Numerous studies have reported a decrease in markers of inflammation in subjects with high coffee intake and suggested that the effects were associated to the large concentrations of antioxidants present in coffee (Table 22.2).

22.4 COFFEE AND GLUCOSE HOMEOSTASIS

Pereira et al. (2002) reported abnormal glucose homeostasis as a fasting plasma insulin and glucose of at least 20 μU/mL and 110 mg/dL, respectively, or the use of medications to control blood glucose. Matthews et al. (1985) described a mathematical relation (homeostasis model assessment, HOMA-IR) between fasting plasma glucose and insulin to predict insulin resistance. Lower HOMA-IR values represent higher insulin sensitivity, and higher values correspond to lower insulin sensitivity; the later finding is known as insulin resistance (IR). IR and hyperinsulinemia contribute to the pathogenesis of T2D (Reaven 1988; Di Filippo et al. 2007).

Studies suggest a negative effect of caffeine on glucose metabolism. Acute caffeine intake impairs glucose homeostasis in healthy (Keijzers et al. 2002; Petrie et al. 2004; Battram et al. 2006; Norager et al. 2006; Dekker et al. 2007), obese, and diabetic individuals (Thong and Graham 2002; Robinson et al. 2004; Lee et al. 2005; Lane et al. 2008). Caffeine consumption before an oral glucose tolerance test (OGTT) (Petrie et al. 2004) reduced the insulin sensitivity index (ISI) in 20%–30% (Greer et al. 2001; Keijzers et al. 2002; Lee et al. 2005; Lane et al. 2008) and decreased the glucose infusion rate during a euglycemic–hyperinsulinemic clamp by a similar extent (Greer et al. 2001; Robinson et al. 2004; Battram et al. 2005; Norager et al. 2006; Battram et al. 2007; Beaudoin et al. 2011).

Although caffeine appears to have a detrimental effect on glucose metabolism, numerous recent studies have reported an inverse relation between coffee intake and T2D. Huxley et al. (2009) performed an extensive systematic review of relevant studies published between 1966 and July 2009 on the association between coffee, decaffeinated coffee, and tea consumption with the risk of diabetes. The authors found evidence of a significant inverse log-linear association between coffee intake and T2D protection, where each additional cup of coffee consumed in a day was associated with a 7% reduction in the excess risk of T2D. Decaffeinated coffee consumption was also related to significantly lower risk of T2D, indicating that coffee components other than caffeine are responsible for the protective effect.

TABLE 22.1
Human Studies Considering Coffee and Obesity

Authors	Study	Population	Conclusion
Riedel et al. (2014)	A double-blind, randomized, controlled crossover intervention study to clarify whether two coffee brews, a market blend (MB) and a study blend (SB), differentially affect blood lipid profiles and glucose concentrations	84 healthy normal-weight subjects (38 female and 46 male). From 20 to 44 years	Caffeine may increase free fatty acid utilization and decrease fat content.
Gavrieli et al. (2011)	A crossover study to investigate the acute effects of caffeinated and decaffeinated coffee consumption on appetite feelings, energy intake, and appetite-, inflammation-, stress-, and glucose metabolism–related markers	16 healthy men (age range, 21–39 years; BMI range, 19.7–28.6 kg/m^2)	No short-term effect on appetite or energy intake.
Yannakoulia et al. (2010)	An epidemiological study to assess the association between coffee drinking and BMI and to evaluate the potential mediating effect of lifestyle factors in a population-based sample from the Mediterranean Islands Study (MEDIS)	553 men and 637 women from 67 to 83 years of age	Heavy coffee drinkers had a significantly higher body mass index than nondrinkers.
Arsenault et al. (2009)	A cross-sectional study from women enrolled in the Dose–Response to Exercise in postmenopausal Women (DREW) trial to examine the relationship between coffee consumption, obesity, and plasma CRP levels	344 postmenopausal, sedentary, overweight/ obese women aged 45–75 years with elevated blood pressure	Coffee consumption appears to attenuate the association between body mass index and C-reactive protein in women not using hormone replacement therapy.
Berkey et al. (2008)	A longitudinal cohort of Growing Up Today Study to examine if excessive recreational Internet time, insufficient sleep, regular coffee consumption, or alcoholic beverages promote weight gain	5,036 girls from the United States, aged from 14 to 21 years	No evidence that coffee consumption promotes weight gain.
Lopez-Garcia et al. (2006a)	A prospective study from 1986 to 1998 to assess the relation between caffeine intake and 12-year weight change	18,417 men and 39,740 women with no chronic diseases at baseline	Increases in caffeine intake may lead to a small reduction in long-term weight gain.
Greenberg et al. (2005)	Prospective cohort study, using data from the First National Health and Nutrition Examination Survey Epidemiologic Follow-Up Study to assess the effect of weight change on the relationship between coffee and tea consumption and diabetes risk	7,006 subjects from the United States with no reported history of diabetes, age 32–88 years	The likelihood of gaining weight decreased as coffee (caffeinated and decaffeinated) consumption increased.
Bracco et al. (1995)	A prospective study to investigate the magnitude of coffee-induced thermogenesis and the influence of coffee ingestion on substrate oxidation	10 lean and 10 obese women	Thermogenesis and lipid oxidation increased but were less stimulated in obese than in lean subjects.

TABLE 22.2

Human Studies Considering Coffee and Inflammatory and Oxidative Stress Markers

Authors	Study	Population	Conclusion
Gavrieli et al. (2011)	A crossover study to investigate the acute effects of caffeinated and decaffeinated coffee consumption on appetite feelings, energy intake, inflammation, stress hormones, and glucose metabolism–related markers.	16 healthy men (age range, 21–39 years; BMI range, 19.7–28.6 kg/m²).	No short-term effect on inflammatory markers.
Pham et al. (2011)	A cohort study on lifestyle-related diseases. The authors examined the relation of coffee consumption on serum CRP considering potential interactions of serum γ-glutamyltransferase (GGT) and bilirubin.	4,455 men and 5,942 Japanese women aged 49–76 years.	Serum CRP concentrations were progressively lower with higher intake of coffee in men with high serum GGT.
Rebello et al. (2011)	Cross-sectional data from the Singapore Prospective study-2 (SP2) cohort to evaluate the associations between habitual coffee and tea consumption and possible mediation by inflammation.	4,139 Singaporeans	No significant association between coffee and inflammatory markers.
Kempf et al. (2010)	A 3-month single-blind (investigator), 3-stage clinical trial to investigate the effects of daily coffee consumption on biomarkers of coffee intake, subclinical inflammation, oxidative stress, glucose, and lipid metabolism.	47 subjects, younger than 65 years with an elevated risk of T2D.	Significant decrease of IL-18 and 8-isoprostane and a significant increase in adiponectin. No significant changes were found for IL-6, MIF, IL-1ra, leptin, CRP, SAA, and nitrotyrosine.
Arsenault et al. (2009)	A cross-sectional study from women enrolled in the Dose–Response to Exercise in postmenopausal Women (DREW) trial to examine the relationship between coffee consumption, obesity, and plasma CRP levels.	344 postmenopausal, sedentary, overweight/obese women aged 45–75 years with elevated blood pressure.	Coffee consumption is negatively associated with CRP.
Williams et al. (2008)	A prospective cohort study from the Nurses' Health Study to test whether the beneficial effects of coffee consumption in metabolism might be explained by changes in circulating levels of adiponectin.	982 women with T2D and 1,058 healthy women.	Consumption of four or more cups of caffeinated coffee was associated with higher adiponectin concentrations on both groups. Inverse association of coffee and inflammatory markers CRP and TNF-α receptor II among diabetic women. No association between consumption of decaffeinated coffee and adiponectin concentration was found.

(*Continued*)

TABLE 22.2 (*Continued*)
Human Studies Considering Coffee and Inflammatory and Oxidative Stress Markers

Authors	Study	Population	Conclusion
Andersen et al. (2006)	A 15-year follow-up study to investigate the relation of coffee drinking with diseases with a major inflammatory component.	27,312 postmenopausal women aged 55–69 years at baseline were followed for 15 years.	Consumption of coffee may inhibit inflammation in postmenopausal women.
Lopez-Garcia et al. (2006b)	A prospective study to assess the relation between long-term coffee and decaffeinated filtered coffee consumption and markers of inflammation and endothelial dysfunction.	730 healthy women and 663 women with T2D.	Inverse association between coffee and E-selectin and CPR on women with T2D and an inverse association between coffee and CPR on healthy women.
Zampelas et al. (2004)	A cross-sectional survey from the ATTICA study to investigate the associations between coffee consumption and inflammatory markers.	1,438 men and 1,482 women aged 18–89 years with no history of CVD.	Subjects who consumed >200 mL coffee/day had higher IL-6, CRP, serum amyloid-A, and TNF-α concentrations than those who did not consume coffee.

Williams et al. (2008) found that a regular intake of four or more cups per day of caffeinated coffee presented approximately 20% higher serum adiponectin concentrations than those with a smaller coffee consumption. Adiponectin, a plasma protein derived from adipose tissue, has several beneficial effects on human health, such as antiatherogenic effects on vascular cells and antidiabetic properties. Low adiponectin levels, also known as hypoadiponectinemia, are related to IR and T2D (Funahashi and Matsuzawa 2006).

Although type 2 diabetes is a complication and not a risk factor for MetS, studies regarding the relationship between coffee daily intake and T2D were included in the summary table, since abnormal glucose homeostasis is a major risk factor for T2D (Table 22.3).

22.5 COFFEE AND HYPERTENSION

Numerous studies have suggested that caffeine in coffee slightly increases blood pressure (BP) shortly after intake in normotensive subjects. Jee et al. (1999) conducted a meta-analysis of 11 controlled clinical trials and found a relationship between coffee intake and higher blood pressure.

Results from various studies regarding blood pressure were not consistent, and recent studies have reported a protective effect against T2D, a strong risk factor for cardiovascular disease, raising the interest again to study the effects of caffeine on the cardiovascular system. Grobbee et al. (1990) studied 45,589 individuals and found no support for the hypothesis that coffee or caffeine consumption increases the risk of coronary heart disease or stroke.

Robertson et al. (1981) found that a tolerance to blood pressure effects was developed after 1–4 days of caffeine ingestion (150 mg/day for 7 days). Additionally, coffee has other components, such as potassium, magnesium, and chlorogenic acid, that may protect the cardiovascular system (Noordzij et al. 2005).

Noordzij et al. (2005) performed a meta-analysis of 16 randomized controlled trials published between January 1966 and January 2003 to study the chronic effect of coffee or caffeine on BP. When comparing the BP effects of caffeine tablets versus coffee drinks, the authors found that the pressure effect is two to three times smaller when caffeine was ingested through coffee.

TABLE 22.3
Human Studies Considering Coffee and Glucose Homeostasis

Authors	Study	Population	Conclusion
Riedel et al. (2014)	A double-blind, randomized, controlled crossover intervention study to clarify whether two coffee brews, a market blend (MB) and a study blend (SB), differentially affect blood lipid profiles and glucose concentrations	84 healthy normal-weight subjects (38 female and 46 male). 20–44 years of age	No significant changes in glucose metabolism.
Gavrieli et al. (2011)	A crossover study to investigate the acute effects of caffeinated and decaffeinated coffee consumption on appetite feelings, energy intake, inflammation, stress hormones, and glucose metabolism–related markers	16 healthy men (age range, 21–39 years; BMI range, 19.7–28.6 kg/m²)	No short-term effect on glucose metabolism.
Rebello et al. (2011)	Cross-sectional data from the Singapore Prospective Study-2 (SP2) cohort to evaluate the associations between habitual coffee and tea consumption and glucose metabolism in a multiethnic Asian population	4,139 Singaporeans	Inverse association between coffee and HOMA-IR.
Zhang et al. (2011)	A prospective cohort study to examine the association between coffee consumption and the incidence of T2D in persons with normal glucose tolerance in a population with a high incidence and prevalence of diabetes	1,141 American Indian subjects. 45–74 years of age	A high level of coffee consumption was associated with a reduced risk of deterioration of glucose metabolism over an average 7.6 years of follow-up.
Kempf et al. (2010)	A 3-month single-blind (investigator), three-stage clinical trial to investigate the effects of daily coffee consumption on biomarkers of coffee intake, subclinical inflammation, oxidative stress, glucose, and lipid metabolism	47 subjects, younger than 65 years with an elevated risk of T2D	No changes in glucose metabolism.
Pereira et al. (2006)	An 11-year prospective cohort study to examine the association between total, caffeinated, and decaffeinated coffee intake and risk of incident T2D	28,812 postmenopausal women free of diabetes and cardiovascular disease	Coffee intake, especially decaffeinated, was inversely associated with the risk of T2D in postmenopausal women.
van Dam et al. (2006)	A prospective cohort study of the Nurses' Health Study II to verify if moderate consumption of both caffeinated and decaffeinated coffee may lower the risk of T2D in younger and middle-aged women	88,259 U.S. women aged 26–46 years without history of diabetes at baseline	Moderate consumption of caffeinated and decaffeinated coffee may lower the risk of T2D in younger and middle-aged women. Coffee constituents other than caffeine may affect the development of T2D.

(Continued)

TABLE 22.3 (*Continued*)
Human Studies Considering Coffee and Glucose Homeostasis

Authors	Study	Population	Conclusion
Greenberg et al. (2005)	Prospective cohort study, using data from the First National Health and Nutrition Examination Survey Epidemiologic Follow-Up Study, to assess the effect of weight change on the relationship between coffee and tea consumption and diabetes risk	7,006 subjects from the United States with no reported history of diabetes, age 32–88 years.	Negative relationship between diabetes risk and consumption of ground coffee and regular tea observed for all nonelderly subjects, who had previously lost weight.
Salazar-Martinez et al. (2004)	Prospective cohort study from the Nurses' Health Study and Health Professionals' Follow-up Study to examine the long-term relationship between consumption of coffee and other caffeinated beverages and incidence of T2D	41,934 men and 84,276 women with no diabetes, cancer, or cardiovascular disease at baseline	Long-term coffee consumption is associated with a statistically significantly lower risk for T2D.
Tuomilehto et al. (2004)	A prospective study to determine the relationship between coffee consumption and the incidence of T2D among Finnish individuals, who have the highest coffee consumption in the world	6,974 Finnish men and 7,655 women aged 35–64 years with no history of stroke, coronary heart disease, or DM at baseline	Coffee intake was inversely associated with the risk of T2D.
van Dam and Feskens (2002)	A prospective study to investigate the association between coffee consumption and risk of clinical T2D in a population-based cohort	17,111 Dutch subjects aged 30–60 years	Coffee consumption was associated with a substantially lower risk of clinical T2D.

Studies have associated a BP-lowering effect of green coffee bean extract (GCE) to chlorogenic acid (CGA) and suggested that hydroxyhydroquinone (HHQ) produced while roasting inhibits the effect of CGA. Therefore, the conflicting information on the effects of coffee on blood pressure may also be related to the different concentrations of caffeine and CGA on the beverage (Suzuki et al. 2002; Ochiai et al. 2009; Kozuma et al. 2005; Yamaguchi et al. 2008; Medina-Remón et al. 2011) (Table 22.4).

22.6 COFFEE AND PLASMA LIPID PROFILE

Jee et al. (2001) conducted a meta-analysis of 14 randomized controlled trials published prior to December 1998 to study the effect of coffee on serum lipids. A dose–response association between coffee intake and LDL and total cholesterol was identified, particularly among hyperlipidemic subjects in trials with caffeinated or boiled coffee.

Studies found that boiled coffee increased the concentration of cholesterol levels in humans (Thelle et al. 1983; Aro et al. 1987; Bak and Grobbee 1989). Aro et al. (1987) studied the effects of boiled coffee, filtered coffee, and tea on serum lipoprotein lipids and found that only boiled coffee increased the concentration of low-density lipoprotein. Therefore, the lipid-raising effect is influenced by the method of brewing. In a later study, van Dusseldorp et al. (1991b) found that most of the cholesterol-raising factor from boiled coffee did not pass a paper filter. Urgert et al. (1997) found

TABLE 22.4

Human Studies Considering Coffee and Hypertension

Authors	Study	Population	Conclusion
Yamaguchi et al. (2008)	A double-blind, randomized controlled trial to investigate the dose–response relationship for CGA in HHQ-free coffee on BP in mildly hypertensive subjects	203 subjects	CGA has an antihypertensive effect in a dose-dependent manner in HHQ-free coffee. Ordinary coffee showed almost no effect on BP.
Kozuma et al. (2005)	A double-blind, randomized, placebo-controlled, parallel group study to evaluate the dose–response relationship of BP to GCE consumption	117 male subjects with mild hypertension	GCE has a blood pressure–lowering effect in patients with mild hypertension.
Kirchhoff et al. (1994)	A population survey to assess the blood pressure in relation to age, sex, weight, height, diabetes, serum lipids, and consumption of coffee, tobacco, and alcohol	3,608 Danish subjects aged 30 to 60 years	The influence of coffee on blood pressure has no potential clinical importance.
Burke et al. (1992)	A cross-sectional study to assess the association between certain lifestyle and personality characteristics and blood pressure in the elderly	843 subjects (338 women and 505 men) aged 60 to 87 years	Higher blood pressure was associated with greater body mass index (BMI), alcohol intake and coffee drinking, and measures of irritability.
Löwik et al. (1991)	A prospective study from the Dutch Nutrition Surveillance System to investigate the associations between blood pressure and nutrition-related variables	255 subjects (138 men and 117 women) aged 65 to 79 years old and who did not use drugs known to affect blood pressure and were not on a diet.	Coffee consumption was positively correlated with blood pressure.
van Dusseldorp et al. (1991a)	A randomized controlled trial to verify the long-term effects of the coffee brewing method on BP levels	64 healthy subjects (33 men and 31 women) aged 17 to 57 years	Boiled and filtered coffee did not affect BP or heart rate. Boiled coffee caused a slight but significant rise in BP.
Salvaggio et al. (1990)	A prospective study to assess the association between habitual coffee consumption and blood pressure levels	9601 subjects (7,506 men and 2,095 women) who were office managers and employees, aged 18–65 years	Blood pressure levels decreased with increasing coffee consumption.

that cafestol, a lipid-soluble diterpene present in coffee beans, is responsible for the cholesterol-raising property of unfiltered coffee (Table 22.5).

22.7 CONCLUSION

Most of the literature found on our extensive database search indicated a potential beneficial effect of coffee consumption over at least one component of the Metabolic Syndrome. Most studies associating coffee with obesity, glucose homeostasis, and inflammatory/oxidative stress markers had either no effect or positive effects on human health. The T2D-protective potential of coffee seems promising and needs to be further studied considering that the rate of diabetes is growing rapidly worldwide.

TABLE 22.5

Human Studies Considering Coffee and Plasma Lipid Profile

Authors	Study	Population	Conclusion
Riedel et al. (2014)	A double-blind, randomized, controlled crossover intervention study to clarify whether two coffee brews, a market blend (MB) and a study blend (SB), differentially affect blood lipid profiles and glucose concentrations.	84 healthy normal-weight subjects (38 female and 46 male). From 20 to 44 years	Increase in HDL cholesterol.
Kempf et al. (2010)	A 3-month single-blind (investigator), three-stage clinical trial to investigate the effects of daily coffee consumption on biomarkers of coffee intake, subclinical inflammation, oxidative stress, glucose, and lipid metabolism	47 subjects, younger than 65 years with an elevated risk of T2D	Increase in HDL cholesterol.
Strandhagen and Thelle (2003)	A prospective, controlled study to assess the effects of the intake and abstention of filtered brewed coffee on blood lipids	121 healthy, nonsmoking subjects aged 29–65 years	Filtered coffee abstention for 3 weeks decreased total serum cholesterol.
Christensen et al. (2001)	A prospective intervention study to assess the effects of filtered coffee consumption on the concentrations of total homocysteine and total cholesterol	191 healthy, nonsmoking, coffee-drinking subjects aged 24–69 years	Abstaining from even commonly consumed amounts of filtered coffee may lower the concentrations of both total homocysteine and total cholesterol.
Fried et al. (1992)	A randomized controlled trial to determine the effect of filtered coffee consumption on plasma lipoprotein cholesterol levels in healthy men	100 healthy male subjects	Consumption of filtered, caffeinated coffee increases the total cholesterol plasma level (HDL/LDL).
Superko et al. (1991)	A randomized controlled trial to study caffeinated and decaffeinated coffee effects on plasma lipoprotein cholesterol, apolipoproteins, and lipase activity.	181 healthy, nonsmoking, coffee-drinking subjects.	Change from caffeinated to decaffeinated coffee increased plasma LDL and apolipoprotein B. Discontinuation of caffeinated coffee produced no change.
van Dusseldorp et al. (1991b)	A randomized controlled trial to verify the long-term effects of the coffee brewing method on BP levels	64 healthy subjects (33 men and 31 women) aged 17 to 57 years	Cholesterol-raising factor from boiled coffee does not pass a paper filter.

Nonetheless, increased blood pressure and LDL cholesterol were reported in some but not all studies and those findings cannot be overlooked. Although studies have suggested that the cholesterol-raising component, cafestol, does not pass the paper filter, and hydroxyhydroquinone-free coffee may even have a hypotensive effect, those results must be confirmed in other studies.

More studies are needed to evaluate the effects of coffee on the components of the MetS. The studies should ideally specify the coffee genotype, brewing, and degree of roasting as well as the concentration of the major components involved in the health effect since these components seem to influence the health outcomes.

REFERENCES

Acheson, K.J., Zahorska-Markiewicz, B., Pittet, P., Anantharaman, K., Jéquier, E. 1980. Caffeine and coffee: Their influence on metabolic rate and substrate utilization in normal weight and obese individuals. *Am J Clin Nutr* 33(5):989–997.

Andersen, L.F., Jacobs Jr, D.R., Carlsen, M.H., Blomhoff, R. 2006. Consumption of coffee is associated with reduced risk of death attributed to inflammatory and cardiovascular diseases in the Iowa Women's Health Study. *Am J Clin Nutr* 83(5):1039–1046.

Aro, A., Tuomilehto, J., Kostiainen, E., Uusitalo, U., Pietinen, P. 1987. Boiled coffee increases serum low density lipoprotein concentration. *Metabolism* 36(11):1027–1030.

Arsenaulti, B.J., Earnest, C.P., Després, J-P, Blair, S.N., Church, T.S. 2009. Obesity, coffee consumption and CRP levels in postmenopausal overweight/obese women: Importance of hormone replacement therapy use. *Eur J Clin Nutr* 63(12):1419–1424.

Bak, A.A., Grobbee, D.E. 1989. The effect on serum cholesterol levels of coffee brewed by filtering or boiling. *N Engl J Med* 321(21):1432–1437.

Ballantyne, C.M., Hoogeveen, R.C., Bang, H. et al. 2004. Lipoprotein-associated phospholipase A2, high-sensitivity C-reactive protein, and risk for incident coronary heart disease in middle-aged men and women in the Atherosclerosis Risk in Communities (ARIC) study. *Circulation* 109:837–842.

Battram, D.S., Arthur, R., Weekes, A., Graham, T.E. 2006. The glucose intolerance induced by caffeinated coffee ingestion is less pronounced than that due to alkaloid caffeine in men. *J Nutr* 136(5):1276–1280.

Battram, D.S., Graham, T.E., Dela, F. 2007. Caffeine's impairment of insulin-mediated glucose disposal cannot be solely attributed to adrenaline in humans. *J Physiol* 583(3):1069–1077.

Battram, D.S., Graham, T.E., Richter, E.A., Dela, F. 2005. The effect of caffeine on glucose kinetics in humans: Influence of adrenaline. *J Physiol* 569(1):347–355.

Beaudoin, M.S., Robinson, L.E., Graham, T.E. 2011. An oral lipid challenge and acute intake of caffeinated coffee additively decrease glucose tolerance in healthy men. *J Nutr* 141(4):574–581.

Berkey, C.S., Rockett, H.R.H., Colditz, G.A. 2008. Weight gain in older adolescent females: The internet, sleep, coffee, and alcohol. *J Pediatr* 153(5):635–639.

Bracco, D., Ferrarra, J.M., Arnaud, M.J., Jéquier, E., Schutz, Y. 1995. Effects of caffeine on energy metabolism, heart rate, and ethylxanthine metabolism in lean and obese women. *Am J Physiol* 269(4 Pt 1):E671–678.

Bertrand, B., Guyot, B., Anthony, F., Lashermes, P. 2003. Impact of the *Coffea canephora* gene introgression on beverage quality of *C. arabica*. *Theor Appl Genet* 107(3):387–394.

Burke, V., Beilin, L.J., German, R. et al. 1992. Association of lifestyle and personality characteristics with blood pressure and hypertension: A cross-sectional study in the elderly. *J Clin Epidemiol* 45(10):1061–1070.

Cavin, C., Holzhaeuser, D., Scharf, G. et al. 2002. Cafestol and kahweol, two coffee specific diterpenes with anticarcinogenic activity. *Food Chem Toxicol* 40(8):1155–1163.

Christensen, B., Mosdol, A., Retterstol, L., Landaas, S., Thelle, D.S. 2001. Abstention from filtered coffee reduces the concentrations of plasma homocysteine and serum cholesterol—A randomized controlled trial. *Am J Clin Nutr* 74(3):302–307.

Davis, A.P., Govaerts, R., Bridson, D.M., Stoffelen, P. 2006. An annotated taxonomic conspectus of the genus *Coffea* (Rubiaceae). *Bot J Linn Soc* 152(4):465–512.

Dekker, M.J., Gusba, J.E., Robinson, L.E., Graham, T.E. 2007. Glucose homeostasis remains altered by acute caffeine ingestion following 2 weeks of daily caffeine consumption in previously non-caffeine-consuming males. *Br J Nutr* 98(3):556–562.

Di Filippo, C., Verza, M., Coppola, L. et al. 2007. Insulin resistance and postprandial hyperglycemia the bad companions in natural history of diabetes: Effects on health of vascular tree. *Curr Diabetes Rev* 3:268–273.

Dórea, J.G., Costa, T.H.M. 2005. Review article: Is coffee a functional food? *Br J Nutr* 93(6):773–782.

Driessen, M.T., Koppes, L.L., Veldhuis, L., Samoocha, D., Twisk, J.W. 2009. Coffee consumption is not related to the metabolic syndrome at the age of 36 years: The Amsterdam Growth and Health Longitudinal Study. *Eur J Clin Nutr* 63(4):536–542.

Dulloo, A.G., Geissler, C.A., Horton, T., Collins, A., Miller, D.S. 1989. Normal caffeine consumption: Influence on thermogenesis and daily energy expenditure in lean and postobese human volunteers. *Am J Clin Nutr* 49(1):44–50.

Farah, A., Monteiro, M., Donangelo, C.M., Lafay, S. 2008. Chlorogenic acids from green coffee extract are highly bioavailable in humans. *J Nutr* 138(12):2309–2315.

Fried, R.E., Levine, D.M., Kwiterovich, P.O. et al. 1992. The effect of filtered-coffee consumption on plasma lipid levels. Results of a randomized clinical trial. *JAMA* 267(6):811–815.

Funahashi, T., Matsuzawa, Y. 2006. Hypoadiponectinemia: A common basis for diseases associated with overnutrition. *Curr Atheroscler Rep* 8(5):433–438.

Gavrieli, A., Yannakoulia, M., Fragopoulou, E. et al. 2011. Caffeinated coffee does not acutely effect energy intake, appetite, or inflammation but prevents serum cortisol concentrations from falling in healthy men. *J Nutr* 141(4):703–707.

Greenberg, J.A., Axen, K.V., Schnoll, R., Boozer, C.N. 2005. Coffee, tea and diabetes: The role of weight loss and caffeine. *Int J Obes Relat Metab Disord* 29(9):1121–1129.

Greer, F., Hudson, R., Ross, R., Graham, T.E. 2001. Caffeine ingestion decreases glucose disposal during a hyperinsulinemic-euglycemic clamp in sedentary humans. *Diabetes* 50(10):2349–2354.

Grobbee, D.E., Rimm, E.B., Giovannucci, E. et al. 1990. Coffee, caffeine, and cardiovascular disease in men. *N Engl J Med* 323(15):1026–1032.

Higdon, J.V., Frei, B. 2006. Coffee and health: A review. *Crit Rev Food Sci Nutr* 46(2):101–123.

Hino, A., Adachi, H., Enomoto, M. et al. 2007. Habitual coffee but not green tea consumption is inversely associated with metabolic syndrome: An epidemiological study in a general Japanese population. *Diabetes Res Clin Pract* 76(3):383–389.

Huxley, R., Lee, C.M., Barzi, F. et al. 2009. Coffee, decaffeinated coffee, and tea consumption in relation to incident type 2 diabetes mellitus a systematic review with meta-analysis. *Arch Intern Med* 169(22):2053–2063.

Hwang, S.J., Kim, Y.W., Park, Y., Lee, H.J., Kim, K.W. 2014. Anti-inflammatory effects of chlorogenic acid in lipopolysaccharide-stimulated RAW 264.7 cells. *Inflamm Res* 63(1):81–90.

Jee, S.H., He, J., Whelton, P.K., Suh, I., Klag, M.J. 1999. The effect of chronic coffee drinking on blood pressure: a meta-analysis of controlled clinical trials. *Hypertension* 33(2):647–652.

Jee, S.H., He, J., Appel, L.J. et al. 2001. Coffee consumption and serum lipids: A meta-analysis of randomized controlled clinical trials. *Am J Epidemiol* 153(4):353–362.

Keijzers, G.B., Galan, B.E., Tack, C.J., Smits, P. 2002. Caffeine can decrease insulin sensitivity in humans. *Diabetes Care* 25(2):364–369.

Kempf, K., Herder, C., Erlund, I. et al. 2010. Effects of coffee consumption on subclinical inflammation and other risk factors for type 2 diabetes: A clinical trial. *Am J Clin Nutr* 91(4):950–957.

Kirchhoff, M., Torp-Pedersen, C., Hougaard, K. et al. 1994. Casual blood pressure in a general Danish population. Relation to age, sex, weight, height, diabetes, serum lipids and consumption of coffee, tobacco and alcohol. *J Clin Epidemiol* 47(5):469–474.

Koenig, W., Sund, M., Fröhlich, M. et al. 1999. C-reactive protein, a sensitive marker of inflammation, predicts future risk of coronary heart disease in initially healthy middle-aged men—Results from the MONICA (Monitoring Trends and Determinants in Cardiovascular Disease) Augsburg Cohort Study, 1984 to 1992. *Circulation* 99(2):237–242.

Kozuma, K., Tsuchiya, S., Kohori, J., Hase, T., Tokimitsu, I. 2005. Antihypertensive effect of green coffee bean extract on mildly hypertensive subjects. *Hypertens Res* 28(9):711–718.

Ky, C.-L., Louarn, J., Dussert, S., Guyot B., Hamon, S., Noirot, M. 2001. Caffeine, trigonelline, chlorogenic acids and sucrose diversity in wild *Coffea arabica* L. and *C. canephora* P. accessions. *Food Chem* 75(2):223–230.

Labonté, M.È., Couture, P., Richard, C., Desroches, S., Lamarche, B. 2013. Impact of dairy products on biomarkers of inflammation: A systematic review of randomized controlled nutritional intervention studies in overweight and obese adults. *Am J Clin Nutr* 97(4):706–717.

LaComb, R.P., Sebastian, R.S., Wilkinson, E.C., Goldman, J.D. 2011. Beverage choices of U.S. adults: What we eat in America, NHANES 2007–2008. Food Surveys Research Group Dietary Data Brief No. 6. http://ars.usda.gov/Services/docs.htm?docid=19476 (retrieved June 1, 2014).

Lane, J.D., Feinglos, M.N., Surwit, R.S. 2008. Caffeine increases ambulatory glucose and postprandial responses in coffee drinkers with type 2 diabetes. *Diabetes Care* 31(2):221–222.

Lee, S., Hudson, R., Kilpatrick, K., Graham, T.E., Ross, R. 2005. Caffeine ingestion is associated with reductions in glucose uptake independent of obesity and type 2 diabetes before and after exercise training. *Diabetes Care* 28(3):566–572.

Lima, F.A., Sant'ana, A.E.G., Ataíde, T.R. et al. 2010. Coffee in human health: A discussion on the substances present in beverages related to cardiovascular diseases (in Portuguese). *Rev Nutr* 23(6):1063–1073.

Lopez-Garcia, E., van Dam, R.M., Lu, Q., Hu, F.B. 2006b. Coffee consumption and markers of inflammation and endothelial dysfunction in health and diabetic women. *Am J Clin Nutr* 84(4):888–893.

Lopez-Garcia, E., van Dam, R.M., Li, T.Y., Rodriguez-Artalejo, F., Hu, F.B. 2008. The Relationship of Coffee Consumption with Total and Disease-Specific Mortality: A Cohort Study. *Ann Intern Med* 148(12):904–914.

Lopez-Garcia, E., van Dam, R.M., Rajpathak, S. et al. 2006a. Changes in caffeine intake and long-term weight change in men and women. *Am J Clin Nutr* 83(3):674–680.

Löwik, M.R., Hofman, Z., Kok, F.J. et al. 1991. Nutrition and blood pressure among elderly men and women (Dutch Nutrition Surveillance System). *J Am Coll Nutr* 10(2):149–155.

Manach, C., Scalbert, A., Morand, C., Rémésy, C., Jiménez, L. Polyphenols: Food sources and bioavailability. *Am J Clin Nutr* 79(5):727–747.

Matthews, D.R., Hosker, J.P., Rudenski, A.S., Naylor, B.A., Treacher, D.F., Turner, R.C. 1985. Homeostasis model assessment: Insulin resistance and beta-cell function from fasting plasma glucose and insulin concentrations in man. *Diabetologia* 28(7):412–419.

Medina-Remón, A., Zamora-Ros, R., Rotchés-Ribalta, M. et al. 2011. Total polyphenol excretion and blood pressure in subjects at high cardiovascular risk. *Nutr Metab Cardiovasc Dis* 21(5):323–331.

Noordzij, M., Uiterwaal, C.S., Arends, L.R. et al. 2005. Blood pressure response to chronic intake of coffee and caffeine: A meta-analysis of randomized controlled trials. *J Hypertens* 23(5):921–928.

Norager, C.B., Jensen, M.B., Weimann, A., Madsen, M.R. 2006. Metabolic effects of caffeine ingestion and physical work in 75-year old citizens. A randomized, double-blind, placebo controlled, cross-over study. *Clin Endocrinol (Oxf)* 65(2):223–228.

Ochiai, R., Chikama, A., Kataoka, K., Tokimitsu, I., Maekawa, Y., Ohishi, M., et al. 2009. Effects of hydroxy-hydroquinone-reduced coffee on vasoreactivity and blood pressure. *Hypertens Res* 32(11):969–974.

Padmapriya, R., Tharian, J.A., Thirunalasundari, T. 2013. Coffee waste management—An overview. *Int J Curr Sci* 9:E83–E91.

Pereira, M.A., Jacobs, Jr., D.R., van Horn, L. et al. 2002. Dairy consumption, obesity, and the insulin resistance syndrome in young adults. The CARDIA study. *JAMA* 287(16):2081–2089.

Pereira, M.A., Parker, E.D., Folsom, A.R. 2006. Coffee consumption and risk of type 2 diabetes mellitus: An 11-year prospective study of 28 812 postmenopausal women. *Arch Intern Med* 166(12):1311–1316.

Petrie, H.J., Chown, S.E., Belfie, L.M., Duncan, A.M., McLaren, D.H. 2004. Caffeine ingestion increases the insulin response to an oral-glucose-tolerance test in obese men before and after weight loss. *Am J Clin Nutr* 80(1):22–28.

Pham, N.M., Wang, Z., Morita, M. et al. 2011. Combined effects of coffee consumption and serum γ-glutamyltransferase on serum C-reactive protein in middle-aged and elderly Japanese men and women. *Clin Chem Lab Med* 49(10):1661–1667.

Reaven, G.M. 1988. Role of insulin resistance in human disease. *Diabetes* 37(12):1595–1607.

Rebello, S.A., Chen, C.H., Naidoo, N. et al. 2011. Coffee and tea consumption in relation to inflammation and basal glucose metabolism in a multi-ethnic Asian population: A cross-sectional study. *Nutr J* 10:61.

Reuter, S., Gupta, S.C., Chaturvedi, M.M., Aggarwal, B.B. 2010. Oxidative stress, inflammation and cancer: How are they linked? *Free Radic Biol Med* 49(11):1603–1616.

Ridker, P.M., Rifai, N., Rose, L., Buring, J.E., Cook, N.R. 2002. Comparison of C-reactive protein and low-density lipoprotein cholesterol levels in the prediction of first cardiovascular events. *N Engl J Med* 347:1557–1565.

Riedel, A., Dieminger, N., Bakuradze, T. et al. 2014. A 4-week consumption of medium roast and dark roast coffees affects parameters of energy status in healthy subjects. Food Research International. Available online April 16, 2014. http://www.sciencedirect.com/science/article/pii/S0963996914002403 (Retrieved June 4, 2014).

Robertson, D., Wade, D., Workman, R., Woosley, R.L., Oates, J.A. 1981. Tolerance to the humoral and hemodynamic effects of caffeine in man. *J Clin Invest* 67:1111–1117.

Robinson, L.E., Savani, S., Battram, D.S. et al. 2004. Caffeine ingestion before an oral glucose tolerance test impairs blood glucose management in men with type 2 diabetes. *J Nutr* 134(10):2528–2533.

Salazar-Martinez, E., Willett, W.C., Ascherio, A. et al. 2004. Coffee consumption and risk for type 2 diabetes mellitus. *Ann Intern Med* 140(1):1–8.

Salvaggio, A., Periti, M., Miano, L., Zambelli, C. 1990. Association between habitual coffee consumption and blood pressure levels. *J Hypertens* 8(6):585–590.

Schwarz, B., Bischof, H.P., Kunze, M. 1994. Coffee, tea, and lifestyle. *Prev Med* 23(3):377–384.

Shields, D.H., Corrales, K.M., Metallinos-Katsaras, E. 2004. Gourmet coffee beverage consumption among college women. *J Am Diet Assoc* 104(4):650–653.

Strandhagen, E., Thelle, D.S. 2003. Filtered coffee raises serum cholesterol: Results from a controlled study. *Eur J Clin Nutr* 57(9):1164–1168.

Superko, H.R., Bortz Jr, W., Williams, P.T., Albers, J.J., Wood, P.D. 1991. Caffeinated and decaffeinated coffee effects on plasma lipoprotein cholesterol, apolipoproteins, and lipase activity: A controlled, randomized trial. *Am J Clin Nutr* 54(3):599–605.

Suzuki, A., Kagawa, D., Ochiai, R., Tokimitsu, I., Saito, I. 2002. Green coffee bean extract and its metabolites have a hypotensive effect in spontaneously hypertensive rats. *Hypertens Res* 25(1):99–107.

Svilaas, A., Sakhi, A.K., Andersen, L.F. et al. 2004. Intakes of antioxidants in coffee, wine, and vegetables are correlated with plasma carotenoids in humans. *J Nutr* 134(3):562–567.

Thelle, D.S., Arnesen, E., Førde, O.H. 1983. The Tromsø heart study. Does coffee raise serum cholesterol? *N Engl J Med* 308(24):1454–1457.

Thong, F.S.L., Graham, T.E. 2002. Caffeine-induced impairment of glucose tolerance is abolished by beta-adrenergic receptor blockade in humans. *J Appl Physiol* 92(6):2347–2352.

Tuomilehto, J., Hu, G., Bidel, S., Lindström, J., Jousilahti, P. 2004. Coffee consumption and risk of type 2 diabetes mellitus among middle-aged Finnish men and women. *JAMA* 291(10):1213–1219.

Urgert, R., van der Weg, G., Kosmeijer-Schuil, T.G., van de Bovenkamp, P., Hovenier, R., Katan, M.B. 1995. Levels of the Cholesterol-Elevating Diterpenes Cafestol and Kahweol in Various Coffee Brews. *J Agric Food Chem* 43(8):2167–2172.

Urgert, R., Essed, N., van der Weg, G., Kosmeijer-Schuil, T.G., Katan, M.B. 1997. Separate effects of the coffee diterpenescafestol and kahweol on serum lipids and liver aminotransferases. *Am J Clin Nutr* 65(2):519–524.

U.S. Department of Agriculture and Agricultural Research Service. 2013. Coffee: World markets and trade. USDA. Washington, DC. http://apps.fas.usda.gov/psdonline/circulars/coffee.pdf (Retrieved June 4, 2014).

U.S. Department of Agriculture and Agricultural Research Service. 2014. Nutrient database for standard reference, Release 26. USDA. Washington, DC. http://ndb.nal.usda.gov/ndb/foods/show/4290 (Retrieved June 10, 2014).

van Dam, R.M., Feskens, E.J. 2002. Coffee consumption and risk of type 2 diabetes mellitus. *Lancet* 360 (9344):1477–1478.

van Dam, R.M., Willett, W.C., Manson, J.E., Hu, F.B. 2006. Coffee, caffeine, and risk of type 2 diabetes: A prospective cohort study in younger and middle-aged U.S. women. *Diabetes Care* 29(2):398–403.

van Dusseldorp, M., Katan, M.B., van Vliet, T., Demacker, P.N., Stalenhoef, A.F. 1991b. Cholesterol-raising factor from boiled coffee does not pass a paper filter. *Arterioscler Thromb Vasc Biol* 11(3):586–593.

van Dusseldorp, M., Smits, P., Lenders, J.W., Thien, T., Katan, M.B. 1991a. Boiled coffee and blood pressure. A 14-week controlled trial. *Hypertension* 18(5):607–613.

Wildman, R.P., McGinn, A.P., Kim, M. et al. 2011. Empirical derivation to improve the definition of the Metabolic Syndrome in the evaluation of cardiovascular disease risk. *Diabetes Care* 34(3):746–748.

Williams, C.J., Fargnoli, J.L., Hwang, J.J. et al. 2008. Coffee consumption is associated with higher plasma adiponectin concentrations in women with or without type 2 diabetes—A prospective cohort study. *Diabetes Care* 31(3):504–507.

Yamaguchi, T., Chikama, A., Mori, K. et al. 2008. Hydroxyhydroquinone-free coffee: A double-blind, randomized controlled dose-response study of blood pressure. *Nutr Metab Cardiovasc Dis* 18(6):408–414.

Yannakoulia, M., Tyrovolas, S., Bountziouka, V. et al. 2010. The mediating effect of physical activity and smoking on the relationship between coffee drinking and body weight in elderly individuals: The Mediterranean Islands study. *J Am Geriatr Soc* 58(6):1208–1210.

Zampelas, A., Panagiotakos, D.B., Pitsavos, C., Chrysohoou, C., Stefanadis, C. 2004. Associations between coffee consumption and inflammatory markers in healthy persons: The ATTICA study. *Am J Clin Nutr* 80(4):862–867.

Zhang, Y., Lee, E.T., Cowan, L.D., Fabsitz, R.R., Howard, B.V. 2011. Coffee consumption and the incidence of type 2 diabetes in men and women with normal glucose tolerance: The Strong Heart Study. *Nutr Metab Cardiovasc Dis* 21(6):418–423.

23 Alcoholic Beverages

Fernanda Aparecida Domenici and Hélio Vannucchi

CONTENTS

23.1 INTRODUCTION

Alcohol beverage is any beverage that contains ethyl alcohol, also called ethanol. It can be considered as the top-selling drug on the planet, and alcoholism as a serious public health problem worldwide. Alcoholism is generally defined as the consistent and excessive consumption of alcoholic beverages to the extent that this behavior interferes with the person's normal, family, social, or professional life. Alcoholism can cause psychological or physiological conditions and also death (Lee et al. 2005).

Alcohol consumption is common in almost all countries and is considered the world's third largest risk factor for diseases and disabilities and the greatest risk factor in middle-income countries (Baan et al. 2007). Alcohol consumption and problems related to alcohol vary widely around the world, but the burden of disease and death remains significant in most countries. Alcohol is a causal factor in 60 types of diseases and injuries and a component cause in 200 others. Almost 4% of all deaths worldwide are attributed to alcohol, greater than deaths caused by HIV/AIDS, violence, or tuberculosis. Alcohol is also associated with many social issues, including violence, child neglect and abuse, and absenteeism in the workplace. The harmful use of alcohol remains a low priority in health policy, whereas many lesser health risks have higher priority (WHO 2011).

According to the World Health Organization, the global consumption of alcohol has increased in recent decades, especially in developing countries. Worldwide, alcohol-related diseases are responsible for approximately 1.8 million deaths and 4% of the global burden of disease. The incidence is highest in the Americas and Europe, where it ranges from 8% to 18% for men and 2% to 4% for women (WHO 2011).

23.2 ALCOHOL METABOLISM

The hepatic metabolism of ethanol is quite dichotomous from that of glucose. Upon oral ingestion of 120 kcal of ethanol, approximately 10% is metabolized by the stomach and intestine in a *first-pass* effect before entry into the portal circulation (Baraona et al. 2001). Another 10% are metabolized by muscle and kidney. Approximately 96 cal reach the liver, accounting for four times the substrate as for glucose. Ethanol enters the hepatocyte through osmosis and does not stimulate insulin secretion.

Once inside the liver, ethanol bypasses glycolysis and is converted by alcohol dehydrogenase 1B (ADH1B) to form acetaldehyde, which, because of its free aldehyde, can generate reactive oxygen species (ROS) and toxic damage (Farfan Labonne et al. 2009) if not quenched by hepatic antioxidants such as glutathione or ascorbic acid (Dey and Cederbaum 2006).

Although the liver is the main organ responsible for metabolizing ingested alcohol, gastric alcohol dehydrogenase (ADH) has been reported to contribute to first-pass metabolism. The relative contribution of the stomach and the liver to first-pass metabolism is controversial. Thus, whereas first-pass metabolism is attributed predominantly to the stomach (Lim et al. 1993; Baraona 2000), other studies stress the role of the liver (Lee et al. 2006). Human ADH, which is present in the liver and stomach, metabolizes alcohol poorly in the liver but may play an important role in first-pass metabolism in the stomach, because gastric alcohol concentrations can reach molar range during alcohol consumption. Alcohol is also metabolized in nonliver tissues that do not contain ADH, such as the brain, by the enzymes cytochrome P450 and catalase. In general, alcohol metabolism is achieved by both oxidative pathways, which either add oxygen or remove hydrogen, and nonoxidative pathways (Baraona et al. 2001; Lee et al. 2003).

23.3   OXIDATIVE PATHWAYS

The enzymes ADH, cytochrome P450 2E1 (CYP2E1), and catalase all contribute to oxidative metabolism of alcohol. ADH, present in the fluid of the cell, converts alcohol to acetaldehyde. This reaction involves an intermediate carrier of electrons, nicotinamide adenine dinucleotide (NAD$^+$), which is reduced by two electrons to form NADH. Acetaldehyde is metabolized mainly by aldehyde dehydrogenase 2 (ALDH$_2$) in the mitochondria to form acetate and NADH. Catalase, located in cell bodies called peroxisomes, requires hydrogen peroxide (H$_2$O$_2$) to oxidize alcohol. CYP2E1, which is present predominantly in the cell's microsomes, assumes an important role in metabolizing ethanol to acetaldehyde at elevated ethanol concentrations (Lieber 1997).

The major pathway of oxidative metabolism of ethanol in the liver involves ADH, an enzyme with many different variants. Metabolism of ethanol with ADH produces acetaldehyde, a highly reactive and toxic by-product that may contribute to tissue damage and the addictive process (Gemma et al. 2006). ADH constitutes a complex enzyme family, and, in humans, five classes have been categorized based on their kinetic and structural properties. At high concentrations, alcohol is eliminated at a high rate because of the presence of enzyme systems with high activity levels, such as class II ADH, β$_3$-ADH, and CYP2E1. This oxidation process involves an intermediate carrier of electrons, nicotinamide adenine dinucleotide (NAD$^+$), which is reduced by two electrons to form NADH. As a result, alcohol oxidation generates a highly reduced cytosolic environment in hepatocytes (Seitz and Becker 2007).

The cytochrome P450 isozymes, including CYP2E1, 1A2, and 3A4, which are present predominantly in the microsomes, or vesicles, of a network of membranes within the cell known as the endoplasmic reticulum, also contribute to alcohol oxidation in the liver. In moderate alcohol consumption, the microsomal ethanol oxidizing system CYP2E1 pathway accounts for a small fraction of alcohol metabolism, ADH representing the more common pathway for alcohol oxidization (Lieber and DeCarli 1972). CYP2E1 is induced by chronic alcohol consumption and have an important role in metabolizing ethanol to acetaldehyde at elevated ethanol concentrations. In addition, CYP2E1-dependent ethanol oxidation may occur in other tissues, such as the brain, where ADH activity is low. It also produces ROS, especially hydroxyethyl, superoxide anion, and hydroxyl radicals, which increase the risk of tissue damage (Seitz and Becker 2007; Lu and Cederbaum 2008).

Ethanol induces hepatocellular damage through several different mechanisms, including mitochondrial damage, membrane effects, hypoxia, cytokine production, and iron mobilization (Dey and Cederbaum 2006). Ethanol is thought to exert toxicity through its metabolism by ADH1B to the intermediary acetaldehyde, which, because of its free aldehyde moiety engages rapidly

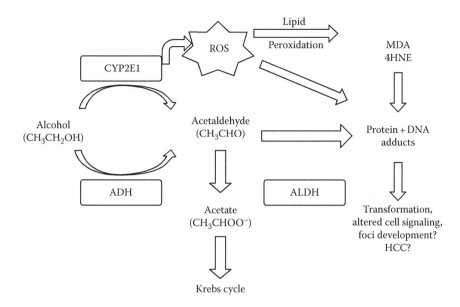

FIGURE 23.1 Pathways of alcohol metabolism. (Data from McKillop, I.H. and Schrum, L.W., *Semin. Liver Dis.*, 29(2), 222, 2009.)

in ROS formation. In the absence of antioxidants, these ROS may lead to lipid peroxidation, fibrogenesis, and cirrhosis (Niemela et al. 1995). ROS can form DNA and protein adducts directly. They can also react with lipid molecules in the cell membrane, resulting in biologically reactive aldehyde molecules, such as 4-hydroxynonenal (4HNE) and malondialdehyde (MDA), compounds that are similar to acetaldehyde (Figure 23.1) (Baan et al. 2007; Seitz and Becker 2007; Lu and Cederbaum 2008).

Catalase, an enzyme located in cell bodies called peroxisomes, is capable of oxidizing ethanol in vitro in the presence of a hydrogen peroxide (H_2O_2)-generating system, such as the enzyme complex NADPH oxidase or the enzyme xanthine oxidase. This is considered a minor pathway of alcohol oxidation, except in the fasted state (Tran et al. 2007; Strumnik and Karski 2012; Heit et al. 2013).

23.4 NONOXIDATIVE PATHWAYS

The nonoxidative metabolism of alcohol is minimal, but its products may have pathological and diagnostic relevance. Alcohol is nonoxidatively metabolized by at least two pathways. One leads to the formation of molecules called fatty acid ethyl esters (FAEEs) from the reaction of alcohol with fatty acids, resulting in weak organic acids that play functional roles in human cells. The other nonoxidative pathway results in the formation of a phospholipid known as phosphatidyl ethanol. FAEEs are detectable in serum and other tissues after alcohol ingestion and persist long after alcohol is eliminated (Werner et al. 2002).

The second nonoxidative pathway requires the enzyme phospholipase D (PLD), which breaks down phospholipids, primarily phosphatidylcholine, to generate phosphatidic acid (PA). This pathway is a critical component in cellular communication. The product of this reaction, phosphatidyl ethanol, is poorly metabolized and may accumulate to detectable levels following chronic consumption of large amounts of alcohol, but its effects on the cell remain to be established (Agarwal 2001; Wilson and Apte 2003).

Oxidative and nonoxidative pathways of alcohol metabolism are interrelated. Inhibition of ethanol oxidation by compounds that inhibit ADH, CYP2E1, and catalase results in an increase in the nonoxidative metabolism of alcohol and increased production of FAEEs in the liver and pancreas (Werner et al. 2002).

23.5   GENETIC ASPECTS OF ALCOHOL METABOLISM

Variations in the rate of alcohol absorption, distribution, and elimination contribute significantly to clinical conditions observed after chronic alcohol consumption. These variations have been attributed to both genetic and environmental factors, gender, drinking pattern, fasting or fed states, and chronic alcohol consumption. Variations in the genes encoding ADH and ALDH produce alcohol- and acetaldehyde-metabolizing enzymes that vary in activity. Polymorphism (SNPs) occurs at the ADH1B and ADH1C gene locations and these different genes are associated with varying levels of enzymatic activity. The ADH1B variations occur at different frequencies in different populations. This genetic variability influences a person's susceptibility to developing alcoholism (Agarwal 2001).

Because SNPs of ADH and ALDH2 play an important role in determining peak blood acetaldehyde levels and voluntary ethanol consumption, they also influence vulnerability to alcohol dependence. A fast ADH or a slow ALDH are expected to elevate acetaldehyde levels and thus reduce alcohol drinking (Quintanilla et al. 2005). ADH and ALDH isozyme activity also influences the prevalence of alcohol-induced tissue damage. Alcoholic cirrhosis is reduced in populations carrying the ALDH2*2 allele (Chao et al. 1994; Nagata et al. 2002).

Elevated acetaldehyde levels induced by ALDH inhibitors were shown to protect against alcohol-induced liver injury in experimental animals (Lindros et al. 1999) and to reduce the release of a signaling molecule, a cytokine, called tumor necrosis factor alpha (TNF-α) from Kupffer cells. This finding is quite contradictory to the belief that acetaldehyde plays a role in liver damage (Nakamura et al. 2004). Studies in the literature found that neither ADH nor ALDH alleles were significantly associated with liver cirrhosis (Zintzaras et al. 2006).

Both acute administration of high doses and chronic administration of ethanol have been reported to produce significant damage to the heart, liver, pancreas, gastrointestinal tract, and brain in humans and experimental animals (Nordmann et al. 1992). Ethanol might be associated with cancer in a variety of ways, including chemical carcinogenesis and a direct contribution in the initiation of cancer. The toxic effects of ethanol may be due to DNA damage, since ethanol itself is not genotoxic, and its metabolism to acetaldehyde is essential for the generation of DNA single-strand breaks (Singh and Khan 1995; Brooks 1997). Ethanol has a mutagenic, carcinogenic, and teratogenic effect in man, and the mechanism by which ethanol exerts its genotoxicity is not understood (Navasumrit et al. 2000). A study (Tavares et al. 2001) showed that chronic administration of ethanol had no clastogenic or cytotoxic effect. The cytochromes P450 activity increased after chronic ethanol consumption, thus possibly preventing the ethanol that has entered the circulation from reaching excessive levels (Tavares et al. 2001).

Alcohol consumption increases the risk of head and neck squamous cell carcinoma. Genotyping data for 64 SNPs in 12 genes were obtained from 1227 African American subjects from North Carolina from 2002 to 2006. Most tested SNPs were not associated with survival, with the exception of the minor alleles of rs3813865 and rs8192772 in CYP2E1. Hazard ratios for eight additional SNPs in CYP2E1, GPx2, SOD1, and SOD2, though not statistically significant, were suggestive of differences in allele hazards for all-cause and cancer death. No consistent associations with survival were found for SNPs in ADH1B, ADH1C, ADH4, ADH7, ALDH2, GPx2, GPx4, and catalase (Hakenewerth et al. 2013).

23.6   CONSEQUENCES OF ALCOHOL METABOLISM

Ethanol metabolism by CYP2E1 and NADH oxidation by the electron transport chain generate ROS that results in lipid peroxidation. This process results in the formation of compounds known as MDA and 4HNE, both of which can form adducts with proteins (Worrall and Thiele 2001;

Wu and Cederbaum 2003). Acetaldehyde and MDA together can react with proteins to generate a stable MDA–acetaldehyde–protein adduct (MAA), as well as induce inflammatory processes in certain types of liver cells (Tuma et al. 1996; Tuma 2002). These and other findings indicate a link between MDA, 4HNE, and MAA adducts and subsequent development of liver disease (Tuma and Casey 2003).

Reactive oxygen species, including superoxide ($O_2^{\bullet-}$), hydrogen peroxide (H_2O_2), hypochlorite ion (OCl^-), and hydroxyl ($^\bullet OH$) radicals, are naturally generated by many reactions in multiple regions of the cell. ROS act by stealing hydrogen atoms from other molecules, thereby converting those molecules into highly reactive free radicals. Also, ROS can combine with stable molecules to form free radicals. Through both of these mechanisms, ROS play an important role in carcinogenesis, atherosclerosis, diabetes, inflammation, aging, and other harmful processes to health. To prevent the damage these reactive compounds can cause, numerous defense systems have evolved in the body involving antioxidants, which can interact with ROS and convert them into harmless molecules. Under normal conditions, a balance between ROS and antioxidants exists in the cells. When this balance is disturbed and an excess of ROS is present, a state known as oxidative stress results (Wu and Cederbaum 2003).

The formation of the free radicals generated by acute ethanol administration has been demonstrated to exert an important role in the pathogenesis of liver injury in rats (Jordao et al. 2004). Administration of ethanol induces an increase in lipid peroxidation both by producing oxygen reactive species and by decreasing the levels of endogenous antioxidants. In a study conducted in 2004, dietary vitamin E caused a dose-dependent increase in liver and plasma concentration of the vitamin, but ethanol administration decreased hepatic vitamin E. Lipid peroxidation was higher in liver of rats that received a deficient diet in vitamin E, independent of ethanol. On the other hand, liver lipid peroxidation was low in control and supplemented groups, but increased with ethanol ingestion. In conclusion, acute administration of ethanol affect vitamin E level, and maintenance of adequate or higher vitamin E levels acts as a protective factor against free radical generation (Jordao et al. 2004).

23.7 METABOLIC SYNDROME

Low to moderate alcohol consumption is associated with increased risk of metabolic syndrome (MetS) and other age-related diseases, including Alzheimer's disease, fractures and osteoporosis, diabetes, ulcer, gallstones, duodenal ulcer, hepatitis A, lymphomas, kidney stones, pancreatic cancer, Parkinson's disease, rheumatoid arthritis, and gastritis (Facchini et al. 1994; Freiberg et al. 2004; Duell et al. 2011).

MetS is a combination of several clinical features, including central obesity, high blood pressure, hyperinsulinemia, impaired fasting and postprandial glucose tolerance, elevated concentrations of triacylglycerols and free fatty acids, low concentrations of HDL cholesterol, and insulin resistance (IR) (Isomaa et al. 2001; Lakka et al. 2002). Microalbuminuria, hyperuricemia, elevated leptin and diminished adiponectin blood level, and plasminogen activator inhibitor type-1 level elevation have also been reported in the MetS (Hanson et al. 2002; Reaven 2005). The clustering of these features has been speculated to increase the risk of cardiovascular disease because each component is associated with the disease. Studies reported that the MetS markedly increases cardiovascular morbidity and mortality (Isomaa et al. 2001; Lakka et al. 2002).

It is believed that a sedentary lifestyle is a key determinant for the occurrence of MetS. Other modifiable risk factors such as diet and cigarette smoking also play an important role in the development of the syndrome in individuals with a genetic predisposition for this group of diseases (Chen et al. 2008).

Recently, an interesting hypothesis to explain the pathophysiology of the MetS has been proposed by Di Chiara et al. (2012) that evaluate the role of inflammation and adipocytokines on the occurrence of the syndrome. In normal conditions, adiponectin carries out its roles for preventing

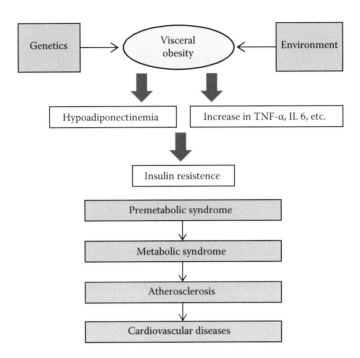

FIGURE 23.2 Progression and outcomes of visceral obesity. (Data from Di Chiara, T. et al., *J. Nutr. Metab.* 2012, 175245, 2012.)

development of vascular changes and the impairment of glucose and lipid metabolism, which may be induced by a variety of attacking factors, such as chemical substances, mechanical stress, or nutritional factors (Di Chiara et al. 2012). Studies on the adiponectin gene showed its important role in the prevention of MetS (Takahashi et al. 2000; Hiuge-Shimizu et al. 2011). In the presence of obesity with visceral fat accumulation and hypertension, hypoadiponectinemia together with the increase of other adipocytokines, such as TNF-α, may be an important background of vascular changes, as well as metabolic disorders, including IR, which characterize the MetS (Figure 23.2). Thus, hypoadiponectinemia is considered a link between visceral obesity and the MetS (Di Chiara et al. 2012).

A study (Simao et al. 2012) that evaluated the components of MetS related to adiponectin levels in overweight and obese patients showed increased inflammatory markers associated with IR and abdominal obesity. Except for an inverse correlation with adiponectinemia, serum levels of uric acid were not correlated with any other inflammatory marker, suggesting a role of uric acid in the etiology of hypoadiponectinemia in the MetS. The authors suggest that further investigations are needed to confirm this probability (Simao et al. 2012) (Figure 23.2).

23.8   ALCOHOL AND METABOLIC SYNDROME

Alcohol has both adverse and protective effects on the components of the MetS. Although some studies associate light to moderate ethanol consumption with improved insulin sensitivity (Facchini et al. 1994; Howard et al. 2004) and wine consumption with reduced cardiovascular risk (Di Castelnuovo et al. 2009), other cross-sectional (Sakurai et al. 1997; Athyros et al. 2007) and prospective studies implicate a dose-dependent effect of chronic consumption of larger doses of ethanol, mainly in beer, in the genesis of IR and the MetS (Athyros et al. 2007).

Alcohol consumption is positively associated with abdominal obesity (Tolstrup et al. 2005; Riserus and Ingelsson 2007; Schroder et al. 2007), high triglyceride levels (Ruixing et al. 2008), high blood pressure (Sesso et al. 2008; Taylor et al. 2009), and hyperglycemia

(Carlsson et al. 2005; Koppes et al. 2005). On the other hand, alcohol consumption has a protective effect on the development of MetS by increasing HDL-C levels (Suh et al. 1992; Linn et al. 1993; Ruixing et al. 2008).

Although beneficial health effects have been reported at lower doses of alcohol consumption, it is important to determine the minimum amount of alcohol necessary to cause beneficial effects (Zhang et al. 2006). Studies have reported an association between alcohol drinking and the prevalent MetS, with inconsistent findings (Park et al. 2003; Freiberg et al. 2004; Lee et al. 2005; Fan et al. 2006). While some authors reported an inversely linear relationship between alcohol consumption and MetS (Djousse et al. 2004; Freiberg et al. 2004), others observed a positively linear relationship (Fan et al. 2006). Such relation appears to differ by types of alcoholic beverage. Compared with nondrinking, light to moderate drinking of wine and beer is favorable for reducing the prevalence odds ratio of MetS (Rosell et al. 2003; Djousse et al. 2004), whereas liquor drinking tends to increase the ratio (Rosell et al. 2003) or has no association with the MetS (Djousse et al. 2004; Freiberg et al. 2004).

Moderate consumption of alcohol appears to have a beneficial effect in the prevention of atherosclerosis. There is also evidence that alcohol may decrease IR and that it also has an antiplatelet effect (Wallerath et al. 2003). Polyphenols from red wines, such as resveratrol, appear to offer significant benefit for cardiovascular disease prevention via its antioxidant activity and increase in nitric oxide concentrations (Baur and Sinclair 2006; Zhang et al. 2009). The increase in endothelial-type nitric oxide synthase expression and activity resulting from induced by red wine, which is a rich source of flavonoids, may be a major mechanism of protection, through a resultant increase in nitric oxide. Flavonoids from red wine may also exert a positive effect in cardiovascular disease prevention by inhibiting LDL oxidation, reducing thrombosis, improving endothelial function, and reducing inflammation (Wallerath et al. 2003; Howard et al. 2004; Maron 2004).

The produced nitric oxide is very sensitive to the presence of free radicals, which react with it and form peroxynitrates, which damage the vascular walls. The endothelial nitric oxide synthase defect plays an important role in the pathogenesis of the MetS. The consequence of the diminished activity of this enzyme is IR, arterial hypertension, and dyslipidemia. The stimulation of the endothelial nitric oxide synthase, which takes part in the HDL transportation, may explain the mechanism of the rise of this fraction due to alcohol influence (Landmesser et al. 2003; Leighton et al. 2006).

The hypothesis that red wine takes part in the MetS control is also confirmed by the fact that oxidative stress plays an important role in the pathogenesis of this syndrome. The oxidative stress reduction causes not only the diminution of biological structures damage, but also a change in metabolic pathways responsible for the syndromes development. The high endothelial nitric oxide synthase activity, which requires an antioxidative protection, limits superoxide production and decreases the oxidative stress (Stoclet et al. 1999).

Studies published during the last years have suggested that moderate alcohol intake might contribute to a lower risk of cardiovascular diseases. Protective mechanism of ethanol involves its influence on lipoprotein synthesis, mainly through the increase in the HDL levels and hepatic apolipoproteins (Hansel et al. 2010; Klatsky 2010; Lindschou Hansen et al. 2011). The blood HDL level rise is observed regardless of the amount of alcohol consumed. A daily dose of 30 g ethanol results in an average HDL level rise of 3.99 mg/dL, and an apolipoproteins A I level rise of 8.82 mg/dL (Rimm et al. 1999). Ethanol also causes an increase of triglyceride lipase activity and a decrease of the HDL removal from the circulation. It has also been found that alcohol influences the reduction in cholesterol ester transformation from the HDL to more atheromatic molecules (Hannuksela et al. 1992; Arriola et al. 2010).

Doses >30 g/day of ethanol can increase the triglycerides level. It has been found that the ethanol intake of 60 g/day increases the triglycerides level by about 0.19 mg/dL per 1 g of alcohol consumed. The triglycerides level augmentation results in the intensification of extra hepatic lipoprotein lipase production. The lipolysis of the triglycerides-rich molecules increases the transformation of cholesterol to the HDL molecules from the circulating VLDL remnants, and increases the total HDL level (Stampfer et al. 1996; Waskiewicz and Sygnowska 2013). Therefore, the balance in favor of mechanisms inhibiting the MetS development, the more so because in individuals drinking up to 15 g/day, a diminution of the triglycerides level and a rise in the HDL level can be observed (Yoon et al. 2004).

23.9 POSSIBLE MECHANISM OF THE EFFECT OF ALCOHOLISM IN METABOLIC SYNDROME

An interaction between genetic and environmental factors, including physical activity, diet, cigarette smoking, and alcohol intake, is possibly involved in the mechanism of the MetS development. Studies concerning the ethanol influence on MetS indicate that it can either enhance or inhibit the disease development (Goude et al. 2002; Yoon et al. 2004). It is related to a variety and multiplicity of MetS components and depends on the amount and type of ethanol consumed (Freiberg et al. 2004).

Ethanol neither elicits an insulin response nor requires a transporter to enter the liver. Once inside the hepatocyte, it bypasses glycolysis and is converted by ADH1B to form acetaldehyde, which promotes ROS formation and toxic damage to the liver if not quenched by hepatic anti-oxidants such as glutathione or ascorbic acid (Dey and Cederbaum 2006). Acetaldehyde is then metabolized by the enzyme $ALDH_2$ to acetic acid, which in turn is metabolized by the enzyme acyl-CoA synthetase short-chain family member 2 to form acetyl-CoA that can then enter the mitochondrial tricarboxylic acid cycle. The excess malonyl-CoA produced from ethanol metabolism inhibits carnitine palmitoyltransferase-1, thereby limiting mitochondrial fatty acid β-oxidation. Ethanol also blocks fatty acid β-oxidation by inhibiting both peroxisome proliferator-activated receptor (PPAR-α) and adenosine monophosphate-activated protein kinase, which lead to increased activity of acetyl-CoA carboxylase and increased levels of malonyl-CoA (Garcia-Villafranca et al. 2008).

PPAR-α is expressed mainly in the liver, kidney, and heart and stimulates the transcription of genes involved in fatty acid uptake and both mitochondrial and peroxisomal fatty acid β-oxidation (Dreyer et al. 1993). The ethanol-induced suppression of PPAR-α also suppresses microsomal triglyceride transfer protein altering the liver lipid export process (Sozio and Crabb 2008). Accumulation of intrahepatic lipid metabolites leads to activation of the enzyme C-jun N-terminal kinase 1 and serine-phosphorylation of insulin receptor substrate-1, leading to further hepatic IR (Lee et al. 2002). Thus, ethanol metabolism results in intrahepatic lipid accumulation and liver injury, inducing hepatic IR, and promoting MetS (Guzman and Castro 1990; Crabb et al. 2004; Yokoyama et al. 2007).

Results from investigations on the relationship between alcohol intake and obesity are not compatible. If alcohol drinking is associated with food consumption, there is a risk of an increase in body mass. However, if there are digestive tract problems, a loss of body mass and even cachexia may be expected, as the use of hepatic glycogen, one of the energetic substrates of the organism, is not being compensated. Although an important correlation between alcohol consumption and body mass index has not been shown, a positive correlation between alcohol intake and waist–hip ratio has been reported (Liu et al. 1994; Sakurai et al. 1997).

The disturbances of carbohydrate metabolism are very frequent in people abusing alcohol. Ethanol induces disturbances of hepatic gluconeogenesis preventing lactate oxidation to pyruvate. The excess of NADH leads to the diminution of pyruvate and oxaloacetate amount, which are being reduced, respectively, to lactate and malate. Christiansen et al. (1996) found that the ability of ethanol to induce hypoglycemia is attenuated or absent in diet-treated type 2 diabetes, and ethanol had no effect in insulin sensitivity. The authors concluded that the risk of acute ethanol-induced aberrations in carbohydrate metabolism in diet-treated type 2 diabetes seems to be less than previously expected, when alcohol is not taken as a part of a meal (Christiansen et al. 1996).

Studies showed that the acute intake of alcohol does not increase the risk of hypoglycemia in patients with type 2 diabetes disease only when sulfonylurea is coadministered (Pietraszek et al. 2010). The alcohol may induce the occurrence of secondary diabetes resulting from the pancreatic B cell islets destruction (Xu et al. 1998).

Alcohol consumption has been associated with endocrine and autonomic changes, including the development of hypertension. However, the sequence of pathophysiological events underlying the emergence of this effect is poorly understood. Numerous studies point to about a 30% risk of arterial hypertension occurrence due to the ethanol intake (Chobanian et al. 2003; Yoon et al. 2004; Correa Leite et al. 2013; Wakabayashi 2013; Waskiewicz and Sygnowska 2013). There is a significant rise in the systolic and diastolic blood pressure. The concept of the repeated withdrawal syndrome, during which time the activity of the sympathetic and the renin–angiotensin–aldosterone systems rises, seems most probable. Another suggested mechanism consists in the rise of systemic resistance as a result of the direct influence of ethanol. It has been found that the risk for hypertension rises with the amount of alcohol consumed (Yoon et al. 2004). It should also be stressed that after the withdrawal from alcohol, the blood pressure values may come back to normal.

Also, the dependence of MetS occurrence frequency on the alcohol intake is more pronounced in whites than in blacks. This concerns the MetS incidence diminution with a moderate, occasional ethanol intake, as well as the increase of the number of the cases due to alcohol abuse (Freiberg et al. 2004).

The pathways delineated in this chapter require further study. An interesting topic for further investigations would be as genetic factors might interact with alcohol consumption in fatty liver disease. The ethanol is one of the factors influencing the MetS development. The action of ethanol may either encourage or limit the development of this syndrome, which depends mainly on the amount and type of alcoholic beverage consumed.

ACKNOWLEDGMENTS

We thank CAPES-PNPD for the financial support.

REFERENCES

Agarwal, D. P. 2001. Genetic polymorphisms of alcohol metabolizing enzymes. *Pathol Biol (Paris)* 49(9): 703–709.

Arriola, L., Martinez-Camblor, P., Larranaga, N. et al. 2010. Alcohol intake and the risk of coronary heart disease in the Spanish EPIC cohort study. *Heart* 96(2): 124–130.

Athyros, V. G., Liberopoulos, E. N., Mikhailidis, D. P. et al. 2007. Association of drinking pattern and alcohol beverage type with the prevalence of metabolic syndrome, diabetes, coronary heart disease, stroke, and peripheral arterial disease in a Mediterranean cohort. *Angiology* 58(6): 689–697.

Baan, R., Straif, K., Grosse, Y. et al. 2007. Carcinogenicity of alcoholic beverages. *Lancet Oncol* 8(4): 292–293.

Baraona, E. 2000. Site and quantitative importance of alcohol first-pass metabolism. *Alcohol Clin Exp Res* 24(4): 405–406.

Baraona, E., Abittan, C. S., Dohmen, K. et al. 2001. Gender differences in pharmacokinetics of alcohol. *Alcohol Clin Exp Res* 25(4): 502–507.

Baur, J. A. and Sinclair, D. A. 2006. Therapeutic potential of resveratrol: The in vivo evidence. *Nat Rev Drug Discov* 5(6): 493–506.

Brooks, P. J. 1997. DNA damage, DNA repair, and alcohol toxicity—A review. *Alcohol Clin Exp Res* 21(6): 1073–1082.

Carlsson, S., Hammar, N., Grill, V. 2005. Alcohol consumption and type 2 diabetes Meta-analysis of epidemiological studies indicates a U-shaped relationship. *Diabetologia* 48(6): 1051–1054.

Chao, Y. C., Liou, S. R., Chung, Y. Y. et al. 1994. Polymorphism of alcohol and aldehyde dehydrogenase genes and alcoholic cirrhosis in Chinese patients. *Hepatology* 19(2): 360–366.

Chen, C. C., Li, T. C., Chang, P. C. et al. 2008. Association among cigarette smoking, metabolic syndrome, and its individual components: The metabolic syndrome study in Taiwan. *Metabolism* 57(4): 544–548.

Chobanian, A. V., Bakris, G. L., Black, H. R. et al. 2003. The seventh report of the joint national committee on prevention, detection, evaluation, and treatment of high blood pressure: The JNC 7 report. *JAMA* 289(19): 2560–2572.

Christiansen, C., Thomsen, C., Rasmussen, O. et al. 1996. The acute impact of ethanol on glucose, insulin, triacylglycerol, and free fatty acid responses and insulin sensitivity in type 2 diabetes. *Br J Nutr* 76(5): 669–675.

Correa Leite, M. L., Moriguchi, E. H., Lima-Costa, M. F. 2013. Effects of interactions between ApoE polymorphisms, alcohol consumption and obesity on age-related trends of blood pressure levels in postmenopausal women: The Bambui cohort study of aging (1997–2008). *Maturitas* 76: 57–63.

Crabb, D. W., Galli, A., Fischer, M. et al. 2004. Molecular mechanisms of alcoholic fatty liver: Role of peroxisome proliferator-activated receptor alpha. *Alcohol* 34(1): 35–38.

Dey, A. and Cederbaum, A. I. 2006. Alcohol and oxidative liver injury. *Hepatology* 43(2 Suppl 1): S63–S74.

Di Castelnuovo, A., Costanzo, S., Di Giuseppe R. et al. 2009. Alcohol consumption and cardiovascular risk: Mechanisms of action and epidemiologic perspectives. *Future Cardiol* 5(5): 467–477.

Di Chiara, T., Argano, C., Corrao, S. et al. 2012. Hypoadiponectinemia: A link between visceral obesity and metabolic syndrome. *J Nutr Metab* 2012: 175245.

Djousse, L., Arnett, D. K., Eckfeldt, J. H. 2004. Alcohol consumption and metabolic syndrome: Does the type of beverage matter? *Obes Res* 12(9): 1375–1385.

Dreyer, C., Keller, H., Mahfoudi, A. et al. 1993. Positive regulation of the peroxisomal beta-oxidation pathway by fatty acids through activation of peroxisome proliferator-activated receptors (PPAR). *Biol Cell* 77(1): 67–76.

Duell, E. J., Travier, N., Lujan-Barroso, L. et al. 2011. Alcohol consumption and gastric cancer risk in the European Prospective Investigation into Cancer and Nutrition (EPIC) cohort. *Am J Clin Nutr* 94(5): 1266–1275.

Facchini, F., Chen, Y. D., Reaven, G. M. 1994. Light-to-moderate alcohol intake is associated with enhanced insulin sensitivity. *Diabetes Care* 17(2): 115–119.

Fan, A. Z., Russell, M., Dorn, J. et al. 2006. Lifetime alcohol drinking pattern is related to the prevalence of metabolic syndrome. The Western New York Health Study (WNYHS). *Eur J Epidemiol* 21(2): 129–138.

Farfan Labonne, B. E., Gutierrez, M., Gomez-Quiroz, L. E. et al. 2009. Acetaldehyde-induced mitochondrial dysfunction sensitizes hepatocytes to oxidative damage. *Cell Biol Toxicol* 25(6): 599–609.

Freiberg, M. S., Cabral, H. J., Heeren, T. C. et al. 2004. Alcohol consumption and the prevalence of the Metabolic Syndrome in the US: A cross-sectional analysis of data from the Third National Health and Nutrition Examination Survey. *Diabetes Care* 27(12): 2954–2959.

Garcia-Villafranca, J., Guillen, A., Castro, J. 2008. Ethanol consumption impairs regulation of fatty acid metabolism by decreasing the activity of AMP-activated protein kinase in rat liver. *Biochimie* 90(3): 460–466.

Gemma, S., Vichi, S., Testai, E. 2006. Individual susceptibility and alcohol effects: Biochemical and genetic aspects. *Ann Ist Super Sanita* 42(1): 8–16.

Goude, D., Fagerberg, B., Hulthe, J. 2002. Alcohol consumption, the metabolic syndrome and insulin resistance in 58-year-old clinically healthy men (AIR study). *Clin Sci (Lond)* 102(3): 345–352.

Guzman, M., Castro, J. 1990. Alterations in the regulatory properties of hepatic fatty acid oxidation and carnitine palmitoyltransferase I activity after ethanol feeding and withdrawal. *Alcohol Clin Exp Res* 14(3): 472–477.

Hakenewerth, A. M., Millikan, R. C., Rusyn, I. et al. 2013. Effects of polymorphisms in alcohol metabolism and oxidative stress genes on survival from head and neck cancer. *Cancer Epidemiol* 37(4): 479–491.

Hannuksela, M., Marcel, Y. L., Kesaniemi, Y. A. et al. 1992. Reduction in the concentration and activity of plasma cholesteryl ester transfer protein by alcohol. *J Lipid Res* 33(5): 737–744.

Hansel, B., Thomas, F., Pannier, B. et al. 2010. Relationship between alcohol intake, health and social status and cardiovascular risk factors in the Urban Paris-Ile-de-France Cohort: Is the cardioprotective action of alcohol a myth? *Eur J Clin Nutr* 64(6): 561–568.

Hanson, R. L., Imperatore G., Bennett, P. H. et al. 2002. Components of the "metabolic syndrome" and incidence of type 2 diabetes. *Diabetes* 51(10): 3120–3127.

Heit, C., Dong, H., Chen, Y. et al. 2013. The role of CYP2E1 in alcohol metabolism and sensitivity in the central nervous system. *Subcell Biochem* 67: 235–247.

Hiuge-Shimizu, A., Maeda, N., Hirata, A. et al. 2011. Dynamic changes of adiponectin and S100A8 levels by the selective peroxisome proliferator-activated receptor-gamma agonist rivoglitazone. *Arterioscler Thromb Vasc Biol* 31(4): 792–799.

Howard, A. A., Arnsten, J. H., Gourevitch, M. N. 2004. Effect of alcohol consumption on diabetes mellitus: A systematic review. *Ann Intern Med* 140(3): 211–219.

Isomaa, B., Almgren, P., Tuomi, T. et al. 2001. Cardiovascular morbidity and mortality associated with the metabolic syndrome. *Diabetes Care* 24(4): 683–689.

Jordao, A. A. Jr., Chiarello, P. G., Arantes, M. R. et al. 2004. Effect of an acute dose of ethanol on lipid peroxidation in rats: Action of vitamin E. *Food Chem Toxicol* 42(3): 459–464.

Klatsky, A. L. 2010. Alcohol and cardiovascular health. *Physiol Behav* 100(1): 76–81.

Koppes, L. L., Dekker, J. M., Hendriks, H. F. et al. 2005. Moderate alcohol consumption lowers the risk of type 2 diabetes: A meta-analysis of prospective observational studies. *Diabetes Care* 28(3): 719–725.

Lakka, H. M., Laaksonen, D. E., Lakka, T. A. et al. 2002. The metabolic syndrome and total and cardiovascular disease mortality in middle-aged men. *JAMA* 288(21): 2709–2716.

Landmesser, U., Dikalov, S., Price, S. R. et al. 2003. Oxidation of tetrahydrobiopterin leads to uncoupling of endothelial cell nitric oxide synthase in hypertension. *J Clin Invest* 111(8): 1201–1209.

Lee, S. L., Chau, G. Y., Yao, C. T., Wu, C. W., Yin, S. J. 2006. Functional assessment of human alcohol dehydrogenase family in ethanol metabolism: Significance of first-pass metabolism. *Alcohol Clin Exp Res* 30(7): 1132–1142.

Lee, S. L., Wang, M. F., Lee, A. I. et al. 2003. The metabolic role of human ADH3 functioning as ethanol dehydrogenase. *FEBS Lett* 544(1–3): 143–147.

Lee, W. Y., Jung, C. H., Park, J. S. et al. 2005. Effects of smoking, alcohol, exercise, education, and family history on the metabolic syndrome as defined by the ATP III. *Diabetes Res Clin Pract* 67(1): 70–77.

Lee, Y. J., Aroor, A. R., S. Shukla, D. 2002. Temporal activation of p42/44 mitogen-activated protein kinase and c-Jun N-terminal kinase by acetaldehyde in rat hepatocytes and its loss after chronic ethanol exposure. *J Pharmacol Exp Ther* 301(3): 908–914.

Leighton, F., Miranda-Rottmann, S., Urquiaga, I. 2006. A central role of eNOS in the protective effect of wine against metabolic syndrome. *Cell Biochem Funct* 24(4): 291–298.

Lieber, C. S. 1997. Ethanol metabolism, cirrhosis and alcoholism. *Clin Chim Acta* 257(1): 59–84.

Lieber, C. S., DeCarli, L. M. 1972. The role of the hepatic microsomal ethanol oxidizing system (MEOS) for ethanol metabolism in vivo. *J Pharmacol Exp Ther* 181(2): 279–287.

Lim, R. T. Jr., Gentry, R. T., Ito, D. et al. 1993. First-pass metabolism of ethanol is predominantly gastric. *Alcohol Clin Exp Res* 17(6): 1337–1344.

Lindros, K. O., Jokelainen, K., Nanji, A. A. 1999. Acetaldehyde prevents nuclear factor-kappa B activation and hepatic inflammation in ethanol-fed rats. *Lab Invest* 79(7): 799–806.

Lindschou Hansen, J., Tolstrup, J. S., Jensen, M. K. et al. 2011. Alcohol intake and risk of acute coronary syndrome and mortality in men and women with and without hypertension. *Eur J Epidemiol* 26(6): 439–447.

Linn, S., Carroll, M., Johnson, C. et al. 1993. High-density lipoprotein cholesterol and alcohol consumption in US white and black adults: Data from NHANES II. *Am J Public Health* 83(6): 811–816.

Liu, S., Serdula, M. K., Williamson, D. F. et al. 1994. A prospective study of alcohol intake and change in body weight among US adults. *Am J Epidemiol* 140(10): 912–920.

Lu, Y., Cederbaum, A. I. 2008. CYP2E1 and oxidative liver injury by alcohol. *Free Radic Biol Med* 44(5): 723–738.

Maron, D. J. 2004. Flavonoids for reduction of atherosclerotic risk. *Curr Atheroscler Rep* 6(1): 73–78.

McKillop, I. H., Schrum, L. W. 2009. Role of alcohol in liver carcinogenesis. *Semin Liver Dis* 29(2): 222–232.

Nagata, N., Hiyoshi, M., Shiozawa, H. et al. 2002. Assessment of a difference in ALDH2 heterozygotes and alcoholic liver injury. *Alcohol Clin Exp Res* 26(8 Suppl): 11S–14S.

Nakamura, Y., Yokoyama, H., Higuchi, S. et al. 2004. Acetaldehyde accumulation suppresses Kupffer cell release of TNF-Alpha and modifies acute hepatic inflammation in rats. *J Gastroenterol* 39(2): 140–147.

Navasumrit, P., Ward, T. H., Dodd, N. J. et al. 2000. Ethanol-induced free radicals and hepatic DNA strand breaks are prevented in vivo by antioxidants: Effects of acute and chronic ethanol exposure. *Carcinogenesis* 21(1): 93–99.

Niemela, O., Parkkila, S., Yla-Herttuala, S. et al. 1995. Sequential acetaldehyde production, lipid peroxidation, and fibrogenesis in micropig model of alcohol-induced liver disease. *Hepatology* 22(4 Pt 1): 1208–1214.

Nordmann, R., Ribiere, C., Rouach, H. 1992. Implication of free radical mechanisms in ethanol-induced cellular injury. *Free Radic Biol Med* 12(3): 219–240.

Park, Y. W., Zhu, S., Palaniappan, L. et al. 2003. The metabolic syndrome: Prevalence and associated risk factor findings in the US population from the Third National Health and Nutrition Examination Survey, 1988–1994. *Arch Intern Med* 163(4): 427–436.

Pietraszek, A., Gregersen, S., Hermansen, K. 2010. Alcohol and type 2 diabetes. A review. *Nutr Metab Cardiovasc Dis* 20(5): 366–375.

Quintanilla, M. E., Tampier, L., Sapag, A. et al. 2005. Polymorphisms in the mitochondrial aldehyde dehydrogenase gene (Aldh2) determine peak blood acetaldehyde levels and voluntary ethanol consumption in rats. *Pharmacogenet Genomics* 15(6): 427–431.

Reaven, G. M. 2005. The metabolic syndrome: Requiescat in pace. *Clin Chem* 51(6): 931–938.

Rimm, E. B., Williams, P., Fosher, K. et al. 1999. Moderate alcohol intake and lower risk of coronary heart disease: Meta-analysis of effects on lipids and haemostatic factors. *BMJ* 319(7224): 1523–1528.

Riserus, U., Ingelsson, E. 2007. Alcohol intake, insulin resistance, and abdominal obesity in elderly men. *Obesity (Silver Spring)* 15(7): 1766–1773.

Rosell, M., De Faire, U., Hellenius, M. L. 2003. Low prevalence of the metabolic syndrome in wine drinkers—Is it the alcohol beverage or the lifestyle? *Eur J Clin Nutr* 57(2): 227–234.

Ruixing, Y., Shangling, P., Hong, C. et al. 2008. Diet, alcohol consumption, and serum lipid levels of the middle-aged and elderly in the Guangxi Bai Ku Yao and Han populations. *Alcohol* 42(3): 219–229.

Sakurai, Y., Umeda, T., Shinchi, K. et al. 1997. Relation of total and beverage-specific alcohol intake to body mass index and waist-to-hip ratio: A study of self-defense officials in Japan. *Eur J Epidemiol* 13(8): 893–898.

Schroder, H., Morales-Molina, J. A., Bermejo, S. et al. 2007. Relationship of abdominal obesity with alcohol consumption at population scale. *Eur J Nutr* 46(7): 369–376.

Seitz, H. K., Becker, P. 2007. Alcohol metabolism and cancer risk. *Alcohol Res Health* 30(1): 38–41, 44–47.

Sesso, H. D., Cook, N. R., Buring, J. E. et al. 2008. Alcohol consumption and the risk of hypertension in women and men. *Hypertension* 51(4): 1080–1087.

Simao, A. N., Lozovoy, M. A., Simao, T. N. et al. 2012. Adiponectinemia is associated with uricemia but not with proinflammatory status in women with metabolic syndrome. *J Nutr Metab* 2012: 418094.

Singh, N. P., Khan, A. 1995. Acetaldehyde: Genotoxicity and cytotoxicity in human lymphocytes. *Mutat Res* 337(1): 9–17.

Sozio, M., Crabb, D. W. 2008. Alcohol and lipid metabolism. *Am J Physiol Endocrinol Metab* 295(1): E10–E16.

Stampfer, M. J., Krauss, R. M., Ma, J. et al. 1996. A prospective study of triglyceride level, low-density lipoprotein particle diameter, and risk of myocardial infarction. *JAMA* 276(11): 882–888.

Stoclet, J. C., Kleschyov, A., Andriambeloson, E. et al. 1999. Endothelial NO release cased by red wine polyphenols. *J Physiol Pharmacol* 50(4): 535–540.

Strumnik, A., Karski, J. 2012. The laboratory diagnostics of alcoholic disease. *Pol Merkur Lekarski* 32(190): 270–273.

Suh, I., Shaten, B. J., Cutler, J. A. et al. 1992. Alcohol use and mortality from coronary heart disease: The role of high-density lipoprotein cholesterol. The Multiple Risk Factor Intervention Trial Research Group. *Ann Intern Med* 116(11): 881–887.

Takahashi, M., Arita, Y., Yamagata, K. et al. 2000. Genomic structure and mutations in adipose-specific gene, adiponectin. *Int J Obes Relat Metab Disord* 24(7): 861–868.

Tavares, D. C., Cecchi, A. O., Jordao, A. A. Jr. et al. 2001. Cytogenetic study of chronic ethanol consumption in rats. *Teratog Carcinog Mutagen* 21(5): 361–368.

Taylor, B., Irving, H. M., Baliunas, D. et al. 2009. Alcohol and hypertension: Gender differences in dose-response relationships determined through systematic review and meta-analysis. *Addiction* 104(12): 1981–1990.

Tolstrup, J. S., Heitmann, B. L., Tjonneland, A. M. et al. 2005. The relation between drinking pattern and body mass index and waist and hip circumference. *Int J Obes (Lond)* 29(5): 490–497.

Tran, M. N., Wu, A. H., Hill, D. W. 2007. Alcohol dehydrogenase and catalase content in perinatal infant and adult livers: Potential influence on neonatal alcohol metabolism. *Toxicol Lett* 169(3): 245–252.

Tuma, D. J. 2002. Role of malondialdehyde-acetaldehyde adducts in liver injury. *Free Radic Biol Med* 32(4): 303–308.

Tuma, D. J., Casey, C. A. 2003. Dangerous byproducts of alcohol breakdown—Focus on adducts. *Alcohol Res Health* 27(4): 285–290.

Tuma, D. J., Thiele, G. M., Xu, D. et al. 1996. Acetaldehyde and malondialdehyde react together to generate distinct protein adducts in the liver during long-term ethanol administration. *Hepatology* 23(4): 872–880.

Wakabayashi, I. 2013. Alcohol intake and triglycerides/high-density lipoprotein cholesterol ratio in men with hypertension. *Am J Hypertens* 26(7): 888–895.

Wallerath, T., Poleo, D., Li, H. et al. 2003. Red wine increases the expression of human endothelial nitric oxide synthase: A mechanism that may contribute to its beneficial cardiovascular effects. *J Am Coll Cardiol* 41(3): 471–478.

Waskiewicz, A., Sygnowska, E. 2013. Alcohol intake and cardiovascular risk factor profile in men participating in the WOBASZ study. *Kardiol Pol* 71(4): 359–365.

Werner, J., Saghir, M., Warshaw, A. L. et al. 2002. Alcoholic pancreatitis in rats: Injury from nonoxidative metabolites of ethanol. *Am J Physiol Gastrointest Liver Physiol* 283(1): G65–G73.

WHO. Global status report on alcohol and health. World Health Organization, Geneva, Switzerland, 2011. http://www.who.int/substance_abuse/publications/global_alcohol_report/en/index.html (accessed June 13, 2013) [cited].

Wilson, J. S., Apte, M. V. 2003. Role of alcohol metabolism in alcoholic pancreatitis. *Pancreas* 27(4): 311–315.

Worrall, S., Thiele, G. M. 2001. Protein modification in ethanol toxicity. *Adverse Drug React Toxicol Rev* 20(3): 133–159.

Wu, D., Cederbaum, A. I. 2003. Alcohol, oxidative stress, and free radical damage. *Alcohol Res Health* 27(4): 277–284.

Xu, D., Dhillon, A. S., Abelmann, A. et al. 1998. Alcohol-related diols cause acute insulin resistance in vivo. *Metabolism* 47(10): 1180–1186.

Yokoyama, H., Hiroshi, H., Ohgo, H. et al. 2007. Effects of excessive ethanol consumption on the diagnosis of the metabolic syndrome using its clinical diagnostic criteria. *Intern Med* 46(17): 1345–1352.

Yoon, Y. S., Oh, S. W., Baik, H. W. et al. 2004. Alcohol consumption and the metabolic syndrome in Korean adults: The 1998 Korean National Health and Nutrition Examination Survey. *Am J Clin Nutr* 80(1): 217–224.

Zhang, H., Zhang, J., Ungvari, Z. et al. 2009. Resveratrol improves endothelial function: Role of TNF{alpha} and vascular oxidative stress. *Arterioscler Thromb Vasc Biol* 29(8): 1164–1171.

Zhang, M., Gong, Y., Corbin, I. et al. 2006. The effects of light and moderate-heavy ethanol exposure on the development of cirrhosis in rats. *Dig Dis Sci* 51(10): 1732–1737.

Zintzaras, E., Stefanidis, I., Santos, M. et al. 2006. Do alcohol-metabolizing enzyme gene polymorphisms increase the risk of alcoholism and alcoholic liver disease? *Hepatology* 43(2): 352–361.

24 Cocoa and Insulin Resistance
Protective Effects on Metabolic Syndrome

Davide Grassi, Giovambattista Desideri, Paolo Di Giosia,
Stefania Di Agostino, Francesca Mai, Angelica Dante,
Federica Patrizi, Letizia Martella, and Claudio Ferri

CONTENTS

24.1 INTRODUCTION

Metabolic syndrome (MetS) is defined by a cluster of cardiovascular disease risk factors that are associated with insulin resistance (Adults Treatment Panel III 2001, Pratley 2007) and is a strong predictor of cardiovascular disease as well as type 2 diabetes (Grassi et al. 2013b). Early detection and treatment of people with MetS may prevent the development of cardiovascular disease and type 2 diabetes.

The rising epidemic of diabetes is a pressing issue in clinical medicine worldwide from both healthcare and economic perspectives. This is fuelled by overwhelming increases in the incidence and prevalence of obesity. Both insulin resistance and endothelial dysfunction that lead to substantial increases in cardiovascular morbidity and mortality characterize obesity and diabetes. Insulin resistance and endothelial dysfunction are also prominent features of important cardiovascular disorders including hypertension, coronary artery disease, and atherosclerosis (Grassi et al. 2013a,b, Shin et al. 2013, Syed Ikmal et al. 2013, Kaur 2014). Accordingly, insulin resistance is thought to be the common binding between metabolic and cardiovascular disorders (Grassi et al. 2011, 2013a).Current treatment strategies include lifestyle modifications such as diet and exercise as the cornerstone of therapy, with eventual additional pharmacologic therapies targeting the individual components of the MetS (Grassi et al. 2013a, van Dam et al. 2013).

Therefore, therapeutic approaches that target either insulin resistance or endothelial dysfunction alone are likely to simultaneously improve both metabolic and cardiovascular pathophysiology and disease outcomes (Grassi et al. 2009, 2013a, van Dam et al. 2013).

Substantial data suggest that flavonoid-rich foods could help to protect from cardiovascular disease (CVD) and cancer (Grassi et al. 2009, van Dam et al. 2013). Kuna Indians of Panama present with low blood pressure levels and little rise in blood pressure with age (Hollenberg et al. 2009). Excluding genetic factors, environmental protective factors were considered, and it was observed that Kuna Indians still residing in their indigenous location in the San Blas Islands (island-dwelling Kuna) drink more than five cups daily of flavonoid-rich cocoa (Hollenberg et al. 2009) as their major source of fluid, thus likely indicating the most rich flavonoid diet of any community. On the contrary, mainland Kuna ingest little commercially available flavanol-poor cocoa (Hollenberg et al. 2009). Regarding this aspect, Bayard et al. (2007) supposed that high flavonoid intake and consequent nitric oxide (NO) system activation—that is, island-dwelling Kuna have a threefold larger urinary nitrate/nitrite ratio than do mainland dwellers (Bayard et al. 2007, Hollenberg et al. 2009)—could be important in reducing ischemic heart disease, stroke, diabetes mellitus, and cancer, all NO-sensitive processes, in this particular populations. The hypothesis was confirmed by showing that in mainland Panama, CVD was the leading cause of death (83.4 ± 0.70 age adjusted deaths/100,000) and cancer was second (68.4 ± 1.6). In contrast, the rate of CVD and cancer among island-dwelling Kuna was much lower (9.2 ± 3.1 and 4.4 ± 4.4, respectively). Further, deaths due to diabetes were much more common in the mainland (24.1 ± 0.74) than in the San Blas (6.6 ± 1.94). This lower risk among Kuna Indians likely reflected a very high flavanol intake and sustained NO synthesis activation (Bayard et al. 2007, Hollenberg et al. 2009). In keeping to this, regulation of hemodynamic and metabolic homeostasis may be coupled by physiological insulin actions in the vascular endothelium to stimulate NO production (Bayard et al. 2007, Hollenberg et al. 2009, Grassi et al. 2011, 2013a).

24.2   INSULIN RESISTANCE: THE RECIPROCAL RELATIONSHIP WITH ENDOTHELIAL FUNCTION

The biological actions of insulin are mediated by specific cell surface receptors that are expressed in nearly every cell in the body. Recently, great progress has been made in understanding the signal transduction pathways controlling classical metabolic actions of insulin to promote glucose uptake in skeletal muscle and adipose tissue through translocation of the insulin-responsive glucose transporter (GLUT) 4 (Abdul-Ghani and DeFronzo 2010, Pansuria et al. 2012).

Among the most important cardiovascular actions of insulin is the stimulation of increased production of the potent vasodilator NO from vascular endothelium (Grassi et al. 2013a, van Dam et al. 2013). In endothelial cells, endothelial NO synthase (eNOS) catalyzes the conversion of the substrate L-arginine to the products NO and L-citrulline (Grassi et al. 2011, van Dam et al. 2013). Classical vasodilators, including acetylcholine, stimulate an increase in intracellular calcium that promotes the binding of calcium/calmodulin to eNOS. In the presence of a variety of cofactors, this results in dissociation of eNOS from caveolin-1 with subsequent dimerization and activation of eNOS (Muniyappa et al. 2008, Abdul-Ghani and DeFronzo 2010, Grassi et al. 2011, Pansuria et al. 2012, van Dam et al. 2013). The insulin signaling pathway in vascular endothelium that regulates activation of eNOS follows a phosphorylation-dependent mechanism that is completely distinct, separable, and independent from classical calcium-dependent mechanisms used by G protein–coupled receptors such as the acetylcholine receptor (Muniyappa et al. 2008, Abdul-Ghani and DeFronzo 2010, Pansuria et al. 2012). In recent years, a complete biochemical signaling pathway leading from the insulin receptor to phosphorylation and activation of eNOS has been elucidated in vascular endothelial cells (Muniyappa et al. 2008, Abdul-Ghani and DeFronzo 2010, Pansuria et al. 2012). This pathway requires activation of the insulin receptor tyrosine kinase, which then phosphorylates the insulin receptor substrate-1 (IRS-1) leading to binding and activation of phosphoinositide 3-kinase (PI3K) and subsequent activation of phosphoinositide-dependent kinase-1 (PDK-1), which then phosphorylates and activates protein kinase B (Akt), which directly phosphorylates and activates eNOS, leading to increased production of NO within a matter of minutes (Muniyappa et al. 2008, Abdul-Ghani and DeFronzo 2010, Pansuria et al. 2012). Insulin-stimulated production of NO leads to capillary recruitment, vasodilatation, and increased blood flow to skeletal muscle improving delivery of glucose and insulin to skeletal muscle (Muniyappa et al. 2008, Abdul-Ghani and DeFronzo 2010, Pansuria et al. 2012, Grassi et al. 2013a). According to this, evaluating the effects of inhibiting eNOS by L-nitro-L-arginine-methyl ester (L-NAME) on total hindlimb blood flow, muscle microvascular recruitment, and hindlimb glucose uptake during euglycemic hyperinsulinemia in rats, Vincent et al. (2003a) reported that insulin significantly increased hindlimb total blood flow (0.69 ± 0.02 to 1.22 ± 0.11 mL/min, $p < 0.05$), glucose uptake (0.27 ± 0.05 to 0.95 ± 0.08 μmol/min, $p < 0.05$), and skeletal muscle microvascular volume (10.0 ± 1.6 to 15.0 ± 1.2 video intensity units, $p < 0.05$). Addition of L-NAME to insulin completely blocked the effect of insulin on both total limb flow and microvascular recruitment and blunted glucose uptake by 40% ($p < 0.05$), thus suggesting that insulin is able to specifically recruit flow to the microvasculature in skeletal muscle via an NO-dependent pathway and that this may be important for insulin action to regulate glucose disposal (Vincent et al. 2003a). In keeping to this, insulin signaling pathways, parallelly involved in distinct tissues with vascular or metabolic functions, may help to tightly couple regulation of vascular function with glucose metabolism playing a fundamental physiological role in coupling hemodynamic and metabolic homeostasis in healthy conditions (Kim et al. 2006, Vincent et al. 2003b). Thus, considering glucose metabolism coupled with blood flow, changes in metabolism could be able to induce alterations in blood flow, while increasing flow will favor changes in metabolism and glucose uptake. It is well known that increased metabolic activity recruits additional blood flow to supply necessary substrates (Vincent et al. 2003b, Kim et al. 2006, Grassi et al. 2011, 2013a). On the contrary, experiments in rats demonstrated that increasing blood flow while maintaining glucose and insulin at constant physiological levels results in flow-dependent increases in glucose disposal (Kim et al. 2006). Elevations in flow also increase the delivery of insulin to skeletal muscle, where insulin directly affects glucose uptake by translocation of GLUT4 (Kim et al. 2006). Therefore, insulin has direct effects (increasing glucose uptake in skeletal muscle) and substantial indirect effects (promoting glucose disposal by increasing blood flow). This cross talk between metabolic and vascular tissues is important for coupling glucose homeostasis and endothelial function (Vincent et al. 2003a,b, Kim et al. 2006).

24.3 INSULIN RESISTANCE: THE SPECIFIC ROLE IN ENDOTHELIAL DYSFUNCTION

Different studies using genetic and diet-induced animal models of obesity reported a direct relationship between impaired metabolism and flow-mediated dilation (FMD) and visceral adipose tissue. Indeed, compromised bioavailability of NO due to oxidative stress emerges as a main cause of endothelial dysfunction in obesity. Inflamed adipose tissue due to hypoxia, and in particular perivascular adipose tissue, secretes larger amounts of ROS and adipokines that deteriorate NO signaling pathways. Abnormal production and activity of the vasoconstrictor-proatherogenic peptide endothelin-1 is also a hallmark of the obesity-associated endothelial dysfunction (Ferri et al. 1997). Accordingly, Ferri et al. (1997) showed that circulating ET-1 levels were significantly higher in obese patients with MetS than in controls ($p < 0.05$) and were directly correlated with fasting insulin levels ($r = 0.564$, $p = 0.015$). In particular, visceral obesity is one of the pivotal causes of insulin resistance, and the pathogenic factors that induce endothelial dysfunction in the earlier stages of obesity will further deteriorate the insulin signaling pathways in endothelial cells, thus leading to blunted vasodilatation and abnormal capillary recruitment and substrate delivery by insulin to the target tissues. According to this, it has been suggested that mechanisms supporting insulin resistance also contribute to endothelial dysfunction. In particular, hyperglycemia leads to glucotoxicity, causing endothelial damage and worsening metabolic disturbances. Similarly, elevated free fatty acid levels in diabetes, obesity, and dyslipidemia lead to lipotoxicity, which favors other mechanisms of insulin resistance and endothelial dysfunction. Proinflammatory and oxidative states associated with metabolic and cardiovascular risk factors represent an additional mechanism negatively affecting the relationship between insulin resistance and endothelial damage (Cersosimo and DeFronzo 2006, Fiorentino et al. 2013).

Insulin resistance and hyperglycemia increase oxidative stress by the ROS production. Increased oxidative stress promotes endothelial dysfunction (Cersosimo and DeFronzo 2006, Erusalimsky and Moncada 2007, Fiorentino et al. 2013) and within the mitochondria, free radicals saturate the oxy-reduction enzymatic capacity deviating NO toward the nitrite formation, impairing the electron transfer chain and promoting cell apoptosis (Cersosimo and DeFronzo 2006, Erusalimsky and Moncada 2007, Fiorentino et al. 2013). Further, also mitochondrial NOS is impaired and the synthesis of NO is compromised (Cersosimo and DeFronzo 2006). The decreased NO synthesis and release, combined with its accelerated consumption during the neutralization of the oxidative stress, decrease NO bioavailability for its normal vasorelaxation (Grassi et al. 2009, 2011). In turn, increased ROS results in insulin resistance with impaired insulin-stimulated translocation of GLUT4 and glucose uptake (Grassi et al. 2009, 2011, Syed Ikmal et al. 2013).

It has been also demonstrated that conditions of insulin resistance are commonly associated with endothelial dysfunction and that the exposure of vascular endothelium to high blood pressure and circulating levels of lipids and glucose is accompanied by reduced NO bioavailability (Panza et al. 1993, Erusalimsky and Moncada 2007, Grassi et al. 2009, 2011, Fiorentino et al. 2013).

These observations supported the hypothesis that endothelial dysfunction is both a cause and a consequence of the metabolic disturbances observed in states of insulin resistance. According to this, de Jongh et al. (2004), injecting insulin directly into the interstitial space and thus bypassing the transendothelial insulin transport step in dogs, showed that defects in insulin transport across the endothelial layer of skeletal muscle contribute to insulin resistance (de Jongh et al. 2004). In turn, insulin resistance with its associated disturbances in glucose and lipid metabolism decreases NO bioavailability leading to impaired endothelial-dependent vasodilatation (Grassi et al. 2013a, Syed Ikmal et al. 2013, Vincent et al. 2003b). The disruption of normal vascular endothelial function, particularly in the arterioles and capillaries, further impairs the metabolic action of insulin, thus establishing a self-perpetuating negative feedback cycle (Kim et al. 2006, Muniyappa et al. 2008, Grassi et al. 2009, 2011, Pansuria. et al. 2012). In addition, a reduction in insulin resistance is accompanied by improved endothelial function and vice versa (Vincent et al. 2003b, Cersosimo and DeFronzo 2006, Kim et al. 2006). Of particular interest, it has been reported that total vasodilator capacity was similar in normoglycemic individuals, whereas it was significantly decreased in normotensive (−17%) and hypertensive (−34%) patients with diabetes (Prior et al. 2005). Compared with insulin sensitivity, endothelium-dependent coronary vasomotion was significantly diminished in insulin resistance (−56%), as well as in impaired glucose tolerant and normotensive and hypertensive diabetic patients (−85%, −91%, and −120%, respectively). Thus, indicating that progressively worsening functional coronary abnormalities of NO-mediated vasomotion occur with increasing severity of insulin resistance and carbohydrate intolerance (Prior et al. 2005). In this regard, although the molecular mechanisms responsible for the metabolic and vascular abnormalities associated with insulin resistance have yet to be entirely elucidated, deficient NO production appears to play a fundamental role. Accordingly, Baron et al. (1995) showed that infusion of L-N monomethyl arginine (L-NMMA), a specific competitive inhibitor of eNOS, into the femoral artery caused a sustained 25% reduction in insulin-stimulated leg glucose uptake. Characterization of molecular mechanisms responsible for the impairment in insulin action and endothelial-mediated vascular responses to the metabolic derangements induced by insulin resistance is of considerable clinical interest in order to have a better understanding of the interrelationship between insulin resistance and endothelial dysfunction in the initiation and progression of atherosclerosis.

Insulin resistance is associated with impaired NOS activity (Kim et al. 2006, Muniyappa et al. 2008, Grassi et al. 2013a) and an abnormal basal NO-mediated dilation in the forearm arterial bed (Calver et al. 1992, Kim et al. 2006, Pansuria et al. 2012).

The insulin-dependent increase of microvascular endothelium-related vasodilation is abolished in insulin resistance conditions such as obesity (de Jongh et al. 2004). Moreover, insulin has been shown to constrict rather than dilate forearm resistance arteries in obese patients (Gudbjörnsdottir et al. 1996). On the other hand, NOS inhibition or endothelium removal reveals a vasoconstrictor effect of insulin on isolated arterioles (Schroeder et al. 1999). Of interest, clarifying the relationship between NO and insulin sensitivity, Shankar et al. (2000) reported that knockout mice that are homozygous null for the eNOS gene present not only with a hemodynamic phenotype of increased basal blood pressure but also of insulin resistance. Therefore, both the mechanisms are coupled in such a manner that endothelial dysfunction can cause insulin resistance, and this, in a vicious circle, negatively affects endothelial function.

24.4 COCOA, FLAVANOLS, AND CARDIOMETABOLIC PROTECTION

A number of studies suggest that flavanols, a major class of flavonoids, might have a causal relationship between flavanol consumption and improvements in cardiovascular mortality and morbidity (Bayard et al. 2007, Grassi et al. 2009, 2013a, Hollenberg et al. 2009). Epidemiological and clinical studies revealed high-flavonoid diet or isolated flavanols, such as (−)-epicatechin, are able to improve the function of the vascular endothelium, as assessed by FMD, through elevation of NO bioavailability and bioactivity (Grassi et al. 2009, 2011). Cocoa and chocolate received attention, because of their high content in flavonoids (Grassi et al. 2009). Karim et al. (2000) demonstrated that procyanidins (i.e., oligomers comprised of epicatechin and catechin subunits) were mostly responsible for aortic ring relaxation and significantly increased eNOS activity (Karim et al. 2000). Consistent with this, we recently observed that epigallocatechin-3-gallate and epicatechin induced a dose-dependent vasorelaxation in phenylephrine precontracted endothelium-intact preparations of rat-isolated aortic rings (Aggio et al. 2013), supporting the pivotal role of flavanols affecting endothelium/NO mechanisms involved in the regulation of arterial basal tone and in both mediating vasorelaxation and counteracting vasoconstriction. Furthermore, we also observed that epigallocatechin-3-gallate and epicatechin did not significantly affect vasorelaxation in precontracted endothelium-denuded preparations (Aggio et al. 2013). Of interest, in endothelium-intact precontracted preparations, Nω-nitro-L-arginine (L-NNA), an inhibitor of eNOS activity, abolished the vasorelaxant effect of epigallocatechin-3-gallate and epicatechin. At high concentrations, epigallocatechin-3-gallate and epicatechin elicited a marked relaxation. This was significantly larger in the presence than in the absence of endothelium or in the presence of L-NNA (Aggio et al. 2013).

In vivo, a large body of evidence suggests that flavonoids and flavonoid-rich products ingestion can improve endothelial function in humans as reported by a significant improvement in NO-dependent FMD. In keeping with this, administration of flavanol-rich cocoa (as cocoa-derived beverage ingested over 5 days) in healthy young and older subjects was observed to improve NO-dependent vasorelaxation, which, in turn, was inhibited by the intravenous administration of an arginine analog blocking NO synthesis (i.e., nitro-L-arginine methyl ester) (Fisher et al. 2003, Fisher and Hollenberg 2006).

Davison et al. (2008) also studied the effects of cocoa flavanols and regular exercise in overweight and obese adults. Authors reported that, compared to low-flavanol (36 mg flavanols), high-flavanol (902 mg flavanols) cocoa acutely increased NO-dependent FMD by 2.4% ($p < 0.01$) and chronically (over 12 weeks; $p < 0.01$) by 1.6% and reduced insulin resistance by 0.31% ($p < 0.05$), independent of exercise (Davison et al. 2008). Expanding on this, we demonstrated that flavanol-rich dark chocolate administration significantly increased the endothelium-dependent FMD of the brachial artery also positively affecting additional cardiovascular risk factors in healthy subjects (Grassi et al. 2005a) as well as in hypertensive patients with and without glucose intolerance (Grassi et al. 2005b, 2008). These data support the hypothesis that flavanols are able to ameliorate the function of not only a normal, but also that of an abnormal, endothelium (Grassi et al. 2005b, 2008).

According to our findings observed in patients with metabolic disturbances, results observed in patients with medicated type 2 diabetes suggested that a single dose of flavanol-rich cocoa was dose dependently associated with significant acute increases in circulating flavanols and FMD (at 2 h, from 3.7% ± 0.2% to 5.5% ± 0.4%, $p < 0.001$) (Balzer et al. 2008). Moreover, the same authors showed that also consumption of cocoa (thrice daily) for a period of 30 days increased baseline FMD by 30% ($p < 0.0001$) (Balzer et al. 2008). Additionally, Faridi et al. (2008), evaluating the acute effects of solid dark chocolate (chocolate bar containing 22 g cocoa powder or a cocoa-free placebo bar containing 0 g cocoa powder) and liquid cocoa intake (sugar-free cocoa containing 22 g cocoa powder, sugared cocoa containing 22 g cocoa powder, or a placebo containing 0 g cocoa powder) on endothelial function and blood pressure in overweight adults, reported that, compared with placebo, solid dark chocolate and liquid cocoa ingestion improved endothelial function (dark chocolate: $4.3\% \pm 3.4\%$ compared to $-1.8\% \pm 3.3\%$; $p < 0.001$; sugar-free and sugared cocoa: $5.7\% \pm 2.6\%$ and $2.0\% \pm 1.8\%$ compared to $-1.5\% \pm 2.8\%$; $p < 0.001$). Endothelial function improved significantly more with sugar-free than with regular cocoa ($5.7\% \pm 2.6\%$ compared to $2.0\% \pm 1.8\%$; $p < 0.001$). The aforementioned data also support the idea that sugar content may attenuate beneficial effects from flavonoids, while sugar-free preparations may augment them. Exactly consequent to this evidence, we observed that compared with flavanol-free white chocolate, flavanol-rich dark chocolate ingestion improved FMD ($p = 0.03$), wave reflections, endothelin-1, and the marker of lipid peroxidation 8-iso prostaglandin F2α [8-iso-PGF(2α)] ($p < 0.05$) (Grassi et al. 2012). Of interest, after white chocolate ingestion, FMD was reduced after an oral glucose tolerance test (OGTT) from 7.88 ± 0.68 to 6.07 ± 0.76 ($p = 0.027$) and to 6.74 ± 0.51 ($p = 0.046$) at 1 and 2 h after the glucose load, respectively. Similarly, after white chocolate but not after dark chocolate, wave reflections, blood pressure, and endothelin-1 and 8-iso-PGF(2α) increased after OGTT (Grassi et al. 2012). Thus, OGTT caused acute, transient impairment of endothelial function and oxidative stress, which was attenuated by flavanol-rich dark chocolate. These results suggest cocoa flavanols may contribute to vascular health by reducing the postprandial impairment of arterial function associated with the pathogenesis of atherosclerosis (Grassi et al. 2012). Accordingly, we showed that, compared to baseline values, short-term administration of flavonoid-rich chocolate significantly lowered insulin resistance as indicated by HOMA-IR and raised insulin sensitivity (QUICKI and ISI), whereas flavonoid-free chocolate was ineffective. In addition, a significant improvement in glucose and insulin responses during oral glucose tolerance tests was observed after flavonoid-rich but not after flavonoid-free chocolate ingestion in healthy volunteers (Grassi et al. 2005a) and hypertensive patients with (Grassi et al. 2008) and without (Grassi et al. 2005b) impaired glucose tolerance. In this context, we also observed a significant increase in insulin sensitivity and pancreatic β-cell function after flavonoid-rich chocolate administration in hypertensive patients with impaired glucose tolerance (Grassi et al. 2008). Changes in insulin sensitivity (Delta ISI—Delta FMD: $r = 0.510, p = 0.001$; Delta QUICKI—Delta FMD: $r = 0.502, p = 0.001$) and beta-cell function [Delta CIR(120)—Delta FMD: $r = 0.400, p = 0.012$] were directly correlated with increases in FMD. Thus, the effects of flavonoids on NO-dependent vascular function and insulin sensitivity might also be linked from a mechanistic point of view (Grassi et al. 2005b, 2008, 2012). In this regard, supporting our data, dietary supplementation with cocoa liquor procyanidins has been observed dose dependently to prevent the development of hyperglycemia in diabetic obese mice (Tomaru et al. 2007). In the diabetic obese mice, a diet containing 0.5% or 1.0% cacao liquor proanthocyanidins decreased the levels of blood glucose and fructosamine compared with that containing 0%, without significant effects on body weight or food consumption (Tomaru et al. 2007). Dorenkott et al. (2014) showed that oligomeric cocoa procyanidins prevented the development of obesity, insulin resistance, and impaired glucose tolerance during high-fat feeding. Further, recently, Cordero-Herrera et al. (2014) showed that (−)-epicatechin and cocoa polyphenolic extract improved insulin sensitivity of human HepG2 cells treated with high glucose, preventing or delaying a potential hepatic dysfunction through the attenuation of the insulin signaling blockade and the modulation of glucose uptake and production (Cordero-Herrera et al. 2014).

We have also recently observed that cocoa flavanols might be effective in improving cognitive function in elderly subjects with mild cognitive impairment (Desideri et al. 2012). The time required to complete Trail Making Test A and Trail Making Test B was significantly ($p < 0.05$) lower in subjects assigned to high flavanols (38.10 ± 10.94 and 104.10 ± 28.73 s, respectively) and intermediate flavanols (40.20 ± 11.35 and 115.97 ± 28.35 s, respectively) in comparison with those assigned to low flavanols (52.60 ± 17.97 and 139.23 ± 43.02 s, respectively). Similarly, verbal fluency test score was significantly ($p < 0.05$) better in subjects assigned to high flavanols in comparison with those assigned to low flavanols (27.50 ± 6.75 versus 22.30 ± 8.09 words per 60 s). Insulin resistance, blood pressure, and lipid peroxidation also decreased among subjects in the high-flavanol and intermediate-flavanol groups. Changes of insulin resistance explained $\approx 40\%$ of composite z score variability through the study period (partial $r(2) = 0.4013$; $p < 0.0001$) (Desideri et al. 2012). Therefore, these data suggest that regular consumption of cocoa flavanols might be effective in improving cognitive function in elderly subjects with mild cognitive impairment and this might be mediated at least in part by an improvement in insulin sensitivity (Desideri et al. 2012).

In agreement with the aforementioned data, a systematic review and meta-analysis of randomized short-term controlled trials (Shrime et al. 2011) reported that flavanol-rich chocolate was able to significantly improve insulin resistance, lipid profiles, blood pressure, and FMD. In particular, regarding insulin resistance, they suggested that HOMA-IR decreased by 0.94 points (95% CI = 0.59, 1.29; $p < 0.001$) with the consumption of flavonoid-rich cocoa (Shrime et al. 2011). Additionally, flavonoid-rich cocoa consumption significantly increased ISI by 4.95 points (95% CI = 2.80, 7.10; $p < 0.001$). This parameter of insulin sensitivity was examined by three studies without significant heterogeneity, while there were not enough data available to analyze fasting insulin levels (Shrime et al. 2011). The same authors described that a nonlinear dose–response relationship was found between FRC and FMD ($p = 0.004$), with maximum effect observed at a flavonoid dose of 500 mg/day.

Aiming to systematically review the effectiveness of different flavonoid subclasses and flavonoid-rich food sources on cardiovascular disease and endothelial function, Hooper et al. (2008) reported that chocolate or cocoa increased FMD by 1.45% (95% confidential interval: 0.62%, 2.28%; two studies). When data were available from ≥ 3 acute studies, only chocolate or cocoa significantly improved FMD (3.99%; 95% confidential interval: 2.86, 5.12; six studies). Only the group represented by chocolate or cocoa was able to show significant effects, both acutely and chronically, on FMD. Considering differences in chemical structures and range of doses, it was observed significant heterogeneity between different flavonoid subgroups (p for heterogeneity <0.01, I2 = $\approx 80\%$ in both acute and chronic studies). This confirmed that different flavonoid groups have different effects on FMD. Additionally, the same group systematically reviewing the effects of chocolate, cocoa, and flavan-3-ols on major cardiovascular risk factors reported consistent acute and chronic benefits of chocolate or cocoa on FMD, with chocolate or cocoa improving FMD regardless of the dose consumed (Hooper et al. 2012). Furthermore, authors showed that insulin resistance (HOMA-IR: -0.67; 95% CI: -0.98, -0.36) was improved by chocolate or cocoa due to significant reductions in serum insulin. Effects on HOMA-IR and FMD remained stable to sensitivity analyses (Hooper et al. 2012). Nevertheless, the authors suggested that the scarce number of studies evaluating the effects of cocoa intake on insulin resistance and metabolic disturbances, as well as the difficulties in studying the metabolic effects of cocoa in diabetes, deserve some caution. Further, experimental studies are required to confirm a potentially beneficial effect of chocolate consumption on metabolic disorders.

24.5 CONCLUSIONS

Increased prevalence of obesity in the world, especially accumulation of abnormal amounts of visceral fat predisposes to insulin resistance, which plays a central role in the definition and expression of the MetS.

Obesity can deregulate the intracellular signaling of insulin due to the production of inflammatory substances triggering hormonal mediator potentials for destabilization of signal transduction, favoring additional metabolic disorders and cardiovascular disease. The endothelium plays a pivotal role in arterial homeostasis and insulin resistance is the most important pathophysiological feature in various prediabetic and diabetic states. Reduced NO bioavailability with endothelial dysfunction is considered the earliest step in the pathogenesis of atherosclerosis. In addition, insulin resistance could account, at least in part, for the endothelial dysfunction (Grassi et al. 2010, 2011,

Pansuria et al. 2012, Kaur 2014). Combination therapies with agents targeting distinct mechanisms are likely to have additive or synergistic benefits.

Large, robust, epidemiologic studies demonstrate beneficial metabolic and cardiovascular health effects for many functional foods containing various polyphenols. Increasing interest has been addressed to the potential of cocoa flavanols in preventing obesity and type 2 diabetes. However, precise molecular mechanisms of action for polyphenols are largely unknown. Moreover, translation of these insights into effective clinical therapies has not been fully performed. Nevertheless, some functional foods are likely sources for safe and effective therapies and preventive strategies for metabolic diseases and their cardiovascular complications. Growing evidence supports a protective effect of cocoa consumption against cardiovascular disease. Cocoa and flavonoids from cocoa have been described to improve endothelial function and insulin resistance. A proposed mechanism could be considered the improvement of the endothelium-derived vasodilator NO by enhancing NO synthesis or by decreasing NO breakdown. Of interest, an in vitro study showed an inhibitory effect of flavanols on angiotensin-converting enzyme (ACE) activity, thus suggesting a possible action of flavanol-rich cocoa on the renin–angiotensin–aldosterone system (Actis-Goretta et al. 2006).

This finding could be of extreme clinical relevance, since renin–angiotensin–aldosterone system activation occurs in many cardiovascular disorders and plays a pivotal role not only in the mechanisms of endothelial dysfunction/activation but also in the onset of insulin resistance (Grassi et al. 2009, 2011). In this context, insulin resistance is a well-known risk factor for cardiovascular disease (Grassi et al. 2009, 2011, 2013a). Thus, flavanols and related polyphenolic antioxidants may counteract insulin resistance by increasing the NO bioavailability and decreasing the formation of ROS and nitrogen species (Grassi et al. 2009, 2010).

Therefore, albeit not all the involved mechanisms have been exhaustively clarified, data from literature seem to suggest that flavonoids present with all the biological potential to positively affect vascular function and insulin resistance via direct and indirect actions. They potentially could be considered as healthy compounds for diet supplementation. Of particular interest, the European Food Safety Authority (EFSA) concluded that a cause and effect relationship has been established between the consumption of cocoa flavanols and maintenance of normal endothelium-dependent vasodilation, suggesting that in order to obtain the claimed effect, cocoa and chocolate (of specific quality for flavonoid content) can be consumed in the context of a balanced diet. After evaluation of all the studies in literature on this issue, they finally stated that 200 mg of cocoa flavanols should be consumed daily in order to obtain the beneficial effect on endothelial function. This amount could be provided by 2.5 g of high-flavanol cocoa powder or 10 g of high-flavanol dark chocolate, and the target population is the general population (European Food Safety Authority (EFSA) 2012)).

REFERENCES

Abdul-Ghani, M.A., DeFronzo, R.A. 2010. Pathogenesis of insulin resistance in skeletal muscle. *J Biomed Biotechnol* 2010:476279.

Actis-Goretta, L., Ottaviani, J.I., Fraga, C.G. 2006. Inhibition of angiotensin converting enzyme activity by flavanol-rich foods. *J Agric Food Chem* 54(1):229–234.

Aggio, A., Grassi, D., Onori, E. et al. 2013. Endothelium/nitric oxide mechanism mediates vasorelaxation and counteracts vasoconstriction induced by low concentration of flavanols. *Eur J Nutr* 52(1):263–272.

Balzer, J., Rassaf, T., Heiss, C. et al. 2008. Sustained benefits in vascular function through flavanol-containing cocoa in medicated diabetic patients a double-masked, randomized, controlled trial. *J Am Coll Cardiol* 51(22):2141–2149.

Baron, A.D., Steinberg, H.O., Chaker, H., Leaming, R., Johnson, A., Brechtel, G. 1995. Insulin-mediated skeletal muscle vasodilation contributes to both insulin sensitivity and responsiveness in lean humans. *J Clin Invest* 96(2):786–792.

Bayard, V., Chamorro, F., Motta, J., Hollenberg, N.K. 2007. Does flavanol intake influence mortality from nitric oxide-dependent processes? Ischemic heart disease, stroke, diabetes mellitus, and cancer in Panama. *Int J Med Sci* 4(1):53–58.

Calver, A., Collier, J., Vallance, P. 1992. Inhibition and stimulation of nitric oxide synthesis in the human forearm arterial bed of patients with insulin-dependent diabetes. *J Clin Invest* 90(6):2548–2554.

Cersosimo, E., DeFronzo, R.A. 2006. Insulin resistance and endothelial dysfunction: The road map to cardiovascular diseases. *Diabetes Metab Res Rev* 22(6):423–436.

Cordero-Herrera, I., Martín, M.Á., Goya, L., Ramos, S. 2014. Cocoa flavonoids attenuate high glucose-induced insulin signalling blockade and modulate glucose uptake and production in human HepG2 cells. *Food Chem Toxicol* 64:10–19.

Davison, K., Coates, A.M., Buckley, J.D., Howe, P.R. 2008. Effect of cocoa flavanols and exercise on cardiometabolic risk factors in overweight and obese subjects. *Int J Obes* (*Lond*) 32(8):1289–1296.

de Jongh, R.T., Serné, E.H., IJzerman, R.G., de Vries, G., Stehouwer, C.D. 2004. Impaired microvascular function in obesity: Implications for obesity-associated microangiopathy, hypertension, and insulin resistance. *Circulation* 109(21):2529–2535.

Desideri, G., Kwik-Uribe, C., Grassi, D. et al. 2012. Benefits in cognitive function, blood pressure, and insulin resistance through cocoa flavanol consumption in elderly subjects with mild cognitive impairment: The Cocoa, Cognition, and Aging (CoCoA) study. *Hypertension* 60(3):794–801.

Dorenkott, M.R., Griffin, L.E., Goodrich, K.M. et al. 2014. Oligomeric cocoa procyanidins possess enhanced bioactivity compared to monomeric and polymeric cocoa procyanidins for preventing the development of obesity, insulin resistance, and impaired glucose tolerance during high-fat feeding. *J Agric Food Chem* 62(10):2216–2227.

Erusalimsky, J.D., Moncada, S. 2007. Nitric oxide and mitochondrial signaling: From physiology to pathophysiology. *Arterioscler Thromb Vasc Biol* 27(12):2524–2531.

European Food Safety Authority (EFSA). 2012. Scientific opinion on the substantiation of a health claim related to cocoa flavanols and maintenance of normal endothelium-dependent vasodilation pursuant to Article 13(5) of Regulation (EC) No 1924/20061. *EFSA J* 10(7):2809.

Executive Summary of the Third Report of the National Cholesterol Education Program (NCEP). 2001. Expert panel on detection, evaluation, and treatment of high blood cholesterol in adults (Adults Treatment Panel III). *JAMA* 285:2486–2497.

Faridi, Z., Njike, V.Y., Dutta, S., Ali, A., Katz, D.L. 2008. Acute dark chocolate and cocoa ingestion and endothelial function: A randomized controlled crossover trial. *Am J Clin Nutr* 88(1):58–63.

Ferri, C., Bellini, C., Desideri, G. et al. 1997. Circulating endothelin-1 levels in obese patients with the metabolic syndrome. *Exp Clin Endocrinol Diabetes* 105(Suppl 2):38–40.

Fiorentino, T.V., Prioletta, A., Zuo, P., Folli, F. 2013. Hyperglycemia-induced oxidative stress and its role in diabetes mellitus related cardiovascular diseases. *Curr Pharm Des* 19(32):5695–5703.

Fisher, N.D., Hollenberg, N.K. 2006. Aging and vascular responses to flavanol-rich cocoa. *J Hypertens* 24(8):1575–1580.

Fisher, N.D., Hughes, M., Gerhard-Herman, M., Hollenberg, N.K. 2003. Flavanol-rich cocoa induces nitric-oxide-dependent vasodilation in healthy humans. *J Hypertens* 21(12):2281–2286.

Grassi, D., Desideri, G., Croce, G., Tiberti, S., Aggio, A., Ferri, C. 2009. Flavonoids, vascular function and cardiovascular protection. *Curr Pharm Des* 15(10):1072–1084.

Grassi, D., Desideri, G., Ferri, C. 2010. Flavonoids: Antioxidants against atherosclerosis. *Nutrients* 2(8):889–902.

Grassi, D., Desideri, G., Ferri, C. 2013a. Protective effects of dark chocolate on endothelial function and diabetes. *Curr Opin Clin Nutr Metab Care* 16(6):662–668.

Grassi, D., Desideri, G., Ferri, C. 2011. Cardiovascular risk and endothelial dysfunction: The preferential route for atherosclerosis. *Curr Pharm Biotechnol* 12(9):1343–1353.

Grassi, D., Desideri, G., Necozione, S. et al. 2012. Protective effects of flavanol-rich dark chocolate on endothelial function and wave reflection during acute hyperglycemia. *Hypertension* 60(3):827–832.

Grassi, D., Desideri, G., Necozione, S. et al. 2008. Blood pressure is reduced and insulin sensitivity increased in glucose-intolerant, hypertensive subjects after 15 days of consuming high-polyphenol dark chocolate. *J Nutr* 138(9):1671–1676.

Grassi, D., Ferri, L., Desideri, G. et al. 2013b. Chronic hyperuricemia, uric acid deposit and cardiovascular risk. *Curr Pharm Des* 19(13):2432–2438.

Grassi, D., Lippi, C., Necozione, S., Desideri, G., Ferri, C. 2005a. Short-term administration of dark chocolate is followed by a significant increase in insulin sensitivity and a decrease in blood pressure in healthy persons. *Am J Clin Nutr* 81(3):611–614.

Grassi, D., Necozione, S., Lippi, C. et al. 2005b. Cocoa reduces blood pressure and insulin resistance and improves endothelium-dependent vasodilation in hypertensives. *Hypertension* 46(2):398–405.

Gudbjörnsdottir, S., Elam, M., Sellgren, J., Anderson, E.A. 1996. Insulin increases forearm vascular resistance in obese, insulin-resistant hypertensives. *J Hypertens* 14(1):91–97.

Hollenberg, N.K., Fisher, N.D., McCullough, M.L. 2009. Flavanols, the Kuna, cocoa consumption, and nitric oxide. *Am Soc Hypertens* 3(2):105–112.

Hooper, L., Kay, C., Abdelhamid, A. et al. 2012. Effects of chocolate, cocoa, and flavan-3-ols on cardiovascular health: A systematic review and meta-analysis of randomized trials. *Am J Clin Nutr* 95(3):740–751.

Hooper, L., Kroon, P.A., Rimm, E.B. et al. 2008. Flavonoids, flavonoid-rich foods, and cardiovascular risk: A meta-analysis of randomized controlled trials. *Am J Clin Nutr* 88(1):38–50.

Karim, M., McCormick, K., Kappagoda, C.T. 2000. Effects of cocoa extracts on endothelium-dependent relaxation. *J Nutr* 130(8S Suppl):2105S–2108S.

Kaur, J. 2014. A comprehensive review on metabolic syndrome. *Cardiol Res Pract* 2014:943162.

Kim, J.A., Montagnani, M., Koh, K.K., Quon, M.J. 2006. Reciprocal relationships between insulin resistance and endothelial dysfunction: Molecular and pathophysiological mechanisms. *Circulation* 113(15):1888–1904.

Muniyappa, R., Iantorno, M., Quon, M.J. 2008. An integrated view of insulin resistance and endothelial dysfunction. *Endocrinol Metab Clin North Am* 37(3):685-x.

Pansuria, M., Xi, H., Li, L., Yang, X.F., Wang, H. 2012. Insulin resistance, metabolic stress, and atherosclerosis. *Front Biosci (Schol Ed)* 4:916–931.

Panza, J.A., Casino, P.R., Kilcoyne, C.M., Quyyumi, A.A. 1993. Role of endothelium-derived nitric oxide in the abnormal endothelium-dependent vascular relaxation of patients with essential hypertension. *Circulation* 87(5):1468–1474.

Pratley, R.E. 2007. Metabolic syndrome: Why the controversy? *Curr Diab Rep* 7:56–59.

Prior, J.O., Quiñones, M.J., Hernandez-Pampaloni, M. et al. 2005. Coronary circulatory dysfunction in insulin resistance, impaired glucose tolerance, and type 2 diabetes mellitus. *Circulation* 111(18):2291–2298.

Schroeder, C.A. Jr., Chen, Y.L., Messina, E.J. 1999. Inhibition of NO synthesis or endothelium removal reveals a vasoconstrictor effect of insulin on isolated arterioles. *Am J Physiol* 276(3 Pt 2):H815–H820.

Shankar, R.R., Wu, Y., Shen, H.Q., Zhu, J.S., Baron, A.D. 2000. Mice with gene disruption of both endothelial and neuronal nitric oxide synthase exhibit insulin resistance. *Diabetes* 49(5):684–687.

Shin, J.A., Lee, J.H., Lim, S.Y. et al. 2013. Metabolic syndrome as a predictor of type 2 diabetes, and its clinical interpretations and usefulness. *J Diabetes Investig* 4(4):334–343.

Shrime, M.G., Bauer, S.R., McDonald, A.C., Chowdhury, N.H., Coltart, C.E., Ding, E.L. 2011. Flavonoid-rich cocoa consumption affects multiple cardiovascular risk factors in a meta-analysis of short-term studies. *J Nutr* 141(11):1982–1988.

Syed Ikmal, S.I., Zaman Huri, H., Vethakkan, S.R., Wan Ahmad, W.A. 2013. Potential biomarkers of insulin resistance and atherosclerosis in type 2 diabetes mellitus patients with coronary artery disease. *Int J Endocrinol* 2013:698567.

Tomaru, M., Takano, H., Osakabe, N. et al. 2007. Dietary supplementation with cacao liquor proanthocyanidins prevents elevation of blood glucose levels in diabetic obese mice. *Nutrition* 23:351–355.

van Dam, R.M., Naidoo, N., Landberg, R. 2013. Dietary flavonoids and the development of type 2 diabetes and cardiovascular diseases: Review of recent findings. *Curr Opin Lipidol* 24(1):25–33.

Vincent, M.A., Barrett, E.J., Lindner, J.R., Clark, M.G., Rattigan, S. 2003a. Inhibiting NOS blocks microvascular recruitment and blunts muscle glucose uptake in response to insulin. *Am J Physiol Endocrinol Metab* 285(1):E123–E129.

Vincent, M.A., Montagnani, M., Quon, M.J. 2003b. Molecular and physiologic actions of insulin related to production of nitric oxide in vascular endothelium. *Curr Diab Rep* 3(4):279–288.

Section VI

Dietary Patterns in Metabolic Syndrome

25 Mediterranean Diet and Metabolic Syndrome

Evanthia Gouveri, Fotios Drakopanagiotakis,
and Emmanuel James Diamantopoulos

CONTENTS

25.1 INTRODUCTION

The Mediterranean diet (MedDiet) represents a dietary pattern that has been associated with multiple health benefits, including lower incidence of various chronic diseases and lower rates of cardiovascular and all-cause mortality (Trichopoulou et al. 2003, Knoops et al. 2004). The MedDiet is the dietary model that was followed by people living in Southern Europe in 1960s and was initially described by Keys (1980). It is characterized by increased antioxidant content and monounsaturated fatty acids (MUFAs) as well as by the consumption of foods with a low glycemic index (Abete et al. 2011). This definition practically means that people who follow this dietary pattern consume large amounts of vegetables, fruits, and nonrefined cereals. Furthermore, consumption of red meat is limited and is substituted for fish and low-fat dairy products instead. Moderate alcohol consumption is also part of the MedDiet, but a hallmark of this dietary pattern is the use of olive oil as the cardinal added lipid. It is suggested that the combination of MedDiet with physical activity plays a beneficial role in modifying cardiovascular risk. In addition, isolated components of the MedDiet have been studied regarding their potential beneficial role in the modification of cardiovascular risk factors (Abete et al. 2011).

Cumulative evidence suggests that the MedDiet has also a beneficial role on the metabolic syndrome (MetS). MetS is a clustering of risk factors that promote atherosclerosis and has been associated with an increased risk for type 2 diabetes mellitus (DM), cardiovascular disease (CVD), and all-cause mortality (Lakka et al. 2002, Wilson et al. 2005). The characteristic features of the syndrome are insulin resistance, abdominal obesity, dyslipidemia, and hypertension. It has been estimated that almost 25% of the global population has MetS, largely due to the obesity epidemic (Zimmet et al. 2005). The reduction of the prevalence and incidence of noncommunicable diseases via the use of simple preventive measures has been the aim of an action plan developed by the World Health Organization (WHO) (WHO 2008). Recognition and identification of individuals with MetS who are at high risk for type 2 DM and CVD and promotion of healthy behaviors such as exercise and a healthy diet (e.g., the MedDiet) for the prevention of these diseases serve the main goals of this action.

Adopting the MedDiet seems to be an effective strategy to reduce the prevalence and incidence of MetS and of its individual components and consequently, the global burden of type 2 diabetes and CVD (Buckland et al. 2008, Pérez-López et al. 2009, Salas-Salvadó et al. 2011). However, the implementation of this dietary pattern in non-Mediterranean populations remains a challenge for public health policies.

25.2 DEFINITION OF THE MEDITERRANEAN DIET

The term *Mediterranean diet* is used mainly to describe the dietary pattern followed by inhabitants of countries bordering the Mediterranean Sea. The MedDiet is a healthy dietary model with multiple variations among countries following this diet, due to cultural or purely geographical reasons. What is considered the prototype of the MedDiet however is the dietary pattern that was followed in South Europe, particularly in the island of Crete in Greece, and South Italy in the 1960s. This dietary habit is usually reported as the *traditional* MedDiet. Initial interest for the MedDiet appeared as a result of potential parameters that could be associated with the unusually high life expectancy that was observed in the populations of Crete and South Italy. Diet as well as physical activity was thought to significantly contribute to the longevity of these populations. Unfortunately, this beneficial lifestyle has not been able to overcome the influence of westernized dietary and lifestyle patterns. Consequently, the *traditional* MedDiet pattern is nowadays followed by significantly fewer people living around the Mediterranean Sea.

Cardinal characteristics of the traditional MedDiet are the increased consumption of fresh and minimally processed vegetables and fruits, nonrefined cereals and products, low-fat dairy products, and the limited consumption of red meat. The MedDiet typically includes alcohol consumption with meals, usually red wine but only in moderation (two glasses per day for men and one for women). Of note, moderate alcohol consumption is optional and only when it is not contraindicated. Furthermore, moderate consumption of fish, poultry, nuts, potatoes, eggs, and sweets is encouraged (Willett et al. 1995). However, the hallmark of the MedDiet is the use of olive oil as the main added lipid and is used both in fresh salads and cooked meals (Trichopoulou 2000) instead of butter or margarine. Salt is also restricted and the use of herbs and spices such as basil, oregano, and thyme serves to flavor foods with the advantage of being practically fat free. Daily consumption of plant foods, such as nuts and olives, is also suggested as part of the MedDiet. However, nuts are rich in calories and therefore, attention should be paid in consuming limited amounts of this food. Additionally, drinking plenty of water is fundamental. Most importantly, it should be kept in mind that the traditional MedDiet is closely associated with regular physical activity as part of the entire healthy Mediterranean lifestyle (Panagiotakos et al. 2005).

Energy intake within the MedDiet is based mainly on consumption of lipids and carbohydrates. Total lipid intake varies among different Mediterranean countries, representing around 40% of total energy intake in Greece and around 30% of total energy intake in Italy (Panagiotakos et al. 2006a). MedDiet is rich in unsaturated and MUFAs. Monounsaturated fats are almost double compared to saturated fats consumed in a MedDiet (Panagiotakos et al. 2006a). The main sources of fat in this dietary model are olive oil, fish, and nuts. Olive oil, the hallmark of MedDiet, is an excellent source of antioxidants and MUFAs. Monounsaturated fat consumption not only results to a decreased consumption of polyunsaturated fats but most significantly, it is associated with a significantly decreased risk of coronary heart disease. Both MUFAs and polyunsaturated fats have been shown to reduce low-density lipoprotein cholesterol (LDL-C) and triglyceride levels with an increase in high-density lipoprotein cholesterol (HDL-C) levels when compared to carbohydrates (Willett 2006).

Indeed, unsaturated fat consumption has been regarded as an effective preventive strategy of coronary heart disease (Gillingham et al. 2011). Olive oil has a beneficial effect to lipid profile, blood pressure (BP), insulin resistance, oxidative stress, endothelial dysfunction, and thrombotic predisposition, and this effect is mediated by its phenolic content (López-Miranda et al. 2010). Therefore, despite the fact that MedDiet is not a low-fat diet, it exerts beneficial effects to the metabolism.

Other fat sources in the MedDiet include fish and nuts. Fish consumption exerts its beneficial effects through the rich content in omega-3 fatty acids. Omega-3 fatty acids are associated with increased insulin sensitivity as well as with BP normalization and triglyceride level reduction (Ebbesson et al. 2007). However, fried fish should be avoided. It is noteworthy that fat consumption in the frame of the MedDiet can be of great benefit regarding cardiovascular risk. In a recently published observational trial regarding the effect of MedDiet for primary prevention of cardiovascular events, it was shown that a MedDiet supplemented with both extra virgin olive oil and with mixed nuts was superior to a control diet with advice to reduce dietary fat, by reducing cardiovascular events by 30%. It is also of importance that this dietary pattern was easier to follow compared to the control diet (Estruch et al. 2013).

Carbohydrate content of the MedDiet is largely provided by fruits, vegetables, legumes, grains, and milk. The advantage of these components is that they are both rich in fibers and that they have a low glycemic index. Fiber content is essential for weight control by reducing the feeling of hunger, as they provide a feeling of satiety for hours. Diets containing rich in fibers carbohydrates have been associated with a reduction in triglyceride serum levels (Abete et al. 2011). The other advantage that carbohydrates in the MedDiet offer is the low glycemic index. The glycemic index depicts the ratio of the blood glucose elevation after the consumption of one grammar of a specific carbohydrate to the blood glucose elevation that occurs after the consumption of pure glucose. The carbohydrate content in the MedDiet derived from vegetables, legumes, and fruits is characterized by a significantly low glycemic index, thus effectively controlling the deleterious anabolic and proliferative effects of postprandial insulin secretion (Abete et al. 2011). Moreover, carbohydrate consumption in MedDiet exerts significant antioxidant and anti-inflammatory properties (Pérez-López et al. 2009).

Furthermore, the polyphenolic components present in wine, such as resveratrol, explain the beneficial effect of moderate alcohol consumption, which is an essential part of the MedDiet. Resveratrol has been shown to act as a potent antioxidant of LDL, to exert anti-inflammatory properties and to reduce platelet aggregation. It is also associated with the potential decrease of carbohydrates absorption (Abete et al. 2011).

The MedDiet is classically depicted as a pyramid (Panagiotakos et al. 2005, 2006a), the base of which constitutes daily consumption of nonrefined cereals and products, such as whole-grain bread and pasta or brown rice, fruits, legumes and vegetables, olive oil, and low-fat dairy products. In the middle level of the pyramid, weekly consumption of fish and poultry, olives, pulses and nuts, potatoes, and eggs is advised. It is worth comment on potatoes being in the middle level of the pyramid, because they have a high glycemic index compared to cereals (Trichopoulou 2000). On the top of the pyramid, rare (once per month) red meat consumption is advised (Panagiotakos et al. 2006a). Daily physical activity and moderate alcohol consumption with meals as well as salt restriction and adequate water uptake are also essential components of the MedDiet and of the Mediterranean lifestyle.

Despite the beneficial effects of each component of the MedDiet, it is not clear whether these components per se or MedDiet as a whole are responsible for the beneficial metabolic effects. In a prospective study of the dietary habits of 22,043 adults in Greece, adherence to MedDiet was found to be associated with lower all-cause and cardiovascular mortality, although no strong associations between individual food groups and all-cause mortality was observed (Trichopoulou et al. 2003). However, people consume meals and not single nutrients and therefore, dietary patterns should better be studied instead of particular food (Trichopoulou 2000, Martínez-González and Sánchez-Villegas 2004). The probability of biologic interactions between different components of MedDiet has been proposed for the healthy benefits of this dietary pattern (Trichopoulou et al. 2003).

25.3 DEFINITION OF THE METABOLIC SYNDROME

MetS is the clustering of several well-known risk factors for the development of CVD: abdominal obesity, hypertension, dyslipidemia, and hyperglycemia. Insulin resistance and abdominal obesity have been considered as the hallmarks of MetS (Grundy et al. 2004, Anonymous 2006). Despite the strong criticism regarding the existence of MetS as a separate syndrome, its definition remains extremely useful for detecting subjects with a high possibility of developing CVD (Reaven 1998). Moreover, although the individual components of MetS are associated with the development CVD and death (Lakka et al. 2002, Wilson et al. 2005, Diamantopoulos et al. 2006), the combination of these factors exerts a much more deleterious effect than the pure sum up of its components (Mottillo et al. 2010, Mitjavila et al. 2013). A recent meta-analysis including 951,083 patients showed that MetS is related to a 2.35-fold increased risk of CVD, a 2.4-fold increase in CVD mortality, and a twice as high the risk for stroke and myocardial infarction. Furthermore, the presence of MetS was associated to a 1.5-fold increase in all-cause mortality (Mottillo et al. 2010).

Definitions of MetS proposed by different Organizations vary. One of the most widely used definition is that of The National Cholesterol Education Program Adult Treatment Panel III (NCEP-ATP III) (Expert Panel on Detection, Evaluation, and Treatment of High Blood Cholesterol in Adults 2001), according to which MetS is defined by the presence of three of the following factors (Expert Panel on Detection, Evaluation, and Treatment of High Blood Cholesterol in Adults 2001, Grundy et al. 2004): increased waist circumference (≥102 cm in men and ≥88 cm in women), elevated fasting plasma glucose levels (≥110 mg/dL-revised criterion ≥100 mg/dL), elevated serum triglyceride levels (≥150 mg/dL), high BP (systolic BP [SAP] ≥130 mmHg or/and diastolic BP (DAP) ≥85 mmHg), and low HDL-C levels (<40 mg/dL in men and <50 mg/dL in women). According to the International Diabetes Federation (IDF) (The IDF consensus worldwide definition of the metabolic syndrome 2006), MetS can be diagnosed when three of the previously mentioned risk factors are present but with the prerequisite that abdominal obesity is one of them. It is noteworthy that different, ethnicity-specific cutoff points for waist circumference are used by the IDF compared to the NCEP-ATP III (Zimmet et al. 2005, the IDF consensus worldwide definition of the metabolic syndrome 2006). Finally, the WHO (WHO 1999) defines MetS when two of the following factors exist: increased body mass index (BMI) or an increased waist-to-hip ratio, increased BP, elevated triglyceride levels, elevated HDL-C levels, and the presence of microalbuminuria in combination with any of the following: DM, impaired fasting glucose (IFG), impaired glucose tolerance (IGT), or insulin resistance.

In accordance to the obesity epidemic, a concomitant rise of MetS has been observed. It is estimated that approximately one-fourth of the global population is affected by MetS. However, higher rates of the syndrome (up to 40%) have also been reported (Ford 2005, Kastorini et al. 2011). Strategies for reducing the obesity and accordingly MetS epidemic are of urgent need. A recent systematic review and meta-analysis showed that lifestyle interventions (diet and/or exercise) and pharmacologic intervention were able to reduce cardiovascular events, to prevent the development of type 2 diabetes, and to reverse MetS (Dunkley et al. 2012). The MedDiet has been proposed as an excellent example of a dietary pattern that, when combined with physical exercise, can reduce MetS.

25.4 EFFECT OF THE MEDITERRANEAN DIET ON THE METABOLIC SYNDROME

Several studies have shown that the MedDiet can offer substantial benefit and reduce the prevalence of MetS, and according to some authors, MedDiet may be the dietary pattern that, most effectively than any other, prevents the development of MetS. This effect is shown to be exerted through modulation of the individual components of MetS. Through implementation of the MedDiet, morbidity and mortality of CVDs may be reduced. Adherence to the MedDiet among adults with MetS has been associated with reduced odds of coronary risk by 35%, after adjustment for potential confounding factors, suggesting that acute coronary events could be prevented when MedDiet is followed by individuals with MetS (Pitsavos et al. 2003).

The prevalence of MetS in relation to the MedDiet was examined in the ATTICA study (Panagiotakos et al. 2004), a health and nutrition survey. Among the 2282 adults (1128 men and 1154 women) from the greater Athens area who participated in the study, without any evidence of CVD or DM, prevalence of MetS was found to be 19.8%. The syndrome was more prevalent in men than women (25.2% vs. 14.6%) and increased accordingly to age. Adherence to the MedDiet was evaluated through a validated nutrient questionnaire. Individuals who followed the MedDiet were found to have a 19% lower risk of having MetS (Panagiotakos et al. 2004).

These results are in striking similarity with the results of the Athens study, a cross-sectional epidemiologic survey of CVD and risk factors that was conducted in the Athens area 20 years before the ATTICA study, in the 1980s, when MetS had not been established as an entity (Gouveri et al. 2011). In the Athens study, 2074 randomly selected adults from the general population were recruited (900 men and 1174 women) and adherence to the MedDiet was evaluated according to a detailed questionnaire about nutrition habits. The MedDiet was followed by almost half of the study population (49.3%). Although women were more likely to adhere to the MedDiet, there was no difference between age groups. Participants with DM or CVD were less likely to follow the MedDiet as their dietary pattern. Adherence to the MedDiet was found to be associated with a 20% lower prevalence of MetS (Gouveri et al. 2011).

Similar results have also been reported by other cohorts conducted in Mediterranean populations. Among 808 individuals with high cardiovascular risk, an inverse association was found between the prevalence of MetS and adherence to the MedDiet. Study participants with the lowest adherence to the MedDiet pattern had a 56% higher possibility of suffering from MetS compared to those with the highest adherence to the MedDiet (Babio et al. 2009).

The inverse relation in prevalence between MetS and MedDiet has not only been reported to adult populations of healthy or high cardiovascular risk individuals but in adolescents as well. In a cross-sectional nutritional study that was conducted in 362 adolescents (age 12–17 years old) living in the Balearic islands, an overall 5.8% prevalence of MetS was reported and the prevalence of MetS was lower in those participants following the MedDiet (Mar Bibiloni et al. 2011).

Adherence to the MedDiet has been associated not only with decreased prevalence but also with decreased incidence of MetS. The SUN cohort (Seguimiento Universidad de Navarra cohort) is a dynamic prospective cohort of Spanish university graduates followed up for 6 years (Tortosa et al. 2007). An initial analysis of 2563 participants who were not obese and did not have MetS, or other risk factors such as DM, hypertension, or hyperlipidemia, examined the relation between adherence to the MedDiet and incidence of MetS. The study showed that adherence to a Mediterranean food pattern for a 6-year duration was associated with 80% lower cumulative incidence of MetS in comparison to those who did not follow the MedDiet (Tortosa et al. 2007).

Furthermore, in a cohort of 3232 French adults enrolled in the SU.VI.MAX study (Supplementation en Vitamines et Mineraux Antioxidants study), the incidence of MetS was prospectively evaluated in a 6-year period in relation to adherence to the MedDiet. Adherence was estimated with the use of three different MedDiet scores. Adherence to the MedDiet was associated with a 50% lower risk of developing MetS in the 6-year follow-up period (Kesse-Guyot et al. 2013).

The beneficial effects of the MedDiet to the development of MetS have also been confirmed in a non-Mediterranean population. Among 1918 participants of the Framingham Heart Study Offspring Cohort without MetS at baseline, adherence to the MedDiet was inversely related to the development of MetS after a 7-year follow-up period (Rumawas et al. 2009). Partial features of MetS as insulin resistance, obesity, and hyperlipidemia were also less frequent in those with the highest adherence to the MedDiet.

25.5 MEDITERRANEAN DIET AND THE INDIVIDUAL COMPONENTS OF THE METABOLIC SYNDROME

The MedDiet seems to favorably affect not only MetS as an entity, but its individual components as well. In the Greek arm of the European Prospective Investigation into Cancer and Nutrition cohort (EPIC) that included 20,343 participants, MedDiet has been found to be inversely associated with systolic and diastolic hypertension, in particular its olive oil, fruit, and vegetable components. Of those components, olive oil was found to play the most prominent role for BP normalization. On the other hand, meat, alcohol, and cereal production was associated with increased arterial pressure (Psaltopoulou et al. 2004).

In a study conducted in Canary Islands (Alvarez León et al. 2006), subjects with a higher adherence to the MedDiet had a 70% lower prevalence of hypertension when compared with the lower adherence, and fruit, vegetable, and monounsaturated fat consumption showed a protective effect on triglycerides, glycemia, and insulin resistance criteria, respectively. Similar results regarding hypercholesterolemia, hypertension, diabetes and obesity, and MetS have been reported in Cypriot older individuals (Panagiotakos et al. 2003). Furthermore, among 4393 participants in the previously mentioned SUN study, the high fruit and vegetable intake was inversely associated with BP compared with low consumption of these items, although fat accounted for more than 37% of the total energy intake in this population (Alonso et al. 2004). In the ATTICA study, adherence to the MedDiet was associated with 26% lower risk of having hypertension, suggesting that this dietary pattern could be an effective dietary intervention to reduce the burden of hypertension. Of note, as the rate of controlled hypertension among those who are treated is not satisfactory (34% in this Greek population), this diet was associated with 36% greater odds of having the BP controlled (Panagiotakos et al. 2003).

Given the fact that the MedDiet is based on foods rich in carbohydrates and lipids, the role of this dietary pattern on weight management has been questioned although the MedDiet has beneficial effects on MetS even without weigh loss (Panagiotakos et al. 2007). However, evidence for several studies and meta-analyses has revealed that the MedDiet can have a beneficial effect on central obesity and weight loss as it is rich in fibers and unsaturated fatty acids (Romaguera et al. 2009). Therefore, this diet beyond the multiple health benefits could also be proposed for weight loss. In the ATTICA study, among 3042 men and women without CVD, an inverse association was observed between adherence to the MedDiet and indexes of obesity (waist-to-hip ratio and BMI). Among participants, those belonging at the highest tertile of MedDiet consumption, lower odds of obesity and central obesity have been observed (51% and 59%, respectively) after adjustment for confounding factors (Panagiotakos et al. 2006b).

Similarly, in a 2-year interventional trial conducted in moderately obese adults (mean BMI=31 kg/m^2) where three different diets were compared (a low-fat restricted-calorie diet, a MedDiet restricted-calorie [with no more than 35% of calories derived from fat], and a low-carbohydrate nonrestricted-calorie diet), mean weight loss was greater among subjects following the low-carbohydrate diet and the MedDiet compared with the low-fat diet (Shai et al. 2008). Furthermore, low-fat diets are not preferred, as it has been demonstrated that a low-fat and high-carbohydrate diet can lower both LDL-C and HDL-C levels (Trichopoulou et al. 2000).

Furthermore, in a large cross-sectional study of 497,308 adult individuals (mainly women) from 10 European countries (Romaguera et al. 2009), higher adherence to a modified (in order to apply across Europe) MedDiet seemed to be associated overall with a lower waist circumference for a given BMI in both sexes and the observed association was stronger in participants from Northern European countries (Romaguera et al. 2009) (although this diet was not significantly associated with BMI).

A meta-analysis of 21 studies (7 cross-sectional, 3 cohorts, and 11 intervention studies) showed that adherence to the MedDiet was associated with a lower prevalence of overweight and obesity in 13 of these studies (Buckland et al. 2008). Similarly, a more recent meta-analysis of 6 trials

(2650 subjects) revealed that the MedDiet is more effective than low-fat diets in reducing body weight and BMI (Shai et al. 2008). These results were further confirmed by a meta-analysis of 16 randomized controlled trials that also concluded that the MedDiet might be suggested as an effective tool for weight loss, when followed for more than 6 months and especially when accompanied with caloric restriction and physical activity (Esposito et al. 2011). Conclusively, although caloric restriction is the cornerstone for weight loss, the composition of a dietary pattern, like the MedDiet, seems to be effective in weight management.

MedDiet has also been shown to have a protective role against the development of diabetes. In a study of 13,380 Spanish university graduates without diabetes at baseline, adherence to the MedDiet was associated with lower risk of type 2 diabetes after 4.4 years of follow-up (Martínez-González et al. 2008). Of note, an incidence rate ratio of 0.17 was observed among participants with the highest adherence to the MedDiet compared with those with the lower adherence to this diet.

Furthermore, in the SU.VI.MAX Study highest adherence to the MedDiet reduced the risk of Mets by half when compared to the lowest adherence and seemed to beneficially affect the individual components of MetS (Kesse-Guyot et al. 2013). After adjusting for BMI, the MedDiet seemed to reduce MetS through favorable effects on BP, lipid profile, insulin resistance, and inflammation.

Results from the EPIC cohort, where only nine components of the MedDiet were recorded, showed that adherence to the MedDiet using this relative MedDiet score was associated only with a small reduction in the incidence of type 2 diabetes (InterAct Consortium et al. 2011). In the Multi-Ethnic Study of Atherosclerosis (MESA) (Abiemo et al. 2013), the dietary habits of 5390 adults of both sexes without diabetes were initially cross-sectionally recorded. Higher adherence to the MedDiet was associated with lower insulin levels at baseline and with lower blood glucose levels before adjusting for obesity. However, the MedDiet was not associated with a lower incidence of diabetes in this study (Abiemo et al. 2013).

Finally, data derived from a recent meta-analysis of 20 randomized controlled diets revealed that the MedDiet significantly reduces glycated hemoglobin (HbA1c) to a greater extend compared with the other diets studied and with the control diets. Therefore, the authors stated that among other beneficial diets, the MedDiet should also be considered an effective tool for the management of diabetes (Ajala et al. 2013).

25.6 MEDITERRANEAN DIET IN THE MANAGEMENT OF THE METABOLIC SYNDROME

The MedDiet seems to be also a useful therapeutic tool for the management of subjects with MetS. In a randomized, single-blind trial, 180 patients with MetS were assigned either to a Mediterranean-style diet plus detailed advice on how to increase daily consumption of olive oil, nuts, grains, fruits, and vegetables or to a cardiac-prudent low-fat diet (fat <30%, protein content 15%–20%, and carbohydrates 50%–60%). Subjects were followed for a period of 2 years: the ones who followed the MedDiet had a 48% reduction in the prevalence of MetS and a greater reduction in body weight. Insulin resistance, endothelial dysfunction, and markers of inflammation were also significantly decreased compared with the control group (Esposito et al. 2004).

In the multicenter PREDIMED 3-arm randomized clinical trial, 1244 subjects at high risk for CVD were randomized to follow the traditional MedDiet that was enriched with virgin olive oil or with nuts, or a low-fat diet. At baseline, 61.4% of the participants met the criteria for MetS and no difference in the prevalence of the syndrome was reported between the three groups. After 1 year of follow-up, individuals who followed the two subtypes of the MedDiet had significantly lower rates of MetS compared to those who followed the low-fat diet. After adjustment for confounding factors, the odds ratios for the reversion of MetS after 1-year adherence to the MedDiet with olive oil or nuts were 1.3 and 1.7, respectively (Salas-Salvadó et al. 2008).

In another randomized controlled trial, 110 women with MetS followed one of two different types of MedDiet (one supplemented with olive oil and the other with nuts) or a low-fat diet for a period of 1 year. Both subtypes of MedDiet were shown to reduce oxidative damage to lipids and DNA compared to the low-fat diet (Mitjavila et al. 2013).

Long-term effects of the MedDiet on the prevention of cardiovascular risk have been clearly shown in a large multicenter trial conducted in Spain, in which 7447 individuals at high cardiovascular risk but without CVD at baseline were randomized to receive a MedDiet supplemented with extra virgin olive oil or nuts without energy restriction, or a low-fat diet. The study was prematurely stopped due to the results of an interim analysis after a median follow-up of 4.8 years, clearly favoring the MedDiet intervention: the incidence of major cardiovascular events was reduced by 30% in subjects who followed the MedDiet with olive oil or nuts, compared with the low-fat diet (Estruch et al. 2013).

Short-term effects after implementation of the MedDiet have also been reported in numerous studies. In a 12-week trial of 89 women with MetS who were randomized either to a Mediterranean-style low-glycemic-load diet or the same diet plus a medical food containing phytosterols, soy protein, and extracts from hops and acacia, both interventions were found to similarly decrease the components of MetS (waist circumference, plasma triglycerides, SAP, and DAP) (Jones et al. 2011). Moreover, even after a 12-week implementation of the MedDiet, atherogenic lipoproteins, which are strongly associated with the development of CVD, were significantly decreased (Jones et al. 2012).

Combination of MedDiet with measures ensuring weight loss is of paramount importance for the management of patients with MetS. These combined effects were examined in a study of 24 men with MetS who underwent a 20-week weight loss period with prior 5-week consumption of the MedDiet, followed by a 5-week MedDiet consumption under weight-stable conditions. It was shown that the combination of the MedDiet with weight reduction led to significant reduction in SAP and DAP, glucose, insulin, plasma triglyceride, and apolipoprotein B levels. The MedDiet without weight loss however was only found to significantly decrease total plasma cholesterol, total/HDL-C, and LDL-C without the other beneficial effects in BP or hyperinsulinemia (Richard et al. 2011). Similar results have been reported with the completion of a 12-week lifestyle intervention program, consisting of 12 weekly sessions of exercise combined with adherence to the MedDiet, resulting in significant weight loss and reduction in waist circumference and in SAP and DAP. Interestingly, this healthy lifestyle pattern led to concomitant reduction of depressive symptoms as well.

Finally, a large meta-analysis of 50 studies with a total of 534,906 subjects has provided strong evidence regarding the effect of MedDiet on MetS. It has been clearly shown that adherence to the MedDiet is associated with a 31% reduction of MetS in both clinical trials and prospective studies. Moreover, adherence to the MedDiet could effectively reduce blood glucose and triglyceride levels, to have a beneficial effect on SAP and DAP, and to increase HDL-C levels (Kastorini et al. 2011).

25.7 RECOMMENDATIONS

Existing evidence suggests that a Mediterranean-style diet is a dietary pattern that can lower the prevalence and incidence of Mets. Although weight management remain the main lifestyle intervention for the prevention and treatment of MetS, the MedDiet, as already discussed, can favorably affect MetS even without weight loss.

A high ratio of unsaturated (MUFA and polyunsaturated) to saturated lipids is recommended according to NCEP-ATP III guidelines (Expert Panel on Detection, Evaluation, and Treatment of High Blood Cholesterol in Adults 2001). Total fat intake should range between 25% and 35% and saturated fat should be limited to less than 7% of total calories. Furthermore, daily cholesterol intake should not exceed 200 mg/dL. These guidelines are compatible with the MedDiet. Unsaturated fats, fiber, and complex carbohydrates are the main characteristics of this healthy dietary pattern. When the MedDiet is followed, total fat has been estimated to represent more than 25%, but less than 35% of total energy intake, with saturated fat covering only 7%–8% of total calories (Zimmet et al. 2005, Bays 2009). Carbohydrates account for 50%–60% of total calories and should be derived from foods rich in complex carbohydrates like whole grains, fruits, and vegetables that have a low glycemic index and can favorably influence the postprandial blood glucose (Riccardi et al. 2003). Of note, Esposito and Giugliano suggested that a moderately altered MedDiet with less carbohydrates (45%) and more dietary lipids (35%–40%, with <10% of saturated fat) could have also beneficial effects on MetS components (Esposito and Giugliano 2010), including insulin sensitivity and lipid profile.

It could be argued that the MedDiet could not be easily adopted by non-Mediterranean populations. Olive oil, for instance, is the main added lipid in this dietary pattern, but it could not easily substitute other dietary fats in different cultures and dietary traditions. However, recommendations on the consumption of less saturated fats and more fresh fruits, vegetables, and legumes, nonrefined cereals, beans, nuts, fish, and low-fat dairy products could be followed by non-Mediterranean populations as well.

25.8 ANTI-INFLAMMATORY AND ANTIOXIDATIVE EFFECTS OF THE MEDITERRANEAN DIET

Evidence suggests that MetS is characterized by a proinflammatory state. Proinflammatory cytokines such as interleukins (IL)-6, IL-7, and IL-8, as well as CRP, have been found to be increased in patients with MetS. These results are consistent with the low-grade inflammation that is associated with endothelial dysfunction. The MedDiet has shown efficacy in reducing the levels of circulating proinflammatory mediators. Healthy subjects without CVD who followed the MedDiet pattern had on average 20% lower CRP levels, 17% lower IL-6 levels, and lower levels of homocysteine and fibrinogen as well as lower white blood cell count (Chrysohoou et al. 2004).

In a randomized controlled trial of subjects with MetS, individuals who were assigned to a MedDiet for a period of 2 years were found to have lower levels of IL-6, IL-7, and IL-8 and CRP, compared to the ones who did not follow this healthy dietary pattern. Endothelial function score did also improve. Moreover, the decrease of the proinflammatory mediators was associated with the decrease in BMI, insulin resistance, levels of glucose, total cholesterol, and triglycerides (Esposito et al. 2011). The negative effect of the MedDiet to the proinflammatory state was assumed to be related to the high-fiber content and the antioxidant properties of omega-3 fatty acids and vitamins, therefore breaking a vicious cycle of inflammation and hyperinsulinemia (Esposito et al. 2011). Olive oil consumption has been shown to acutely decrease inflammatory and oxidative stress markers such as urinary hydrogen peroxide and thromboxane 2 (Bogani et al. 2007). This effect is mainly attributed to the high MUFA content and to the phenolic compounds of olive oil, although the pharmacological properties of olive oil are a very active research area (Pérez-Martínez et al. 2011).

Interestingly enough, even subjects with the Mets who do not benefit from weight loss when following the MedDiet, the degree of overall inflammation is significantly decreased (Richard et al. 2012).

Although different variations of the MedDiet exist, there is evidence that these variants exert similar antioxidative action. In a study comparing the effect of a MedDiet variant rich in olive oil content or nuts with a diet with low fat content, both variants were effective in reducing CRP, IL-6, and endothelial and monocytary adhesion molecules, while in the low-fat diet these proinflammatory mediators were increased (Urpi-Sarda et al. 2012). Of note, the effect of MedDiet may be more beneficial in subjects more prone to develop atherosclerosis. Homozygotes and heterozygotes for methylenetetrahydrofolate reductase C677T mutation, which is associated with oxidative modification of LDL-C, had greater benefit regarding reduction in oxidized LDL-C compared with subjects not carrying this mutation (Pitsavos et al. 2006).

Conclusively, anti-inflammatory and antioxidant properties of the MedDiet might in part explain the beneficial effects of this dietary model on MetS and its components.

25.9   COMMENTS AND PERSPECTIVE

MetS and its components (central obesity, insulin resistance, hyperglycemia, hypertension, and dyslipidemia) have emerged as a public health issue as they have detrimental health- and economic-related implications. Consequently, public health policies should focus on the implementation of intervention strategies that could be widely adopted. Lifestyle changes have already been considered the cornerstone for the prevention and treatment of MetS. Weight management, a healthy diet, and physical activity are suggested. The MedDiet has been proved an effective tool for both the prevention and treatment of MetS. Questions arise regarding the possibility of implementing this healthy dietary pattern among non-Mediterranean populations (Trichopoulou 2000). Even among individuals living in countries bordering the Mediterranean basin, the rates of following the MedDiet have dropped in the last decades following the westernized way of living and eating (Gouveri et al. 2011). Therefore, promoting this dietary model and persuading people to follow it for the rest of their lives is a challenging goal for health policies.

Furthermore, although many dietary items characterizing the MedDiet have been considered effective for the prevention and treatment of cardiometabolic risk factors and CVD, for instance, olive oil, nuts, and red wine, the study of food groups and healthy diets is more intriguing, as people consume meals and not only single nutrients, and therefore, prospective studies are needed to confirm existing data (Trichopoulou 2000).

The beneficial effect of the MedDiet on oxidative stress and inflammation has already been supported; however, the exact mechanisms by which the individual components of the MedDiet or this dietary pattern as a whole exert their protective role on cardiovascular system and on metabolism are not completely understood. Great interest has been shown in this field and continued research is expected to clarify the previously mentioned underlying mechanisms.

25.10   CONCLUSIONS

Cumulative evidence suggests that not only single healthy foods but rather entire dietary patterns can play a key role on metabolic risk factors and on cardiometabolic diseases. Therefore, healthy dietary interventions could reduce the prevalence and incidence of MetS. The MedDiet has demonstrated favorable effect both on MetS as a syndrome and on its individual features and could be therefore recommended as a promising lifestyle strategy for the prevention and treatment of MetS. Given the increasing prevalence of MetS worldwide and the subsequent increase in type 2 DM and CVD, the promotion of a healthy lifestyle is considered the first-line intervention that should be urgently widely implemented.

The adoption of the MedDiet combined with adequate physical activity is a challenge, particularly among non-Mediterranean populations and among younger individuals. Nevertheless, although a Mediterranean-style diet might seem difficult to follow by non-Mediterranean populations, a balanced increase in consumption of fresh foods rich in fiber and antioxidants and a reduction in saturated fats are considered the main changes toward a healthier dietary model that could be easily achieved. Health professionals should inform people on the multiple benefits that could be derived from this dietary pattern and encourage them to adopt it not as a kind of *diet* but as a healthy habit that could be followed for a lifetime.

REFERENCES

Abete, I., Goyenechea, E., Zulet, M.A., Martínez, J.A. 2011. Obesity and metabolic syndrome: Potential benefit from specific nutritional components. *Nutr Metab Cardiovasc Dis* 21(Suppl. 2): B1–B15.

Abiemo, E.E., Alonso, A., Nettleton, J.A. et al. 2013. Relationships of the Mediterranean dietary pattern with insulin resistance and diabetes incidence in the Multi-Ethnic Study of Atherosclerosis (MESA). *Br J Nutr* 109: 1490–1497.

Ajala, O., English, P., Pinkney, J. 2013. Systematic review and meta-analysis of different dietary approaches to the management of type 2 diabetes. *Am J Clin Nutr* 97: 505–516.

Alonso, A., de la Fuente, C., Martín-Arnau, A.M., de Irala, J., Martínez, J.A., Martínez-González, M.A. 2004. Fruit and vegetable consumption is inversely associated with blood pressure in a Mediterranean population with a high vegetable-fat intake: The Seguimiento Universidad de Navarra (SUN) Study. *Br J Nutr* 92: 311–319.

Alvarez León, E., Henríquez, P., Serra-Majem, L. 2006. Mediterranean diet and metabolic syndrome: A cross-sectional study in the Canary Islands. *Public Health Nutr* 9: 1089–1098.

Anonymous. 2006. The IDF consensus worldwide definition of the metabolic syndrome. http://www.idf.org/webdata/docs/IDF_Meta_def_final.pdf. Accessed on July 17, 2013.

Babio, N., Bulló, M., Basora, J. et al. 2009. Adherence to the Mediterranean diet and risk of metabolic syndrome and its components. *Nutr Metab Cardiovasc Dis* 19: 563–570.

Bays, H.E. 2009. "Sick fat," metabolic disease, and atherosclerosis. *Am J Med* 122: S26–S37.

Bogani, P., Galli, C., Villa, M., Visioli, F. 2007. Postprandial anti-inflammatory and antioxidant effects of extra virgin olive oil. *Atherosclerosis* 190: 181–186.

Buckland, G., Bach, A., Serra-Majem, L. 2008. Obesity and the Mediterranean diet: A systematic review of observational and intervention studies. *Obes Rev* 9: 582–593.

Chrysohoou, C., Panagiotakos, D.B., Pitsavos, C., Das, U.N., Stefanadis, C. 2004. Adherence to the Mediterranean diet attenuates inflammation and coagulation process in healthy adults: The ATTICA Study. *J Am Coll Cardiol* 44: 152–158.

Diamantopoulos, E.J., Andreadis, E.A., Tsourous, G.I. et al. 2006. Metabolic syndrome and prediabetes identify overlapping but not identical populations. *Exp Clin Endocrinol Diabetes* 114: 377–383.

Dunkley, A.J., Charles, K., Gray, L.J., Camosso-Stefinovic, J., Davies, M.J., Khunti, K. 2012. Effectiveness of interventions for reducing diabetes and cardiovascular disease risk in people with metabolic syndrome: Systematic review and mixed treatment comparison meta-analysis. *Diabetes Obes Metab* 14: 616–625.

Ebbesson, S.O., Tejero, M.E., Nobmann, E.D. et al. 2007. Fatty acid consumption and metabolic syndrome components: The GOCADAN study. *J Cardiometab Syndr* 2: 244–249.

Esposito, K., Giugliano, D. 2010. Mediterranean diet and the metabolic syndrome: The end of the beginning. *Metab Syndr Relat Disord* 8: 197–200.

Esposito, K., Kastorini, C.M., Panagiotakos, D.B., Giugliano, D. 2011. Mediterranean diet and weight loss: Meta-analysis of randomized controlled trials. *Metab Syndr Relat Disord* 9: 1–12.

Esposito, K., Marfella, R., Ciotola, M. et al. 2004. Effect of a mediterranean-style diet on endothelial dysfunction and markers of vascular inflammation in the metabolic syndrome: A randomized trial. *JAMA* 292: 1440–1446.

Estruch, R., Ros, E., Salas-Salvadó, J. et al. 2013. Primary prevention of cardiovascular disease with a Mediterranean diet. *N Engl J Med* 368: 1279–1290.

Executive Summary of the Third Report of The National Cholesterol Education Program (NCEP). 2001. Expert panel on detection, evaluation, and treatment of high blood cholesterol in adults (Adult Treatment Panel III). *JAMA* 285(16): 2486–2497.

Ford, E.S. 2005. Prevalence of the metabolic syndrome defined by the International Diabetes Federation among adults in the U.S. *Diabetes Care* 28: 2745–2749.

Gillingham, L.G., Harris-Janz, S., Jones, P.J. 2011. Dietary monounsaturated fatty acids are protective against metabolic syndrome and cardiovascular disease risk factors. *Lipids* 46: 209–228.

Gouveri, E.T., Tzavara, C., Drakopanagiotakis, F. et al. 2011. Mediterranean diet and metabolic syndrome in an urban population: The Athens Study. *Nutr Clin Pract* 26: 598–606.

Grundy, S.M., Brewer, H.B. Jr., Cleeman, J.I., Smith, S.C. Jr., Lenfant, C., American Heart Association, National Heart, Lung, and Blood Institute. 2004. Definition of metabolic syndrome: Report of the National Heart, Lung, and Blood Institute/American Heart Association conference on scientific issues related to definition. *Circulation* 109: 433–438.

InterAct Consortium, Romaguera, D., Guevara, M. et al. 2011. Mediterranean diet and type 2 diabetes risk in the European Prospective Investigation into Cancer and Nutrition (EPIC) study: The InterAct project. *Diabetes Care* 34: 1913–1918.

Jones, J.L., Comperatore, M., Barona, J. et al. 2012. A Mediterranean-style, low-glycemic-load diet decreases atherogenic lipoproteins and reduces lipoprotein (a) and oxidized low-density lipoprotein in women with metabolic syndrome. *Metabolism* 61: 366–372.

Jones, J.L., Fernandez, M.L., McIntosh, M.S. et al. 2011. A Mediterranean-style low-glycemic-load diet improves variables of metabolic syndrome in women, and addition of a phytochemical-rich medical food enhances benefits on lipoprotein metabolism. *J Clin Lipidol* 5: 188–196.

Kastorini, C.M., Milionis, H.J., Esposito, K. et al. 2011. The effect of Mediterranean diet on metabolic syndrome and its components: A meta-analysis of 50 studies and 534,906 individuals. *J Am Coll Cardiol* 57: 1299–1313.

Kesse-Guyot, E., Ahluwalia, N., Lassale, C., Hercberg, S., Fezeu, L., Lairon, D. 2013. Adherence to Mediterranean diet reduces the risk of metabolic syndrome: A 6-year prospective study. *Nutr Metab Cardiovasc Dis* 23: 677–683.

Keys, A. 1980. *Seven Countries: A Multivariate Analysis of Death and Coronary Heart Disease.* Harvard University Press, Cambridge, MA.

Knoops, K.T., deGroot, L.C., Kromhout, D. et al. 2004. Mediterranean diet, lifestyle factors, and 10-year mortality in elderly European men and women: The HALE project. *JAMA* 292: 1433–1439.

Lakka, H.M., Laaksonen, D.E., Lakka, T.A. et al. 2002. The metabolic syndrome and total and cardiovascular disease mortality in middle-aged men. *JAMA* 288: 2709–2716.

López-Miranda, J., Pérez-Jiménez, F., Ros, E. et al. 2010. Olive oil and health: Summary of the II international conference on olive oil and health consensus report, Jaén and Córdoba (Spain) 2008. *Nutr Metab Cardiovasc Dis* 20: 284–294.

Mar Bibiloni, M., Martínez, E., Llull, R. et al. 2011. Metabolic syndrome in adolescents in the Balearic Islands, a Mediterranean region. *Nutr Metab Cardiovasc Dis* 21: 446–454.

Martínez-González, M.A., de la Fuente-Arrillaga, C., Nunez-Cordoba, J.M. et al. 2008. Adherence to Mediterranean diet and risk of developing diabetes: Prospective cohort study. *BMJ* 336: 1348–1351.

Martínez-González, M.A., Sánchez-Villegas, A. 2004. The emerging role of Mediterranean diets in cardiovascular epidemiology: Monounsaturated fats, olive oil, red wine or the whole pattern? *Eur J Epidemiol* 19: 9–13.

Mitjavila, M.T., Fandos, M., Salas-Salvadó, J. et al. 2013. The Mediterranean diet improves the systemic lipid and DNA oxidative damage in metabolic syndrome individuals. A randomized, controlled, trial. *Clin Nutr* 32: 172–178.

Mottillo, S., Filion, K.B., Genest, J. et al. 2010. The metabolic syndrome and cardiovascular risk a systematic review and meta-analysis. *J Am Coll Cardiol* 56: 1113–1132.

Panagiotakos, D.B., Chrysohoou, C., Pitsavos, C., Stefanadis, C. 2006a. Association between the prevalence of obesity and adherence to the Mediterranean diet: The ATTICA study. *Nutrition* 22: 449–456.

Panagiotakos, D.B., Pitsavos, C., Chrysohoou, C. et al. 2004. Impact of lifestyle habits on the prevalence of the metabolic syndrome among Greek adults from the ATTICA study. *Am Heart J* 147: 106–112.

Panagiotakos, D.B., Pitsavos, C., Stefanadis, C. 2006b. Dietary patterns: A Mediterranean diet score and its relation to clinical and biological markers of cardiovascular disease risk. *Nutr Metab Cardiovasc Dis* 16: 559–568.

Panagiotakos, D.B., Pitsavos, C., Zampelas, A., Chrysohoou, C., Stefanadis, C. 2005. The relationship between fish consumption and the risk of developing acute coronary syndromes among smokers: The CARDIO2000 case-control study. *Nutr Metab Cardiovasc Dis* 15: 402–409.

Panagiotakos, D.B., Pitsavos, C.H., Chrysohoou, C. et al. 2003. Status and management of hypertension in Greece: Role of the adoption of a Mediterranean diet: The Attica study. *J Hypertens* 21: 1483–1489.

Panagiotakos, D.B., Polystipioti, A., Polychronopoulos, E. 2007. Prevalence of type 2 diabetes and physical activity status in elderly men and women from Cyprus (the MEDIS Study). *Asia Pac J Public Health* 19: 22–28.

Pérez-López, F.R., Chedraui, P., Haya, J., Cuadros, J.L. 2009. Effects of the Mediterranean diet on longevity and age-related morbid conditions. *Maturitas* 64: 67–79.

Pérez-Martínez, P., García-Ríos, A., Delgado-Lista, J., Pérez-Jiménez, F., López-Miranda, J. 2011. Mediterranean diet rich in olive oil and obesity, metabolic syndrome and diabetes mellitus. *Curr Pharm Des* 17: 769–777.

Pitsavos, C. et al. 2006. Interaction between Mediterranean diet and methylenetetrahydrofolate reductase C677T mutation on oxidized low density lipoprotein concentrations: The ATTICA study. *Nutr Metab Cardiovasc Dis.*16(2):91–9.

Pitsavos, C., Panagiotakos, D.B., Chrysohoou, C. et al. 2003. The adoption of Mediterranean diet attenuates the development of acute coronary syndromes in people with the metabolic syndrome. *Nutr J* 2: 1.

Psaltopoulou, T., Naska, A., Orfanos, P., Trichopoulos, D., Mountokalakis, T., Trichopoulou, A. 2004. Olive oil, the Mediterranean diet, and arterial blood pressure: The Greek European Prospective Investigation into Cancer and Nutrition (EPIC) study. *Am J Clin Nutr* 80: 1012–1018.

Reaven, G.M. 1988. Banting lecture 1988. Role of insulin resistance in human disease. *Diabetes* 37: 1595–1607.

Riccardi, G., Clemente, G., Giacco, R. 2003. Glycemic index of local foods and diets: The Mediterranean experience. *Nutr Rev* 61: S56–S60.

Richard, C., Couture, P., Desroches, S., Charest, A., Lamarche, B. 2011. Effect of the Mediterranean diet with and without weight loss on cardiovascular risk factors in men with the metabolic syndrome. *Nutr Metab Cardiovasc Dis* 21: 628–635.

Richard, C., Couture, P., Desroches, S., Lamarche, B. 2012. Effect of the Mediterranean diet with and without weight loss on markers of inflammation in men with metabolic syndrome. *Obesity* (*Silver Spring*) 21(1): 51–57.

Romaguera, D., Norat, T., Mouw, T. et al. 2009. Adherence to the Mediterranean diet is associated with lower abdominal adiposity in European men and women. *J Nutr* 139: 1728–1737.

Rumawas, M.E., Meigs, J.B., Dwyer, J.T., McKeown, N.M., Jacques, P.F. 2009. Mediterranean-style dietary pattern, reduced risk of metabolic syndrome traits, and incidence in the Framingham Offspring Cohort. *Am J Clin Nutr* 90: 1608–1614.

Salas-Salvadó, J., Bulló, M., Babio, N. et al. 2011. Reduction in the incidence of type 2 diabetes with the Mediterranean diet: Results of the PREDIMED-Reus nutrition intervention randomized trial. *Diabetes Care* 34: 14–19.

Salas-Salvadó, J., Fernández-Ballart, J., Ros, E. et al. 2008. Effect of a Mediterranean diet supplemented with nuts on metabolic syndrome status: One-year results of the PREDIMED randomized trial. *Arch Intern Med* 168: 2449–2458.

Shai, I., Schwarzfuchs, D., Henkin, Y. et al. 2008. Weight loss with a low-carbohydrate, Mediterranean, or low-fat diet. *N Engl J Med* 359: 229–241.

Tortosa, A., Bes-Rastrollo, M., Sanchez-Villegas, A., Basterra-Gortari, F.J., Nuñez-Cordoba, J.M., Martinez-Gonzalez, M.A. 2007. Mediterranean diet inversely associated with the incidence of metabolic syndrome: The SUN prospective cohort. *Diabetes Care* 30: 2957–2959.

Trichopoulou, A. 2000. From research to education: The Greek experience. *Nutrition* 16: 528–531.

Trichopoulou, A., Vasilopoulou, E. 2000. Mediterranean diet and longevity. *Br J Nutr* 84(2):205–209.

Trichopoulou, A., Costacou, T., Bamia, C., Trichopoulos, D. 2003. Adherence to a Mediterranean diet and survival in a Greek population. *N Engl J Med* 348: 2599–2608.

Urpi-Sarda, M., Casas, R., Chiva-Blanch, G. et al. 2012. Virgin olive oil and nuts as key foods of the Mediterranean diet effects on inflammatory biomarkers related to atherosclerosis. *Pharmacol Res* 65: 577–583.

Willett, W.C. 2006. The Mediterranean diet: Science and practice. *Public Health Nutr* 9: 105–110.

Willett, W.C., Sacks, F., Trichopoulou, A. et al. 1995. Mediterranean diet pyramid: A cultural model for healthy eating. *Am J Clin Nutr* 61: 1402S–1406S.

Wilson, P.W., D'Agostino, R.B., Parise, H., Sullivan, L., Meigs, J.B. 2005. Metabolic syndrome as a precursor of cardiovascular disease and type 2 diabetes mellitus. *Circulation* 112: 3066–3072.

World Health Organization. 1999. Definition, diagnosis and classification of diabetes mellitus and its complications. Part 1: Diagnosis and classification of diabetes mellitus. WHO, Geneva, Switzerland.

World Health Organization. 2008. 2008–2013 Action plan for the global strategy for the prevention and control of noncommunicable diseases. WHO, Geneva, Switzerland.

Zimmet, P., Magliano, D., Matsuzawa, Y., Alberti, G., Shaw, J. 2005. The metabolic syndrome: A global public health problem and a new definition. *J Atheroscler Thromb* 12: 295–300.

26 Dietary Approaches to Stop Hypertension

José Henrique da Silvah, Cristiane Maria Mártires de Lima,
Roberta Deh Souza Santos, Vivian Marques Miguel Suen,
Roberta Soares Lara Cassani, and Júlio Sérgio Marchini

CONTENTS

26.1 INTRODUCTION

The data discussed here will be presented along with the clinical case below, related to the topic.

A 28-year-old patient seeks medical care for evaluation because he is worried about his health. The patient has no complaints, does not report any diseases or the chronic use of medications. His father died of acute myocardial infarction at 54 years of age. The patient eats his meals outside the home and his diet is poorly fractionated, poor in fruits and vegetables, rich in saturated fatty acids and with an energy content exceeding ideal levels. Physical examination reveals blood pressure of 134×88 mmHg, abdominal circumference of 110 cm and acanthosis nigricans in the occipital region. He reports that his weight was 79 kg 10 years ago and now is about 98 kg. The patient returns 1 week later with the following blood test results: fasting glycemia = 110 mg/dL, triglycerides = 280 mg/dL, HDL-cholesterol = 30 mg/dL.

Considering a diagnosis of metabolic syndrome (MetS) for this patient, the decision made was to institute the DASH diet among other measures for a change in life style. Questions about the efficacy of this dietary approach for the treatment of MetS, as well as acceptance by the patients, certainly are causes of constant concern.

The DASH diet (Sacks et al. 2001) derives from a multicenter, controlled, randomized study that determined the effect of different dietary patterns and not of specific nutrients on blood pressure levels. In the mentioned study, the period of intervention consisted of 8 weeks, during which the volunteers were randomized to one of the three diets:

1. Control group: diet with the typical nutritional composition of North American eating habits
2. Group receiving a control diet rich in fruit and vegetables (with a potassium and magnesium content close to the 75th percentile of intake by North American people and with a large amount of fiber)
3. Group receiving the DASH diet (diet rich in fruit and vegetables, skim milk, and dairy products and with reduced amounts of total fats and cholesterol)

The amount of sodium offered was the same for all diets (close to 3 g/day), and four energetic levels were offered according to individual needs for weight maintenance. Both the diet rich in fruit and vegetables and the DASH diet were able to reduce blood pressure values compared to the control diet, a fact that encouraged their inclusion in various recommendations, such as those of the American Heart Association (Kraus et al. 2000). On this basis, the aim of the DASH diet (Table 26.1) is to reduce the intake of saturated fat, total fat, sodium (Table 26.2), and cholesterol and to increase the intake of fruit, vegetables, potassium, calcium, magnesium, fiber, and proteins.

The aim of the clinical use of the DASH diet (Racine et al. 2011) is to treat patients with cardiovascular diseases characterized by arterial hypertension (Blumenthal et al. 2010a, Edwards et al. 2011), dyslipidemia (Obarzanek et al. 2001), and all other conditions that increase the cardiovascular risk factors. The reduction of sodium intake (<100 mmol or 2300 mg), especially in combination with the DASH diet (Sharma and Schoor 1997), seems to reduce arterial pressure (AP) in a substantial manner (Appel et al. 1997, Chen et al. 2010). Besides, it is positively associated with weight loss, reduction of abdominal fat, sympathetic activity in the central nervous system, and arterial stiffness and peripheral vascular resistance, and with improvement of renal function and arterial dysfunction.

The DASH diet, even when combined with sodium restriction, still has a content of more than 2 g/day of this nutrient, a fact that makes it reasonably accepted by the population. If combined to the regular practice of exercises and weight loss, this diet has significant effects on the control of AP. However, these beneficial effects for the population depend on the ability of the therapist to transmit

---

TABLE 26.1
Nutrient Composition: DASH

Nutrient	Quantity	Nutrient	Quantity
Total fat	27% of the TCV	Sodium	2300 mg
Saturated fat	6% of the TCV	Potassium	4700 mg
Protein	18% of the TCV	Calcium	1250 mg
Carbohydrates	55% of the TCV	Magnesium	500 mg
Cholesterol	150 mg	Fiber	30 g

TCV, total energy value offered by the diet per day.

TABLE 26.2

Useful Information for the Reduction of the Amount of Sodium in the Diet

1. Choose seasonings (condiments) that do not contain sodium such as fresh herbs, fresh or powdered garlic, onion, coriander, lemon, basil, parsley, etc. Limit the consumption of readymade salad dressings.[a]
2. Try not to consume sausages or canned foods.[a] They contain large amounts of sodium for conservation.
3. Avoid excessive consumption of soft drinks,[a] even in the light/diet forms,[b] since they contain large amounts of sodium in their composition. A lower and sporadic consumption (one to two 200 mL glasses/day) corresponds to about 3% of the daily amount of sodium recommended.[c]
4. Always read food labels and try to eat foods with a maximum of 7% of the daily amount of sodium recommended.
5. Prefer whole to common foods since they contain smaller amounts of sodium.
6. Avoid fast foods.[d] Even a sandwich defined as healthy may contain a high amount of sodium.

[a] Check the sodium content on the label of industrialized products.
[b] Light, a smaller amount of a nutrient. Diet, absence of one or more nutrients.
[c] Percentage based on the information on the label of a cola-flavored soft drink of low energy value.
[d] Fast food, food that can be prepared quickly in a standardized manner for fast serving in snack bars.

to the patient the necessity to accept and follow the diet and on the ability of the patient to adhere to this plan for long periods of time (Racine et al. 2011). Although not yet conclusive, other factors also enhance the effects of the DASH diet, such as increased intake of foods containing calcium and magnesium and reduced ethanol intake (Edwards et al. 2011).

In the present text, for didactic purposes, food intake is defined as the ingestion of food by healthy people, with no concern about preventing, treating, or recovering from diseases. The term *diet* is the modification of food intake in order to prevent, treat, and recover from diseases. The various aims of the DASH diet are defined and discussed in the following and examples of their distribution in food intake will be presented.

26.2 DASH: ACCUMULATED EVIDENCE

1. DASH and systemic arterial hypertension
   a. Nonpharmacological treatment of systemic arterial hypertension (level A of evidence).
   b. Prehypertension and stage I of hypertension, with overweight or obesity. DASH + physical activity, both for weight loss (level B of evidence B).
   c. DASH diet with a low sodium content results in more effective pressure reductions (level of evidence B).
   d. Blood pressure reduction with the DASH diet is observed in the Afro-American population, both among hypertensive and normotensive individuals (level B of evidence).
   e. Patients with MetS seem to obtain greater reduction of systolic AP when submitted to the DASH + established recommendations consisting of weight loss, reduced sodium intake, and physical activity (level B of evidence).
2. DASH for the treatment of dyslipidemia and the reduction of cardiovascular risk (level A of evidence)
   a. A small reduction of total cholesterol levels and of LDL-c, with no changes in triglycerides with the DASH to maintain weight (level B of evidence).
   b. DASH + weight loss resulted in greater LDL-c reduction among diabetics (level B of evidence).
   c. Conflicting results regarding HDL-c (level B of evidence).
   d. Reduced cardiovascular and cerebrovascular risk among women on a prolonged use of, and good adherence to, the DASH style diet (level B of evidence).

     e. Reduction of cardiovascular risk within 10 years with the DASH diet (level B of evidence).

     f. The addition of the DASH diet to established recommendations induces a reduction of cardiovascular risk similar to that obtained with the recommendations alone (level B of evidence).

3. DASH and weight loss (level B of evidence)

     a. DASH possibly results in greater weight loss compared to control (level B of evidence).

     b. In addition to low adherence, the introduction of a DASH style diet with digital guidance (*Internet*) results in a small weight loss (level B of evidence).

4. DASH for diabetes mellitus and MetS

     a. Weight loss by means of the DASH diet with energy restriction + physical activity is superior to DASH alone and to common diets for the improvement of insulin sensitivity, glycemic levels, and lipid profile (level B of evidence).

     b. DASH diet for more than 16 weeks seems to improve fasting insulinemia regardless of weight loss (level B of evidence).

     c. Among individuals with MetS, the DASH diet in combination with other changes in life style, including weight loss, seems to be superior to each of the measures alone (level B of evidence).

5. Adherence to treatment

     a. DASH diet with 2300 mg or 100 mmol of sodium/day shows good acceptance (level B of evidence).

     b. Patients may require a long period to reach the goals regarding the intake of fruit, vegetables, and dairy products (level B of evidence).

26.2.1 DASH AND SYSTEMIC ARTERIAL HYPERTENSION

A controlled randomized assay, the ENCORE Study (Blumenthal et al. 2010a), compared three groups of overweight or obese people, prehypertensive or stage I hypertensive, respectively, submitted to the DASH diet alone, the DASH diet in combination with a weight loss diet, and a common diet (control). In addition to the known differences from the DASH diet regarding a greater quantity of fibers, potassium, magnesium, and calcium, the common diet contained about 30% more sodium. In addition to AP, the main outcome, biomarkers of cardiovascular risk were evaluated. An appropriate quantity of energy was prescribed to the DASH and common diet groups for weight maintenance. In contrast, for the DASH diet plus weight loss group, the total energy value was reduced by about 500 kcal/day in order to obtain a weight loss of 1 lb/week. The reduction of systolic AP was 16.1 (95% CI, 13.0–19.2) mmHg after treatment with the DASH diet plus weight loss, 11.2 (8.1–14.3) mmHg for the group treated with the DASH diet alone, and 3.4 (0.4–6.4) mmHg for the group receiving a common diet. The reduction of diastolic AP was 9.9 (8.1–11.6) mmHg for the group treated with the DASH diet plus weight loss, 7.5 (5.8–9.3) mmHg for the group treated with the DASH diet alone, and 3.8 (2.2–5.5) mmHg for the group receiving a common diet. The group treated with the DASH diet plus a program of weight loss also showed lower left ventricular mass values after treatment compared to the groups receiving the DASH diet alone and a common diet.

    In another multicenter and randomized trial, Sacks et al. (2001) evaluated the effects of the DASH diet and of reduced sodium intake on the systolic and diastolic blood pressure of 412 normotensive and stage 1 hypertensive volunteers. The subjects were divided into two groups, respectively, receiving a control diet (n = 204) and the DASH diet (n = 208). Each group ingested in random order the assigned diet with high (150 mmol), intermediate (100 mmol), and low (50 mmol) daily sodium levels for 30 days each. Energy consumption was adjusted for the maintenance of body weight of the volunteers. Both the control and DASH diet groups showed a progressive reduction of systolic blood pressure in parallel to the reduced consumption of salt (from high to intermediate 2.1 mmHg [control], 1.3 mmHg [DASH]; from intermediate to low 4.6 mmHg [control], 1.7 mmHg [DASH]). When the dietary interventions were compared for each level of salt consumption, the DASH group showed a significantly lower systolic blood pressure than the control group. In addition to reducing systolic arterial pressure, the DASH diet was also important by reducing diastolic AP in patients who ingested large amounts of sodium. Therefore, compared to the control diet with high sodium levels, the DASH diet plus a lower sodium level induced a greater reduction of systolic blood pressure (7.1 mmHg in normotensives and 11.5 mmHg in hypertensives) than each intervention applied individually. Among hypertensive subjects, the combined effects of the DASH and sodium reduction were comparable to those of pharmacological therapy with a single drug. A possible determinant of this greater blood pressure withdrawal could be the higher potassium consumption with the DASH diet. The DASH study itself demonstrated that, with a greater consumption of fruits and vegetables, the intake of potassium increased from 37 to 71 mmol/day. Even with sodium ingestion around 130 mmol/day, the DASH diet, with higher potassium intake, induced a greater reduction of blood pressure (Appel et al. 1997). In the Afro-American population, the DASH study demonstrated greater reduction of systolic and diastolic blood pressures than observed in the white population, both among hypertensive and normotensive subjects (Sacks et al. 2001).

In the PREMIER study, volunteers with MetS, compared to healthy volunteers, obtained a lower reduction of systolic AP (−8 vs. −12 mmHg) when only recommendations regarding life style (weight loss, reduced sodium intake and physical activity) were followed. However, in the group following the DASH diet + established recommendations, the reduction of blood pressure was similar in patients with and without MetS (−9.8 vs. −11.2 mmHg; p = 0.231). There was no difference in other indicators such as diastolic blood pressure, lipid profile, or HOMA-IR (Obarzanek et al. 2001).

26.2.2 DASH for Dyslipidemia and for the Reduction of Cardiovascular Risk

The DASH study showed a 0.35 mmol/L or 13.7 mg/dL reduction in total cholesterol, a 0.28 mmol/L or 10.7 mg/dL reduction in LDL-c, but also a 0.09 mmol/L or 3.7 mg/dL reduction in HDL-c. There were no important changes in triglycerides compared to the control diet or differences in ethnic origin, but males obtained greater reductions in total cholesterol and LDL-c. In that study, the participants had a body mass index~28 kg/m^2 and received an energy value for the maintenance of weight. The authors concluded that the DASH diet resulted in little changes in lipid profile but with the potential to reduce the cardiovascular risks. This antagonism, which means, reduction of HDL-c, needs to be better studied (Obarzanek et al. 2001). The reduction of the Framingham risk was observed between DASH and the control diet (RR = 0.82, 95% CI: 0.75–0.90) and between DASH and the fruits and vegetables diet (RR = 0.89, 95% CI: 0.81–0.97) (Chen et al. 2010). In contrast, a randomized crossover Iranian clinical trial evaluating the DASH diet versus control in type 2 diabetics showed that the DASH diet promoted a greater increase in HDL-c, a greater withdrawal in LDL-c, and a similar reduction in triglycerides compared to the control diet (Azadbakht et al. 2011). The adherence to the interventions could not be guaranteed since it was evaluated by self-reported intake and the patients were instructed to keep a dietary pattern instead of receiving a ready diet.

A cohort study with duration of 24 years revealed a reduction in the relative risk of fatal and non-fatal cardiovascular and cerebrovascular disease with the use of a DASH-style diet but not with the DASH diet itself. The study was conducted only with women, evaluating them seven times during the 24 years of the study (1980–2004) by means of a dietary survey. The women were stratified into quintiles according to their adherence for consumption of eight possible food groups of the DASH diet. The reductions in the relative risk were potentiated with greater adherence to the DASH-style diet (Fung et al. 2008). When the Framingham risk score at baseline was compared to that at 6 months of the study, data of the PREMIER study showed a relative risk in cardiovascular disease of 0.86 (95% CI: 0.81–0.91, p < 0.001) in the group submitted to the established recommendations and of 0.88 (95% CI: 0.83–0.94, p < 0.001) in the DASH + recommendations group. The authors concluded that the reductions obtained were substantial and, when achieved, they could be of benefit for public health (Maruthur et al. 2009).

Some studies have suggested other beneficial effects of greater potassium intake with the DASH diet, that is, reduction of the risk for cerebrovascular disease; a preventive effect on renal disease at the vascular, glomerular, and tubular levels; reduction of urinary calcium and, consequently, of the generation of stones in the urinary tract, as well as helping the prevention of bone demineralization.

26.2.3 DASH and Weight Loss

The Iranian study of diabetic patients mentioned previously demonstrated a greater weight loss with the DASH diet compared to control (−5.0 ± 0.9 kg vs. −2.0 ± 0.3 kg). The patients received each diet in a random order for 8 weeks, with a washout of 4 weeks. The total daily energy intake did not differ, but there was a difference in energy density, which was lower in the DASH diet. This may explain the greater weight loss for patients on a DASH diet. There was also a greater reduction in abdominal circumference in the DASH diet group (−6.7 ± 1.2 cm vs. −1.9 ± 0.4 cm). The study, however, had no information about the energetic deficit provoked by the intervention that promoted the weight loss, and both interventions provided about 2100 kcal/day (Chen et al. 2010). Recent studies have demonstrated an important association between the reduction in abdominal fat and the reduction in risk factors related to the MetS, such as AP and serum triglyceride and cholesterol concentrations (Cassani et al. 2009a). In parallel, a study about the utilization of energy substrates by women in the climacteric period demonstrated that the rate of lipid oxidation was inversely proportional to total energetic intake, body mass index, and abdominal circumference, demonstrating that energy intake seems to be associated with the accumulation of intra-abdominal fat (Santos et al. 2008).

In addition to the low adherence observed (only 26%), a DASH-style diet followed through the Internet only produced a small weight loss in overweight or obese subjects compared to baseline at the end of a clinical trial of 12-month duration (−4.2 lb or −1.9 kg; 95% CI: −2.2 to −6.2) (Moore et al. 2008).

26.2.4 DASH for Diabetes Mellitus and Risk Factors

In a controlled randomized study, hypertensive overweight or obese subjects showed improved insulin sensitivity when submitted to the DASH diet + energy restriction + physical activity. The intention was to promote energy deficit of 500 kcal/day compared to subjects receiving only the DASH diet or the usual control diets. In the group whose intervention was DASH diet + energy restriction + physical activity, 18 subjects were initially glucose intolerant to glucose or diabetic. Of these, 72% obtained an improvement of their glycemic status during the intervention versus 54% of the group receiving DASH only and 42% of the group receiving a control diet. In other words, diabetic subjects developed glucose intolerance and intolerant subjects obtained normal glycemia values 2 h after the 75 g glucose test.

Lipid profile, total cholesterol and triglycerides values were lower in the DASH diet + energy restriction + physical activity group compared to the other two groups. However, in the same study, these benefits were not observed when the DASH diet alone was compared to the control or common diet (Blumenthal et al. 2010b). A systematic review that only evaluated the DASH diet as an intervention without considering weight loss demonstrated a reduction of fasting insulinemia only when the DASH was prescribed for a period of more than 16 weeks (mean reduction: −0.16, 95% CI, −0.23 to −0.08, p < 0.0001) (Shirani et al. 2013). It was observed that only one study contributed to this association of DASH intervention with the reduction of fasting insulinemia and when this study was removed from the analysis, this effect was no longer observed. Still, in the same study, no improvement in fasting glycemia or HOMA-IR was observed. The authors pointed out that the beneficial effects occur in association with weight loss, as shown in a study of type 2 diabetics, in which the DASH group obtained a greater weight loss than control and also better indicators such as fasting glycemia (−29.4±6.3 mg/dL vs. −12.8±6.7 mg/dL) and glycosylated hemoglobin (−1.7%±0.1% vs. −0.5%±0.02%) (Chen et al. 2010). Recent review studies have shown that diets containing carbohydrates with a lower glycemic load and a greater quantity of polyphenols, present in the DASH diet, favor a better control of glucose metabolism (Cassani 2012). Other studies have demonstrated that glucose metabolism is impaired in hypokalemic states, with a reduction of insulin secretion due to hyperglycemia (He et al. 2001).

26.2.5 ADHERENCE TO TREATMENT

In the DASH-sodium trial, questionnaires were applied to all the participants at different times in order to determine the more acceptable level of daily salt consumption (high = 150 mmol; intermediate = 100 mmol; low = 50 mmol) and which diet (DASH vs. control) could be followed after the study. Each person consumed each level of sodium randomly for 30 days. The intermediate level was the most acceptable in both interventions, and the DASH diet was considered likely to maintain its use. People of black ethnicity, however, showed greater preference for the control diet. An Australian study comparing the WELL strategy (weight loss, exercise, lower blood pressure, and longevity) with established goals regarding the consumption of fruits, vegetables, and dairy products based on the DASH diet with a diet with fat restriction and with advice for an increased intake of these groups revealed equivalent weight loss. The WELL group consumed more portions of the above foods. However, it should be pointed out that adherence to the protocol was assessed by patient self-report, which is subjected to bias. It is interesting to note that the participants in the WELL group reached the goals of consumption after 8 weeks (Booth et al. 2003).

The PREMIER study used cognitive-behavioral strategies of group counseling weekly during the first 8 weeks, every 2 weeks during the subsequent 6 months, and monthly during the last 12 months (Maruthur et al. 2009). Seven individual sessions were also held along the 18 months of the study. This approach was considered to favor adherence to the DASH pattern and to the recommendations of dietary reference intakes (DRIs). Most of the subjects in the DASH + established interventions group (modifications of life style) achieved two-thirds of the DRIs for most nutrients within up to 6 months (Lin et al. 2007). Even stronger emphasis on food selection and on the consumption of fruits and vegetables would improve adherence.

26.3 DETAILED GOALS OF THE DASH DIET

26.3.1 TOTAL FAT

Total fat is defined as the energy proportion referring to lipids supplied by the total diet. It is important to consume lipids through the diet, since they play important and essential roles in the organism. Lipids are involved in the supply and storage of energy, are hormone precursors, components of the bile and of the cell membrane (phospholipids), and participate in intracellular signaling systems (Lottenberg 2009). Since lipids are hydrophobic molecules, their circulation in blood depends on the formation of lipoproteins (chylomicrons, very-low-density lipoprotein [VLDL], low-density lipoprotein [LDL], and high-density lipoprotein [HDL]) (Gillingham et al. 2011, Cunha 2012). The DASH diet recommends the intake of a maximum of 27% of the total daily energy value of fat.

However, the diet of Western countries provides about 30%–40% of energy intake from fat. Examples of total fat–rich foods are avocado, bacon, fried foods in general, fat meats (fatty Brazilian Zebu cattle hump, sirloin steak), and yellow cheeses, among others. It is important to be aware of the type of fat predominantly ingested; thus, the recommendation is to consume more monounsaturated and polyunsaturated fats and the lowest possible amount of saturated fat (Cassani et al. 2012), as discussed in detail in the following texts.

26.3.2 SATURATED FAT

Saturated fat is defined as the one with complete hydrogenation of the carbon chain occurs, with no double bond between the carbon atoms. At room temperature, saturated fat is in the solid form. In general, saturated fats are from animal origin and rarely of vegetable source. Examples of sources of saturated fat are coconut oil, palm oil, butter, pork lard, and cheddar cheese, among other foods (Table 26.3). The DASH diet, as demonstrated earlier, recommends the consumption of up to 6% of the total energy value of a meal from saturated fat.

26.3.3 MONOUNSATURATED FAT

Monounsaturated fatty acids (MUFAs) (Gillingham et al. 2011) have only one double bond in their carbon chain. MUFAs have a higher freezing point than polyunsaturated fatty acids (PUFAs). Both MUFAs and PUFAs are liquid at room temperature. Oleic acid (18:1 n-9) and palmitoleic acid (16:1 n-7) are examples of MUFAs frequently found in nature. Oleic acid is the most abundant MUFA, corresponding to about 90% of *cis* MUFA. Important sources of MUFA are olive oil (*Olea europaea*) (73% fat content), hazelnut oil (*Corylus*) (78%), canola oil (rape, *Brassica napus*) (63%), avocado oil (*Persea gratissima*) (71%), and apricot oil (*Prunus armeniaca, Linnaeus*) (60%).

The intake of these oils is encouraged because this type of fat reduces the plasma concentration of LDL-cholesterol and does not provoke oxidation of this cholesterol fraction. One of the reasons

TABLE 26.3
Fat Content of Raw Foods (*in Natura*) per 100 g Food, in Decreasing Order

Food	Cholesterol (mg)	Total Fat (g)	Saturated Fat (g)	Fibers (g)	Proteins (g)
Coconut oil	0	100	86.5	0	0.0
Butter	215	81	51.4	0	0.9
Lard	95	100	39.2	0	0.0
Cheddar cheese	105	33	21.0	0	24.9
Soy oil	0	100	15.0	0	0.0
Mozzarella cheese	79	22	13.2	0	22.2
Beef	209	24	11.7	0	15.0
Cocoa (powder)	0	14	8.1	33	19.6
Pork	72	21	7.9	0	16.7
Egg	372	10	3.1	0	12.6
Chicken	86	8	2.3	0	17.4
Human milk	14	4	2.0	0	1.0
Whole cow's milk	209	26	16.7	0	26.3
Salmon	46	4	0.8	0	20.5
Pasta	0	2	0.3	11	7.5
Beans	0	1	0.2	16	21.4
Rice	0	0.5	0.1	3	6.5
Okra	0	8	0.0	3	1.9

Source: Data from the U.S. Department of Agriculture. Agricultural Research Service. 2012.

why oleic acid does not increase LDL-c is that it is a better substrate for acetyl-coA cholesterol acyltransferase (ACAT) in the liver. Thus, excess cholesterol, in the free form, is esterified, without inducing the suppression of LDL-c receptors. The recommendation is a daily intake of up to 20% of the dietary total energy value from monounsaturated fats.

26.3.4 POLYUNSATURATED FAT

Polyunsaturated fatty acids have more than one double bond between carbons in their chemical constitution and belong to different series depending on the location of the first double bond in the carbon chain starting from the methyl terminal (identified with the letter Ω). On this basis, PUFA are classified as series Ω-3, Ω-6, and Ω-9. The PUFA most commonly found is the Ω-6 series, which means, linoleic acid (C18:2), followed by arachidonic acid (C20:4). The main sources of PUFA are corn and sunflower oils (Ω-6), linseed and soy oils (Ω-9), and the fat of cold- and deep-water fish (Ω-3).

Despite the beneficial actions of PUFA in the modulation of the pathways that interfere with hypercholesterolemia, Ω-6 PUFA, when consumed in large quantities, may have negative effects such as a reduction of HDL-c levels. However, recent studies have demonstrated that reduced quantities of Ω-6 PUFA seem to contribute to greater cardiovascular risk than increased quantities. Thus, it has been suggested to ingest about 6%–10% of the total energy value in the form of this fatty acid (Cassani et al. 2012). Table 26.4 lists the PUFA and MUFA contents of the vegetable oils most frequently consumed by the population.

26.3.4.1 Cholesterol

Cholesterol is a polycyclic long-chain alcohol with an essential and fundamental role as a precursor of vitamin D, glucocorticoids, mineralocorticoids, estrogen, testosterone, bile salts, and cell membrane. Human beings are able to synthesize all the cholesterol necessary for the maintenance of health, that is, 250 mg/day. However, in view of the multiple dietary sources of cholesterol, the population, especially the Western one, is consuming excessive amounts of this fat (see Table 26.5). All

TABLE 26.4
Monosaturated and Polyunsaturated Fat Content of Crude Oils (*in Natura*), in g/100 g Food

Food	Saturated Fat	MUFA	PUFA
Coconut oil	86.5	5.8	1.8
Hazelnut oil	7.4	78.0	10.2
Safflower oil	7.5	75.2	12.8
Olive oil	13.8	73.0	10.5
Avocado oil	11.6	70.5	13.5
Almond oil	8.2	69.9	17.4
Canola oil	7.4	63.7	28.1
Poppy seed oil	13.5	19.7	62.4
Wheat germ oil	18.8	15.1	61.7
Soy oil	15.6	22.8	57.7
Corn oil	12.9	27.6	54.7
Cottonseed oil	25.9	17.8	51.9

Source: Data from the U.S. Department of Agriculture. Agricultural Research Service. 2012.

TABLE 26.5
Cholesterol Content of Foods (*in Natura*), in g/100 g Food

Food	Total Fat	Cholesterol
Egg	9.5	372.0
Butter	81.1	215.0
Beef	23.5	209.0
Whole cow's milk	26.1	97.0
Chicken with skin	8.1	86.0

Source: Data from the U.S. Department of Agriculture. Agricultural Research Service. 2012.

animal foods contain cholesterol, whereas foods with no animal fat contain very small or no quantities of this molecule. In studies with the DASH diet, the objective is a cholesterol consumption of around 150 mg/day (Dash Guide 2006).

26.3.4.2 Fibers

Food fibers form a set of substances originating from vegetables and are resistant to the action of human digestive enzymes. They are classified as soluble and insoluble according to their solubility in water. The DASH diet recommends the daily intake of 30 g of fibers.

Examples of soluble fibers are pectin, the β-glucans (Cloetens et al. 2012), and inulin. Pectins are present in apples, carrots, beets, bananas, cabbage, peas, orange peel, and okra. As fruits ripen, pectin becomes more soluble. In contrast, β-glucans are soluble fibers found in the cell wall of cereals such as oats and barley, and their total quantity is influenced both by genetic and environmental conditions. Inulin is a food fiber with a prebiotic effect. It acts as bacterial substrate from intestinal flora and it is found in chicory and artichokes (Saad 2006).

Examples of insoluble fibers are cellulose, hemicellulose, and lignin. Cellulose is the main constituent of the cell wall of plants, especially in the outer layer of fruits and vegetables and it is found in whole grains, dry legumes, apples, pears, plums, almonds, etc. Hemicellulose is also part of the cell wall of plants and its main food sources are apples, beets, whole grains, cabbage, bananas, legumes, corn, etc. Finally, lignin is the harder and more resistant fibrous tissues of plants cells walls. It is found in carrots, peas, whole grains, peaches, tomatoes, strawberries, and potatoes.

26.3.4.3 Proteins

The amino acids, which are components of proteins, are classified as essential and nonessential. In some pathological conditions or in young developing organisms, amino acids may become *conditionally essential*. The essential amino acids are isoleucine, histidine. leucine, lysine, methionine, phenylalanine, threonine, tryptophan, and valine.

The biological value of a protein is related to its amino acid profile and corresponds to its efficency of utilization by the human organism. The greater the biological value of a protein, the larger the number of amino acids and the greater the amount of nitrogen retained by the organism. Eggs, for example, contain proteins of high biological value with 94% utilization by the human organism. Other foods containing high biological value protein are cow's milk, fish, beef, chicken, and beans.

The protein intake recommended by the DASH diet is 18% of the total energy value. It is important to emphasize that it is necessary to include proteins of high biological value in the diet. The total quantity of protein is relevant, but the equilibrium and distribution of its nutrients among different meals permits the activation of protein synthesis and increase thermogenesis, as well as the supply of protein levels needed for the release of the PYY hormone by L cells in the ileum after each meal for the control of satiety. The increased thermogenesis and the control of satiety are effects of adequate protein content in the diet, which favors weight loss and is highly significant for the reduction of cardiovascular risk and the control of MetS (Cassani et al. 2009b).

26.3.5 SODIUM

Sodium is an essential mineral that participates in the water–electrolyte homeostasis of the human organism. The body of a human adult contains approximately 250 g of salt. In developed countries, the estimated sodium intake tends to exceed the limit recommended by the World Health Organization (WHO), which is 2 g sodium or 5 g salt/person/day. In developing countries, information about sodium intake is still scarce. A Brazilian study based on the 2002/2003 Survey of Family Budgets revealed that the quantity of sodium available for consumption in Brazilian households exceeds more than twice the maximum recommended intake (Sarno et al. 2009).

Sodium is mainly found in kitchen salt and in industrialized foods. *In natura*, higher amounts of sodium are found in celery, milk, and seafood (IOM 2005). Among the industrialized foods containing high quantities of sodium are salami, sausages, smoked meats, processed cheese, canned foods in general, and condiments.

26.3.6 POTASSIUM

Potassium is the most abundant intracellular cation in the human organism. Among other functions, it participates in the conduction of electrical stimuli on heart and nervous system. A low intake of this mineral can lead to muscle weakness, glucose intolerance, increased AP, and increased risk of developing kidney stones, arrhythmias, and even cardiac arrest.

The recommended potassium intake is 4.7 g/day for adults (IOM 2005). This level maintains lower blood pressure levels, reduces the risk of kidney stones, and possibly reduces bone loss. The main sources of this nutrient are fruits and vegetables such as spinach, melon, almonds, Brussels sprouts, mushrooms, bananas, oranges, and potatoes, among others.

26.3.7 CALCIUM

Calcium represents 1%–2% of the body mass of an adult, and almost all of it is found in teeth and bones. However, it is also present in smaller quantities in blood, extracellular fluid, muscle, and other tissues, mediating vascular contraction and vasodilatation, nerve transmission, and gland secretion. Chronic calcium deficiency resulting from inadequate intake or from impaired intestinal absorption for long periods is an important cause of the reduction of bone mass and of osteoporosis. A study of patients with short bowel syndrome did not detect increased urinary calcium excretion, and intestinal loss seems to be responsible for the reduction of bone mass (Rodella et al. 2012).

The main dietary sources of calcium are milk and dairy products and foods of animal origin (Table 26.6). The recommended daily intake for adults is 1000 mg for women and 800 mg for men (IOM 1997).

26.3.8 MAGNESIUM

The total quantity of magnesium in the human body is approximately 25 g, 50%–60% of which is located in the bones. This mineral is a cofactor for more than 300 enzymatic systems involved in the generation of energy both in aerobic and anaerobic forms, and in glycolysis and the remaining systems, such as potassium transport.

TABLE 26.6

Quantity of Calcium in Foods (*in Natura*), in mg/100 g Food

Food	Quantity of Calcium
Human milk	32
Whole cow's milk	276
Whole goat's milk	134
Skimmed cow's milk	125
Parmesan cheese	1184
Cheddar cheese	721
Mozzarella cheese	505
Tofu (soy cheese)	350
Ricotta cheese	207
Canned sardines	382
Broccoli	47
Kale	40

Source: Data from the U.S. Department of Agriculture. Agricultural Research Service. 2012.

The main sources of magnesium are green leaves, but the mineral is also found in whole grains and nuts. The recommended intake is 320 mg for women and 420 mg for men (DASH Guide 2006).

26.4 EXAMPLE OF A DASH MENU

Menu of a typical DASH diet for an adult male with a BMI of 24 kg/m² according to a 2000 kcal diet are shown in Tables 26.7 and 26.8. Table 26.7 shows household food measurements, and Table 26.8 shows the nutrient intake.

26.5 FINAL CONSIDERATIONS

Nontransmissible chronic diseases are one of the most important causes of morbidity and mortality in the world population. The MetS, defined as a set of entities potentially triggering cardiac and cerebrovascular diseases and type 2 diabetes mellitus, definitely attracts the interest of the scientific community. This will continue to be important in the near future because of the close correlation between its prevalence and the lifestyle that has been adopted by the population over the last decades regarding its diet but also the practice of physical, work, and leisure activities. Thus, the discussion of the treatment of this disease or group of diseases must also consider all the aspects of the daily routine of the patient. The person must be evaluated as a whole, not only regarding his or her physical health but also within his or her social, economic, psychological, and even geographical environment. For example, in some regions of the world, it is difficult to eat fruits and vegetables. Similarly, for economic reasons, the acquisition of these foods and of skimmed dairy products may become unlikely. In this case, a greater participation of society would be important, in addition to political interventions in order to facilitate access to these foods. A patient with MetS must be periodically evaluated by a doctor, who should preferentially have experience in the area of diseases related to food intake (Dutra-de-Oliveira and Marchini 1997). However, knowledge about this syndrome and its treatment should be an objective of all medical specialties, since MetS

TABLE 26.7

Household Food Measurements for an Example of Dash Diet for an Adult Male

Foods	Quantity in Household Measures
Breakfast	
Skimmed milk	1 cream cheese cup
Whole wheat bread	1 slice
White cheese	2 thick slices
Papaya	1 unit
Morning snack	
Apple	1 unit
Lunch	
Rice	5 tablespoons
Beans	1 ladle
Grilled chicken	1 medium slice
Boiled carrot	2 tablespoons
Boiled beet	2 tablespoons
Lettuce	1 dessert plate
Tomato	4 slices
Pineapple	1 slice
Afternoon snack	
Toast	4 units
Banana	1 unit
Dinner	
Cucumber	½ unit
Tomato	4 slices
Raw carrot	3 tablespoons
Cooked zucchini	3 tablespoons
Grilled chicken	1 medium slice
Grapes	1 small bunch
Supper	
Skimmed yogurt	1 pot

may develop in any patient. This can be easily understood if we consider patients with chronic renal failure or rheumatologic diseases such as systemic lupus erythematosus, diseases that include cardiovascular conditions among the most important causes of mortality (Silvah 2012). The same reason applies to all professionals in the health area and, whenever possible, it is important that a multidisciplinary team evaluate this kind of patient. It should be emphasized that the overall care of patients in the hospital environment should count with a multiprofessional team including physician, psychologist, nurse, pharmacist-biochemist, and a nutritionist among other health professionals, each being responsible for sectors specifically related to his/her knowledge. The DASH diet presented here and used for the treatment of MetS seems to be potentially beneficial mainly with respect to arterial hypertension, but also involving a reduced risk of cardiovascular diseases. However, we observed that, in the various studies surveyed, adherence to diet therapy was only based on self-reported intake. In most cases, the patients were only counseled about the diet and did not receive it ready for consumption. This approach, commonly used in intervention

TABLE 26.8
Nutritional Composition of the Menu Presented in Table 26.7

Nutrients	Quantity
Energy (kcal/day)	1988
Carbohydrate (%TCV)	57
Lipid (%TCV)	19
Protein (% TCV)	21
Calcium (mg/day)	965
Phosphorus (mg/day)	1467
Magnesium (mg/day)	377
Sodium (mg/day)	4200
Potassium (mg/day)	4519
Fibers (g/day)	29
Cholesterol (mg/day)	226

Source: Data from the U.S. Department of Agriculture. Agricultural Research Service. 2012.
TCV, total energetic value of the meal per day.

studies, especially those related to the nutrition area, is subjected to bias. Although it is impossible to conduct all investigations in a specific unit, with meal delivery and observation of intake, the approach of Fung et al. (2008) is a model to be followed. In their study, for analysis of the results, the volunteers were stratified into quintiles regarding adherence to treatment, with consequent better clarity regarding the association detected.

REFERENCES

Appel, L.J., Moore, T.J., Obarzanek, E. et al. 1997. A clinical trial of the effects of dietary patterns on blood pressure. DASH collaborative research group. *N Engl J Med* 336:1117–1124.

Azadbakht, L., Fard, N.R., Karimi, M. et al. 2011. Effects of the Dietary Approaches to Stop Hypertension (DASH) eating plan on cardiovascular risks among type 2 diabetic patients: A randomized crossover clinical trial. *Diabetes Care* 34:55–57.

Blumenthal, J.A., Babyak, M.A., Hinderliter, A. et al. 2010a. Effects of the DASH diet alone and in combination with exercise and weight loss on blood pressure and cardiovascular markers in men and women with high blood pressure: The ENCORE study. *Arch Intern Med* 170:126–135.

Blumenthal, J.A., Babyak, M.A., Sherwood, A. et al. 2010b. Effects of the dietary approaches to stop hypertension diet alone and in combination with exercise and caloric restriction on insulin sensitivity and lipids. *Hypertension* 55:1199–1205.

Booth, A.O., Nowsen, C.A., Worsley, T., Margerison, C., Jorna, M.K. 2003. Dietary approaches for weight loss with increased fruit, vegetables and dairy. *Asia Pac J Clin Nutr* 12(Suppl.):S10.

Cassani, R. 2012. O que é uma dieta saudável para prevenção da doença cardiovascular: O papel dos nutrientes sobre lípides, sobrepeso, hipertensão arterial e inflamação subclínica. *Rev Soc Cardiol Estado de São Paulo* 22:9–13.

Cassani, R.S., Nobre, F., Pazin-Filho, A., Schmidt, A. 2009a. Relationship between blood pressure and anthropometry in a cohort of Brazilian men: A cross-sectional study. *Am J Hyperten* 22:980–984.

Cassani, R.S.L., Nobre, F., Pazin-Filho, A., Schmidt, A. 2009b. Prevalência de fatores de risco cardiovascular em trabalhadores de uma indústria brasileira. *Arq Bras Cardiol* 92:16–22.

Chen, S.T., Maruthur, N.M., Appel, L.J. 2010.The effect of dietary patterns on estimated coronary heart disease risk: Results from the Dietary Approaches to Stop Hypertension (DASH) trial. *Circ Cardiovasc Qual Outcomes* 3:484–489.

Cloetens, L., Ulmius, M., Johansson-Persson, A. et al. 2012. Role of dietary beta-glucans in the prevention of the metabolic syndrome. *Nutr Rev* 70:444–458.

Cunha, S.F.C. 2012. Nutrologia conceitual. In: D.F. Ribas, V.M.M. Suen (eds.). *Tratado de Nutrologia*, 1st edn. Manole: São Paulo, Brazil, pp. 1–34.

Dash Guide. 2006. Your guide to lowering your blood pressure with DASH. U.S. Department of Health and Human Services. National Institutes of Health. National Heart, Lung, and Blood Institute. NIH Publication No. 06-4082. Revised April 2006 http://www.nhlbi.nih.gov/health/public/heart/hbp/dash/new_dash.pdf. Accessed on April 23, 2012.

Dutra-de-Oliveira, J.E., Marchini, J.S. 1997. Primary care physicians and clinical nutrition: Can good medical nutrition care be offered without well-trained physicians in the area? *Am J Clin Nutr* 65(6 Suppl.):2010S–2012S.

Edwards, K.M., Wilson, K.L., Sadja, J., Ziegler, M.G., Mills, P.J. 2011. Effects on blood pressure and autonomic nervous system function of a 12-week exercise or exercise plus DASH-diet intervention in individuals with elevated blood pressure. *Acta Physiol (Oxford)* 203:343–350.

Fung, T.T., Chiuve, S.E., McCullough, M.L., Rexrode, K.M., Logroscino, G., Hu, F.B. 2008. Adherence to a DASH-style diet and risk of coronary heart disease and stroke in women. *Arch Intern Med* 168:713–720.

Gillingham, L.G., Harris-Janz, S., Jones, P.J. 2011. Dietary monounsaturated fatty acids are protective against metabolic syndrome and cardiovascular disease risk factors. *Lipids* 46:209–228.

He, F.J., MacGregor, G.A. 2001. Fortnightly review: Beneficial effects of potassium. *BMJ* 323:497–501.

Institute of Medicine (IOM). 1997. *Dietary Reference Intakes for Calcium, Phosphorus, Magnesium, Vitamin D, and Fluoride*. Washington, DC: National Academy Press.

Institute of Medicine (IOM). 2005. *Dietary Reference Intakes for Water, Potassium, Sodium, Chloride, and Sulfate*. Washington, DC: National Academy Press.

Krauss, R.M., Eckel, R.H., Howard, B. et al. 2000. AHA dietary guidelines: Revision 2000: A statement of health care professionals from the Nutrition Committee of the American Heart Association. *Circulation* 102:2284–2299.

Lin, P.H., Appel, L.J., Funk, K. et al. 2007. The PREMIER intervention helps participants follow the Dietary Approaches to Stop Hypertension dietary pattern and the current Dietary Reference Intakes recommendations. *J Am Diet Assoc* 107:1541–1551.

Lottenberg, A.M. 2009. Importância da gordura alimentar na prevenção e no controle de distúrbios metabólicos e da doença cardiovascular. *Arq Bras Endocrinol Metab* 53:595–607.

Maruthur, N.M., Wang, N.Y., Appel, L.J. 2009. Lifesty le interventions reduce coronary heart disease risk: Results from the PREMIER Trial. *Circulation* 119:2026–2031.

Moore, T.J., Alsabeeh, N., Apovan, C.A. et al. 2008. Weight, blood pressure, and dietary benefits after 12 months of a web-based nutrition education program (DASH for health): Longitudinal observational study. *J Med Internet Res* 10(4): e52.

Obarzanek, E., Sacks, F.M., Vollmer, W.M. et al. 2001. Effects on blood lipids of a blood pressure-lowering diet: The Dietary Approaches to Stop Hypertension (DASH) trial. *Am J Clin Nutr* 74:80–89.

Racine, E., Troyer, J.L., Warren-Findlow, J., McAuley, W.J. 2011. The effect of medical nutrition therapy on changes in dietary knowledge and DASH diet adherence in older adults with cardiovascular disease. *J Nutr Health Aging* 15:868–876.

Rodella, F., Marchini, J.S., Ribas, D.F., Padovan, G.J., Santos, A.F.S., Suen, V.M.M. 2012. Urinary calcium excretion in short bowel syndrome patients receiving cyclic parenteral nutrition: Case report. *Int J Nutrology* 5:103–105.

Saad, S.M.I. 2006. Prebióticos e probióticos: O estado da arte. *Rev Bras Cien Farm* 42:1–16.

Sacks, F.M., Svetkey, L.P., Vollmer, W.M. et al. 2001. Effects on blood pressure of reduced dietary sodium and the dietary approaches to stop hypertension (DASH) diet. DASH-Sodium Collaborative Research Group. *N Engl J Med* 344:3–10.

Santos, R.D.S., Suen, V.M.M., Iannetta, O., Marchini, J.S. 2008. Climacteric, physically active women ingesting their routine diet oxidize more carbohydrates than lipids. *Climacteric* 11:454–460.

Sarno, F., Claro, R.M., Levy, R.B., Bandoni, D.H., Ferreira, S.R., Monteiro, C.A. 2009. Estimativa de consumo de sódio pela população brasileira, 2002–2003. *Rev Saúde Públ* 43:219–225.

Sharma, A.M., Schorr, U. 1997. Dietary patterns and blood pressure. *N Engl J Med* 337:637–638.

Shirani, F., Salehi-Abargouei, A., Azadbakht, L. 2013. Effects of dietary approaches to stop hypertension (DASH) diet on some risk for developing type 2 diabetes: A systematic review and meta-analysis on controlled clinical trials. *Nutrition* 29:939–947.

Silvah, J.H. 2012. Terapia Nutrológica nas Insuficiências Renal Aguda e Crônica em adultos. In: D.F. Durval, V.M.M. Suen (eds.). *Tratado de Nutrologia*, 1st edn. Manole: São Paulo, Brazil, pp. 365–381.

U.S. Department of Agriculture, Agricultural Research Service. 2012. USDA National Nutrient Database for Standard Reference, Release 25. Nutrient Data Laboratory Home Page, http://www.ars.usda.gov/ba/bhnrc/ndl. Accessed on April 23, 2012.

27 Low-Caloric Diets

Lucilene Rezende Anastácio and
Maria Isabel Toulson Davison Correia

CONTENTS

27.1 INTRODUCTION

Metabolic syndrome is highly prevalent worldwide and is considered a public health concern due to its impact on morbidity and mortality as well as on health care costs. Obesity, insulin resistance, hypertension, and atherogenic lipemia are altogether grouped in this entity, which, per se, is a strong risk factor for diabetes and cardiovascular events. The estimated prevalence in the general population is up to 34% (Ford et al. 2010), but it may be higher among vulnerable patients who are in post–liver transplantation stage (Anastacio et al. 2011) and with systemic lupus (Moura dos Santos et al. 2013). It is noteworthy that not only the common associated morbid conditions impact on the subjects' quality of life but also other not so mentioned conditions, such as periodontal diseases, lead to worse outcomes (Nibali et al. 2013).

Lifestyle modifications are key to alter the course of the syndrome and, among these, diet plays an essential and fundamental role. Therefore, in this chapter, we will highlight the basis as well as the important aspects of dietary aspects, such as caloric restriction.

27.2 WEIGHT LOSS AND CALORIC RESTRICTION

Weight loss (at least 5%–10% of initial body weight) and long-term maintenance of the weight loss are primary targets to reverse the components of the metabolic syndrome (Ferland and Eckel 2011). Obese patients need not achieve ideal body weight to improve their metabolic profile (Muzio et al. 2005), since weight loss *per se* can reduce abdominal obesity, one of the main causes for the appearance of all the components of the syndrome. Adipose tissue plays an important role in maintaining blood pressure levels and lipid and glucose metabolism, and is responsible for the production of various cytokines influencing the development of the syndrome (Cameron et al. 2008).

Weight loss maintenance is a challenge, since 30%–35% of the lost weight is regained within the first year (Wadden et al. 2004). Only about 20% of the overweight and obese individuals who undergo weight-loss therapy and who lose at least 10% of their initial weight are able to maintain such a loss after 1 year (Wing and Hill 2001). Studies on nutritional intervention and weight loss are focused on decreasing hunger and promoting satiety in order to improve adherence and facilitate weight loss as well as weight maintenance (Paddon-Jones et al. 2008).

The best diet to promote weight loss remains controversial. An individual's personal preferences and his/her metabolic parameters should be considered when developing a personalized dietary intervention (Ferland and Eckel 2011). However, the suggested dietary treatment must take into consideration, as a primary goal, caloric restriction, in order to promote negative energy balance and weight loss. Therefore, some authors emphasize that low-calorie diets result in clinically meaningful weight loss regardless of which macronutrient proportion they have (Sacks et al. 2009). Therefore, the type of diet seems to matter less than the diet adherence. A trial that enrolled 160 overweight or obese individuals with known hypertension, dyslipidemia, or fasting hyperglycemia randomized them into the Atkins (with carbohydrate restriction), Zone (with macronutrient balance), Weight Watchers (with calorie restriction), or Ornish (with fat restriction) diet groups. The amount of weight loss was modest, and it was more related with self-reported dietary adherence rather than with the diet type (Dansinger et al. 2005). On the other hand, some authors defend that energy deficit is really the key factor to promote weight loss, but macronutrient composition could influence changes in body composition and long-term compliance (Abete et al. 2010, Larsen et al. 2010).

Severe caloric restriction (600–800 kcal/day) was capable of inducing weight loss (average of 7% of their initial weight) with marked improvement in glucose, insulin, leptin, and triglycerides after 4–6 weeks, in obese individuals with metabolic syndrome (Xydakis et al. 2004). However, although this diet does promote a rapid weight loss, it is very difficult to maintain such restriction and the possibility of regaining weight is greater (Bantle et al. 2008).

Five percent loss of initial weight by restriction of 600 calories/day throughout 6 months led to reduction on oxidative stress and enhancement of antioxidant status in patients with metabolic syndrome (Angelico et al. 2012). Other authors have achieved weight loss and improvement of lipid-related risk factors and fasting insulin levels with 750 kcal of caloric restriction (Sacks et al. 2009). Generally, an energy deficit of 500–1000 kcal/day will result in a loss of approximately 0.5–1 kilo/week and an average total weight loss of about 8% after 6 months (Klein et al. 2004).

Energy restriction could be carried out in a continuous or intermittent fashion. A randomized comparison of energy restriction as intermittent restriction (650 kcal/day for 2 days/week) or a continuous restriction (1500 kcal/day for 7 days/week) showed an equal effectiveness for weight loss and improvement in metabolic syndrome markers among young overweight women throughout a period of 6 months (Harvie et al. 2011).

27.3 MACRONUTRIENT COMPOSITION IN CALORIC RESTRICTION

27.3.1 Carbohydrate

Low-carbohydrate diets have often been recommended as effective tools for weight loss over short-term periods. Glucose is the major insulin secretagogue, and insulin resistance has been tied to the hyperinsulinemic state or the effect of such a state on lipid metabolism (Volek and Feinman 2005). Carbohydrate restriction reduces insulin secretion, allowing greater rates of lipid oxidation and management of the incoming dietary lipids (Volek et al. 2009). Also, carbohydrate restriction improves glycemic control, blood pressure, and lipid profile (Accurso et al. 2008).

A comparison between two hypocaloric diets (containing each one 1500 kcal)—a carbohydrate-restricted diet (% carbohydrate–fat–protein = 12:59:28) and a low-fat diet (56:24:20)—for 12 weeks revealed that both interventions led to improvements in several metabolic markers. However, subjects following the carbohydrate-restricted diet had consistently reduced glucose and insulin concentration, as well as they had a greater weight loss and adiposity decrease, with concomitant more favorable lipid profile when compared with patients from the low-fat diet group (Volek et al. 2009).

The American Diabetes Association (ADA) traditionally recommends against less than 130 g of carbohydrates/day (IOM 2002). This value represents the recommended dietary allowance (RDA) for carbohydrate and is based on providing adequate glucose as the required fuel for the central nervous system without reliance on glucose production from ingested protein or fat (Bantle et al. 2008). According to the ADA, long-term metabolic effects of very-low-carbohydrate diets (such as increased level of ketone bodies, high losses of body water, headache, and constipation) are unclear, and such diets could eliminate fiber and micronutrients from many food sources (Bantle et al. 2008, Abete et al. 2010).

Studies with less severe carbohydrate restriction also have shown encouraging results. Low glycemic index carbohydrates as 40%–50% of total diet calories seem to increase satiety levels; improve insulin regulation; and reduce blood pressure, triglycerides, and low-density lipoproteins, oxidative stress, and inflammatory markers (Abete et al. 2010). High glycemic index carbohydrate sources (as sugar drinks, sweets, starchy foods, refined grain products, and potatoes) produce high glycemic responses that elicit a sequence of hormonal changes that alter fuel partitioning and cause overeating (Brand-Miller et al. 2002).

It is also important to highlight the importance of limiting fructose in the treatment of metabolic syndrome. Excessive intake of products containing added sugar, in particular, fructose, is one of the suggested causes of obesity and metabolic syndrome (Lim et al. 2010). Reduction of energy and added fructose intake may represent an important therapeutic target to reduce the frequency of obesity and diabetes (Madero et al. 2011). A meta-analyses with 19,431 participants showed that individuals who consumed most often one to two serving/day, sugar-sweetened beverages had a 20% greater risk of developing metabolic syndrome (Malik et al. 2010).

27.3.2 PROTEIN

Moderate-protein-content diets (20%–30%) have been recommended. They may lead to early satiety, improve adherence, enhance weight and fat mass loss, increase lean mass retention, decrease blood pressure and triglycerides, improve insulin regulation as well as they may also be associated with energy expenditure reduction (Abete et al. 2010). Due to the dietary restriction, it is advisable that protein requirements are calculated considering protein/kg of body weight. A randomized control trial showed that the lower threshold intake for protein must be set at 1.2/g/kg/day to maintain blood protein homeostasis (Dutheil et al. 2012). This study was conducted with 28 elderly subjects with metabolic syndrome undergoing energy imbalance of 500 kcal and physical activity (3.5 h/week). They were randomly assigned to two groups: normal protein (1.0 g/kg/day) and high protein (1.2 g/kg/day). Patients in the normal protein diet developed decreased albuminemia after 3 months, whereas albuminemia remained stable in patients on a higher protein diet (Dutheil et al. 2012).

Although a greater protein intake is recommended for the treatment of metabolic syndrome, it should be considered that excessive protein intake could overexert the kidney and increase the end products of protein metabolism (urea end uric acid) (Fouque and Guegre-Egziabherl 2009). It could also increase the intake of undesirable saturated fatty acids via proteins of animal origin. Therefore, it is wise and prudent to observe the diet as a whole.

27.3.3 FAT

Extreme restriction of fat has not been recommended lately, for the treatment of metabolic syndrome components. However, the consumption of some types of fat should be discouraged (cholesterol, saturated fatty acids, and trans fatty acids), while others should be encouraged (polyunsaturated and monounsaturated fatty acids). High dietary fat is expected to be deleterious if there is sufficient carbohydrate to provide the hormonal status in which fat will be stored rather than oxidized (Volek et al. 2009).

The Expert Panel on Detection, Evaluation, And Treatment of High Blood Cholesterol In Adults (Adult Treatment Panel III) allows an increase of total fat of 30%–35% of total calories, and up to 20% of the calorie intake should come from monounsaturated fatty acids, up to 10% from polyunsaturated and saturated fatty acids, and up to 1% from trans fatty acids (NCEP 2001).

The American Dietetic Association recommends less than 7% of total calories on saturated fat and less than 200 mg/dL of cholesterol intake (Bantle et al. 2008). High intakes of saturated fatty acids and cholesterol directly raise LDL-cholesterol concentrations and worsen insulin sensitivity (NCEP 2001, Bantle et al. 2008).

High monounsaturated fatty acid diet can decrease fasting insulin levels and improve insulin resistance as well as the LDL-cholesterol/HDL-cholesterol ratio (Due et al. 2008) and triglycerides (Esposito et al. 2004). Monounsaturated fatty acids can be found in olive oil, canola oil, nuts, and avocado, and they are a major component of the Mediterranean diet. The latter is based on olive oil, fruits and vegetables, whole grains, nuts and fish and limited on red meat, eggs, and whole fat dairy products as well as sugar/refined grains. Generally, this diet is composed of 15% protein; 40%–50% complex carbohydrates; and 30%–40% fat—at least half from monounsaturated fatty acids (MUFA) and less than 10% of saturated fatty acids (SAT) (Ambring et al. 2004, Gerhard et al. 2004, Rodriguez-Villar et al. 2004). A meta-analysis of 50 studies including 534,906 individuals on the effect of the Mediterranean diet on metabolic syndrome and its components revealed that adherence to this diet was associated with reduced risk of metabolic syndrome as well as a protective role on its components (Kastorini et al. 2011).

Polyunsaturated fatty acids should include the provision of adequate amounts of n-3 polyunsaturated fatty acids. Two or more servings of fish per week (with the exception of commercially fried fish filets) provide the minimum recommended n-3 polyunsaturated fatty acids (Bantle et al. 2008). The adequate intake of n-3 recommended by the Institute of Medicine (Washington, USA) is 1.6 g for adult men and 1.1 g for adult women (IOM 2002). The same organ also recommends that n-6 polyunsaturated fatty acids should be consumed; this gives 5%–10% of total calories (IOM 2002).

The most common dietary n-3 polyunsaturated fatty acids are alpha-linolenic acid (ALA—18:3 n-3), eicosapentaenoic acid (EPA—22:5 n-3), and docosahexaenoic acid (DHA—22:6 n-3). ALA is found in vegetable sources (as flaxseeds, canola, and soybean oil and nuts) and is a precursor for the EPA and DHA (found in fatty fish and fish oil). Studies assessing all these fatty acids have shown the lower efficacy of dietary ALA when compared with EPA + DHA with respect to long-chain n-3 polyunsaturated fatty acids levels in rats (Talahalli et al. 2010).

An isoenergetic and high-complex carbohydrate diet supplemented with 1.2 g of long-chain n-3 polyunsaturated fatty acids promoted decreased triacylglycerol and nonesterified fatty acid concentrations in subjects with metabolic syndrome, after 12-week intervention (Tierney et al. 2011). A review of randomized controlled trials on the effect of EPA and DHA supplementation with doses greater than 1 g for at least 3 months has shown a significant reduction of triglycerides, ranging from 7% to 25% (Lopez-Huertas 2012). In this review, the author concluded that high doses of n-3 polyunsaturated fatty acids (≥3 g/day) may lead to further triglycerides reduction which may increase other risk factors, such as low-density lipoprotein (LDL) levels. Beyond its proven effects in reducing triglycerides, n-3 polyunsaturated fatty acids can also modulate adipocytokines (reducing TNF-α levels; IL-6 and leptin and increasing adiponectin levels) that cause inflammation, glucose and lipid disorders, and reduce platelet aggregation as well as blood pressure levels (Barre 2007). Omega-3 polyunsaturated fatty acids may also affect weight loss by increasing satiety (Parra et al. 2008) and fatty acid oxidation (Couet et al. 1997).

27.3.4 Fibers

Soluble fibers can decrease energy intake by promoting appetite control (Wanders et al. 2011). They may also improve glycemic index of meals; therefore, they positively influence glucose metabolism (Schulze et al. 2004). They also can exert a blood-pressure-lowering effect in hypertensive subjects (Streppel et al. 2005) and may alter gut microbiota, due to their prebiotic function (Costabile et al. 2008). Soluble fibers lead to better cholesterol control and might positively affect other lipid parameters such as triglyceridemia.

TABLE 27.1

Summary of Recommendations for Nutritional Intervention on Metabolic Syndrome

Calorie/Nutrient	Recommendation	Observation
Calorie restriction	500–1000 kcal/day	
Carbohydrates	40%–50%	Low glycemic index
		Fructose restricted
Proteins	20%–30% and/or 1.2 g/kg/day	
Total fat	30%–40%	
Saturated fatty acids	<7%	
Polyunsaturated fatty acids	<10%	
n-3 PUFA	1.1–1.6 g	Fatty fish sources
n-6 PUFA	5%–10%	
Monounsaturated fatty acids	15%–20%	High in extra-virgin olive oil
Fiber	30 g	

Whole grain cereals, fruits, vegetables, and beans are excellent sources of soluble fibers, such as beta-glucans, glucomannans, guar, pysilium, pectins, and mucilages. Guidelines for dietary treatment of metabolic syndrome recommend fiber intake of 30 g/day (NCEP 2001). A daily dose of 2.3–10 g of beta-glucan—a soluble fiber found in oat bran and barley—has been recommended to give health benefits related to the treatment of metabolic syndrome (Cloetens et al. 2012) (Table 27.1).

27.4 FINAL CONSIDERATIONS AND PERSPECTIVES

Metabolic syndrome is highly prevalent worldwide and is related to an increased risk of cardiovascular diseases. Diet and exercise play key roles in both the prevention and treatment of such entity. Mediterranean diet, or better, lifestyle, characterized by the intake of larger amounts of fruits, vegetables, and legumes together with good-quality olive oil and red wine, as well as adequate intake of lean protein has been associated with the prevention and improvement of metabolic syndrome. Therefore, this should be aimed by the health care givers and administrators as a low-cost strategy to fight such syndrome. Moreover, education campaigns should be developed and spread worldwide.

Lifestyle modifications are not easy once they are firmly rooted in one's life, especially when living in the current western world. Therefore, expecting people to improve eating habits and adopt routine physical activity is extremely challenging. This makes it important to stimulate governmental health and educational policies to spread and implement strategies that can help save lives and decrease health care costs.

REFERENCES

Abete, I., Astrup, A., Martinez, J.A. et al. 2010. Obesity and the metabolic syndrome: Role of different dietary macronutrient distribution patterns and specific nutritional components on weight loss and maintenance. *Nutr Rev* 68:214–231.

Accurso, A., Bernstein, R.K., Dahlqvist, A. et al. 2008. Dietary carbohydrate restriction in type 2 diabetes mellitus and metabolic syndrome: Time for a critical appraisal. *Nutr Metab* 5:9.

Ambring, A., Friberg, P., Axelsen, M. et al. 2004. Effects of a Mediterranean-inspired diet on blood lipids, vascular function and oxidative stress in healthy subjects. *Clin Sci* 106:519–525.

Anastacio, L.R., Ferreira, L.G., Ribeiro, H. et al. 2011. Metabolic syndrome after liver transplantation: Prevalence and predictive factors. *Nutrition* 27:931–937.

Angelico, F., Loffredo, L., Pignatelli, P. et al. 2012. Weight loss is associated with improved endothelial dysfunction via NOX2-generated oxidative stress down-regulation in patients with the metabolic syndrome. *Intern Emerg Med* 7:219–227.

Bantle, J.P., Wylie-Rosett, J., Albright, A.L. et al. 2008. Nutrition recommendations and interventions for diabetes: A position statement of the American Diabetes Association. *Diabetes Care* 31(Suppl 1): S61–S78.

Barre, D.E. 2007. The role of consumption of alpha-linolenic, eicosapentaenoic and docosahexaenoic acids in human metabolic syndrome and type 2 diabetes—A mini-review. *J Oleo Sci* 56:319–325.

Brand-Miller, J.C., Holt, S.H., Pawlak, D.B., McMillan, J. 2002. Glycemic index and obesity. *Am J Clin Nutr* 76:281S–285S.

Cameron, A.J., Boyko, E.J., Sicree, R.A. et al. 2008. Central obesity as a precursor to the metabolic syndrome in the AusDiab study and Mauritius. *Obesity* 16:2707–2716.

Cloetens, L., Ulmius, M., Johansson-Persson, A., Akesson, B., Onning, G. 2012. Role of dietary beta-glucans in the prevention of MetS. *Nutr Rev* 70:444–458.

Costabile, A., Klinder, A., Fava, F. et al. 2008. Whole-grain wheat breakfast cereal has a prebiotic effect on the human gut microbiota: A double-blind, placebo-controlled, crossover study. *Br J Nutr* 99:110–120.

Couet, C., Delarue, J., Ritz, P., Antoine, J.M., Lamisse, F. 1997. Effect of dietary fish oil on body fat mass and basal fat oxidation in healthy adults. *Int J Obes Relat Metab Disord* 21:637–643.

Dansinger, M.L., Gleason, J.A., Griffith, J.L. et al. 2005. Comparison of the Atkins, Ornish, Weight Watchers, and Zone diets for weight loss and heart disease risk reduction: A randomized trial. *JAMA* 293(5):43–53.

Due, A., Larsen, T.M., Hermansen, K. et al. 2008. Comparison of the effects on insulin resistance and glucose tolerance of 6-mo high-monounsaturated-fat, low-fat, and control diets. *Am J Clin Nutr* 87:855–862.

Dutheil, F., Lac, G., Courteix, D. et al. 2012. Treatment of metabolic syndrome by combination of physical activity and diet needs an optimal protein intake: A randomized controlled trial. *Nutr J* 11:72.

Esposito, K., Marfella, R., Ciotola, M. et al. 2004. Effect of a mediterranean-style diet on endothelial dysfunction and markers of vascular inflammation in the metabolic syndrome: A randomized trial. *JAMA* 292:1440–1446.

Expert Panel on Detection, Evaluation, and Treatment of High Blood Cholesterol in Adults. 2001. Executive summary of the third report of the national cholesterol education program (NCEP) expert panel on detection, evaluation, and treatment of high blood cholesterol in adults (Adult Treatment Panel III). *JAMA* 285:2486–2497.

Ferland, A., Eckel, R.H. 2011. Does sustained weight loss reverse the metabolic syndrome? *Curr Hypertens Rep* 13:456–464.

Ford, E.S., Li, C., Zhao, G. 2010. Prevalence and correlates of metabolic syndrome based on a harmonious definition among adults in the US. *J Diabetes* 2:180–193.

Fouque, D., Guebre-Egziabher, F. 2009. Do low-protein diets work in chronic kidney disease patients? *Semin Nephrol* 29:30–38.

Gerhard, G.T., Ahmann, A., Meeuws, K. et al. 2004. Effects of a low-fat diet compared with those of a high-monounsaturated fat diet on body weight, plasma lipids and lipoproteins, and glycemic control in type 2 diabetes. *Am J Clin Nutr* 80:668–673.

Harvie, M.N., Pegington, M., Mattson, M.P. et al. 2011. The effects of intermittent or continuous energy restriction on weight loss and metabolic disease risk markers: A randomized trial in young overweight women. *Int J Obes* 35:714–727.

IOM. 2002. *Dietary Reference Intakes: Energy, Carbohydrate, Fiber, Fat, Fatty Acids, Cholesterol, Protein, and Amino Acids*. Washington, DC: National Academies Press.

Kastorini, C.M., Milionis, H.J., Esposito, K., Giugliano, D., Goudevenos, J.A., Panagiotakos, D.B. 2011. The effect of Mediterranean diet on metabolic syndrome and its components: A meta-analysis of 50 studies and 534,906 individuals. *J Am Coll Cardiol* 57:1299–1313.

Klein, S., Sheard, N.F., Pi-Sunyer, X. et al. 2004. Weight management through lifestyle modification for the prevention and management of type 2 diabetes: Rationale and strategies: A statement of the American Diabetes Association, the North American Association for the Study of Obesity, and the American Society for Clinical Nutrition. *Diabetes Care* 27:2067–2073.

Larsen, T.M., Dalskov, S.M., van Baak, M. et al. 2010. Diets with high or low protein content and glycemic index for weight-loss maintenance. *N Engl J Med* 363(25):2102–2113.

Lim, J.S., Mietus-Snyder, M., Valente, A. et al. 2010. The role of fructose in the pathogenesis of NAFLD and the metabolic syndrome. *Nat Rev Gastroenterol Hepatol* 7:251–264.

Lopez-Huertas, E. 2012. The effect of EPA and DHA on metabolic syndrome patients: A systematic review of randomised controlled trials. *Br J Nutr* 107(Suppl 2):S185–S194.

Madero, M., Arriaga, J.C., Jalal, D. et al. 2011. The effect of two energy-restricted diets, a low-fructose diet versus a moderate natural fructose diet, on weight loss and metabolic syndrome parameters: A randomized controlled trial. *Metabolism* 60:1551–1559.

Malik, V.S., Popkin, B.M., Bray, G.A. et al. 2010. Sugar-sweetened beverages and risk of metabolic syndrome and type 2 diabetes: A meta-analysis. *Diabetes Care* 33:2477–2483.

Moura dos Santos, F., Borges, M.C., Telles, R.W. et al. 2013. Excess weight and associated risk factors in patients with systemic lupus erythematosus. *Rheumatol Int* 33:681–688.

Muzio, F., Mondazzi, L., Sommariva, D. et al. 2005. Long-term effects of low-calorie diet on the metabolic syndrome in obese nondiabetic patients. *Diabetes Care* 28:1485–1486.

Nibali, L., Tatarakis, N., Needleman, I. et al. 2013. Clinical review: Association between metabolic syndrome and periodontitis: A systematic review and meta-analysis. *J Clin Endocrinol Metab* 98:913–920.

Paddon-Jones, D., Westman, E., Mattes, R.D. et al. 2008. Protein, weight management, and satiety. *Am J Clin Nutr* 87:1558S–1561S.

Parra, D., Ramel, A., Bandarra, N. et al. 2008. A diet rich in long chain omega-3 fatty acids modulates satiety in overweight and obese volunteers during weight loss. *Appetite* 51:676–680.

Rodriguez-Villar, C., Perez-Heras, A., Mercade, I. et al. 2004. Comparison of a high-carbohydrate and a high-monounsaturated fat, olive oil-rich diet on the susceptibility of LDL to oxidative modification in subjects with Type 2 diabetes mellitus. *Diabet Med* 21:142–149.

Sacks, F.M., Bray, G.A., Carey, V.J. et al. 2009. Comparison of weight-loss diets with different compositions of fat, protein, and carbohydrates. *N Engl J Med* 26(360):859–873.

Schulze, M.B., Liu, S., Rimm, E.B. et al. 2004. Glycemic index, glycemic load, and dietary fiber intake and incidence of type 2 diabetes in younger and middle-aged women. *Am J Clin Nutr* 80:348–356.

Streppel, M.T., Arends, L.R., van't Veer, P. et al. 2005. Dietary fiber and blood pressure: A meta-analysis of randomized placebo-controlled trials. *Arch Intern Med* 165:150–156.

Talahalli, R.R., Vallikannan, B., Sambaiah, K., Lokesh, B.R. 2010. Lower efficacy in the utilization of dietary ALA as compared to preformed EPA + DHA on long chain n-3 PUFA levels in rats. *Lipids* 45:799–808.

Tierney, A.C., McMonagle, J., Shaw, D.I. et al. 2011. Effects of dietary fat modification on insulin sensitivity and on other risk factors of the metabolic syndrome—LIPGENE: A European randomized dietary intervention study. *Int J Obes* 35:800–809.

Volek, J.S., Feinman, R.D. 2005. Carbohydrate restriction improves the features of Metabolic Syndrome. Metabolic Syndrome may be defined by the response to carbohydrate restriction. *Nutr Metab* 2:31.

Volek, J.S., Phinney, S.D., Forsythe, C.E. et al. 2009. Carbohydrate restriction has a more favorable impact on the metabolic syndrome than a low fat diet. *Lipids* 44:297–309.

Wadden, T.A., Butryn, M.L., Byrne, K.J. 2004. Efficacy of lifestyle modification for long-term weight control. *Obes Res* 12(Suppl.):151S–162S.

Wanders, A.J., van den Borne, J.J., de Graaf, C. et al. 2011. Effects of dietary fibre on subjective appetite, energy intake and body weight: A systematic review of randomized controlled trials. *Obes Rev* 12:724–739.

Wing, R.R., Hill, J.O. 2001. Successful weight loss maintenance. *Annu Rev Nutr* 21:323–341.

Xydakis, A.M., Case, C.C., Jones, P.H. et al. 2004. Adiponectin, inflammation, and the expression of the metabolic syndrome in obese individuals: The impact of rapid weight loss through caloric restriction. *J Clin Endocrinol Metab* 89:2697–2703.

Index